D1298441

Clinical Breast Imaging

A Patient Focused Teaching File

Gilda Cardeñosa, M.D.

Professor of Radiology
Director of Breast Imaging
Department of Radiology
Virginia Commonwealth University Health System
Medical College of Virginia Hospitals
Richmond, Virginia

Clinical Breast Imaging

A Patient Focused Teaching File

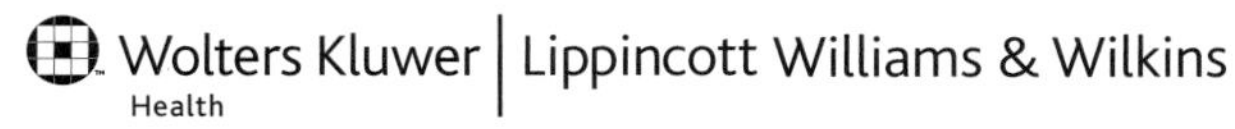
Wolters Kluwer Health | Lippincott Williams & Wilkins
Philadelphia • Baltimore • New York • London
Buenos Aires • Hong Kong • Sydney • Tokyo

Acquisitions Editor: Lisa McAllister
Managing Editor: Kerry Barrett
Production Manager: Nicole Walz
Senior Manufacturing Manager: Ben Rivera
Marketing Manager: Angela Panetta
Creative Director: Doug Smock
Cover Designer: Larry Didona
Production Services: TechBooks, Inc.
Printer: Maple-Press

530 Walnut Street
Philadelphia, PA 19106 USA
LWW.com

Printed in the USA

Library of Congress Cataloging-in-Publication Data

Cardenosa, Gilda.
Clinical breast imaging : a patient focused teaching file / Gilda Cardenosa.
p. ; cm.
Includes bibliographical references and index.
ISBN-10:0-7817-6267-7 (alk. paper)
ISBN-13:978-0-7817-6267-0
1. Breast—Imaging—Atlases. 2. Breast—Radiography—Atlases. 3. Breast—Cancer—Diagnosis—Atlases. I. Title.
[DNLM: 1. Breast Diseases—radiography—Atlases. 2. Mammography—methods—Atlases. 3. Ultrasonography, Mammary—methods—Atlases. WP 17 C266c 2007]
RC280 B8C3744 2007
618.1'907572—dc22

2006029274

Care has been taken to confirm the accuracy of the information presented and to describe generally accepted practices. However, the authors, editors, and publisher are not responsible for errors or omissions or for any consequences from application of the information in this book and make no warranty, expressed or implied, with respect to the currency, completeness, or accuracy of the contents of the publication. Application of this information in a particular situation remains the professional responsibility of the practitioner.

The author, editors, and publisher have exerted every effort to ensure that drug selection and dosoge set forth in this text are in accordance with current recommendations and practice at the time of publication. However, in view of ongoing research, changes in government regulations, and the constant flow of information relating to drug therapy and drug reactions, the reader is urged to check the package insert for each drug for any change in indications and dosage and for added warnings and precautions. This is particularly important when the recommended agent is a new or infrequently employed drug.

Some drugs and medical devices presented in this publication have Food and Drug Administration (FDA) clearance for limited use in restricted research settings. It is the responsibility of the health care provider to ascertain the FDA status of each drug or device planned for use in their clinical practice.

To purchase additional copies of this book, call our customer service department at (800) 638-3030 or fax orders to (301) 223-2320. International customers should call (301) 223-2300.

Visit Lippincott Williams & Wilkins on the Internet: http://www.LWW.com. Lippincott Williams & Wilkins customer service representatives are available from 8:30 am to 6:00 pm, EST.

10 9 8 7 6 5 4 3 2 1

To Mary Jones and Roxanne Aton

Your courage is inspirational, your impact profound. You light the path and motivate so many of us to work relentlessly with gentle passion, quiet strength, steadfast commitment, and serene humility to make a difference, one patient at a time.

Thank you.

Contents

Preface

Winston Churchill described writing a book as an adventure: "To begin with, it is a toy and an amusement; then it becomes a mistress and then it becomes a master, and then a tyrant. The last phase is that just as you are about to be reconciled to your servitude, you kill the monster and fling him out to the public." This is so! Writing a book is solitary work that grabs hold of you and quickly consumes your every waking moment and frequently haunts your dreams. In the end, as "you kill the monster and fling him out to the public," you can only hope fervently that what you thought needed to be written, and the manner in which you chose to present your ideas, is useful but, most important, challenges others to think critically about the concepts presented.

The effect of breast imaging, and the role of radiologists, in the management of women with breast cancer goes unstated and, in many ways, misrepresented. There is continued skepticism and criticisms relative to our contributions to patient care and the significance of what has already been accomplished: the routine identification of small, lymph node–negative, stage 0 and stage I invasive cancers and ductal carcinoma in situ. Prior to the advent of high-quality mammography, some breast diseases such as ductal carcinoma in situ (DCIS) were considered "rare" and our understanding of these diseases was limited. As a direct result of screening mammography, DCIS is routinely diagnosed and our knowledge, relative to the heterogeneity of this disease, has exploded. Recently reported decreases in breast cancer mortality rates are attributed by many to more effective treatment, ignoring or relegating to a secondary role our ability to detect DCIS, stage 0, and stage I lesions in many patients. Is early detection possibly the more important factor, and does not our ability to identify small lesions increase available treatment options for patients and render them more effective?

Clinical Breast Imaging: A Patient Focused Teaching File presents a clinically oriented, common-sense approach to screening, diagnostic evaluation, and the management of patients with breast conditions encountered commonly by breast-imaging radiologists. What is presented reflects a philosophical approach to breast imaging, centered on empathy for patients, who deserve complete evaluations and prompt answers, never forgetting that we are first and foremost physicians and clinicians, albeit with focused training in radiology and breast imaging. The concept of the clinical breast imager is rooted in the firm conviction that as breast imagers we make an incredibly valuable contribution to patient care—and yet, by virtue of our pivotal position in potentially bridging clinical and pathologic findings, with expanding imaging capabilities, there is so much more that we can do to revolutionize patient care and the manner in which that care is delivered. We must first, however, recognize our unique position, embrace the challenges, and spearhead the journey. Clinical breast imaging is a movement that is hard to stop, because it is the right thing to do.

I have arbitrarily divided the book into four chapters: "My Aunt Minnie," "Screening," "Diagnostic Breast Imaging," and "Management." Chapter 2, "Screening," discusses our approach to screening studies and potential abnormalities detected on screening mammograms. Because I wanted each patient presented to stand independently, there is repetition of basic concepts, but my aim was to build a strong infrastructure from which you can advance the care of your patients and the field of breast imaging. It is also important to emphasize that although this book is divided into chapters, the division is arbitrary. Presenting screening mammograms without the diagnostic evaluation, when one is indicated, makes little sense to me; I cannot squander invaluable opportunities to teach and carry the discussion to appropriate completion. Consequently, there is overlap: Diagnostic and management issues are discussed in the chapter on screening, and screening studies are presented in the diagnostic and management chapters. Management issues are discussed in the diagnostic chapter. The differentials listed are not intended to be exhaustive lists but rather, reasonable possibilities for one or multiple findings. It is also important to recognize that the situation presented here is, by necessity, artificial: Unlike what is presented here, in a screening population, most mammograms are normal; and although the incidence of cancer is higher in a diagnostic patient population, many patients are also normal or have benign changes and not cancer.

In an era when high technology dominates the interest of radiology residents, I can only encourage them strongly to consider breast imaging as a wonderful opportunity to make a powerful and significant difference in the lives of their patients.

Gilda Cardeñosa

Acknowledgments

Over the years I have been helped, supported, encouraged, and inspired by many colleagues. In particular, I would like to acknowledge Drs. Christine Quinn, Michael Linver, Ellen Mendelson, Gillian Newstead, Regina O'Brien, Edward Hendrick, G. W. Eklund, Peter Dempsey, Robert Schmidt, Cindy Lorino, Barbara Schepps, Martha Mainiero, Phillip Murphy, Stephen Feig, Jacqueline Hogge, Rebecca Zuurbier, Anne Roberts, Celia Parodi, Mirta Lanfranchi, Felix Leborgne, Deborah Hall, Teresa McCloud, John Pile-Spellman, William Chilcote, Arlene Libby, Gus Magrinat, Matthew Manning, Robert Murray, Peter Young, Ericka Coates, Jerome Gehl, Minta Phillips, Randy Jackson, and Stuart Geller. I would also like to specifically acknowledge two exceptional women who have been instrumental in advancing the importance of high-quality mammography at the national and international level, as well as through their outstanding courses for technologists and physicians, Rita Heinlein and Debra Deibel. It has been a privilege to work and learn with them, and I thank them for their friendship. Lastly, I owe a special debt of gratitude to Drs. Ann S. Fulcher and Mary Ann Turner, Chair and Vice Chair, Department of Radiology, Virginia Commonwealth University, for their support and patience as I worked to complete this project.

On a personal note, I acknowledge the support of Amy Davis, Leigh Kuhnly, Cara Sams, and Diana Shepherd, four very special women whose relentless commitment to patient care is inspirational. They toil selflessly behind the scenes, making an incredible difference to so many of us. I am also particularly indebted to Kathleen M. Connelly, who, over the years, through many projects and personal trials, has steadfastly, and without ever casting judgment, supported and believed in my life's work and me.

When asked what the three most important things for parents to do when raising children are, Alfred Schweitzer responded, "Example, example and example." This is what my mother, Gilda Paniza Cardeñosa, provided many times over: I owe everything I am to her. Always with a smile on her face and a joke up her sleeve, she was tenacious in her efforts to give me as much of a chance in life as possible. With an incredible work ethic and her silently persistent and resourceful ways, she helped make dreams a reality when others mocked them as foolish fantasies. Although she is no longer here, her spirit lives and I continue to be guided by the strong principles and work ethic she instilled in me.

Ultimately, it was Lisa McAllister at Lippincott Williams & Wilkins who made this dream come true. I can only hope this book is as useful as I believed in its need to be published. She has been incredibly supportive, gracious, and patient with me, as I struggled and made requests for more figure space and time. I will forever be grateful to her. Kerry Barrett and Louise Bierig have been instrumental to this project. Their many suggestions and meticulous work are reflected in the final product, and I thank them for their commitment.

Lastly, to all of the others including Nicole Walz, Ben Rivera, Angela Panetta, Doug Smock, Larry Didona at Lippincott Williams & Wilkins and Max Leckrone and the team at TechBooks, Inc. who worked behind the scenes to bring this to fruition, many thanks for your hard work and dedication.

Clinical Breast Imaging

A Patient Focused Teaching File

Chapter 1

My Aunt Minnie

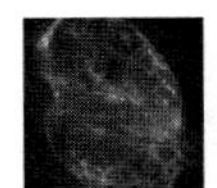
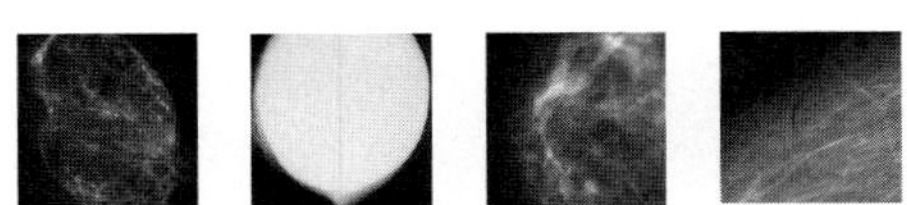
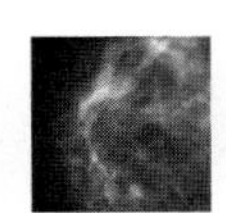
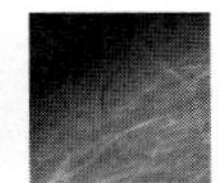

TERMS

- Amorphous calcifications
- Artifacts
- Calcified parasites
- Cysts
- Dystrophic calcifications
- Extracapsular implant rupture
- Fibroadenolipomas
- Gel bleed
- Hair
- Hickman catheter
- Hyalinizing fibroadenomas
- Implants
- Intracapsular implant rupture
- Keloids
- Lipomas
- Lucent centered calcifications
- Lymph nodes
- Milk of calcium
- Negative density artifacts
- Nipple rings
- Oil cysts
- Plus density artifacts
- Radiolucent mass
- Rod-like calcifications
- Seborrheic keratoses
- Skin folds
- Sternalis muscle
- Vascular calcifications
- Wire fragments
- Wire localization

INTRODUCTION

The term "Aunt Minnie" is used in radiology to characterize lesions that have a distinctive, unique appearance. Most radiology residents learn about Aunt Minnie early in their careers. While planning this book, I thought a chapter on Aunt Minnie would be easy to put together. I have discovered that this is not so! At least in mammography, the concept of Aunt Minnie is difficult to apply and I have struggled in selecting what should be included in this chapter. Does Aunt Minnie really always look the same? If for the same entity there is some variation in appearance, can it still be Aunt Minnie? Is your Aunt Minnie the same as my Aunt Minnie?

By this point you are probably wondering why I am dwelling on this. Probably this is by way of a disclaimer! I have elected to illustrate entities I define as Aunt Minnie. Some of you may not recognize my Aunt Minnie; however, the entities presented are distinctive and should be recognized as benign or iatrogenic. Rarely do these require additional evaluation, short-interval follow-up, or intervention.

FOR PATIENT DISCUSSIONS

In approaching "patient" (as opposed to "case") discussions, consider the 4 D's. The first is *detection.* Is there a potential abnormality? The second is a *description* of a confirmed finding based on complete information (e.g., additional clinical and imaging evaluations). Your description should lead you and the listener to a differential and the likely diagnosis you will propose. The third D is your *differential.* When considering the possibilities, remember that all findings have benign and malignant considerations and you should move through the list in a logical manner. Try not to jump back and forth from benign to malignant. Tell the listener what you think the lesion could be, not what it is not. Also, try to be specific; saying that "this is likely a malignancy or cancer" is not very insightful. The last D is what you think the *diagnosis* is most likely to be.

PATIENT 1

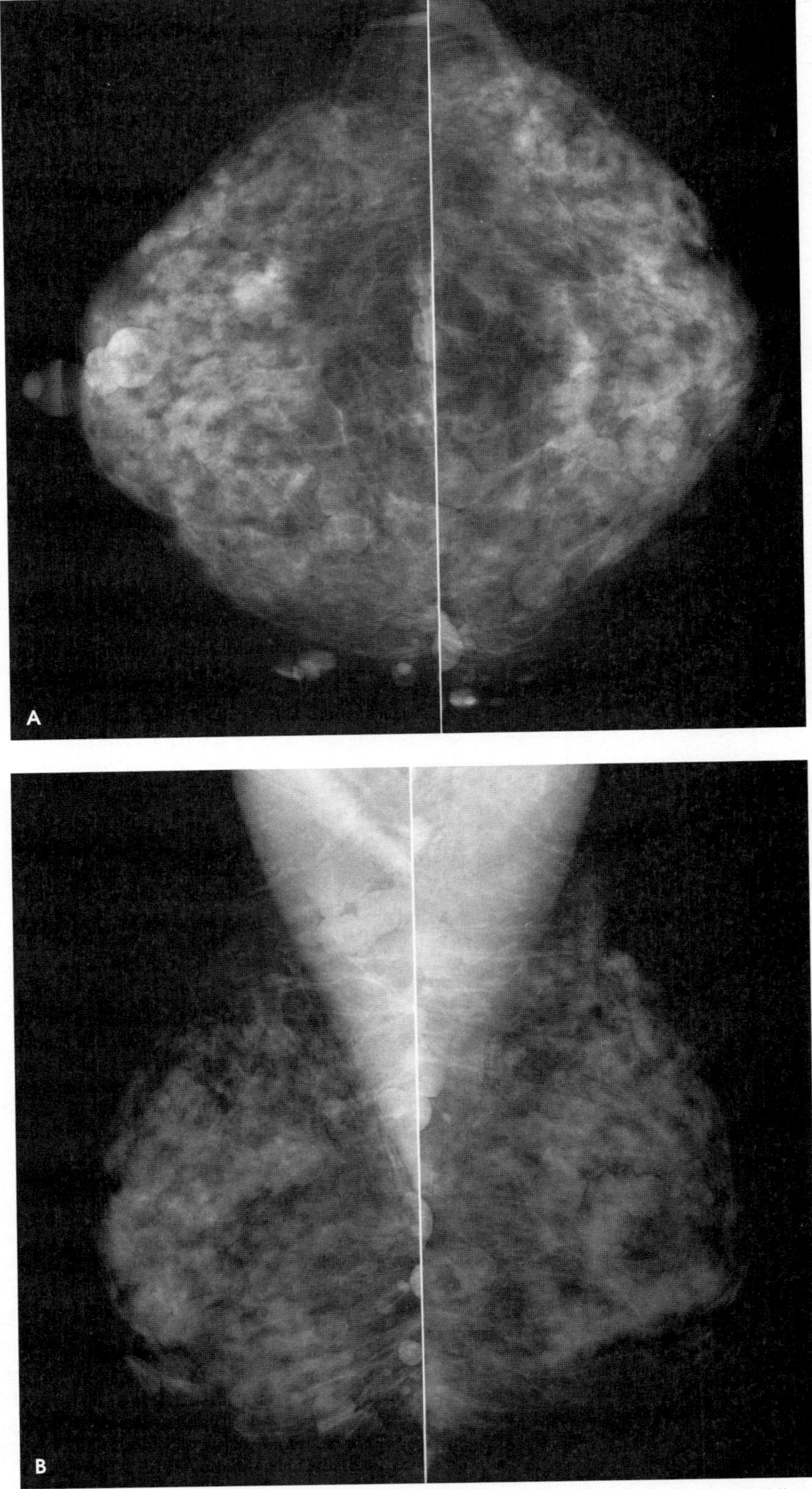

Figure 1.1. Screening study, 42-year-old woman: craniocaudal **(A)** and mediolateral oblique **(B)** views.

What is your diagnosis?
If you are not sure, what can you do to be 100% sure?

Multiple masses are projecting on the breast parenchyma bilaterally. On close inspection, air is seen as a thin radiolucency, partially or completely outlining the margins of several of the masses (Fig. 1.1C, thicker arrows). Those in tangent to the x-ray beam are seen extending beyond the breast (Fig. 1.1C, thin arrows). Bilateral skin lesions may be seen in otherwise healthy women or, when this numerous, in women with neurofibromatosis. These patients can be challenging. We are often mesmerized by benign findings and neglect more subtle findings that potentially reflect breast cancer. So, do not let benign, obviously malignant, or clinical findings distract you from reviewing the mammogram completely. *You need to be even more focused in looking for potential signs of early breast cancer around and in between obvious findings.* If there is any question about a mass being on the skin you can examine the patient and, if still not sure, place a metallic BB on the identified skin lesion and obtain follow-up images with the BB (and skin lesion) in tangent to the x-ray beam.

BI-RADS® category 1: negative. BI-RADS® category 2: benign finding is used if the skin lesions are described in the body of the report. Next screening mammography is recommended in 1 year.

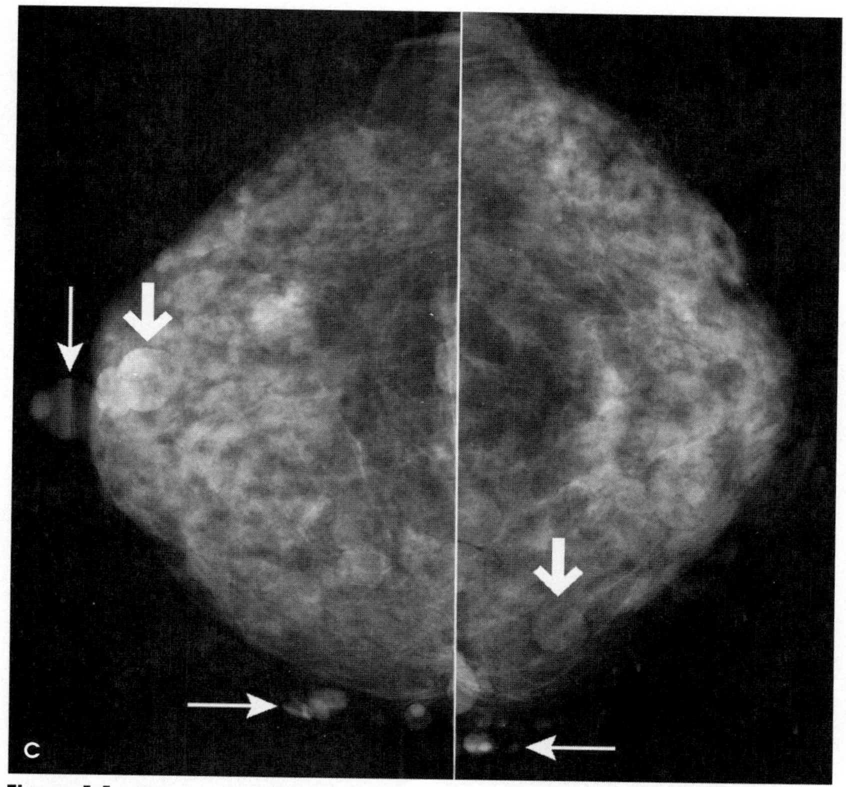

Figure 1.1. (*Continued*) **(C)** Craniocaudal view. Skin lesions projecting beyond the skin (*thin arrows*) are easily identified. Skin lesions superimposed on the parenchyma (*thick arrows*) can often be identified by a sharply defined lucency (air) partially or completely outlining their margins.

PATIENT 2

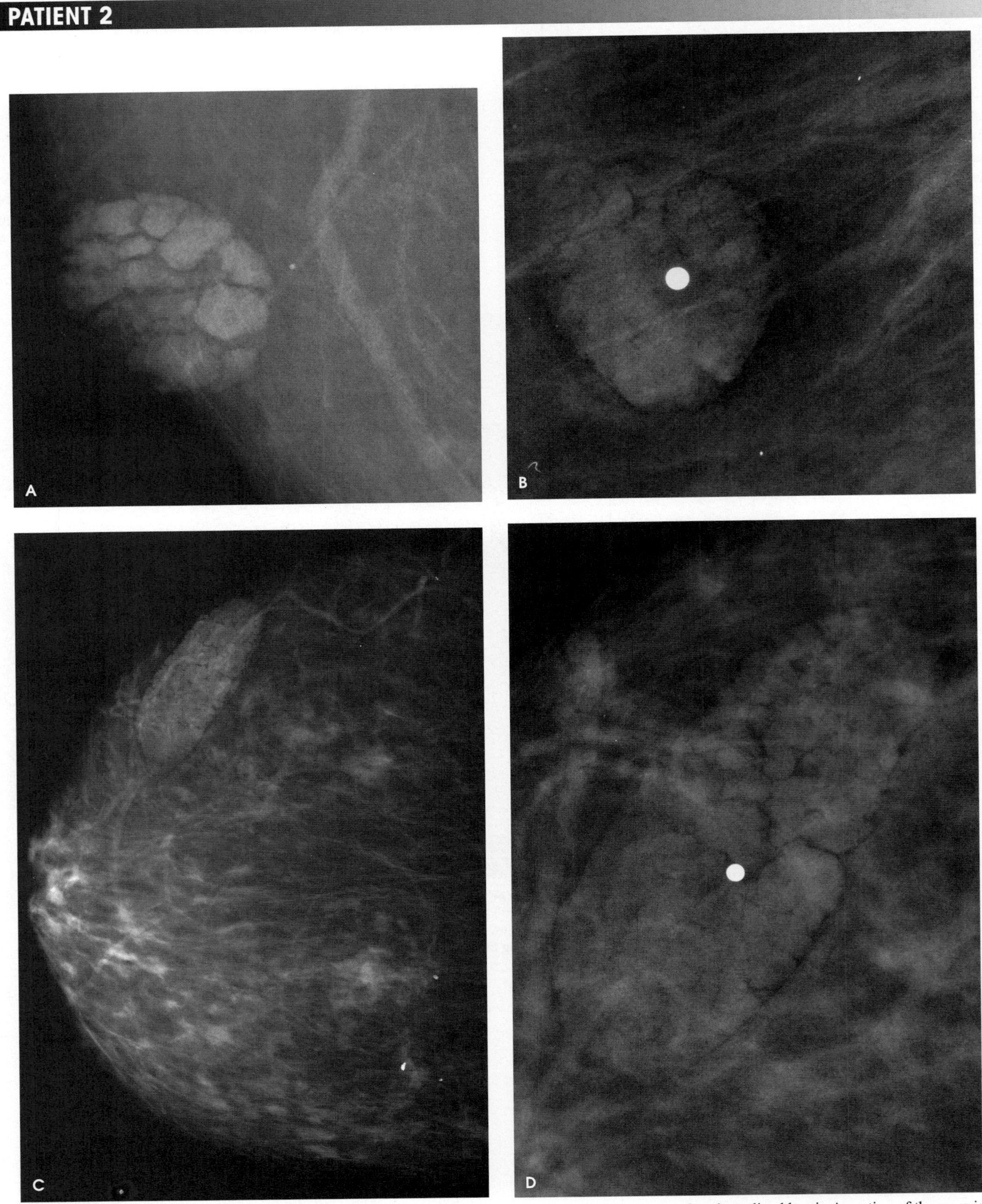

Figure 1.2. **A:** Skin lesion, right breast, photographically coned view. The interstices of the lesion are sharply outlined by air. A portion of the mass is seen extending beyond the breast. **B:** Skin lesion, left breast, photographically coned view. Metallic BB placed on the skin lesion. A thin, sharply defined lucency (air) outlines the margins of the mass as well as some of the interstices of the lesion. Craniocaudal **(C)** and photographically coned **(D)** views of skin lesion, laterally in the right breast. Metallic BB placed on skin lesion. The margins and interstices of the lesion are sharply defined by a surrounding lucency (air).

What is the diagnosis in these three patients, and how can you be certain?
What else could you do?

Seborrheic keratoses: Characteristic mammographic appearance is demonstrated with these three patients. When superimposed on the breast parenchyma, skin lesions are often partially, or completely, outlined by a thin radiolucency (air), as are the interstices of the verrucous lesions. When they are in tangent to the x-ray beam, their extension beyond the skin is outlined by air (radiolucent). Although metallic BBs are often used to mark these skin lesions, the mammographic appearance of the verrucous lesions is distinctive. Metallic BBs are more helpful on smooth skin lesions, because these are more likely to simulate a breast lesion when superimposed on the breast parenchyma on the two standard views of the breast (e.g., craniocaudal and mediolateral oblique views). When a technologist uses a BB, she indicates the reason on the woman's history form and affixes a sticker on the films (e.g., "BB on mole" or "BB on lump") indicating the reason for the use of the BB. Unless the skin lesions are too numerous to mark, the routine use of BBs to mark skin lesions can avert some callbacks.

Seborrheic keratoses are common benign epidermal tumors distributed on skin that bears hair. They do not develop on mucosal surfaces and are infrequent under the age of 30 years. They are common, typically multiple, and continue to develop as patients age. A familial predilection with a possible autosomal dominant form of inheritance has been described. Seborrheic keratoses are typically flat when they first develop and over time can become more verrucous, polypoid, and pedunculated in appearance. Rarely, rapid proliferation or increases in the size of pre-existing lesions may be an indication of an internal malignancy (Leser-Trélat sign).

PATIENT 3

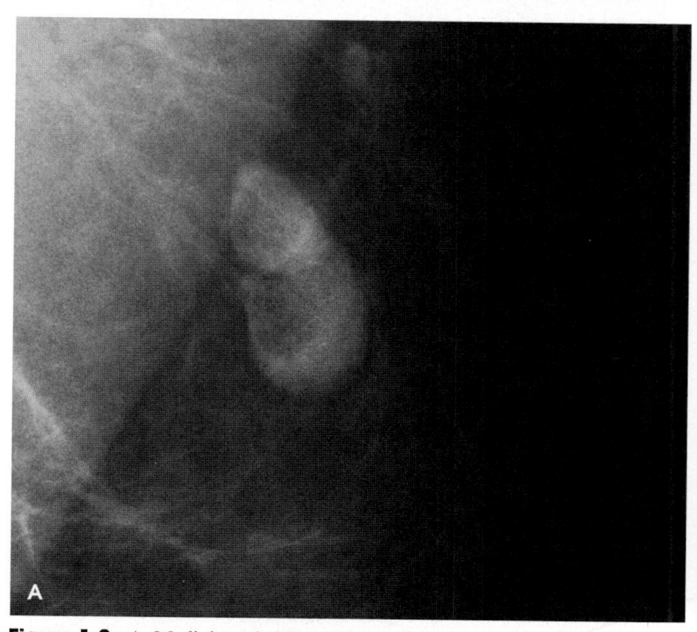

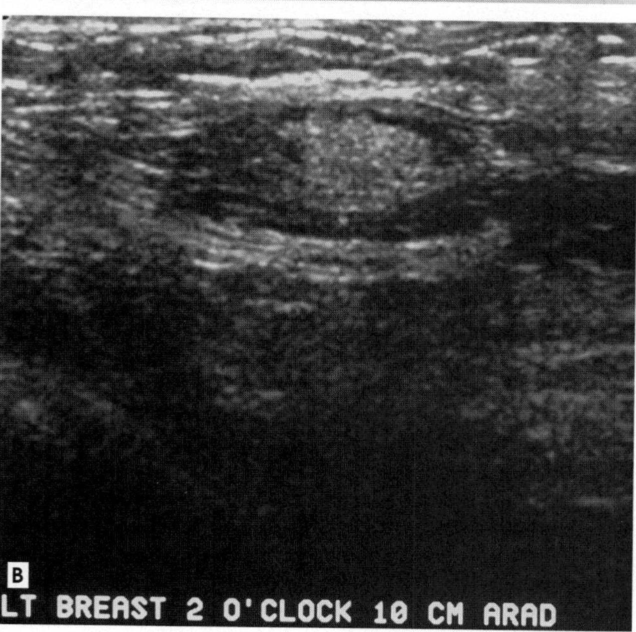

Figure 1.3. **A:** Mediolateral oblique, photographically coned view of an oval, mixed-density (fat containing) mass. **B:** Ultrasound image, antiradial (ARAD) projection of a hypoechoic mass with a focus of central echogenicity corresponding to the mass shown in **(A)** at the 2 o'clock position, 10 cm from the left nipple.

What are imaging findings of intramammary lymph nodes?

The mammographic appearance of lymph nodes is variable (Fig. 1.3A, C). Most commonly, intramammary lymph nodes are well circumscribed, oval (reniform), mixed-density (fat containing) masses localized to the upper outer quadrants. However, they can be found anywhere, including the inner quadrants, and may fluctuate in size and density. They may have a prominent fatty component relative to the water-density portion or vice versa. Rarely, lymph nodes disappear, only to reappear on subsequent mammograms. The mammographic appearance of "normal" lymph nodes is usually distinctive enough that no additional imaging is indicated.

Ultrasound is used adjunctively in patients in whom a lymph node is suspected but a fatty hilum is not definitely seen mammographically. Ultrasound is also the primary imaging modality used in patients who are under the age of 30 years, pregnant, or lactating, who present with a palpable finding. On ultrasound, lymph nodes are typically well-circumscribed masses with a hypoechoic cortical area and a hyperechoic central, or eccentric focus, corresponding to the fatty hilar region seen mammographically (Fig. 1.3B, D, E, F, G, H). If power Doppler is used, blood flow is seen associated with the hyperechoic region.

On T2-weighted magnetic resonance images, lymph nodes demonstrate high signal intensity. Following contrast administration, lymph nodes are characterized by rapid contrast uptake on

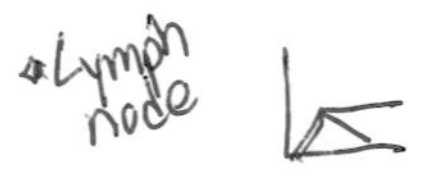

T1-weighted images. This uptake is followed by either a plateau or rapid washout. Contrast enhancement may appear rimlike when the hilar region is centrally located (Fig. 1.31, J). Vessels can sometimes be seen in the hilar region.

Mammographically, if a lymph node increases in size and density and there is associated loss of the fatty hilum with indistinct or spiculated margins, biopsy may be indicated; in many women, however, these changes are reactive and do not reflect a malignant process. Similarly, on ultrasound, biopsy is considered if there is thickening and bulging of the cortical area, often asymmetric and microlobulated, with concomitant thinning and apparent mass effect, or complete loss, of the hyperechoic hilar region. Increased blood flow can be seen in some of these lymph nodes.

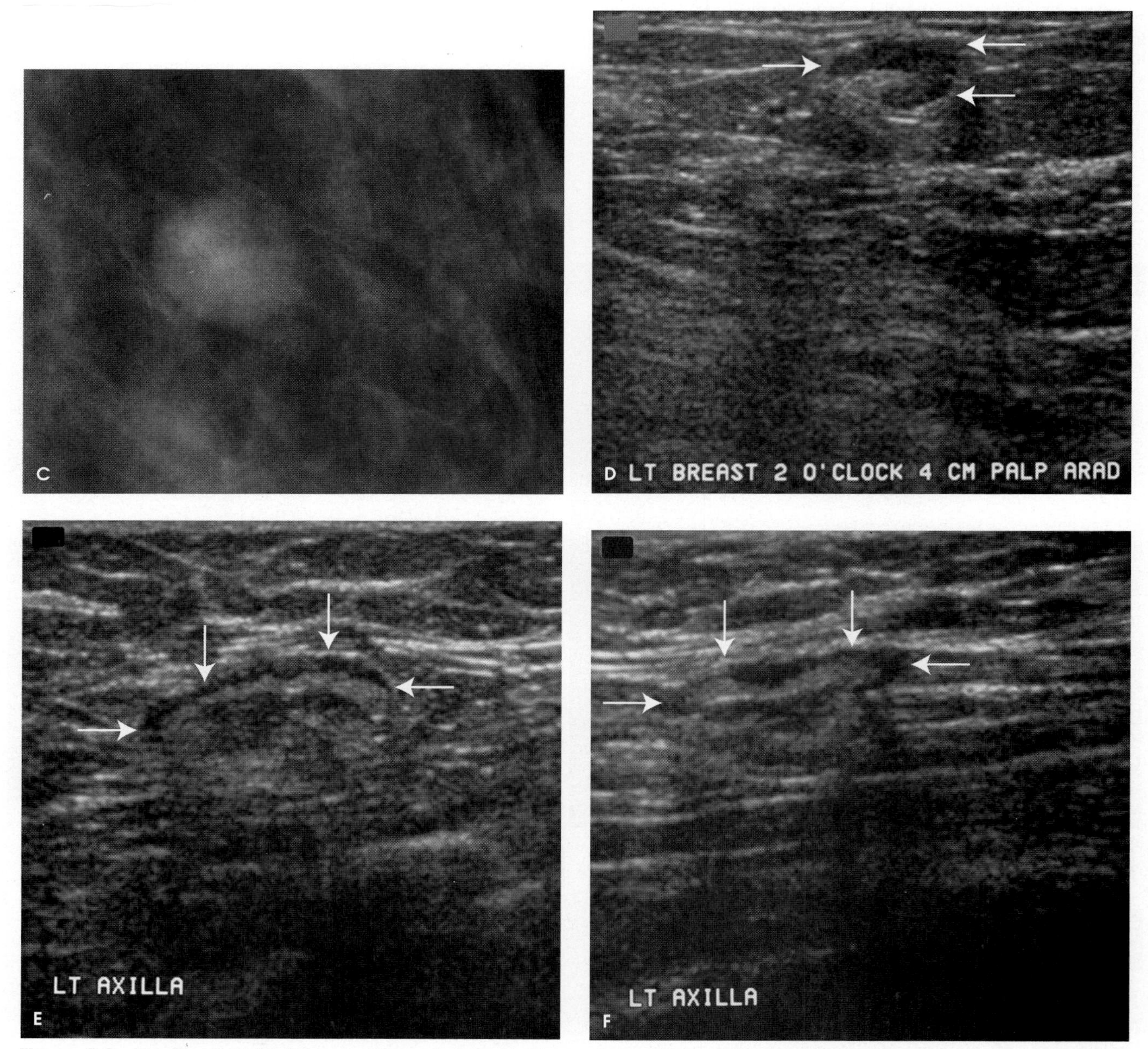

Figure 1.3. (*Continued*) **C:** Mediolateral oblique, photographically coned view of a round mass with what may be an eccentric fatty hilum. **D:** Ultrasound image, antiradial (ARAD) projection of palpable (PALP) hypoechoic mass (arrows), with an eccentric focus of echogenicity corresponding to the mass shown in **(C)** at the 2 o'clock position, 4 cm from the left nipple. **E:** Ultrasound image, left axilla, demonstrating an oval lymph node (*arrows*) characterized by a thin hypoechoic cortex and central area of echogenicity corresponding to the fatty hilum seen on mammograms. **F:** Ultrasound image, left axilla, demonstrating an oval mass (*arrows*) with a thin hypoechoic cortex and a central oval area of echogenicity.

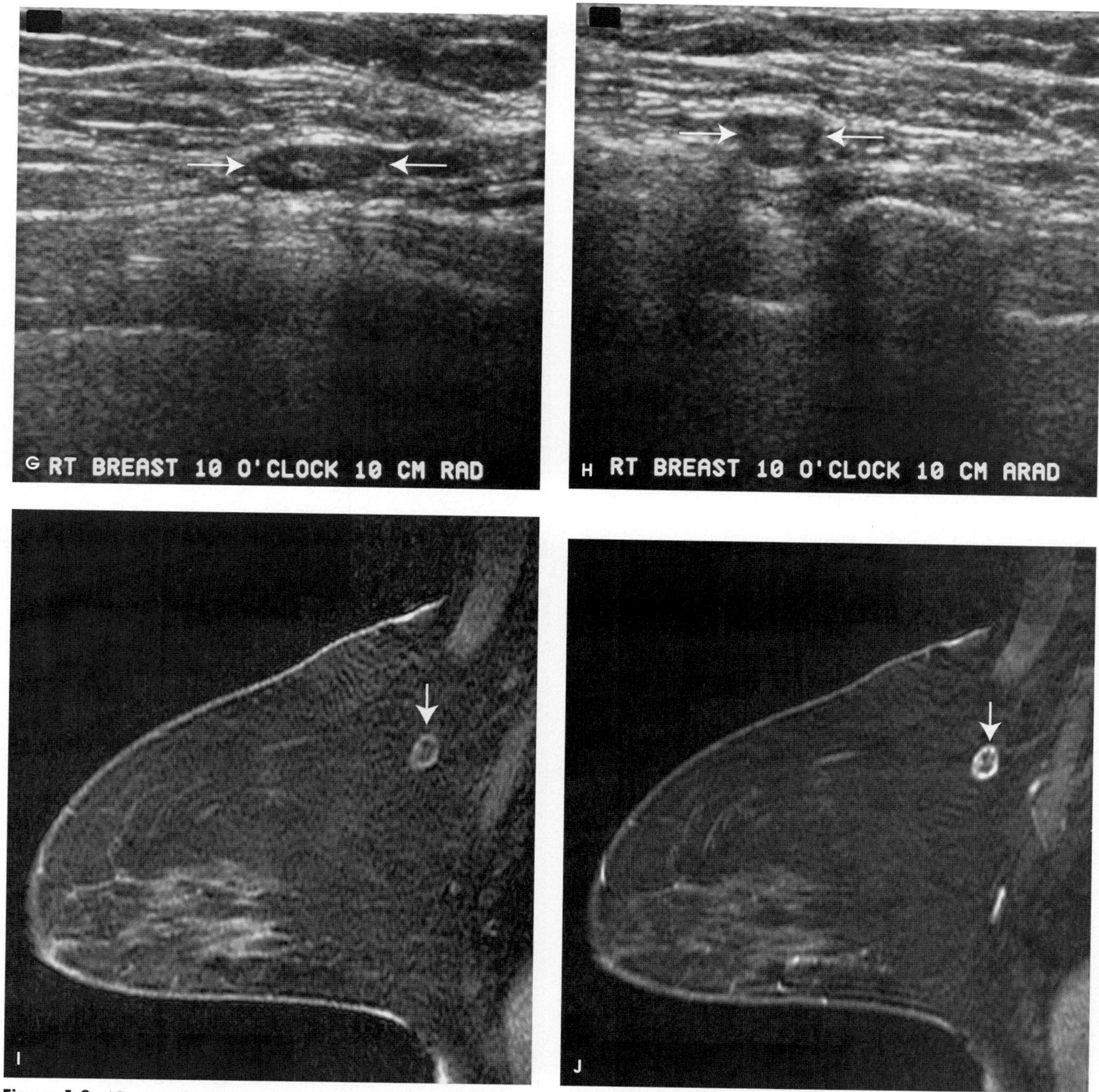

Figure 1.3. (*Continued*) Ultrasound images, in radial (RAD) **(G)** and antiradial (ARAD) **(H)** projections, of an oval mass (*arrows*) characterized by a hypoechoic cortex and a central focus of echogenicity, at the 10 o'clock position, 10 cm from the right nipple. **I:** T1-weighted sagittal image, precontrast, demonstrating a mass with a central focus of lower signal intensity. **J:** T1-weighted sagittal image, immediately postcontrast, at the same tabletop position shown in **(I)**, demonstrates rapid enhancement of the cortical rim of the mass.

PATIENT 4

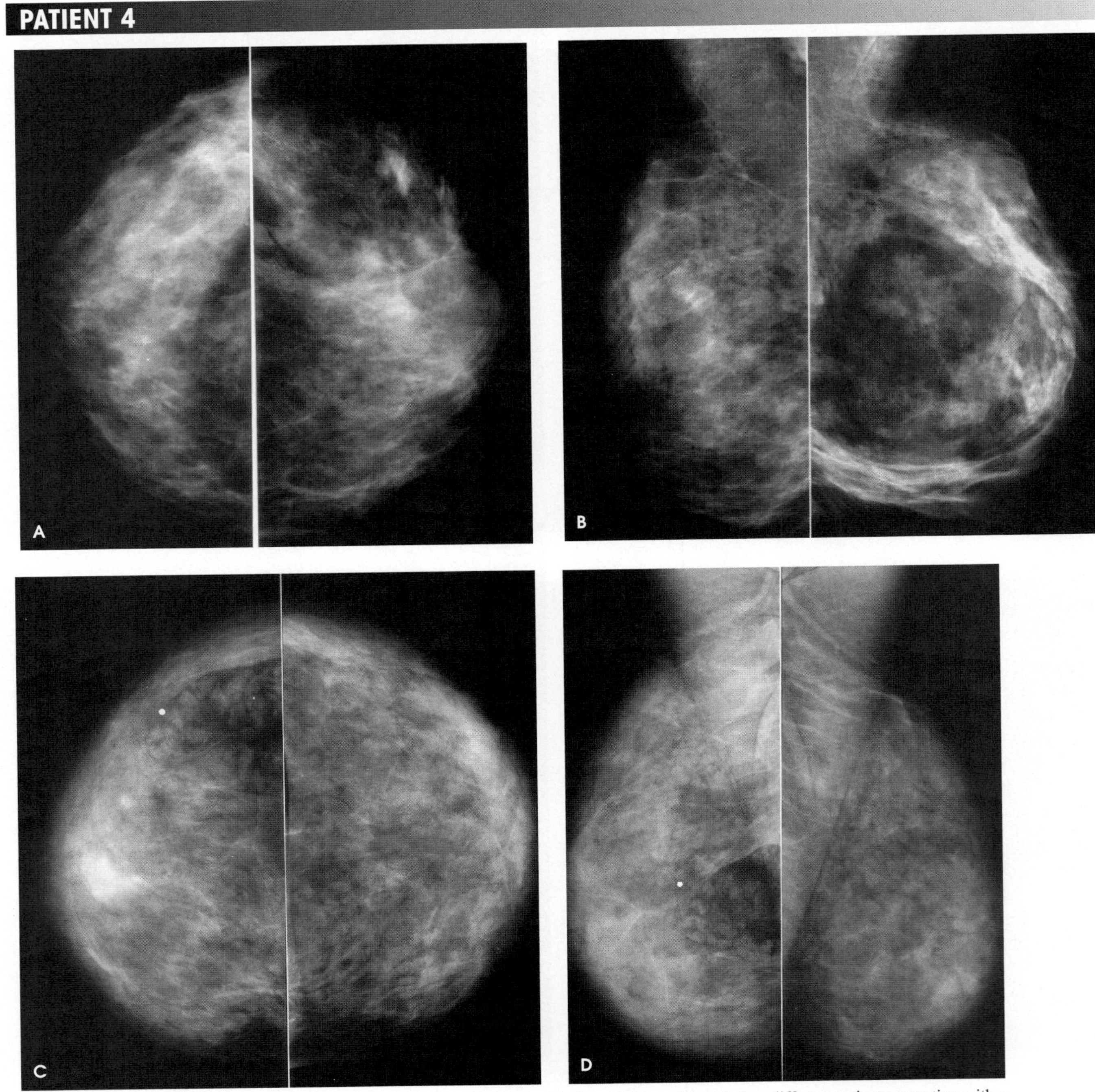

Figure 1.4. Screening study. Craniocaudal **(A)** and mediolateral oblique **(B)** views. Diagnostic study in a different patient presenting with a "lump" in the right breast. Craniocaudal **(C)** and mediolateral oblique **(D)** views (metallic BB marking palpable finding).

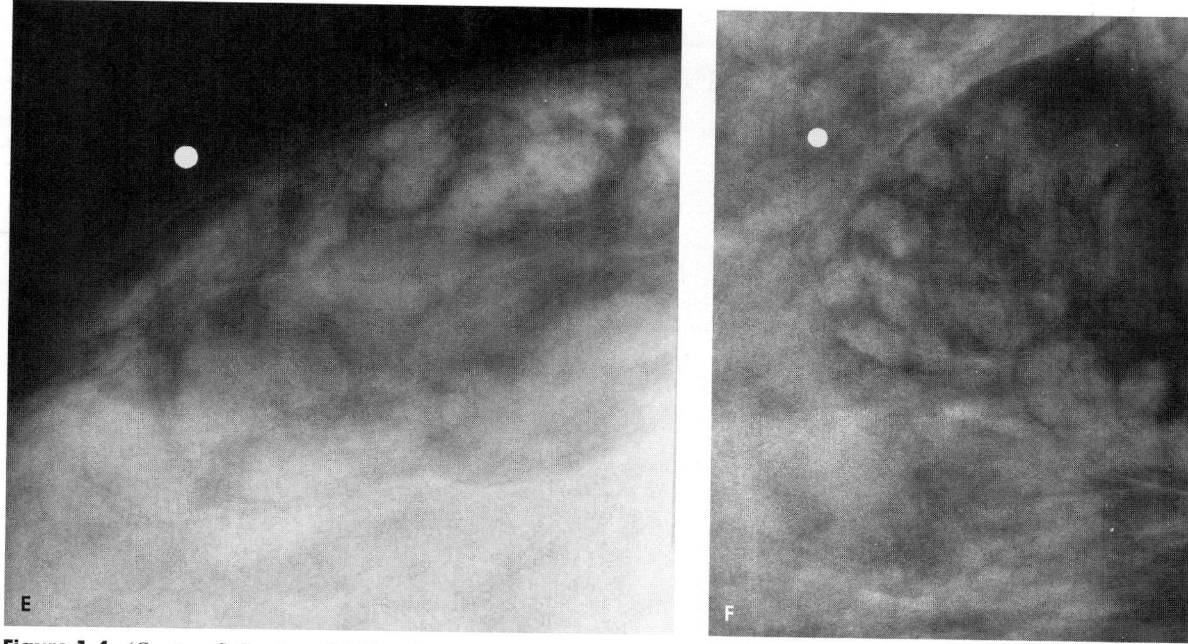

Figure 1.4. (*Continued*) Craniocaudal **(E)** and mediolateral oblique **(F)** spot compression views of the palpable finding in the right breast.

How would you describe the findings? What is your diagnosis?

Mixed-density (fat containing) masses are imaged mammographically in these two patients consistent with fibroadenolipomas (also called hamartoma, breast-within-a-breast). Fatty, glandular and fibrous tissues are surrounded, and separated, from the remainder of the breast tissue by a fibrous pseudocapsule. As illustrated by these two patients, the proportions of each tissue type vary from patient to patient. In some women the lesions are mostly fatty, in others glandular tissue predominates. They can be detected on screening studies (Fig. 1.4A, B, left breast) or, in some patients can present as a palpable finding (Fig. 1.4C, D, right breast). Rarely, they occur in accessory axillary glandular tissue and may enlarge rapidly.

On ultrasound, fibroadenolipomas are usually separable from surrounding normal tissue and characterized by an admixture of hypo- and hyperechoic areas with disruption of normal tissue architecture. The posterior acoustic features of these lesions are variable and include no posterior acoustic features, enhancement, shadowing, or a combined pattern (areas of enhancement and areas of shadowing).

Variable combinations of adipose tissue, fibrous stroma, and lobular structures are seen histologically and, although separable from the adjacent breast tissue, hamartomas lack a true capsule. Rarely, myxoid and chondroid hamartomas are reported histologically when the lesions contain muscle and cartilage, respectively. A myxoid hamartoma has been reported in a 36-year-old male presenting with a slowly growing breast mass. Breast cancer can arise in fibroadenolipomas, so the tissue in these lesions should be evaluated for the development of any mass, distortion, or calcifications as thoroughly as breast tissue anywhere else.

BI-RADS® category 2: benign finding. Next screening mammogram is recommended in 1 year.

PATIENT 5

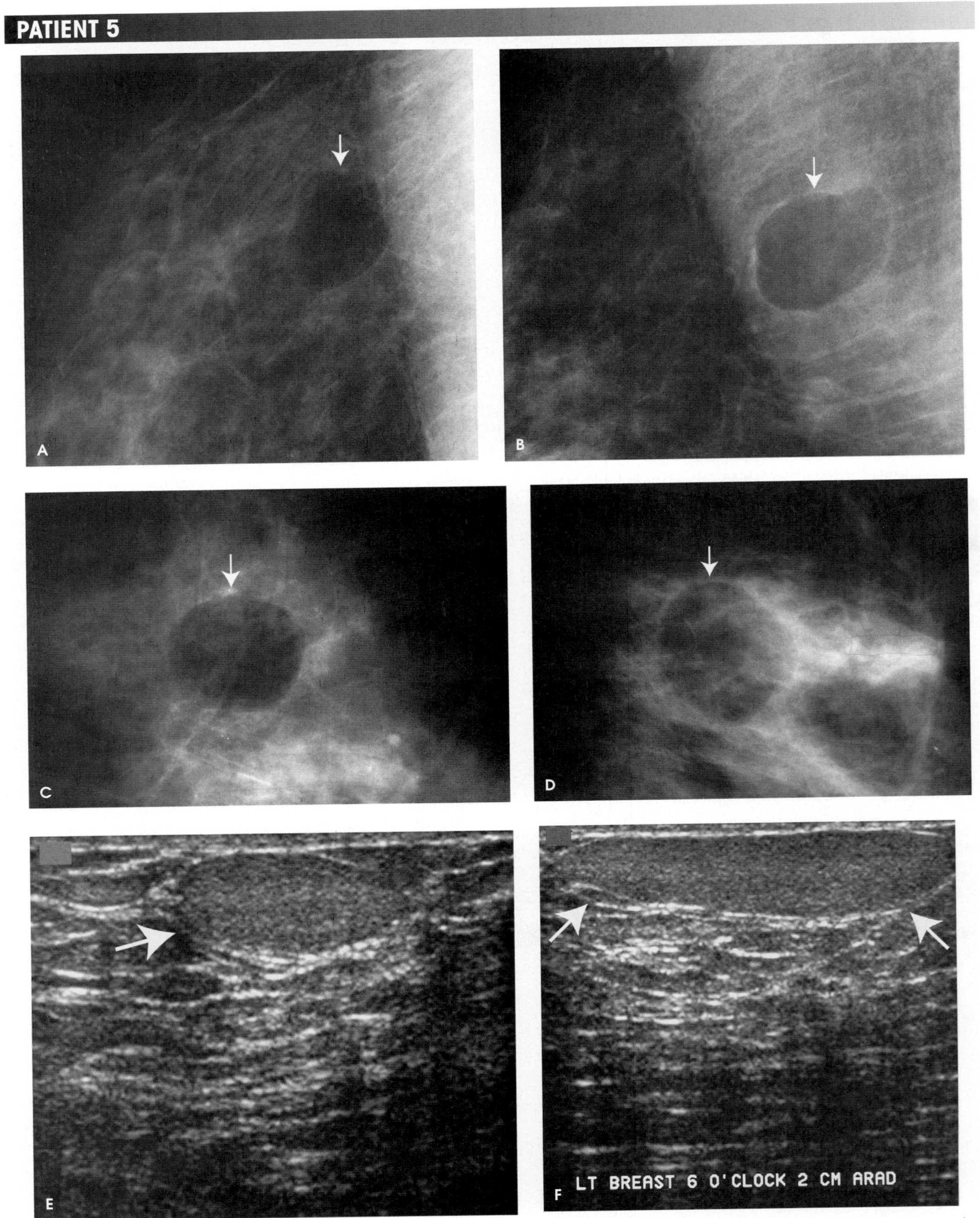

Figure 1.5. Screening study. Craniocaudal **(A)** view exaggerated laterally and mediolateral oblique **(B)** view, photographically coned. Screening study, different patient. Craniocaudal **(C)** and mediolateral oblique **(D)** views, photographically coned. Ultrasound images in radial **(E)** and antiradial (ARAD) **(F)** projections of a palpable mass at the 6 o'clock position, 2 cm from the left nipple, radiolucent on the mammogram (not shown).

How would you describe the findings?
What is your diagnosis?

Radiolucent, well-circumscribed masses (*small arrows*) with a thin fibrous capsule consistent with lipomas; these rarely calcify. Unlike oil cysts, which have a variable sonographic appearance but often simulate cysts, lipomas are well circumscribed, solid, slightly hypo- or isoechoic masses on ultrasound (*large arrows*). In some women, lipomas can be slightly hyperechoic and a small amount of posterior acoustic enhancement may be noted (Fig. 1.5E, F). A gentle mass effect on surrounding tissue and Cooper ligaments can also be seen with some lipomas. Rarely, lipomas can be seen within the pectoral muscle.

BI-RADS® category 2: benign finding. Next screening mammography is recommended in 1 year.

PATIENT 6

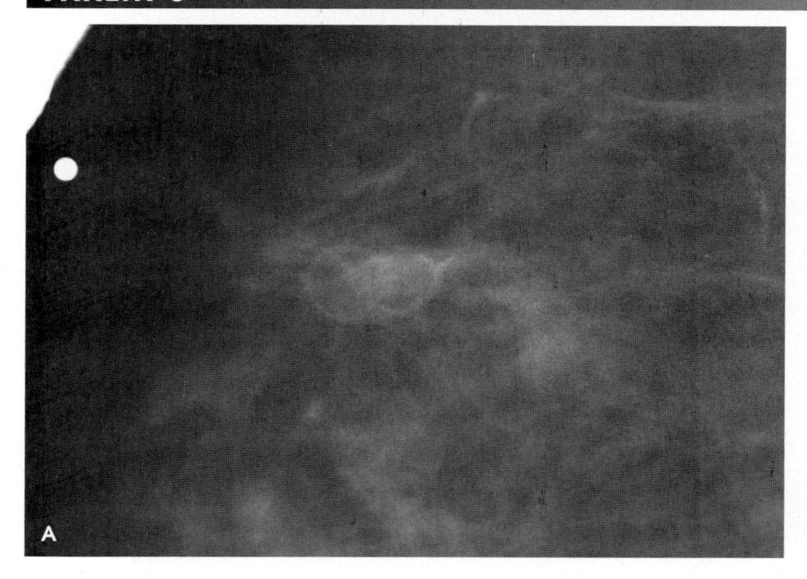

Figure 1.6. Diagnostic study in a 60-year-old patient presenting with a "lump" in her right breast. Spot tangential **(A)** view of the "lump" with a metallic BB placed at the site of concern. The patient has had a reduction mammoplasty.

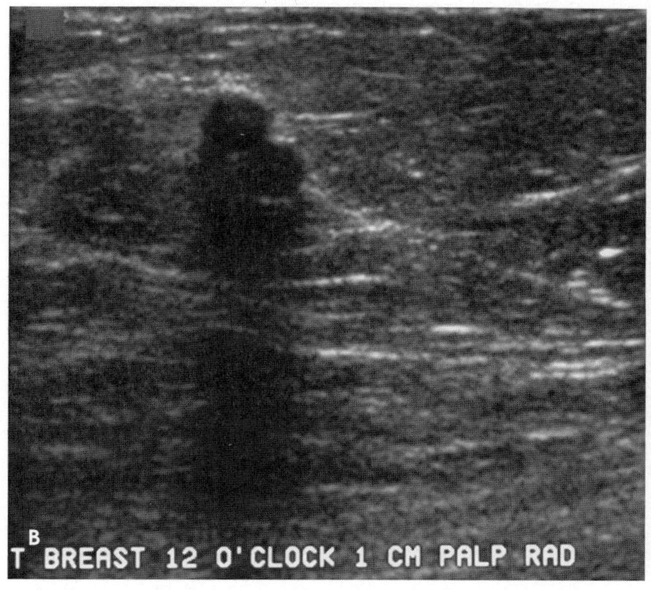

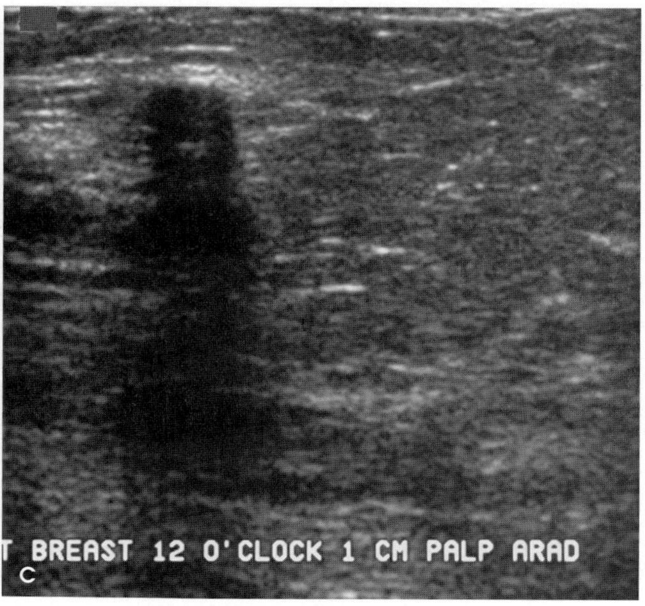

Figure 1.6. Ultrasound images, radial (RAD) **(B)** and antiradial (ARAD) **(C)** projections of palpable finding, right breast.

How would you describe the findings? What is your diagnosis?

Two adjacent 5-mm round, well-circumscribed radiolucent masses are seen mammographically, corresponding to the "lump" described by the patient. Given the history of a reduction mammoplasty, these are consistent with oil cysts. The diagnosis is established mammographically. Radiolucent masses in the breast are benign. The benign nature of the palpable finding is discussed with the patient, and she is reassured that this is not breast cancer and that it will not become cancerous. A definitive report is issued to avoid unnecessary surgery.

BI-RADS® category 2: benign finding. Next screening mammography is recommended in 1 year.

On physical examination, there is a discrete, hard, lobulated mass palpated at the 12 o'clock position, 1 cm from the right nipple. A macrolobulated, nearly anechoic mass with significant shadowing is imaged, corresponding to the palpable finding. Although the ultrasound is included for illustrative purposes, the diagnosis is made on the mammographic findings (i.e., ultrasound is not indicated when a radiolucent mass is seen mammographically). Oil cysts can have a variable appearance on ultrasound, ranging from simulating a simple cyst to a complex cystic mass or a mass with significant shadowing as seen here.

PATIENT 7

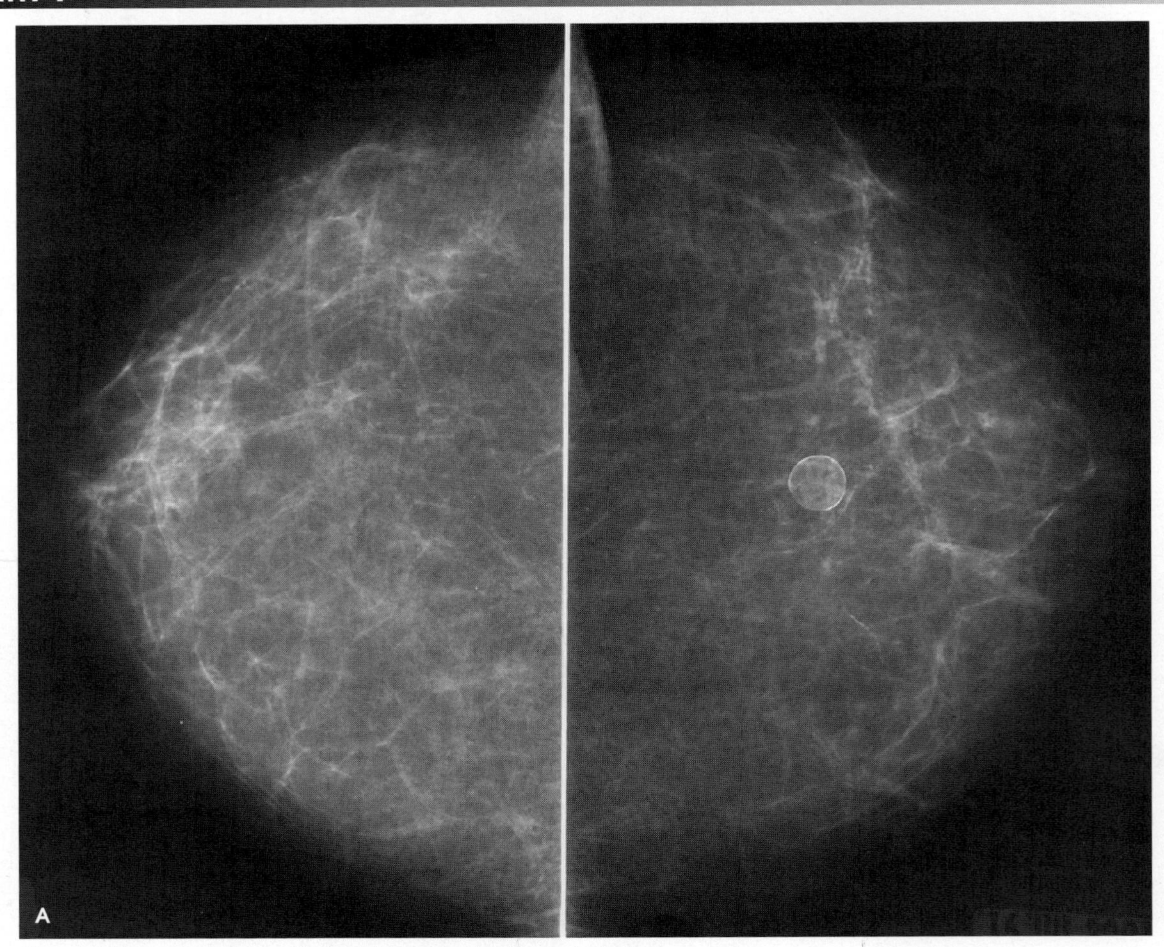

Figure 1.7. Screening study, 49-year-old woman. Craniocaudal **(A)** view.

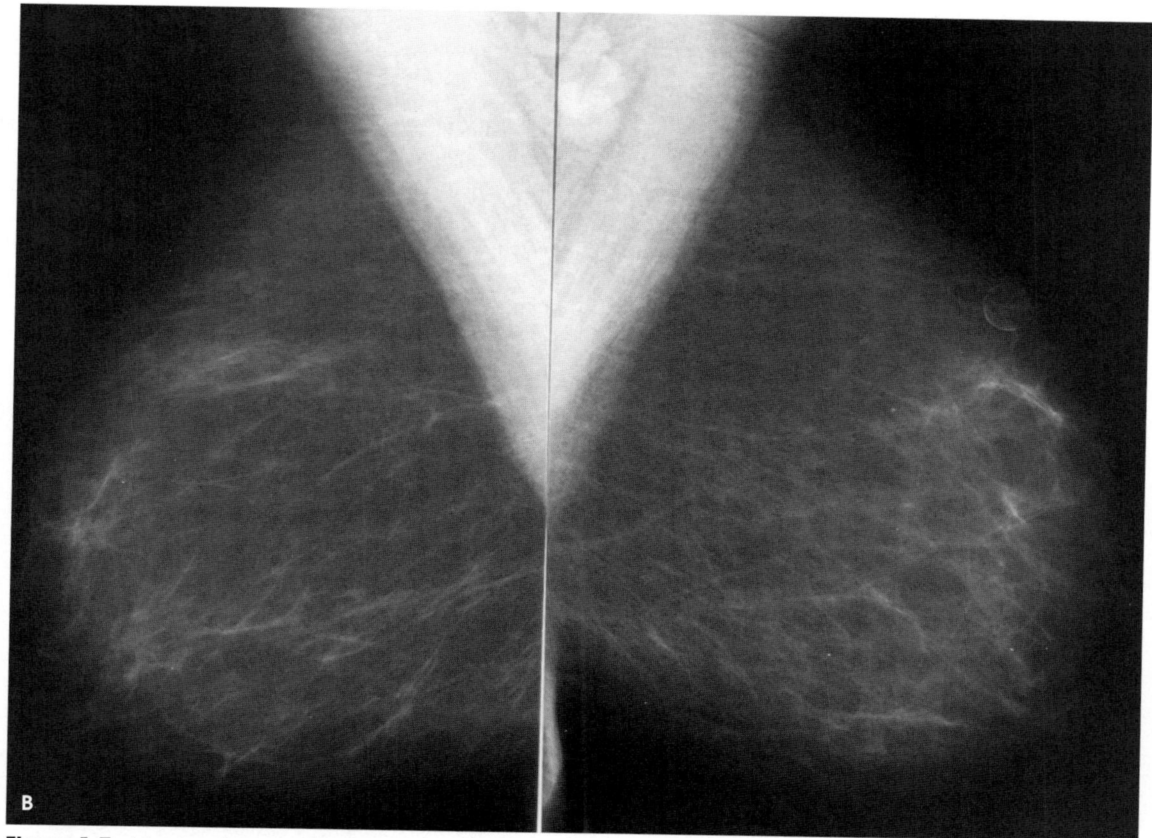

Figure 1.7. (*Continued*) Mediolateral oblique view.

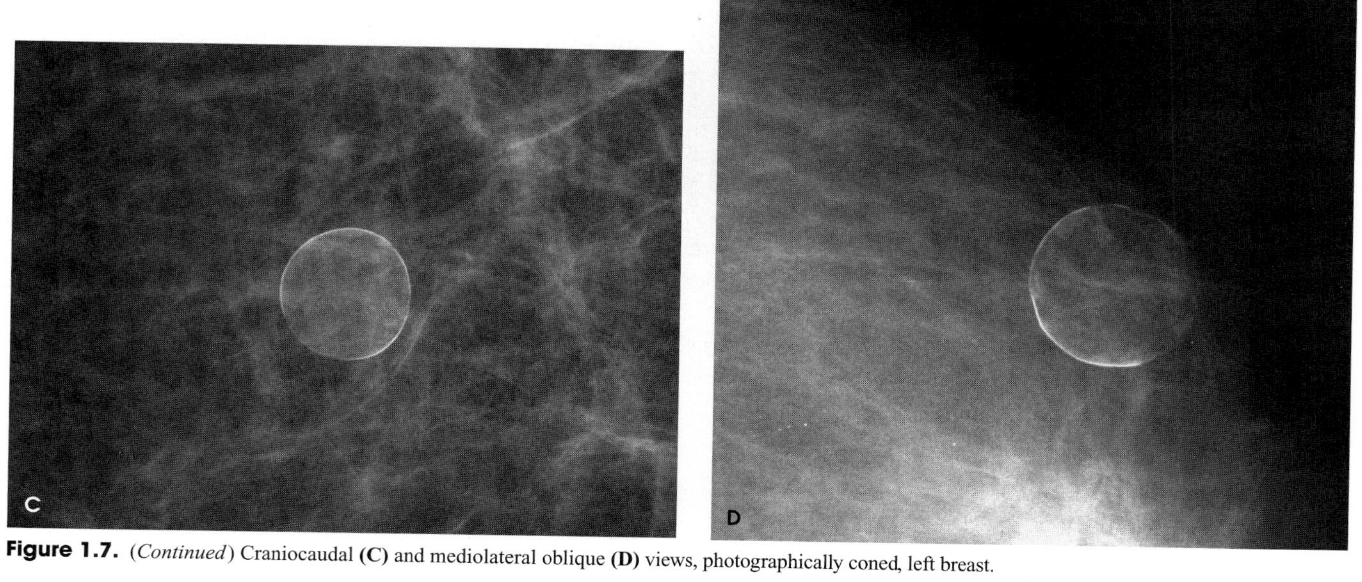

Figure 1.7. (*Continued*) Craniocaudal **(C)** and mediolateral oblique **(D)** views, photographically coned, left breast.

How would you describe the findings?

These are oil cysts with eggshell or rim calcification. Oil cysts commonly develop following trauma or surgery; however, most patients do not recall the trauma (and may not recall surgery). These are round or oval, well-circumscribed, radiolucent masses. As illustrated here, thin calcifications can develop in the wall of the cyst. With time these may stabilize or decrease progressively in size (Fig. 1.7E, F) and, in some patients, eventually resolve completely.

Steatocystoma multiplex is a rare, autosomal dominant condition characterized by the presence of multiple cutaneous cysts appearing during adolescence and increasing progressively with age involving the anterior trunk, back, proximal extremities, and external genitalia. Multiple oil cysts are seen mammographically.

BI-RADS® category 1: negative. BI-RADS® category 2: benign finding is used if the findings are described in the body of the report. Next screening mammogram is recommended in 1 year.

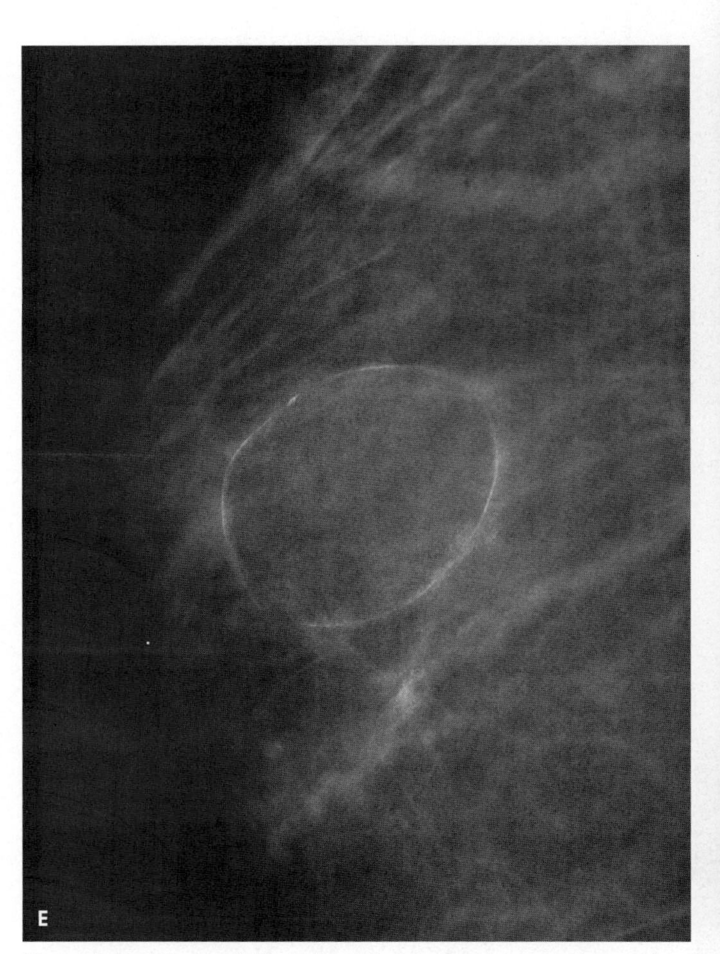

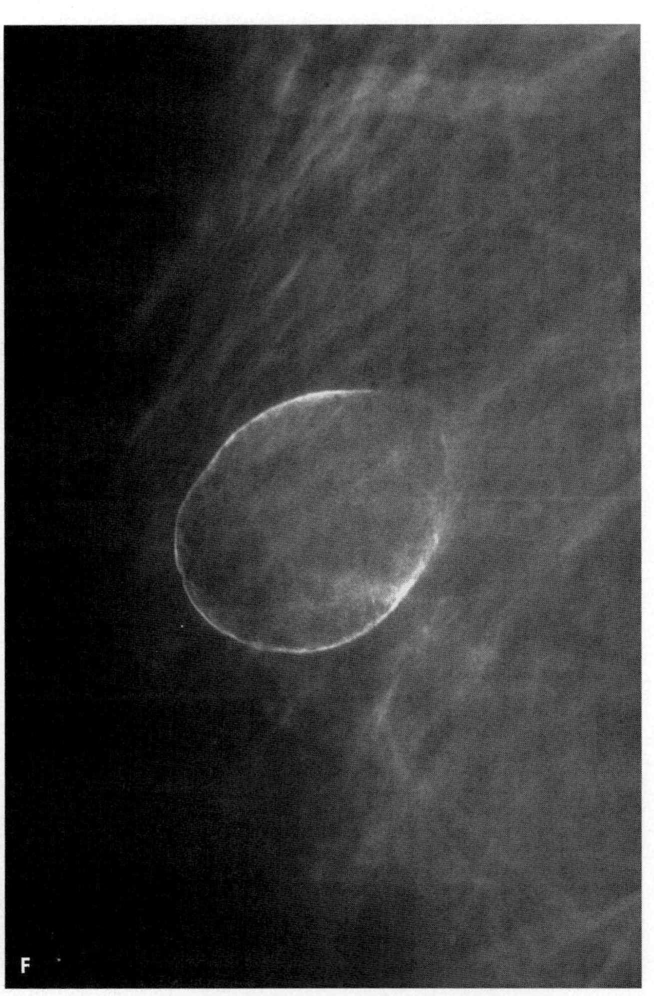

Figure 1.7. *(Continued)* Screening study, 46-year-old woman. Photographically coned images **(E, F)** of same area in the right breast, 2 years apart.

PATIENT 8

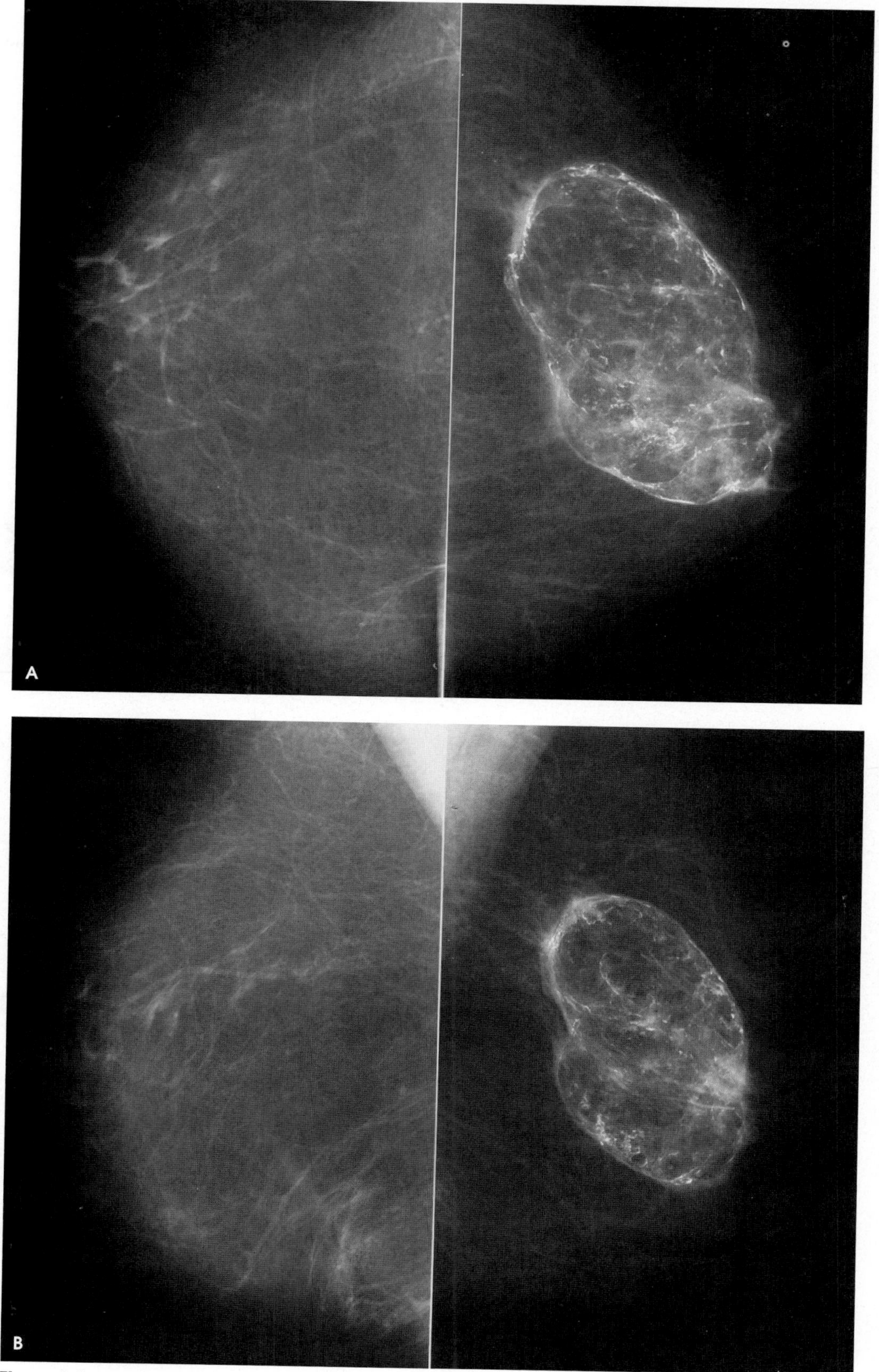

Figure 1.8. Screening study, 63-year-old woman. Craniocaudal **(A)** and mediolateral oblique **(B)** views, left breast.

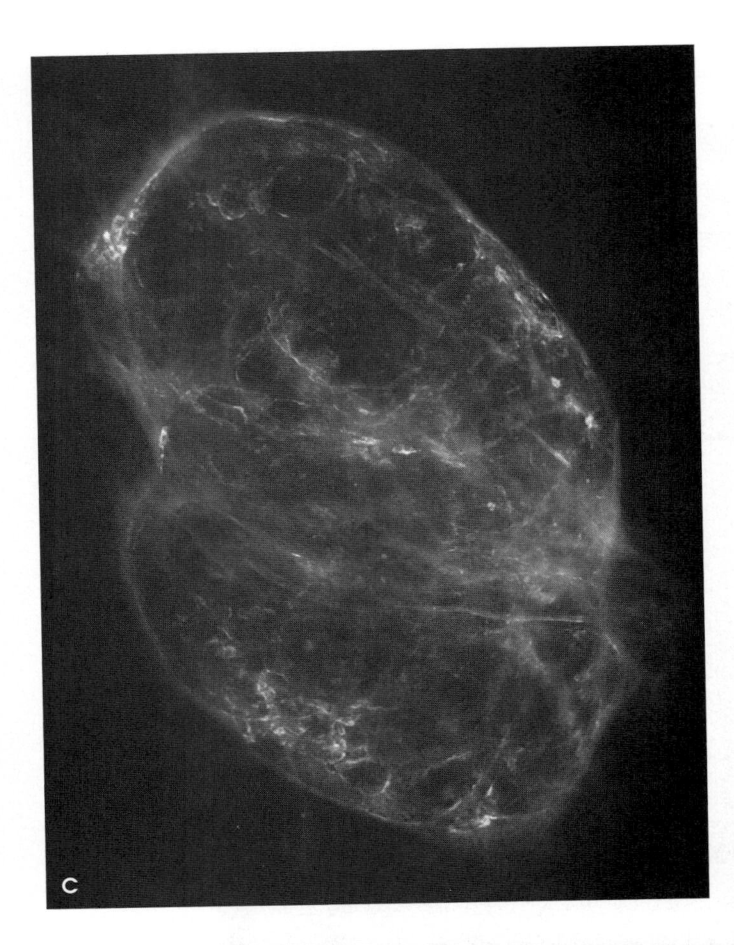

Figure 1.8. (*Continued*) Mediolateral oblique **(C)** view, left breast, photographically coned.

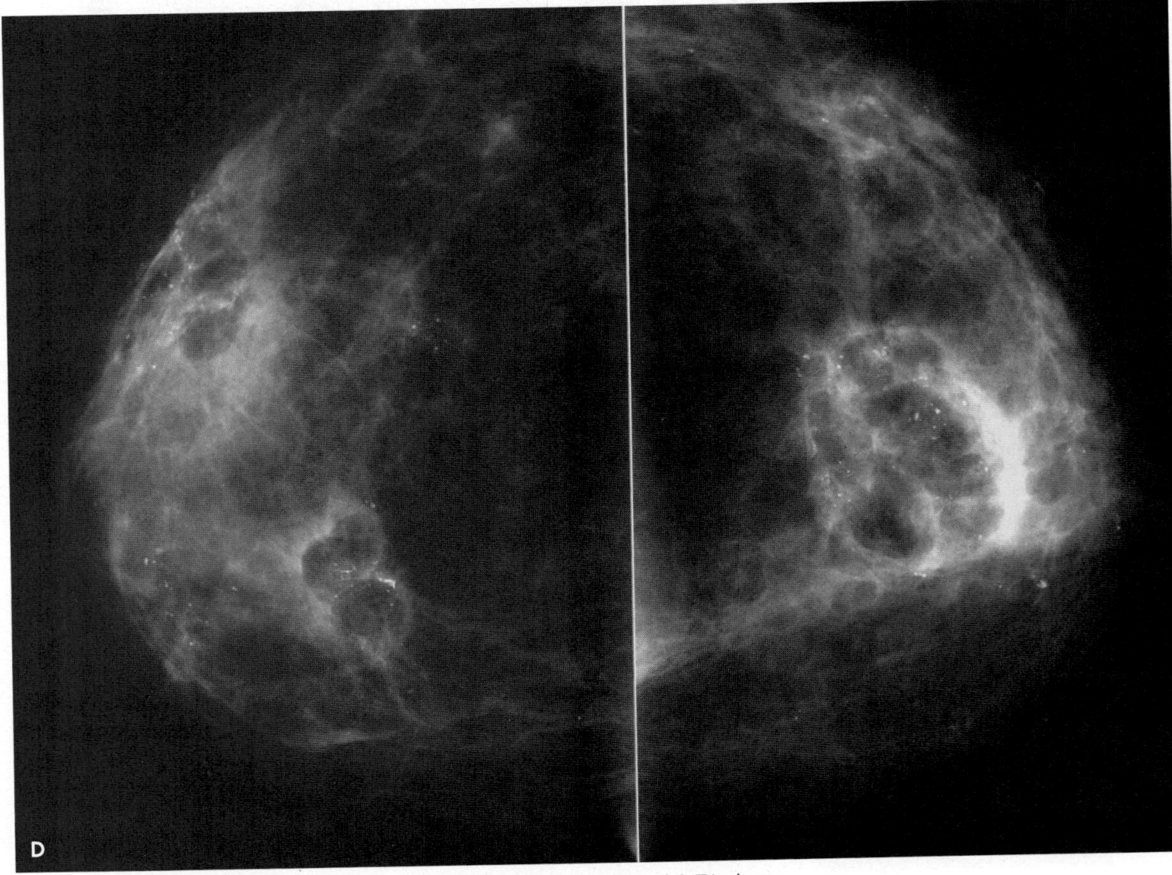

Figure 1.8. (*Continued*) Screening study, 40-year-old woman. Craniocaudal **(D)** views.

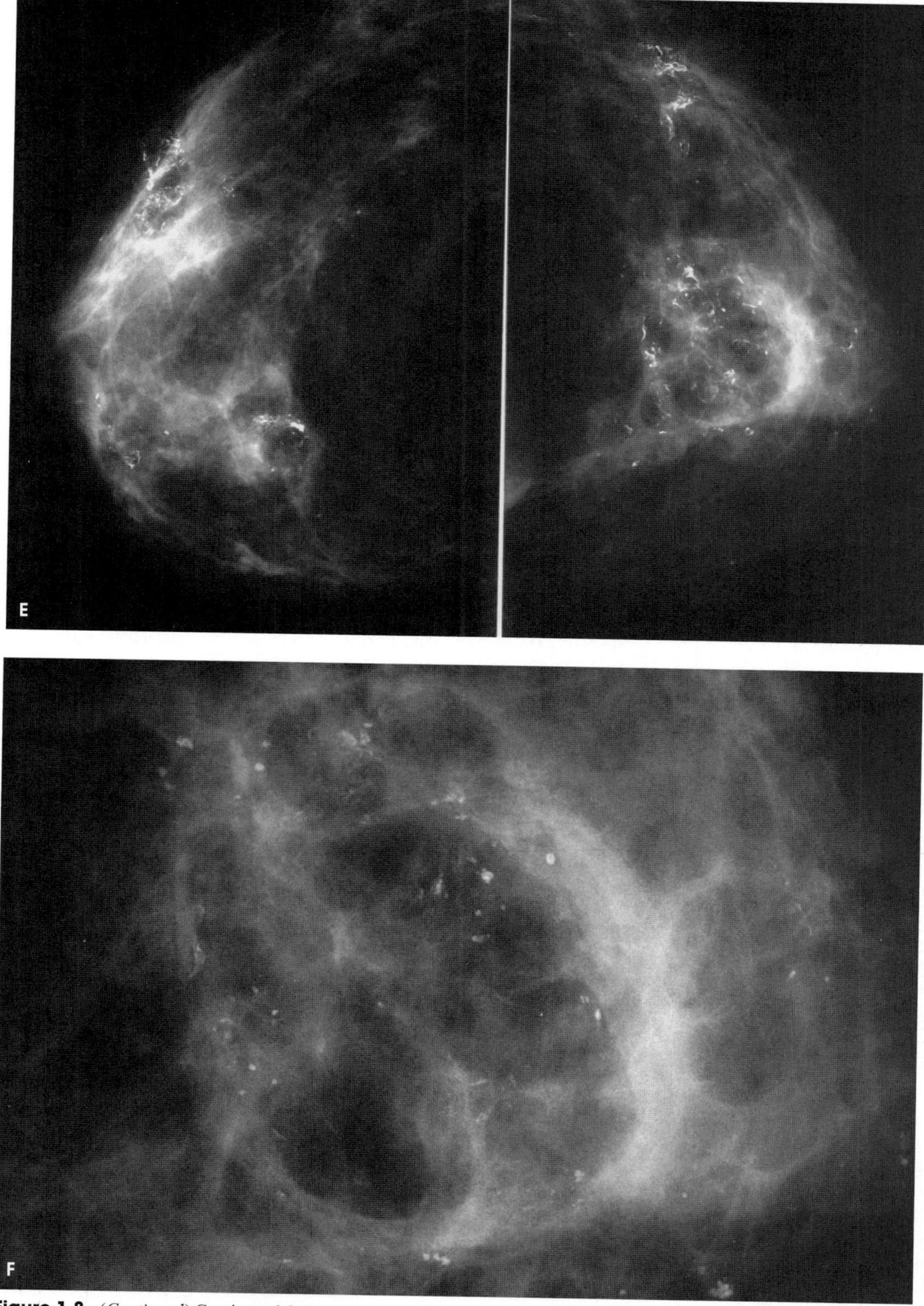

Figure 1.8. (*Continued*) Craniocaudal **(E)** views, 1 year following **(D)**. Craniocaudal **(F)** view, left breast, photographically coned.

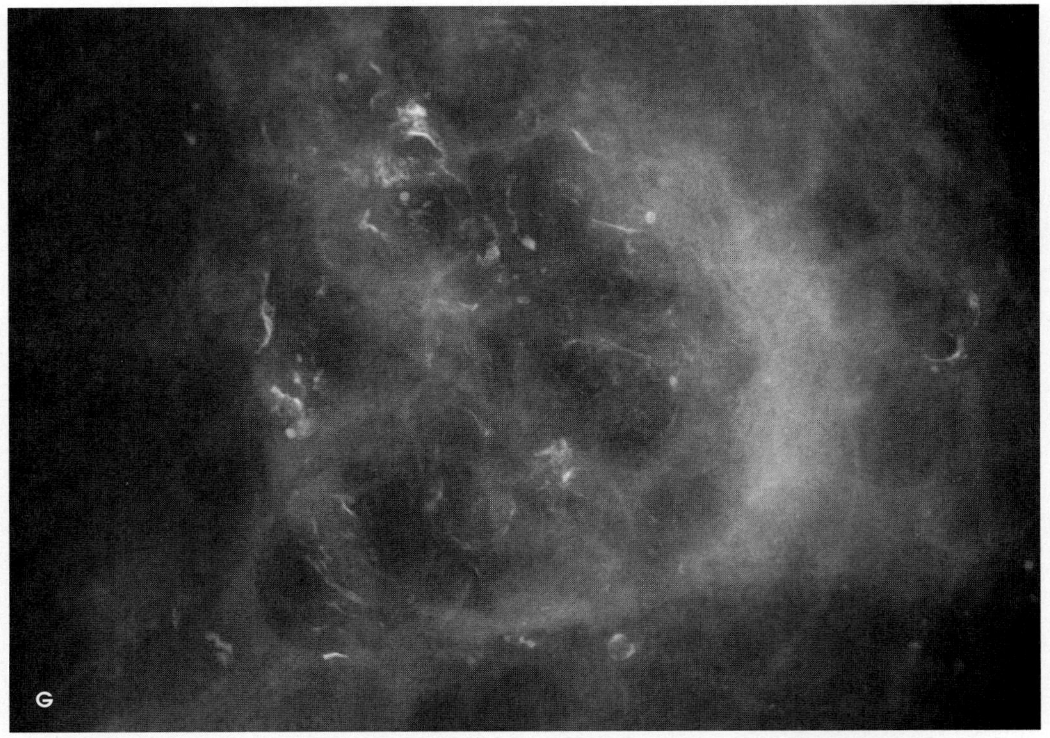

Figure 1.8. (*Continued*) Craniocaudal **(G)** view, left breast, photographically coned, 1 year following **(F)**.

How would you describe the findings? What procedure have both of these patients undergone?

A radiolucent mass with mural and internal curvilinear calcifications is seen in the left breast in Fig. 1.8A–C. The appearance of some of the internal calcifications suggests the presence of smaller lucent masses within the dominant mass. Also noted is asymmetric tissue inferiorly on the right mediolateral oblique view demonstrating a swirling pattern (Fig. 1.8B). The left breast is smaller than the right. The findings suggest a history of reduction mammoplasty, which is confirmed on the patient's history sheet.

In the second patient, multiple mixed-density masses of varying sizes are present bilaterally (Fig. 1.8D). A few dense calcifications are associated with some of the masses (Fig. 1.8D, F). A year later, many more coarse calcifications are noted associated with the mixed-density (fat containing) masses (Fig. 1.8E). The calcifications are now more curvilinear in appearance, seemingly outlining a cluster of lucent masses (Fig. 1.8G). As the calcifications have increased, the overall size and associated soft tissue component of some of the masses has decreased. The presence of multiple, bilateral oil cysts may reflect a history of trauma or, as in this patient, reduction mammoplasty. Comparison films, if available, will be helpful in establishing a change in overall breast size following the surgery, as well as the development of the oil cysts.

What are the imaging findings associated with fat necrosis?

In the acute setting, fat necrosis following reduction mammoplasty may present with one or multiple, mixed-density masses; some may be spiculated. As the inflammatory process associated with fat necrosis resolves, single or multiple, uni- or bilateral oil cysts of varying sizes may remain. Although some may develop rim calcifications, most develop coarser, curvilinear calcifications, as demonstrated in these two patients. With time, these may stabilize, continue to calcify, or some eventually resolve completely. In some patients, these become palpable as they calcify 1 or 2 years following the surgery. When they are palpable, it is important to reassure the patient that the palpable finding is benign and requires no further intervention. It is also important that a definitive report be issued.

BI-RADS® category 1: negative. BI-RADS® category 2: benign finding is used if the findings are described in the body of the report. Next screening mammogram is recommended in 1 year.

PATIENT 9

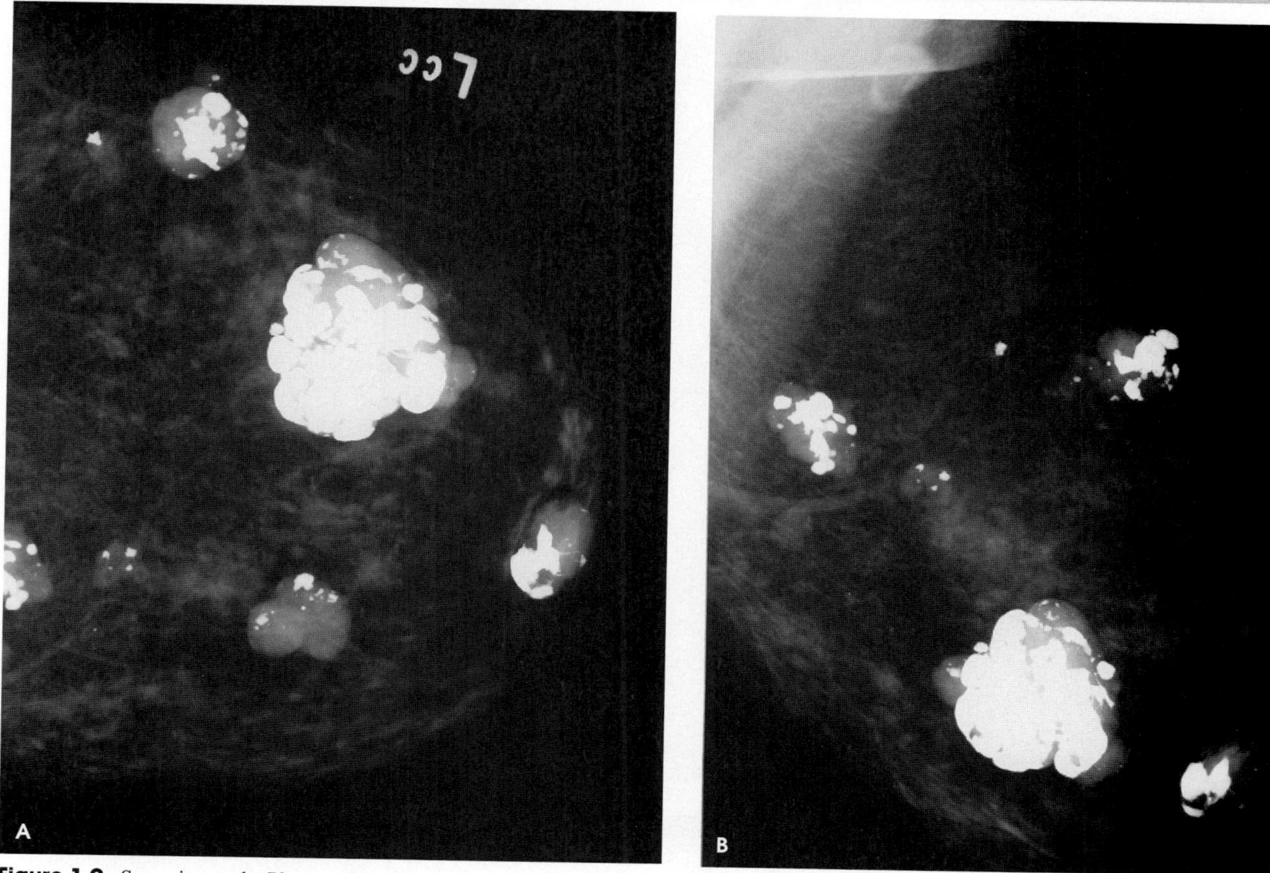

Figure 1.9. Screening study, 70-year-old woman. Craniocaudal **(A)** and mediolateral oblique **(B)** views, left breast.

What is the diagnosis and what BI-RADS® category would you assign?

Multiple, well-circumscribed, dense masses, some with macrolobulations and varying amounts of associated dense, coarse calcifications, are present in the left breast. These are hyalinizing fibroadenomas with associated dystrophic calcifications (i.e., popcorn-type calcifications). As estrogen levels decrease, the epithelial component in fibroadenomas atrophies and is replaced by dense, hyalinized fibrous tissue. These changes may be characterized mammographically by a decrease in size, an increase in density, and the development of dense, dystrophic calcifications in a pre-existing well-circumscribed mass. Because these calcifications develop in hyalinized fibrous tissue, they are variable in size, shape, and density (i.e., there is no preformed space molding the developing calcifications). Also noted is a well-circumscribed, mixed-density oval mass superimposed on the pectoral muscle on the mediolateral oblique view, consistent with a lymph node.

BI-RADS® category 2: benign finding. Next screening mammogram is recommended in 1 year.

PATIENT 10

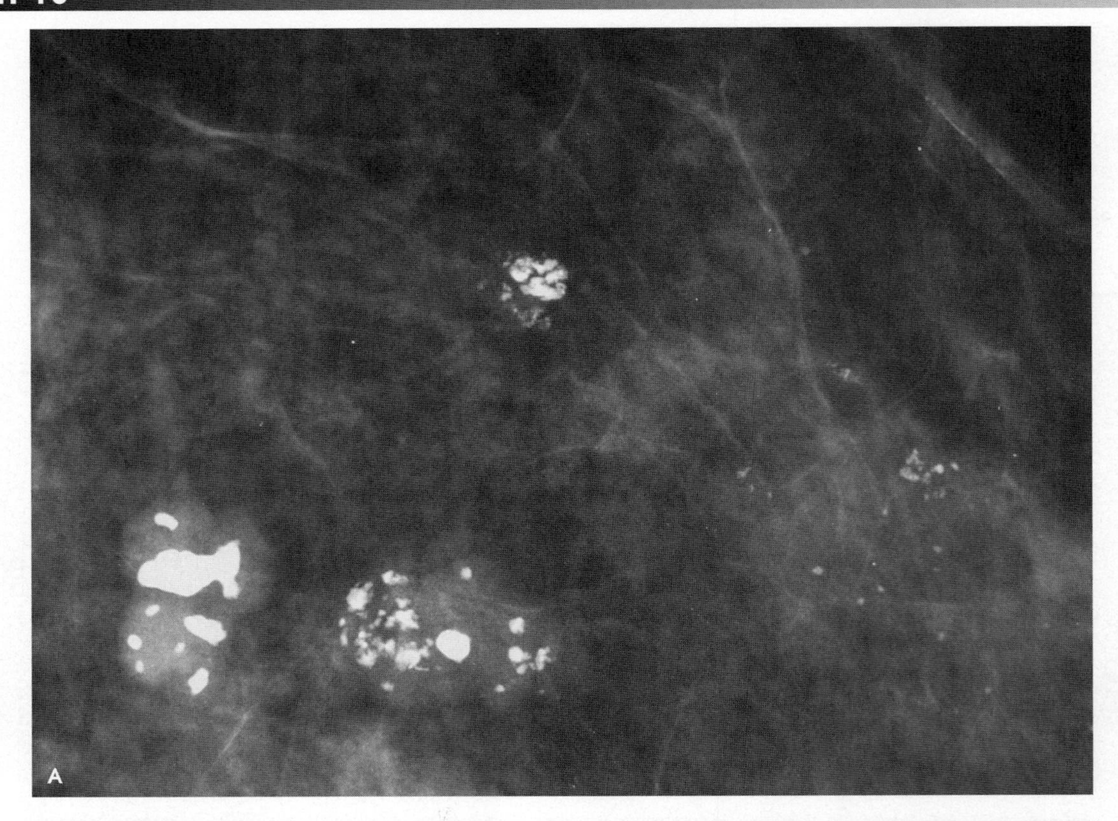

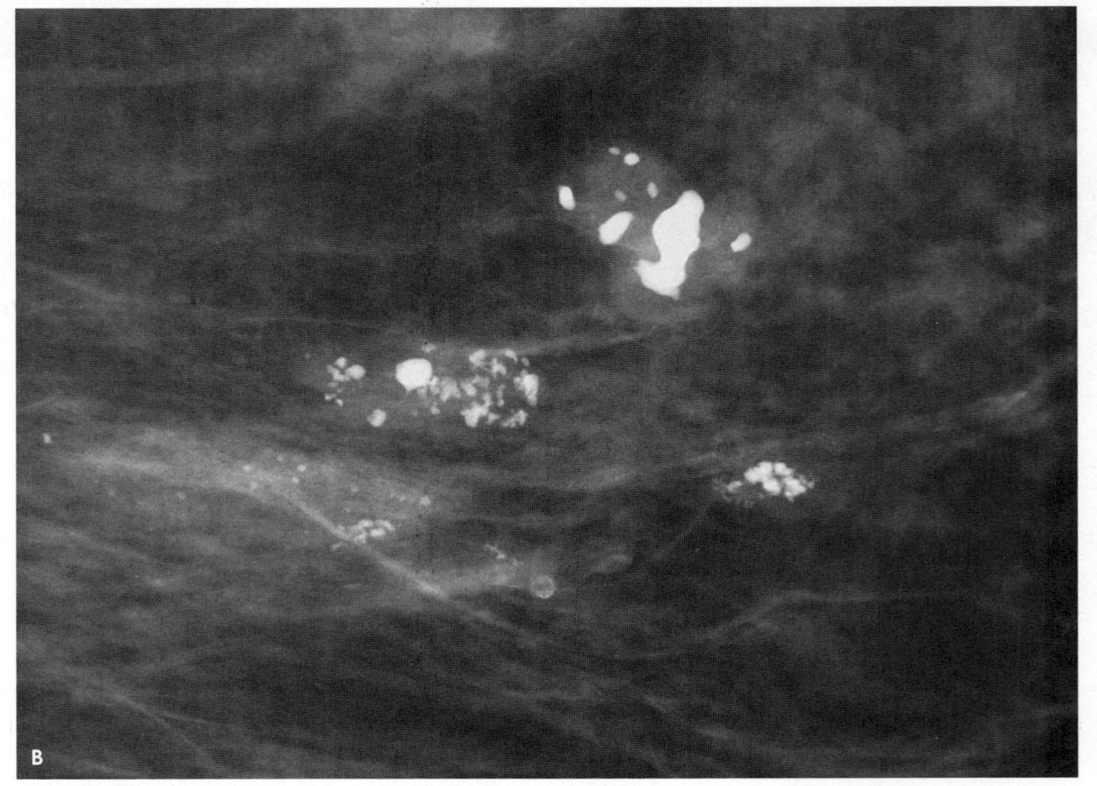

Figure 1.10. Screening study, 65-year-old woman. Craniocaudal **(A)** and mediolateral oblique **(B)** views, left breast, photographically coned.

What observations can you make, and do you think this woman needs to be called back for additional evaluation?

Two macrolobulated, dense masses with partially well circumscribed margins and coarse, dense calcifications are imaged in the left breast. A cluster of dense, tightly packed calcifications is also present (Fig. 1.10C, arrow), with no associated soft tissue component. Scattered benign calcifications and arterial calcification (Fig. 1.10C arrowheads) are incidentally noted. These are all hyalinizing fibroadenomas. It is important to recognize that a mass is not always seen in association with the dystrophic calcifications of a fibroadenoma (i.e., a cluster of calcifications alone can represent a hyalinizing fibroadenoma). These findings require no additional evaluation or short-interval follow-up. However, don't be lulled by obviously benign findings; make sure to focus your attention on the remainder of the mammogram.

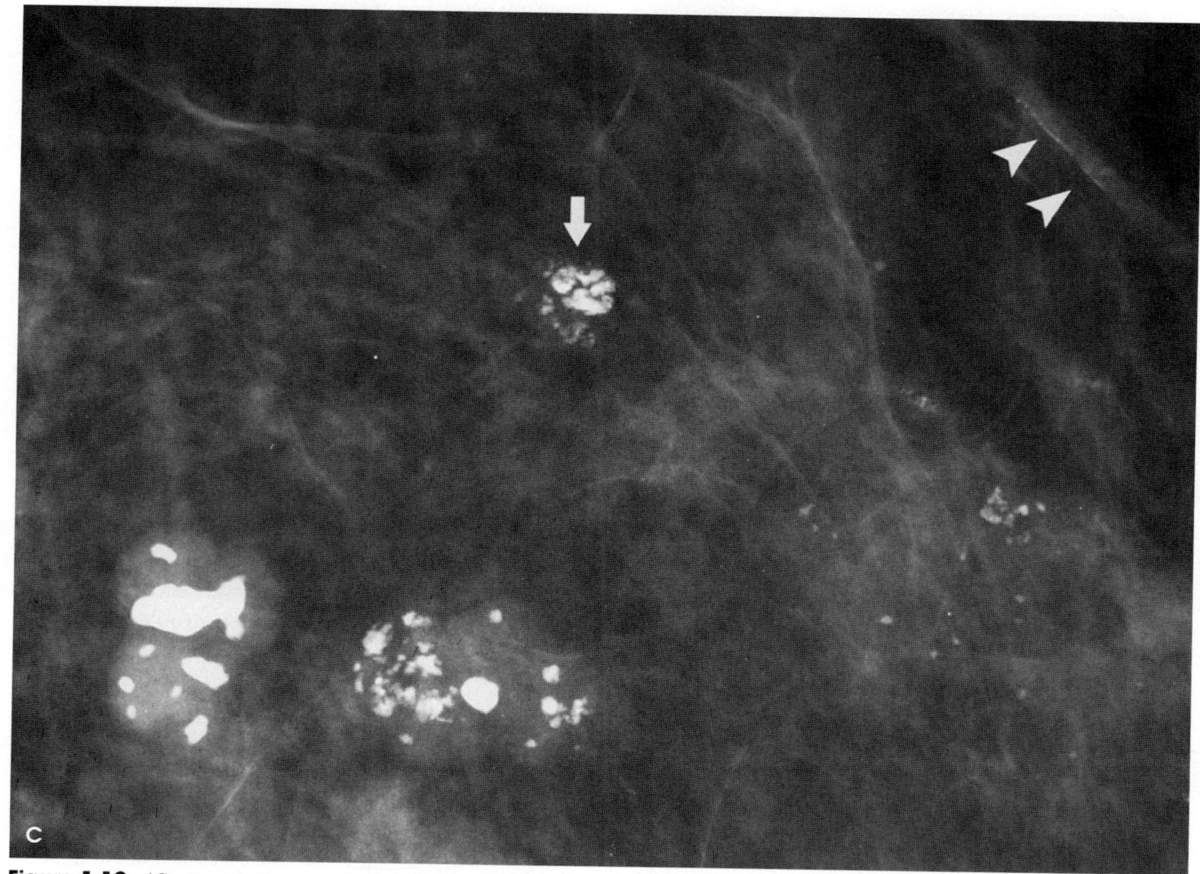

Figure 1.10. (*Continued*) Craniocaudal **(C)** view, left breast. Macrolobulated masses with dense, coarse calcifications represent hyalinizing fibroadenomas. Although no soft tissue component is present, a cluster of dense tightly packed calcifications (arrow) also represents a hyalinizing fibroadenoma. Arterial calcification (arrowheads) is present.

PATIENT 11

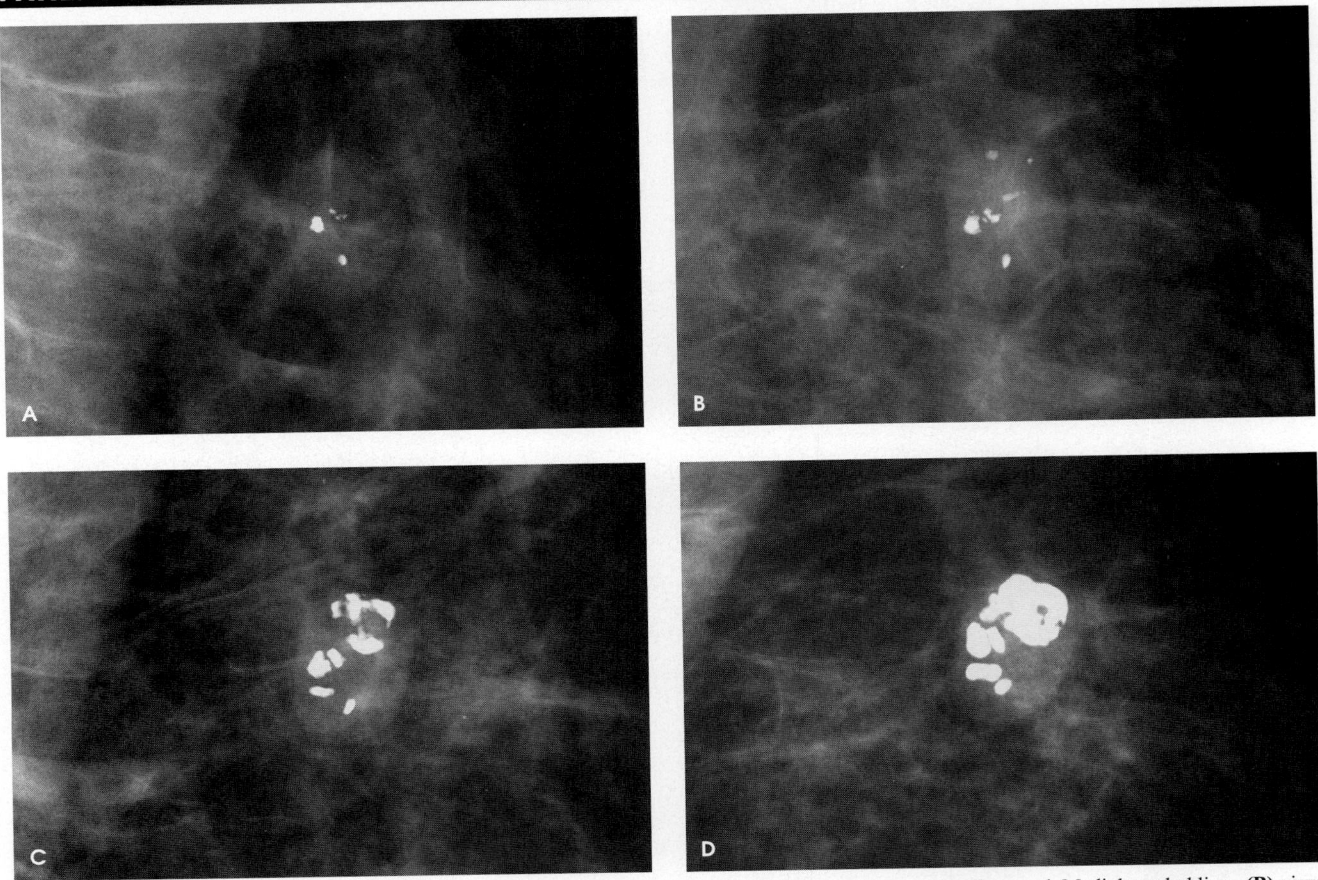

Figure 1.11. Screening studies, 43-year-old woman. Mediolateral oblique **(A)** view left breast, photographically coned. Mediolateral oblique **(B)** view, left breast, 1 year after **(A)**, photographically coned. Mediolateral oblique **(C)** view, left breast, 3 years after **(A)**, photographically coned. Mediolateral oblique **(D)** view, left breast, 5 years after **(A)**, photographically coned.

What is your diagnosis?

An oval mass, with partially obscured and well-circumscribed margins and associated dense coarse calcifications, is imaged anterior to the pectoral muscle. On subsequent screening studies, the mass decreases slightly in size, becomes denser, and the calcifications increase in number, size, and density. These findings are diagnostic of a hyalinizing fibroadenoma with dystrophic calcifications (i.e., developing popcorn calcification). This finding is benign and requires no additional evaluation or short-interval follow-up.

PATIENT 12

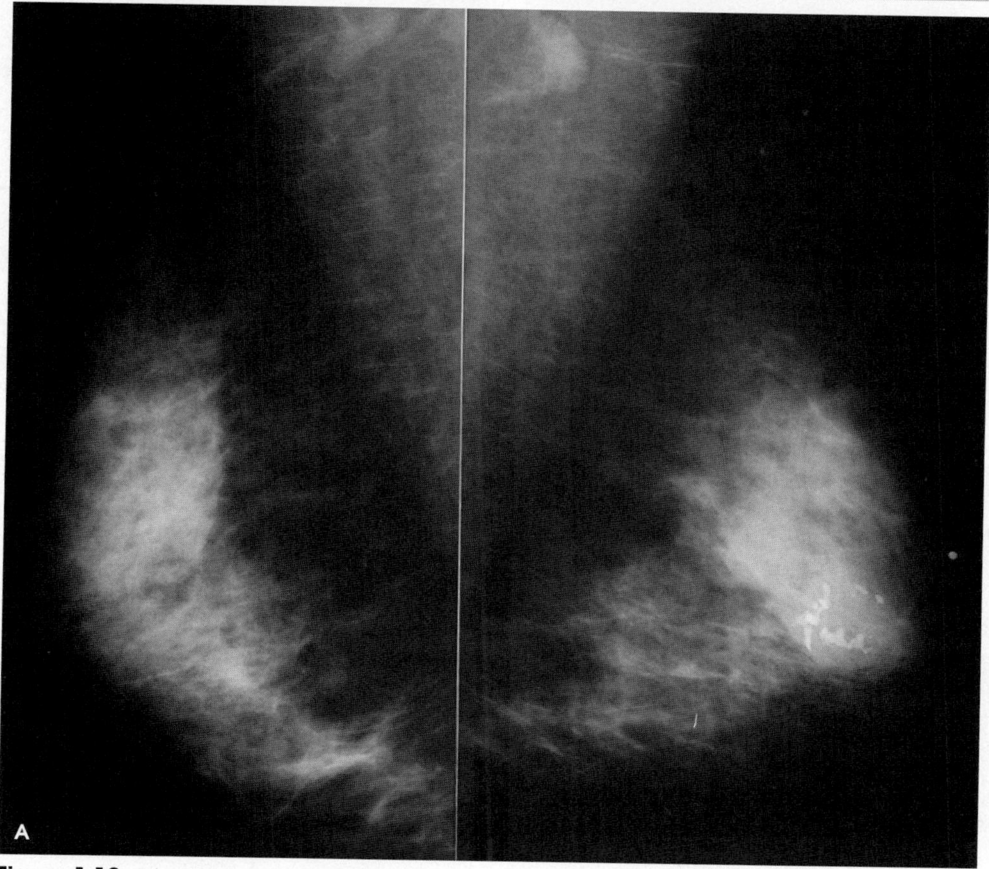

Figure 1.12. Diagnostic study, 48-year-old patient presenting with a "lump" in the left breast. Mediolateral oblique (**A**) views with metallic BB on the "lump" described by the patient in the left breast.

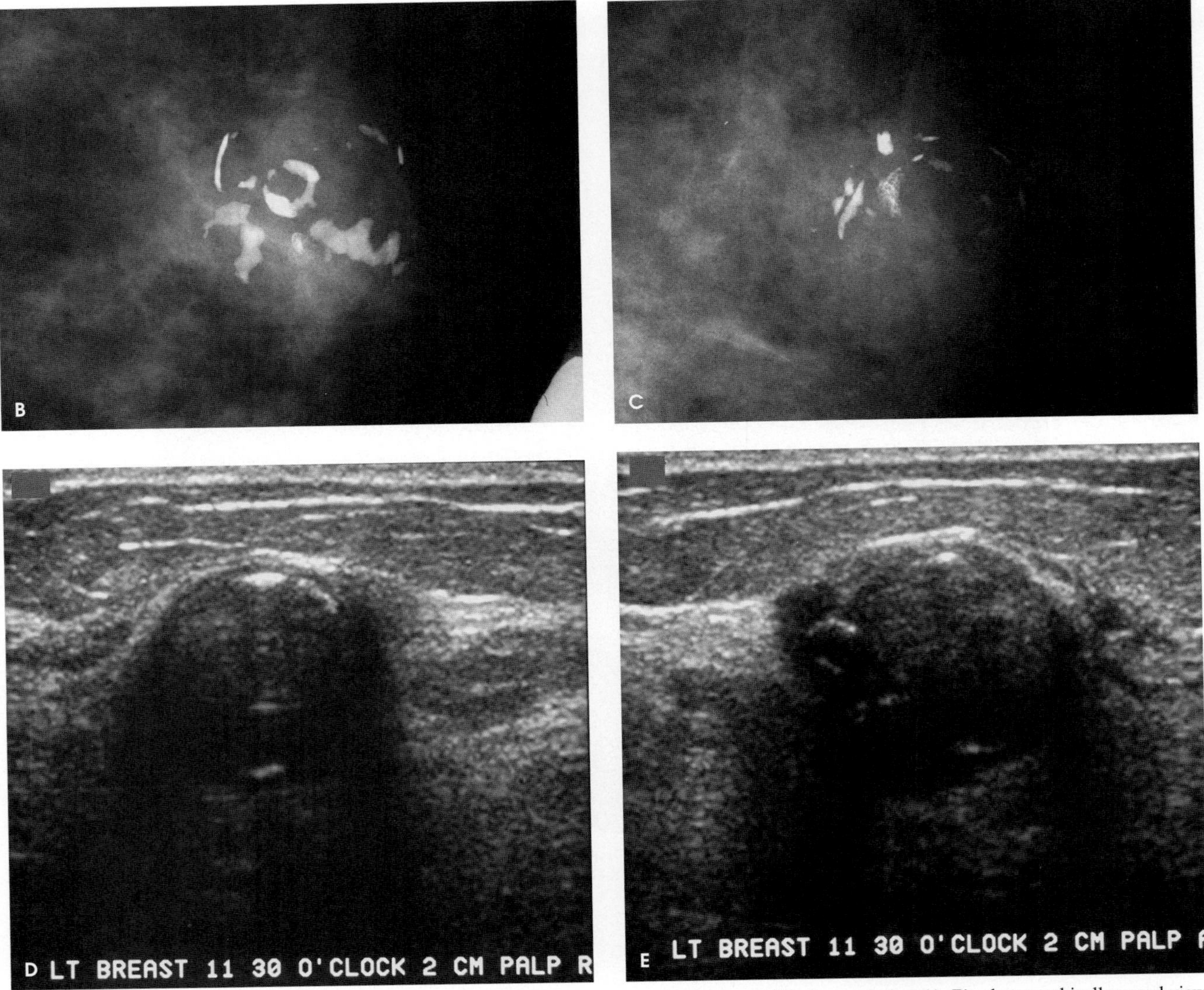

Figure 1.12. (*Continued*) Spot compression **(B)** view of palpable finding. Left subareolar area **(C)**, 5 years before **(A, B)**, photographically coned view. Ultrasound images, radial (RAD) **(D)** and antiradial (ARAD). **(E)** projections of palpable (PALP) finding.

How would you describe the mammographic and ultrasound findings, and what is your recommendation for this patient?

Lymph nodes are present in both axillary regions. A 2-cm mass with obscured margins and associated coarse calcifications is seen in the left subareolar area on the mediolateral oblique views. On the spot compression view, the margins are irregular and indistinct. Compared with the study from 5 years previously, the mass is now more dense and the calcifications are larger.

On physical examination, a readily mobile, hard, nontender mass is palpated at the 11:30 o'clock position, 2 cm from the left nipple. On ultrasound, a round mass with heterogeneous echotexture and shadowing is imaged corresponding to the palpable finding. Several areas of hyperechogenicity (Fig. 1.12F, G, arrows), some curvilinear, others with associated shadowing (Fig. 1.12F, G, arrowheads), are noted consistent with the calcifications seen mammographically. The mammographic findings are diagnostic of a hyalinizing fibroadenoma with associated dystrophic calcifications. Although an ultrasound is shown here for completeness, the diagnosis is made on the mammographic findings. This is explained to the patient; she is reassured that what she feels is a benign lesion that will not turn into cancer and has been present for 5 years with no significant changes. A definitive report is issued describing the palpable finding as a hyalinizing fibroadenoma requiring no further intervention or short-interval follow-up.

As the estrogen levels decrease, the epithelial elements in fibroadenomas atrophy and are replaced by an increasing amount of fibrous tissue. Mammographically, hyalinizing fibroadenomas may decrease slightly in size and become more dense so that, in some women, they become more readily apparent while some undergo calcification, as demonstrated in this patient.

BI-RADS® category 2: benign finding. Next screening mammogram is recommended in 1 year.

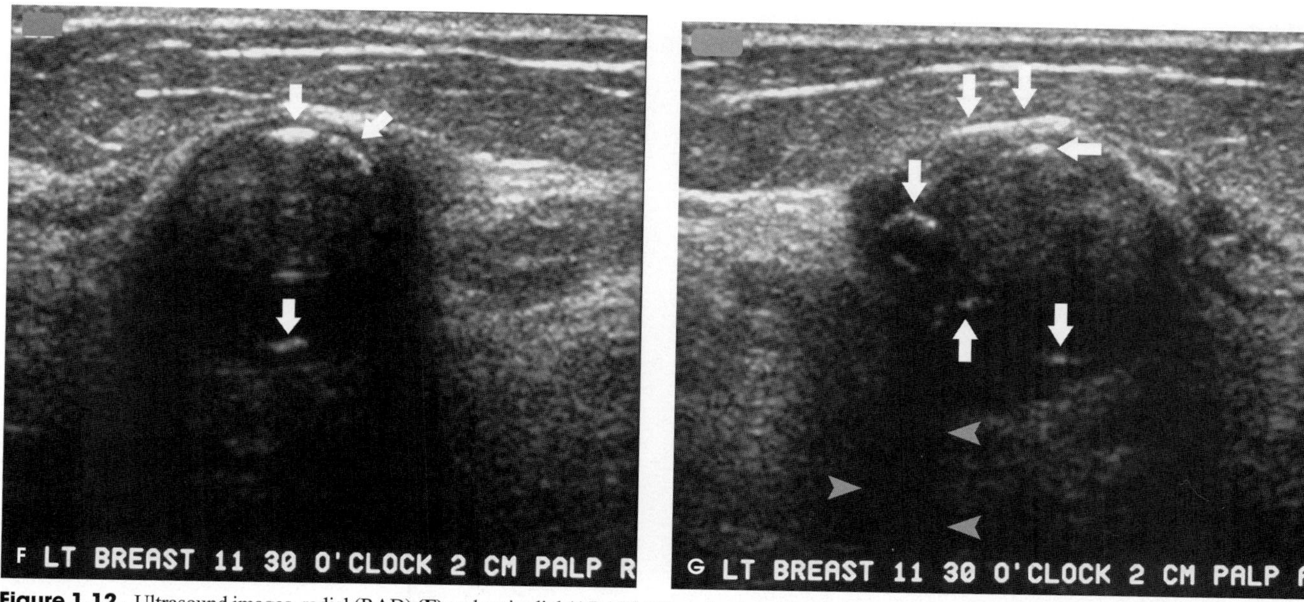

Figure 1.12. Ultrasound images, radial (RAD) **(F)** and antiradial (ARAD) **(G)** projections of palpable (PALP) finding in the left breast at the 11:30 o'clock position, 2 cm from the nipple. A round, hypoechoic mass with heterogeneous echotexture, dense calcifications (*arrows*), and shadowing are imaged, corresponding to the palpable area of concern to the patient. Shadowing (*arrowheads*) is intermittently seen associated with some of the calcifications.

PATIENT 13

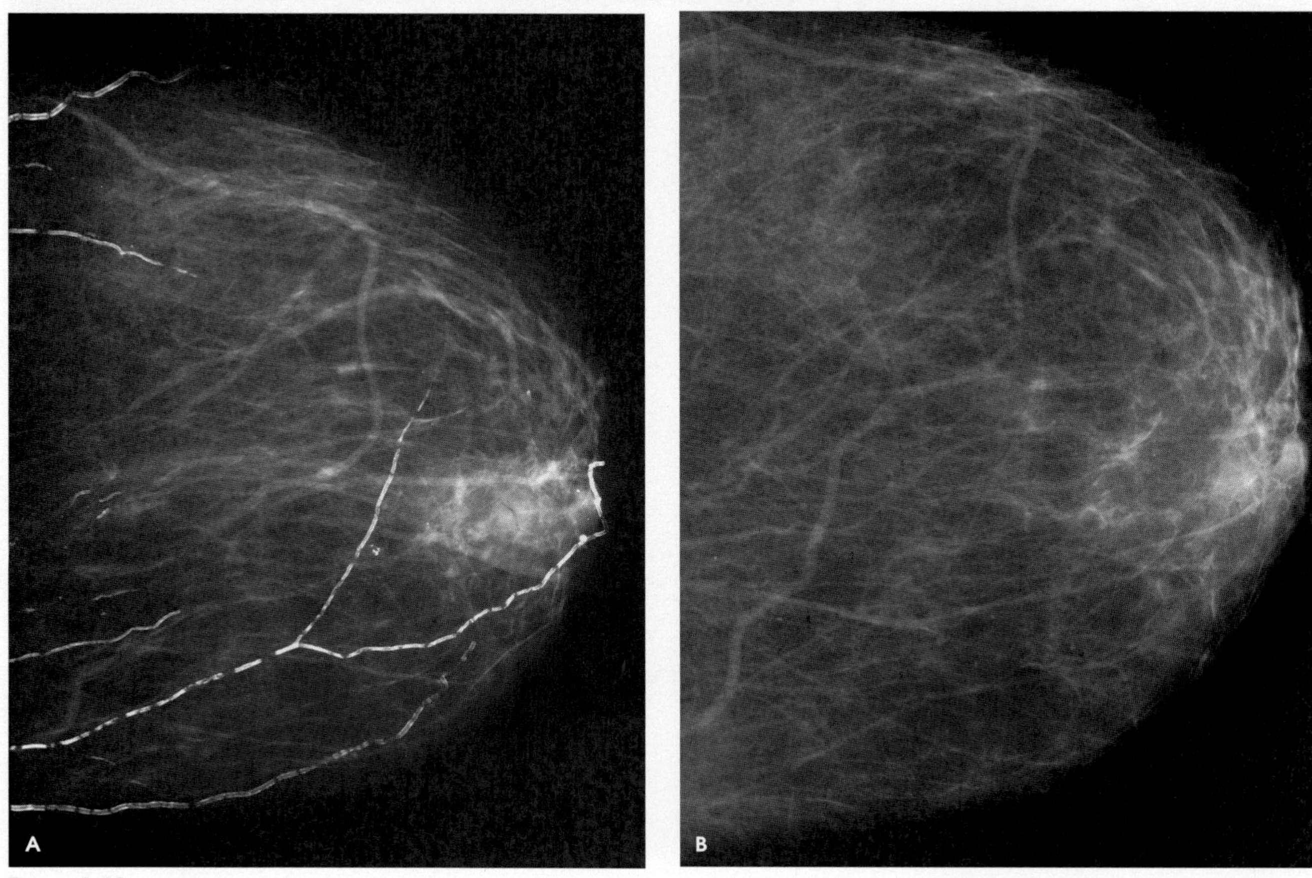

Figure 1.13. Screening mammogram, 63-year-old woman. Craniocaudal **(A)** view, left breast. Craniocaudal **(B)** view, left breast, 3 years previously.

How would you describe the findings?

Linear, parallel, tram-track-like calcifications represent vascular (arterial) calcifications. This patient has developed dense vascular calcifications in the span of 3 years, suggesting the possibility of diabetes or atherosclerotic disease that may be significant. In this patient, I describe the development of vascular calcifications in the mammographic report. It is reasonable to contact the referring physician directly, particularly if the patient provides no information relative to underlying diabetic, cardiac, or renal disease (e.g., what medications is the patient taking?), to discuss the findings.

Reportedly, arterial calcifications are more common in postmenopausal women who are not on hormone replacement therapy (HRT). The rapid development of arterial calcifications in some perimenopausal women might serve as an indication for considering HRT; also, mammography may prove helpful in monitoring the effectiveness of HRT. The prevalence of arterial calcifications increases with age among all women. However, it is important to recognize that arterial calcifications are reportedly four times more likely in diabetic patients (i.e., those on insulin or oral hypoglycemic agents) and three times more likely in hypertensive patients (i.e., those on oral antihypertensives) compared to women with no history of diabetes or hypertension.

Arterial calcifications in young women, particularly when in conjunction with skin thickening (specifically axillary skin) and breast microcalcifications, have also been reported in women with pseudoxanthoma elasticum (PXE). This is an autosomal recessive disorder characterized by fragmentation, clumping, and calcification of elastic fibers in skin, eyes, and arteries. Yellowish skin papules and redundant skin folds at flexural sites (e.g., axilla, groin) are common cutaneous findings. Angioid streaks in the retina affect almost 100% of patients after the age of 30 years and can result in loss of visual acuity. Peripheral vascular disease, resulting from calcification of medium-sized arteries, can lead to claudication, hypertension, angina, myocardial infarction, cerebrovascular accidents, bowel angina with resulting gastrointestinal bleeding, and complicated pregnancies, often resulting in miscarriages. Although skin changes commonly develop during childhood, the disorder is not usually diagnosed until the third or fourth decade, when systemic complications become apparent.

BI-RADS® category 2: benign finding. Next screening mammogram is recommended in 1 year.

PATIENT 14

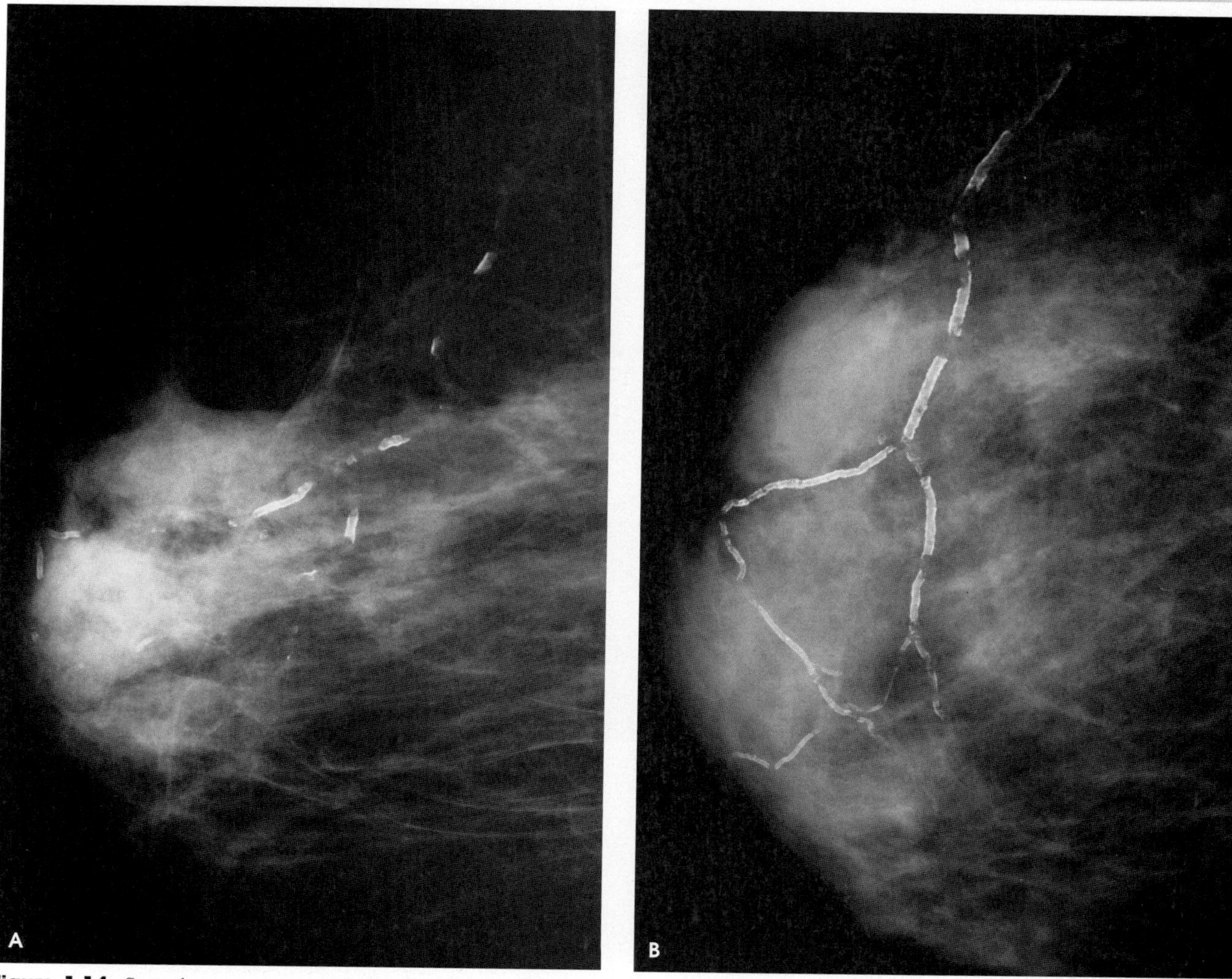

Figure 1.14. Screening mammogram, 55-year-old woman. Mediolateral oblique **(A)** view, right breast. Mediolateral oblique **(B)** view, right breast, 4 years previously.

How would you describe the findings?

Dense, linear, parallel, tram-track-like calcifications represent vascular (arterial) calcification. In this patient, the arterial calcification is resolving. Typically, vascular calcifications develop and can be seen mammographically as women age. As illustrated by this patient, if the underlying cause(s) of atherosclerosis is (are) treated successfully, vascular calcifications can resolve partially or completely, but this is the rare case.

Reportedly, arterial calcifications are more common in postmenopausal women who are not on hormone replacement therapy (HRT). The rapid development of arterial calcifications in some perimenopausal women might serve as an indication for considering HRT; also, mammography may prove helpful in monitoring the effectiveness of HRT. The prevalence of arterial calcifications increases with age among all women. However, it is important to recognize that arterial calcifications are reportedly four times more likely in diabetic patients (i.e., those on insulin or oral hypoglycemic agents) and three times more likely in hypertensive patients (i.e., those on oral antihypertensives) compared to women with no history of diabetes or hypertension.

Arterial calcifications in young women, particularly when in conjunction with skin thickening (specifically axillary skin) and breast microcalcifications, have also been reported in women with pseudoxanthoma elasticum (PXE). This is an autosomal recessive disorder characterized by fragmentation, clumping and calcification of elastic fibers in skin, eyes, and arteries. Yellowish skin papules and redundant skin folds at flexural sites (e.g., axilla, groin) are common cutaneous findings. Angioid streaks in the retina affect almost 100% of patients after the age of 30 years and can result in loss of visual acuity. Peripheral vascular disease, resulting from calcification of medium-sized arteries, can lead to claudication, hypertension, angina, myocardial infarction, cerebrovascular accidents, bowel angina with resulting gastrointestinal bleeding, and complicated pregnancies, often resulting in miscarriages. Although skin changes commonly develop during childhood, the disorder is not usually diagnosed until the third or fourth decade, when systemic complications become apparent.

BI-RADS® category 2: benign finding. Next screening mammogram is recommended in 1 year.

PATIENT 15

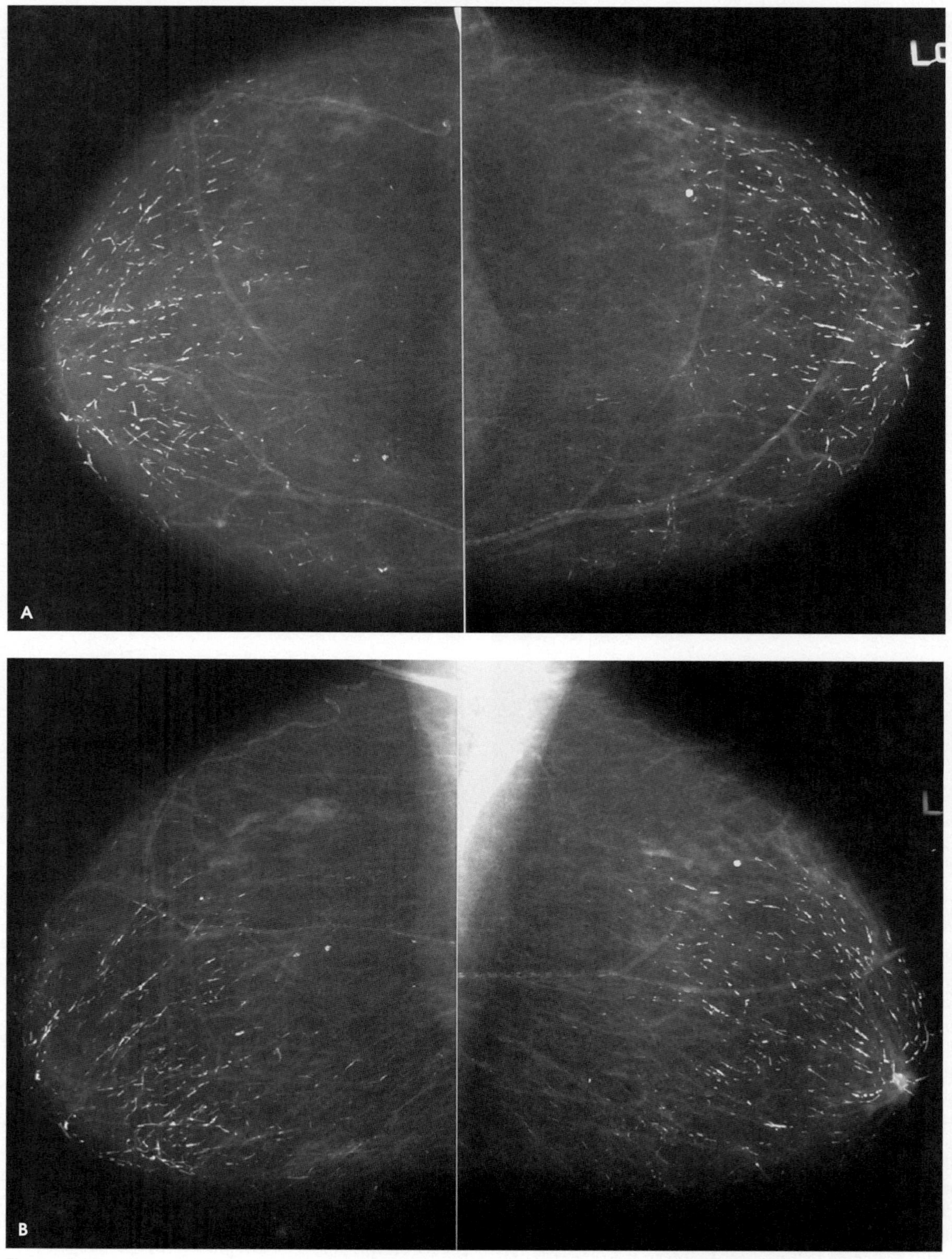

Figure 1.15. (*Continued*) Screening study, 80-year-old woman. Craniocaudal **(A)** and mediolateral oblique **(B)** views.

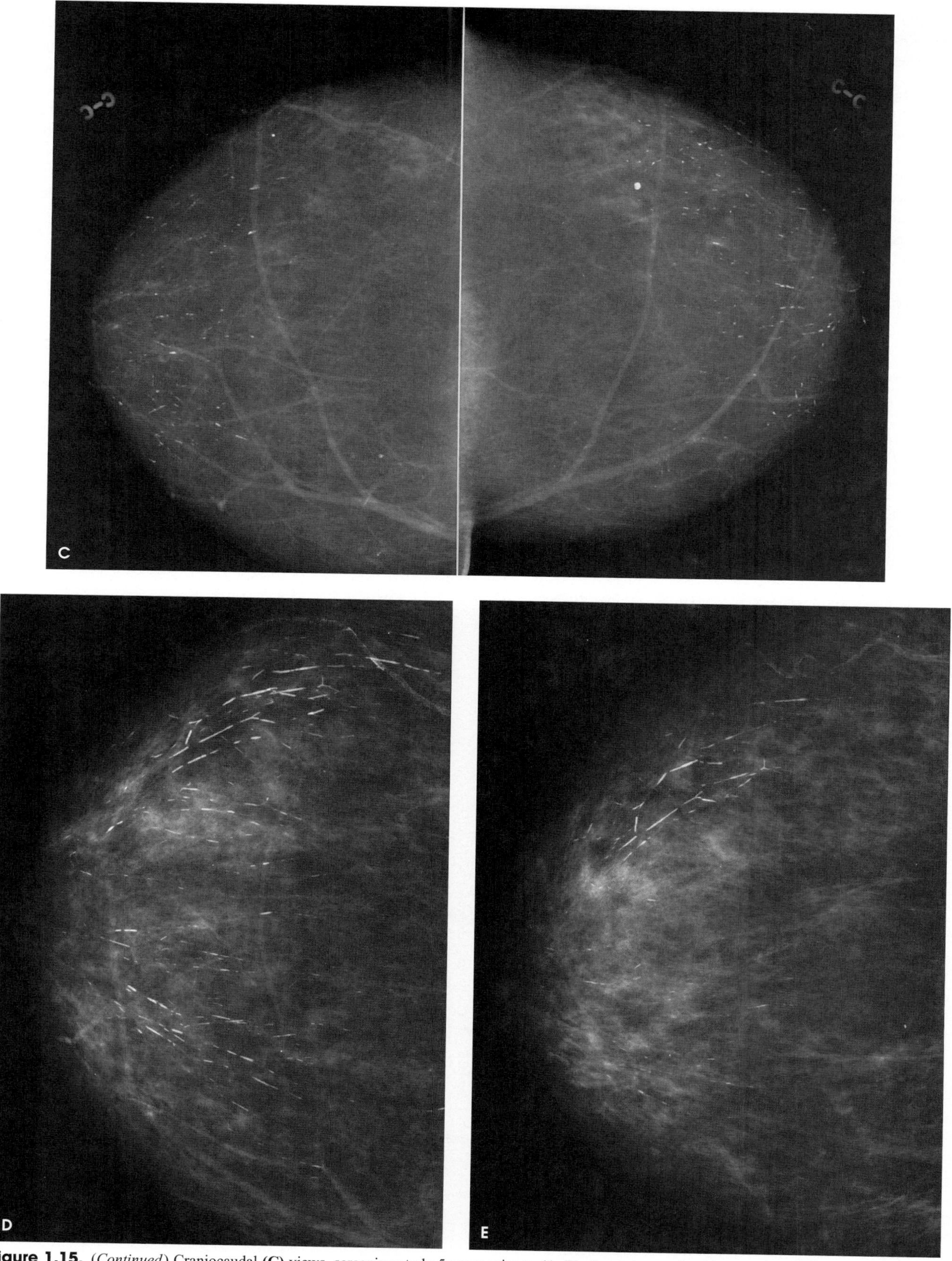

Figure 1.15. (*Continued*) Craniocaudal **(C)** views, screening study 5 years prior to **(A, B)**. Screening study, 76-year-old woman. Craniocaudal **(D)** view, right breast. Craniocaudal **(E)** view, right breast, 2 years prior to **(D)**.

How would you describe the findings, and what would you recommend next?

Large rodlike calcifications are present bilaterally (Fig. 1.15A, B). These calcifications are typically coarse, dense, and rod shaped. As demonstrated, they develop progressively (compare Fig. 1.15A with Fig. 1.15C), are often oriented toward the nipple, and the process is commonly bilaterally. Branching may be seen, and when the calcifications develop periductally, a central lucency may be noted. These calcifications have been described as being associated with duct ectasia; a variety of terms have been used to describe the process, including periductal mastitis, secretory disease, comedo mastitis, plasma cell mastitis, and mastitis obliterans. Also noted is the progressive development of arterial calcifications.

Progressive development of large rodlike calcifications is noted in the right craniocaudal views shown in Fig. 1.15D. These are benign and require no additional evaluation or intervention. Also noted is vascular calcification. Annual screening mammography is recommended for these two patients. However, a word of caution is indicated when large rodlike calcifications develop focally in a patient, particularly if the calcifications are not oriented toward the nipple and there are no other calcifications in either breast. Rarely, ductal carcinoma in situ (DCIS) with central necrosis can present with calcifications that may be mistaken for the type of calcification illustrated here.

BI-RADS® category 1: negative. BI-RADS® category 2: benign finding is used if the calcifications are described in the body of the report. Next screening mammogram is recommended in 1 year.

PATIENT 16

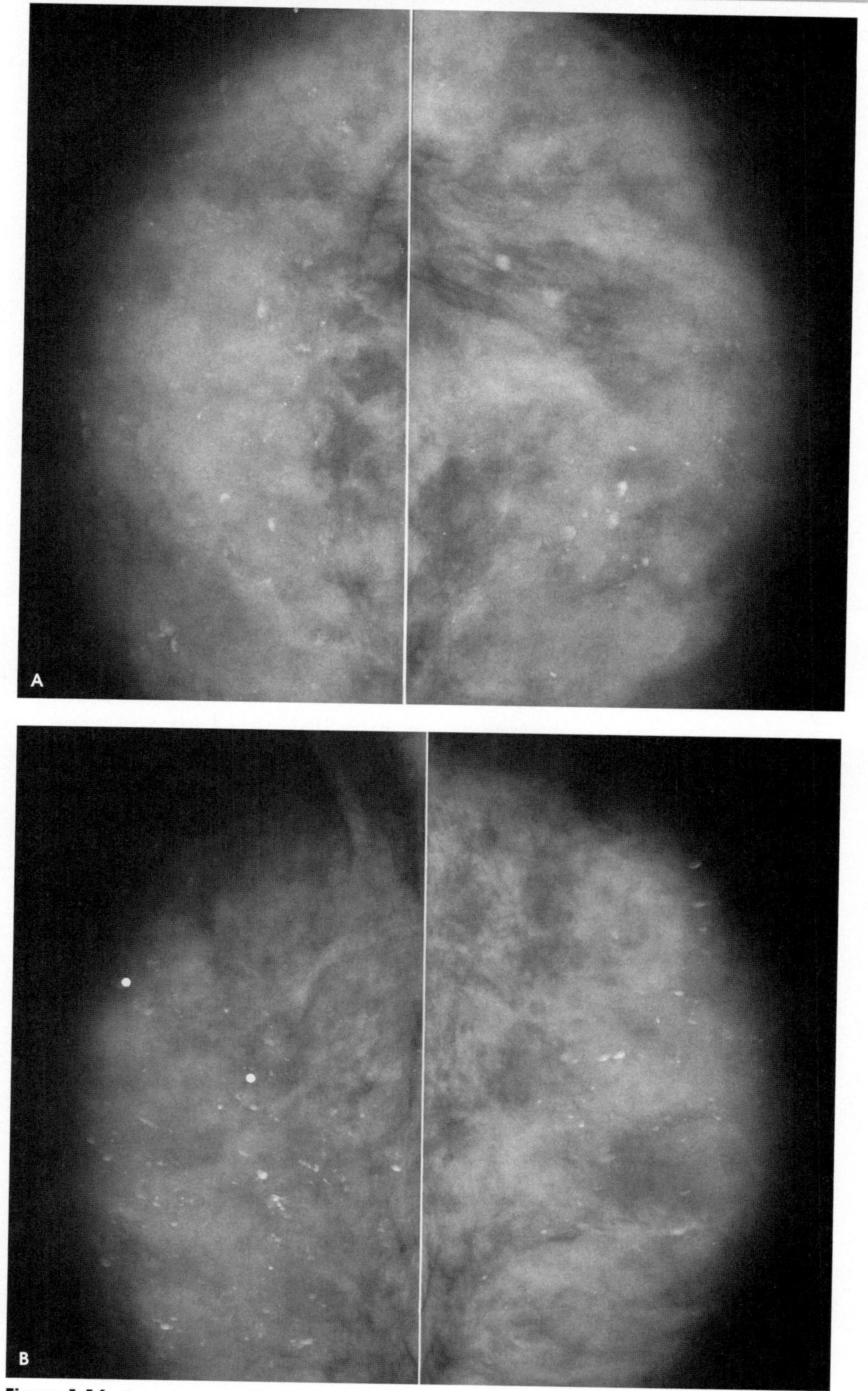

Figure 1.16. Screening study, 42-year-old woman. Craniocaudal **(A)** and mediolateral oblique **(B)** views.

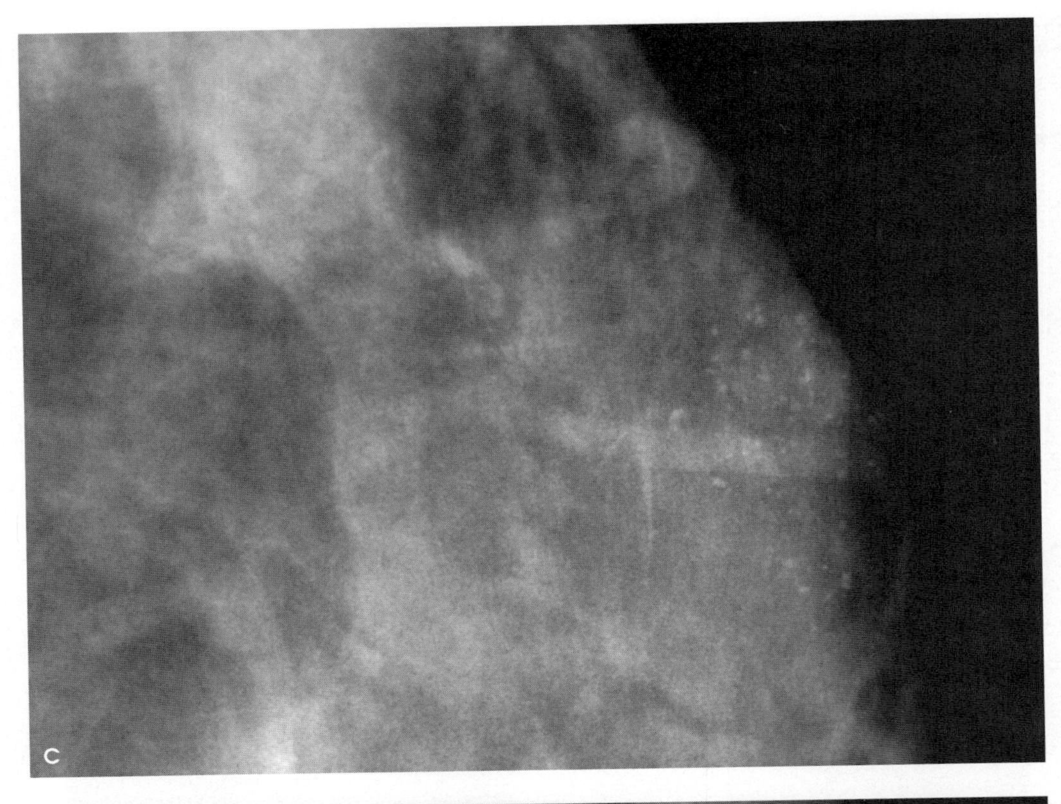

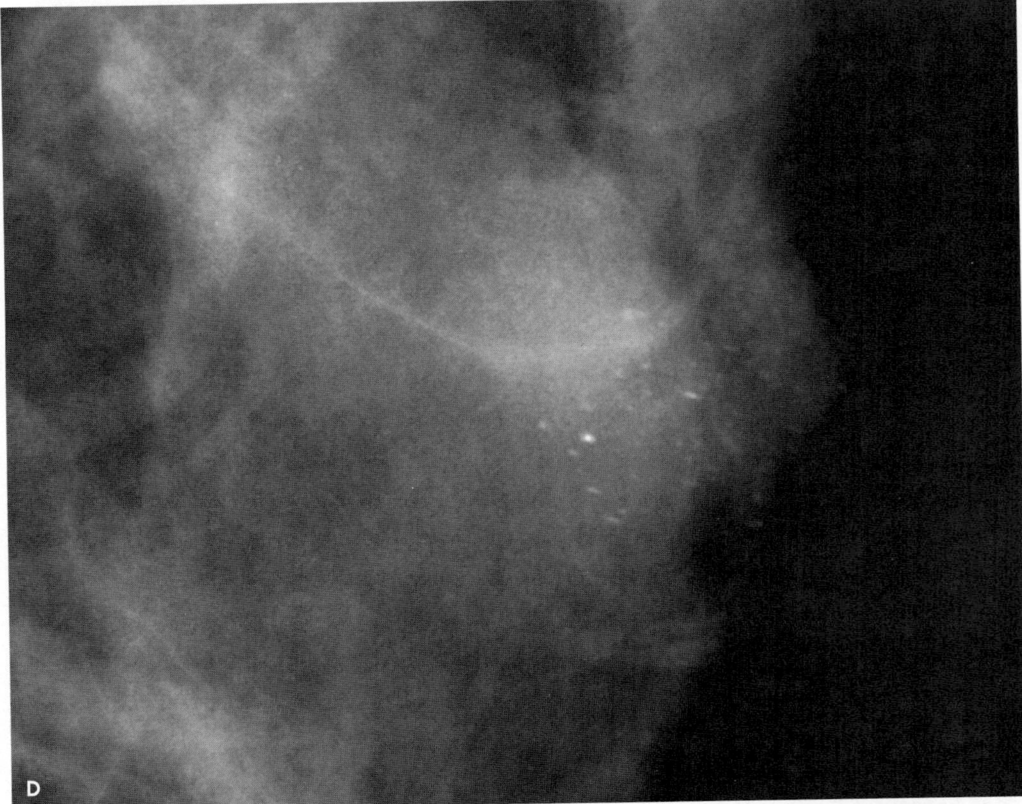

Figure 1.16. (*Continued*) Digital screening study, 40 year-old woman. Craniocaudal **(C)** and mediolateral oblique **(D)** views of the left breast, photographically coned.

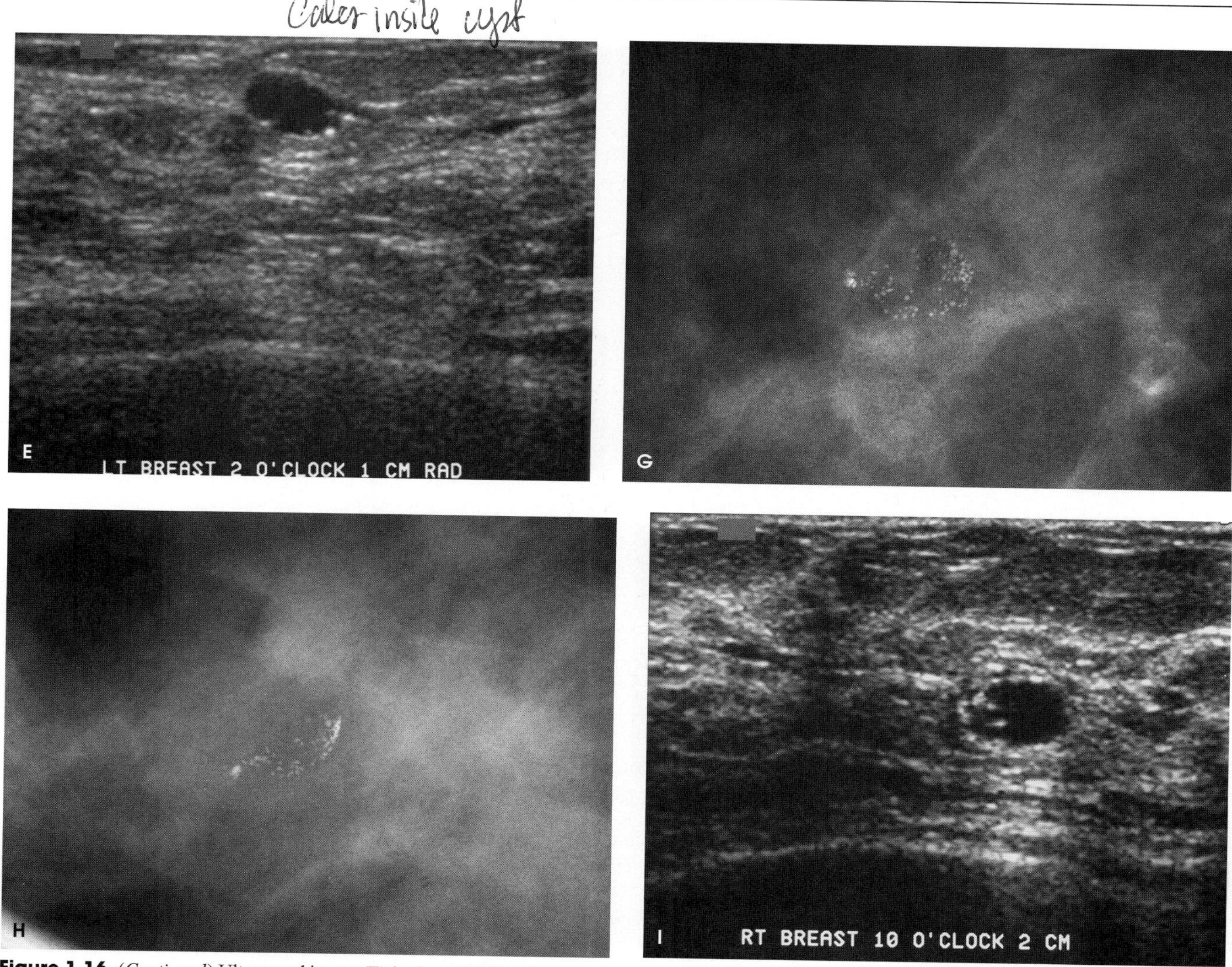

Figure 1.16. (*Continued*) Ultrasound image **(E)** in the radial (RAD) projection at the 2 o'clock position, 1 cm from the left nipple. Screening study, 72-year-old woman. Craniocaudal **(G)** and mediolateral oblique **(H)** views, photographically coned. Ultrasound Image **(I)** at the 10 o'clock position, 2 cm from the left nipple.

For each mammogram shown, describe the findings. What is the diagnosis in all three patients, and is a biopsy or short-interval follow-up indicated for any of these patients?

Amorphous calcifications of varying size and shapes are diffusely scattered throughout the dense parenchyma on the craniocaudal views (Fig. 1.16A). On the mediolateral oblique views, the calcifications are well defined, higher in density compared to the craniocaudal view, and most demonstrate a curvilinear or linear appearance (Fig. 1.16B).

A cluster of amorphous calcifications is seen laterally in the left breast on the craniocaudal view (Fig. 1.16C). The individual calcifications are better defined, denser, and demonstrate a more linear appearance on the mediolateral oblique view (Fig. 1.16D). On ultrasound (Fig. 1.16E), a cluster of subcentimeter cysts is imaged at the 2 o'clock position, 1 cm from the nipple (only one of which is shown), corresponding to the area of the clustered calcifications seen mammographically. Discrete echogenic foci (Fig 1.16F, arrows) and a linear area of echogenicity (Fig 1.16F, arrowheads) are noted in the dependent portion of the cyst, corresponding to some of the layering calcifications identified mammographically (Fig. 1.16F).

A cluster of round and oval calcifications is imaged in the right craniocaudal view (Fig. 1.16G). The calcifications shift in position and their overall distribution suggests that they are contained within a nonvisualized round mass on the mediolateral oblique view (Fig. 1.16H). On ultrasound (Fig. 1.16I), a cyst is imaged at the 10 o'clock position of the right breast, 2 cm from the nipple, the expected location of the calcifications seen mammographically. Discrete echogenic foci (Fig 1.16J, arrows) and an irregular curvilinear focus of echogenicity (Fig 1.16J, arrowheads) are imaged in the cyst, reflecting the calcifications seen mammographically (Fig. 1.16J). As expected, the calcifications are contained in a cyst.

These three patients demonstrate the variable appearance of milk of calcium. The diagnosis is established on the mammographic features of the calcifications. This reflects calcium in suspension within microcysts, less commonly in macrocysts. Amorphous calcifications are seen on the craniocaudal view. On mediolateral oblique and 90-degree lateral views, the calcium layers creating sharply defined, curvilinear calcifications ("teacups"). The characteristic mammographic feature of this type of calcification, therefore, is a differential appearance between craniocaudal and 90-degree lateral views, although it can also be seen on mediolateral oblique views in many patients. If the diagnosis is in question on the screening study, the patient is called back to confirm the diagnosis with a 90-degree lateral view. This process can be diffuse and bilateral, unilateral or focal. Although it is most common for the calcium to be in suspension, in some patients there are individual calcifications (often with somewhat geometric shapes) in suspension that can be seen changing appearances between craniocaudal and mediolateral oblique or 90-degree lateral views. If an ultrasound is done, cystic changes, some with associated calcifications, are often identifiable.

BI-RADS® category 1: negative. BI-RADS® category 2: benign finding is used if the calcifications are described in the body of the report. Next screening mammogram is recommended in 1 year.

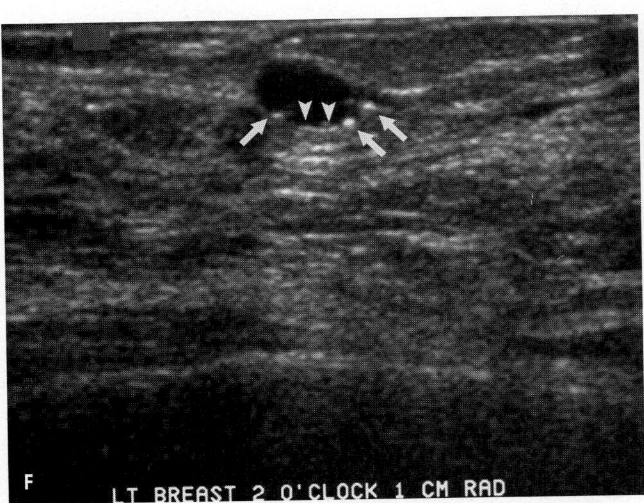

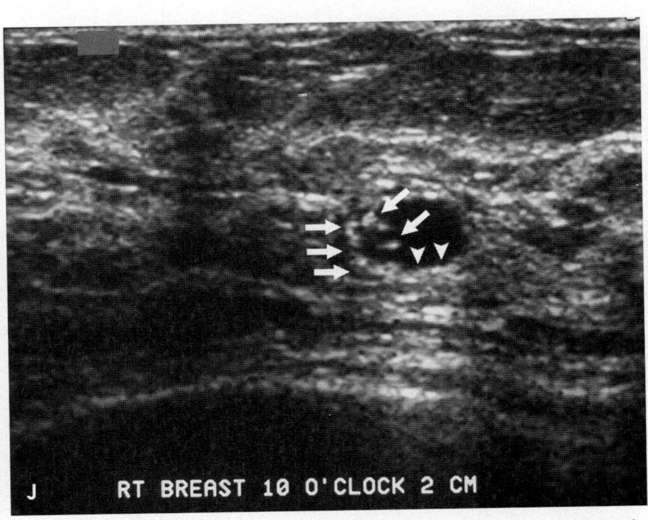

Figure 1.16. (*Continued*) Ultrasound image **(F)** in the radial (RAD) projection at the 2 o'clock position, 1 cm from the left nipple. One of several sub-centimeter cysts in the upper outer quadrant of the left breast. Echogenic foci (*arrows*) and a linear focus of echogenicity (*arrowheads*) are noted in the dependent portion of the cyst. This is milk of calcium. **(J)** Ultrasound image **(J)** at the 10 o'clock position, 2 cm from the left nipple. A cyst with calcifications (*arrows*) and a curvilinear focus of echogenicity consistent with calcium out of suspension in the dependent portion of the cyst (*arrowheads*).

PATIENT 17

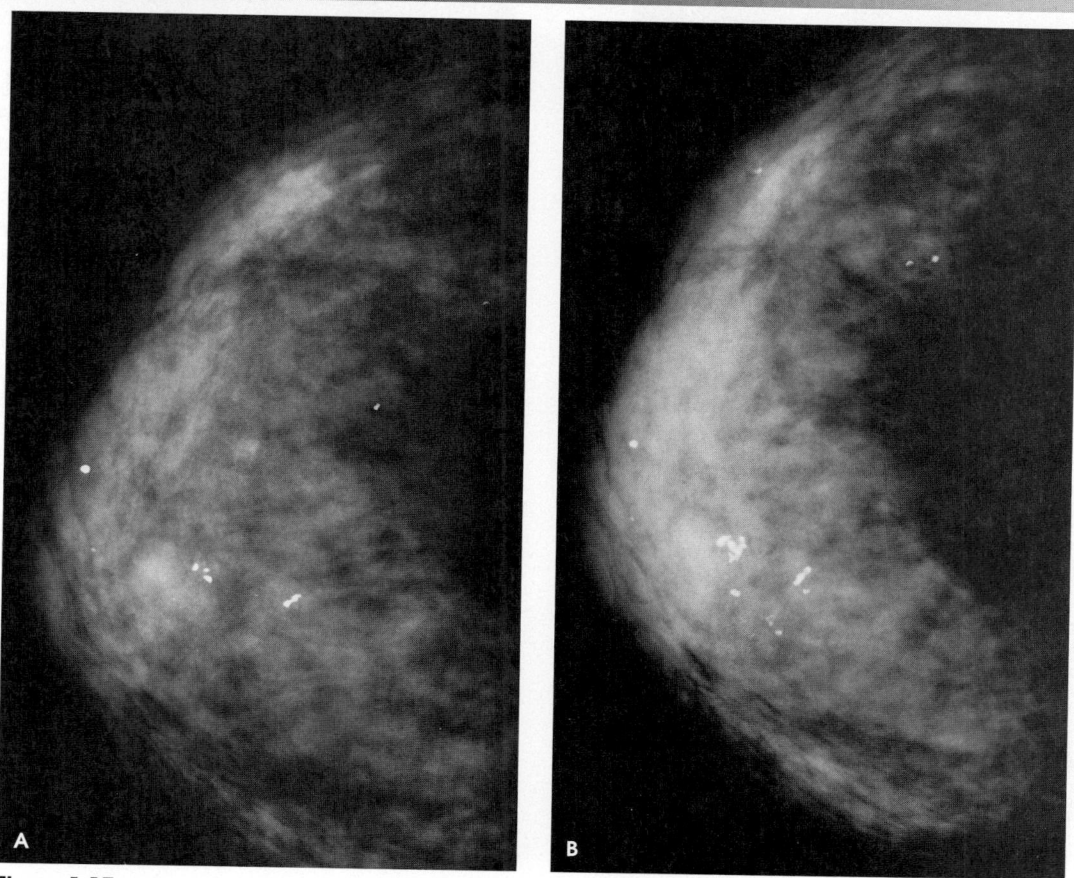

Figure 1.17. Screening study, 67-year-old patient. Craniocaudal **(A)** view, right breast. Craniocaudal **(B)** view, right breast, 2 years after **(A)**.

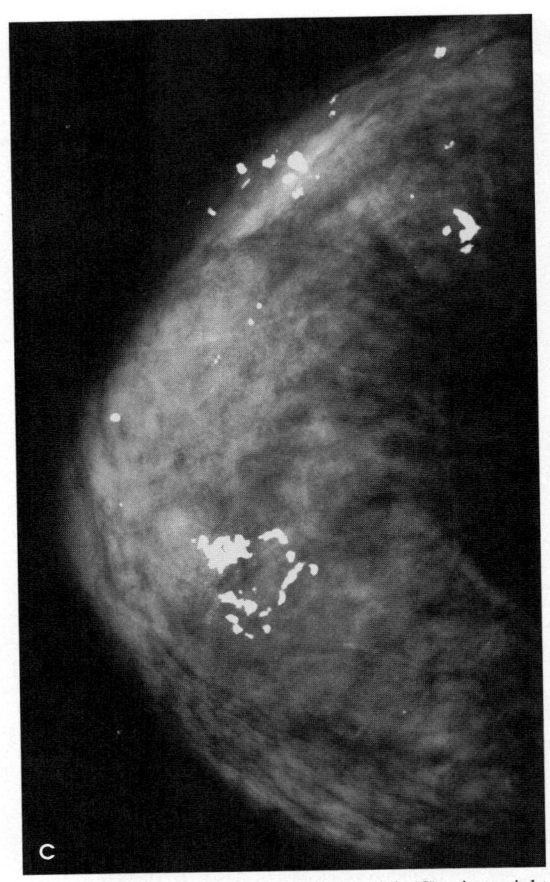

Figure 1.17. (*Continued*) Craniocaudal **(C)** view, right breast, 4 years after **(A)**.

How would you describe the findings, and what is your diagnosis?

This patient illustrates the progressive development of dystrophic calcifications. These calcifications develop in stromal fibrous tissue and not in predefined anatomic spaces or structures (e.g., acini, ducts, or vasculature). Consequently, they are variable in size, shape, and density. When diffuse and bilateral, they can reflect the presence of an underlying metabolic (e.g., renal failure, hyperparathyroidism), inflammatory, or degenerative process. When focal, they can be associated with hyalinizing fibroadenomas, sclerosed papillomas, or fat necrosis (posttrauma, postsurgical). In most women, no etiology is identified.

BI-RADS® category 1: negative. BI-RADS® category 2: benign finding, is used if the calcifications are described in the body of the report. Next screening mammogram is recommended in 1 year.

PATIENT 18

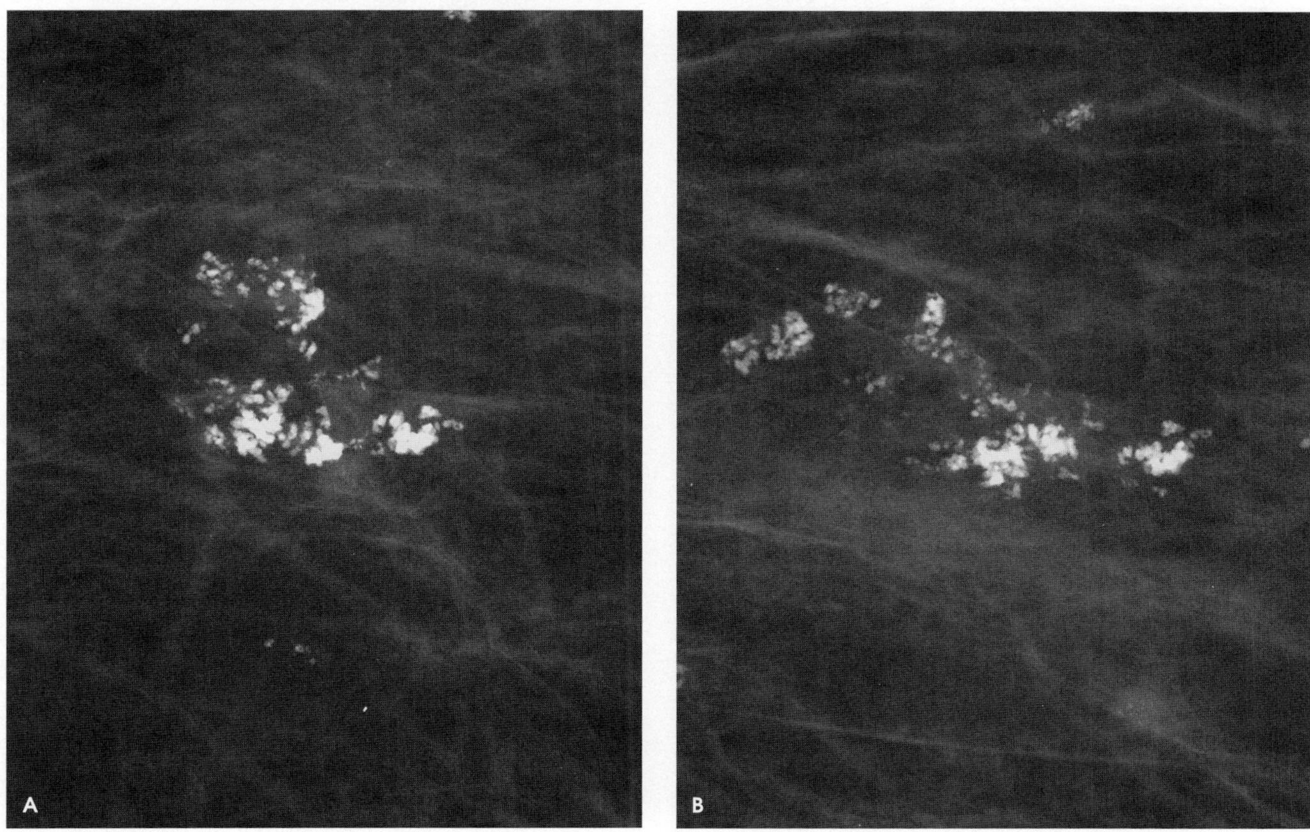

Figure 1.18. Screening study, 72-year-old woman. Craniocaudal **(A)** and mediolateral oblique **(B)** views, photographically coned.

What is the most likely diagnosis?

A focus of coarse, dystrophic calcifications is noted in this patient's mammogram. Although no mass is seen, these most likely reflect a hyalinized fibroadenoma. The bottom line is that these are benign and require no additional evaluation, short-interval follow-up, or intervention.

BI-RADS® category 1: negative. BI-RADS® category 2: benign finding is used if the calcifications are described in the body of the report. Next screening mammogram is recommended in 1 year.

PATIENT 19

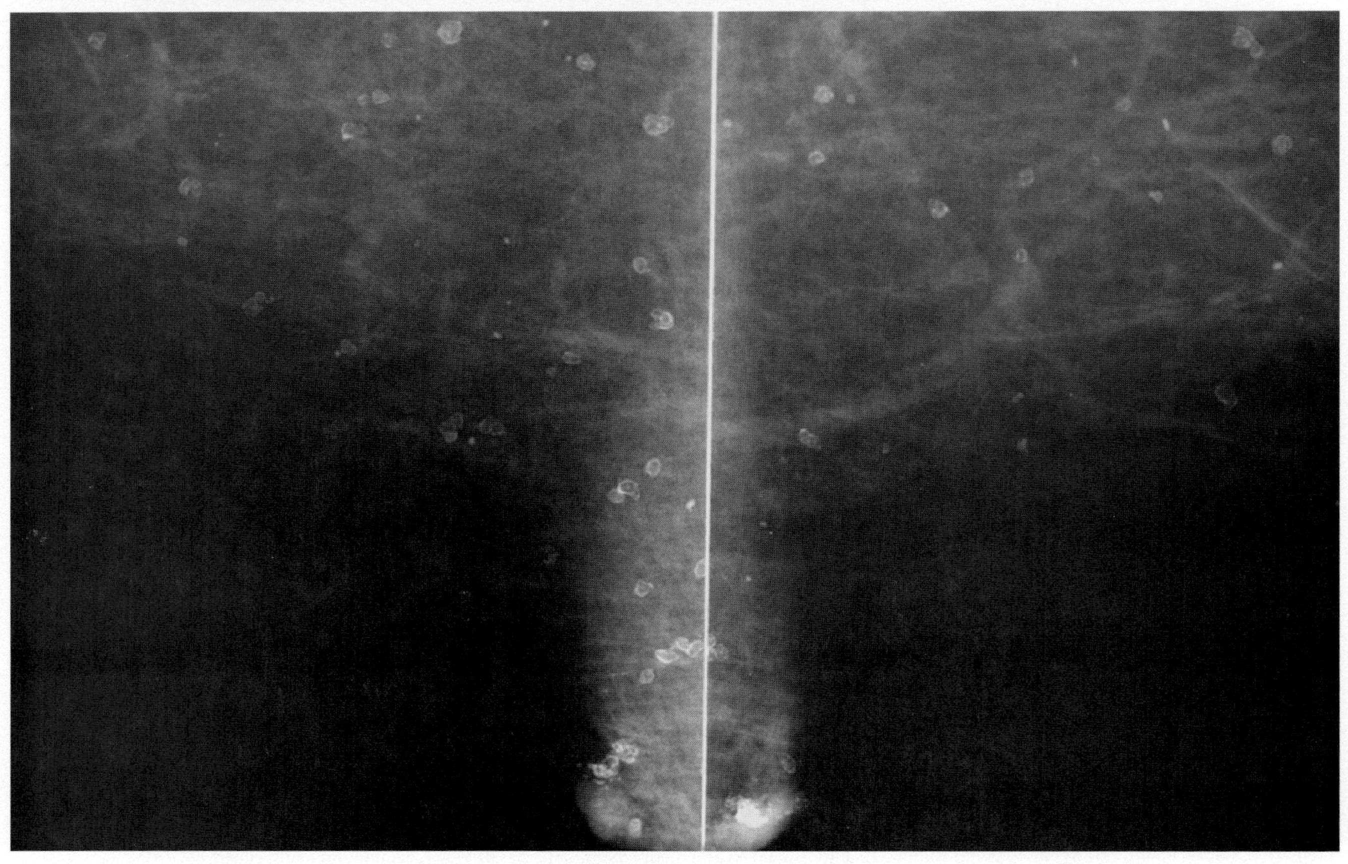

Figure 1.19. Screening study, 53-year-old woman. Craniocaudal views, photographically coned.

How would you describe the findings, and do you think additional evaluation is indicated?

Clusters of round and oval, lucent-centered calcifications are imaged in the posteromedial aspect of the breasts. These are skin calcifications in a common location and require no additional evaluation. Regardless of size, lucent-centered calcifications are benign.

BI-RADS® category 1: negative. Next screening mammogram is recommended in 1 year.

PATIENT 20

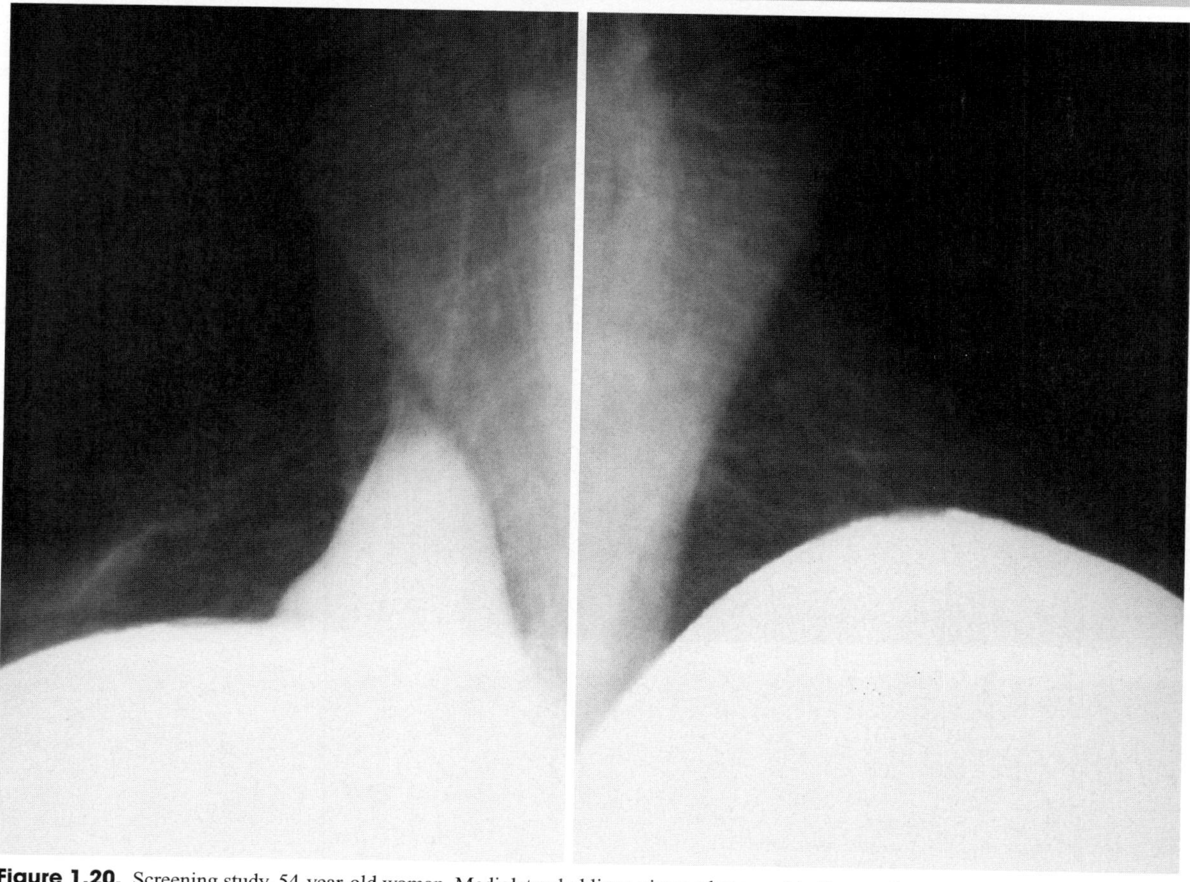

Figure 1.20. Screening study, 54-year-old woman. Mediolateral oblique views, photographically coned.

What is your impression?

Silicone implants are present in a subglandular location. A triangular density is imaged, extending superiorly from the right implant along the anterior edge of the pectoral muscle. This is consistent with silicone and an extracapsular implant rupture. Extravasated silicone is noted as a high-density material that can assume a variety of shapes and sizes. In some women, silicone is seen as round high-density masses or triangular globs in the breast, whereas in others it is within the lymphatic system extending into the axilla.

What is gel bleed?

Relative to silicone implants, consider three different concepts: gel bleed, intracapsular implant rupture, and extracapsular implant rupture. Gel bleed is a natural phenomenon associated with silicone implants. The implant shell, made of silicone, is a semipermeable membrane that allows for the egress or bleed of silicone naturally. This bleed may be low or high grade, depending on the amount of cross-linking of the silicone elastomere shell. Gel bleed is not imaged on mammograms or ultrasound. On magnetic resonance images, gel bleed is characterized by the filling of wrinkles ("keyhole") present in otherwise intact implants. This is in contrast with the extravasation of silicone resulting from a disruption of the implant shell.

What types of implant ruptures are there, and how are they diagnosed?

After an implant is placed in the body, a fibrous capsule forms around the implant. If rupture of the implant shell occurs and there is an intact "native" fibrous capsule, the extravasated silicone is contained by the capsule (i.e., intracapsular implant rupture). This type of implant rupture is not apparent on a mammogram; it may be identified on ultrasound and it is easily diagnosed with magnetic resonance imaging (MRI). If the patient's own capsule is disrupted, rupture of the implant can result in extracapsular extension of the extravasated silicone. This type of rupture can be diagnosed mammographically, on ultrasound, and with MRI.

PATIENT 21

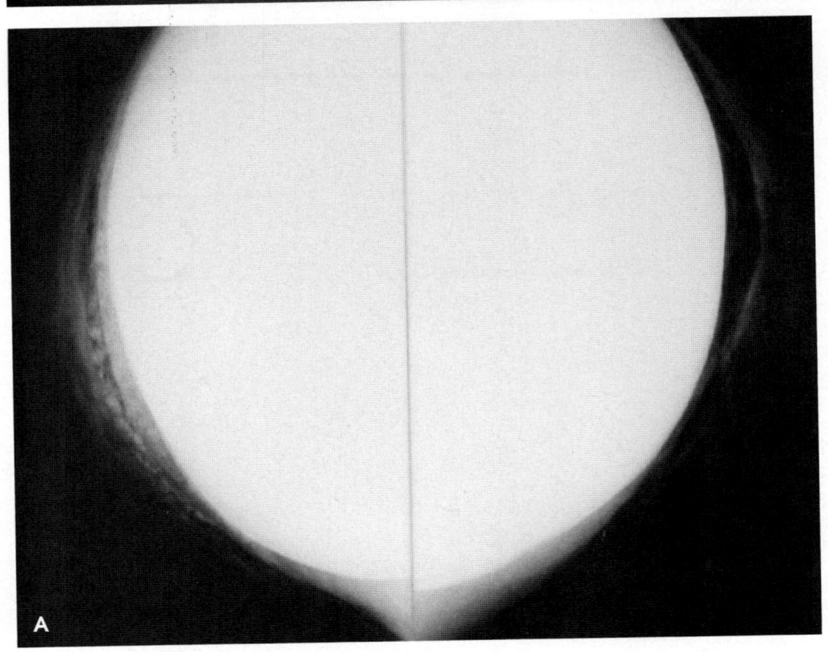

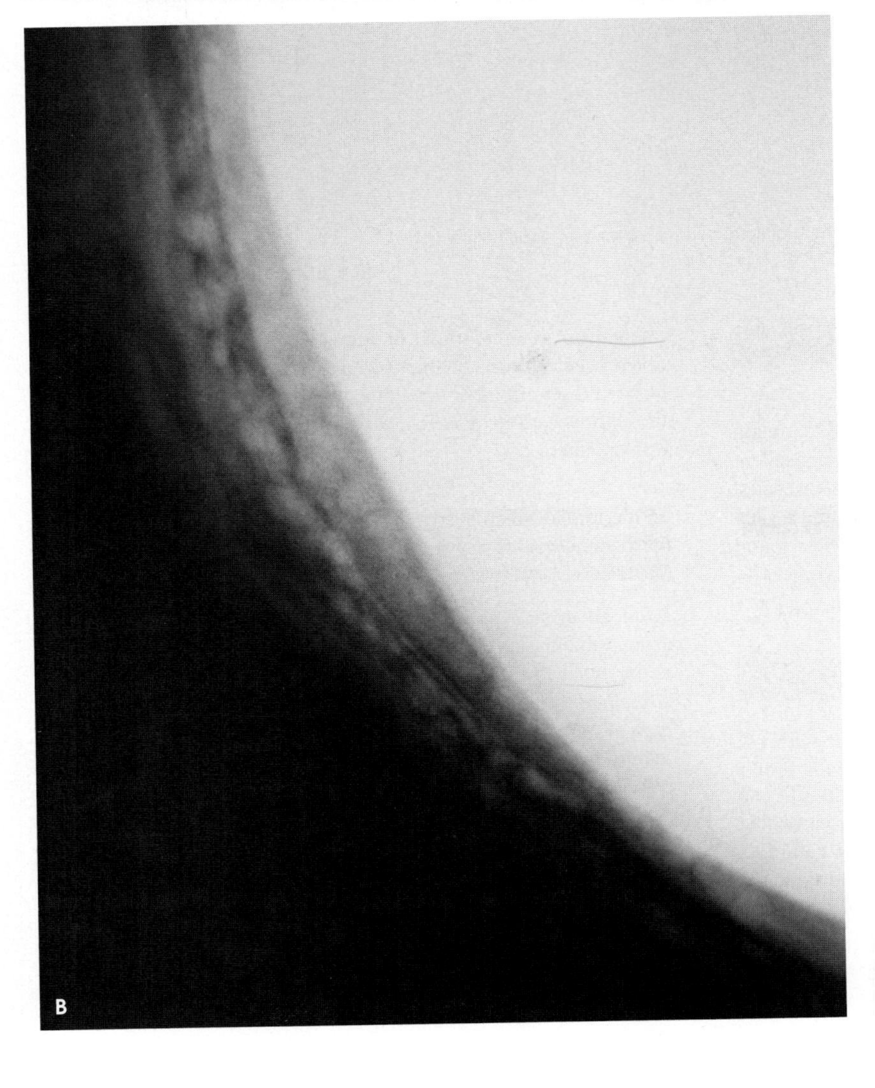

Figure 1.21. Screening study, 40-year-old woman. Craniocaudal **(A)** views, photographically coned. Craniocaudal **(B)** view, right breast medially, photographic cone down.

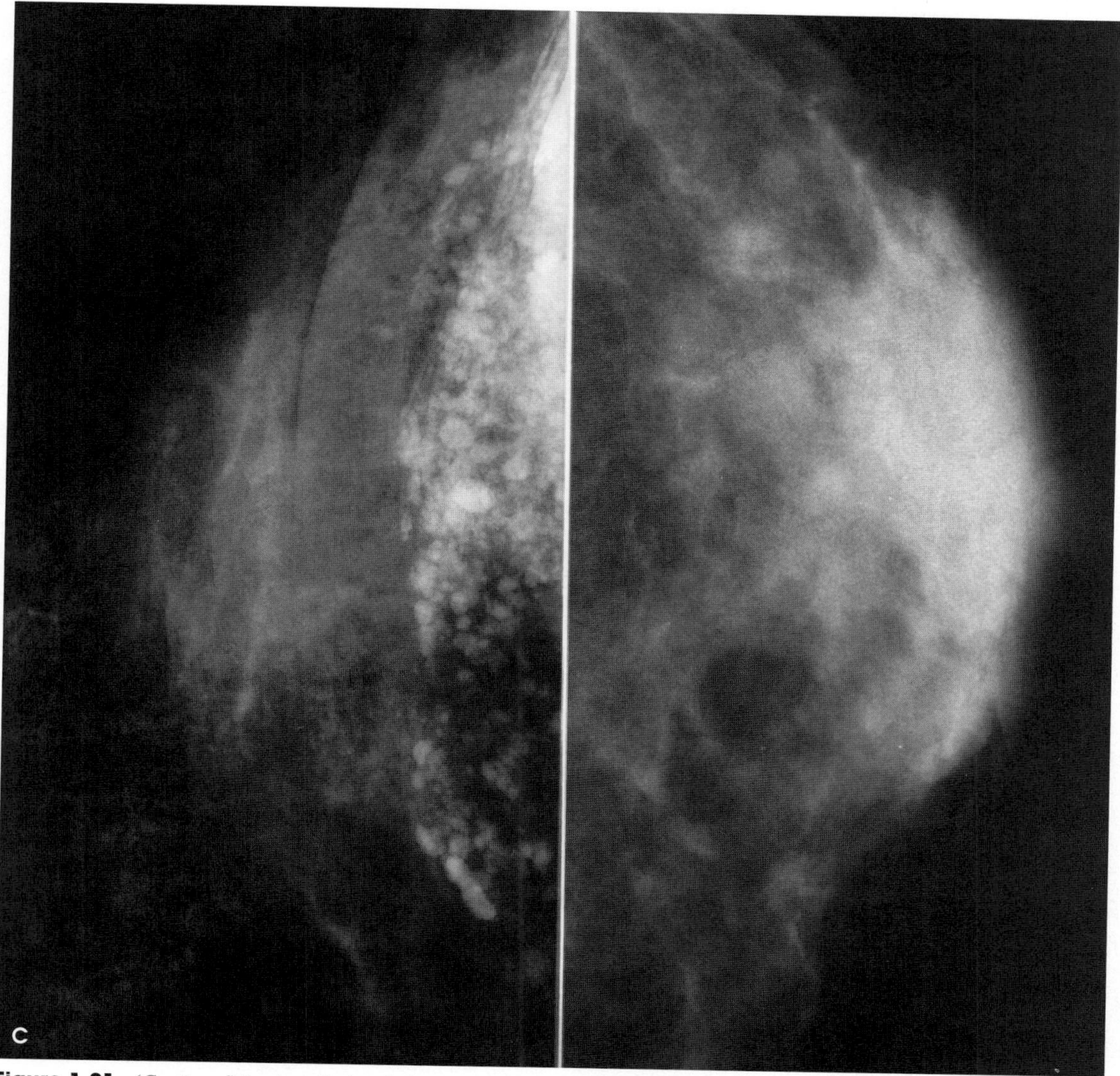

Figure 1.21. (*Continued*) Implant displaced views **(C)**, craniocaudal projection.

What is your diagnosis?

Round, high-density globules of silicone are imaged at the edge of the silicone implant, medially on the right. These are better imaged on the implant-displaced view (Fig. 1.21C). This finding is consistent with extracapsular implant rupture.

PATIENT 22

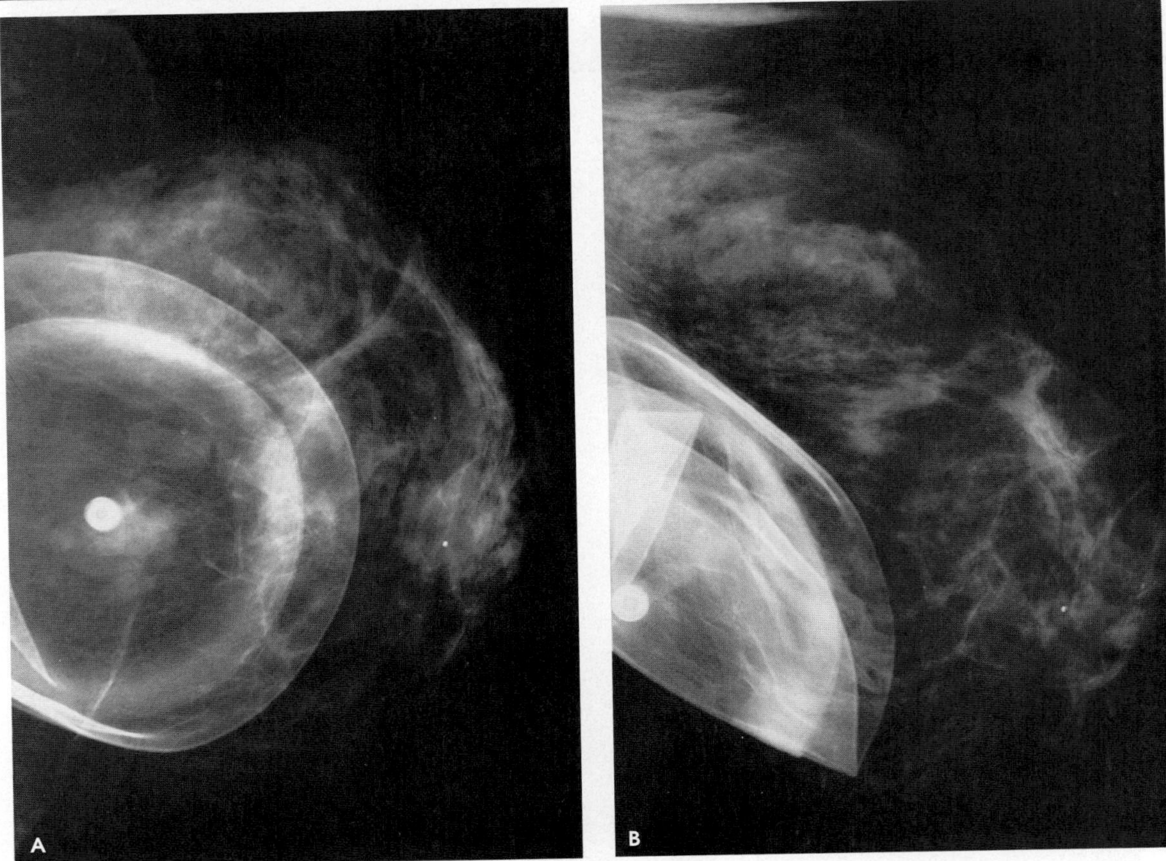

Figure 1.22. Screening study, 75-year-old woman. Craniocaudal **(A)** and mediolateral oblique **(B)** views, left breast.

What is your impression?

Saline implants are present in a subglandular location. The significant folding of the implant on the oblique view and the relative lack of opacity in the craniocaudal view is consistent with partial (nearly complete) collapse of a saline implant.

PATIENT 23

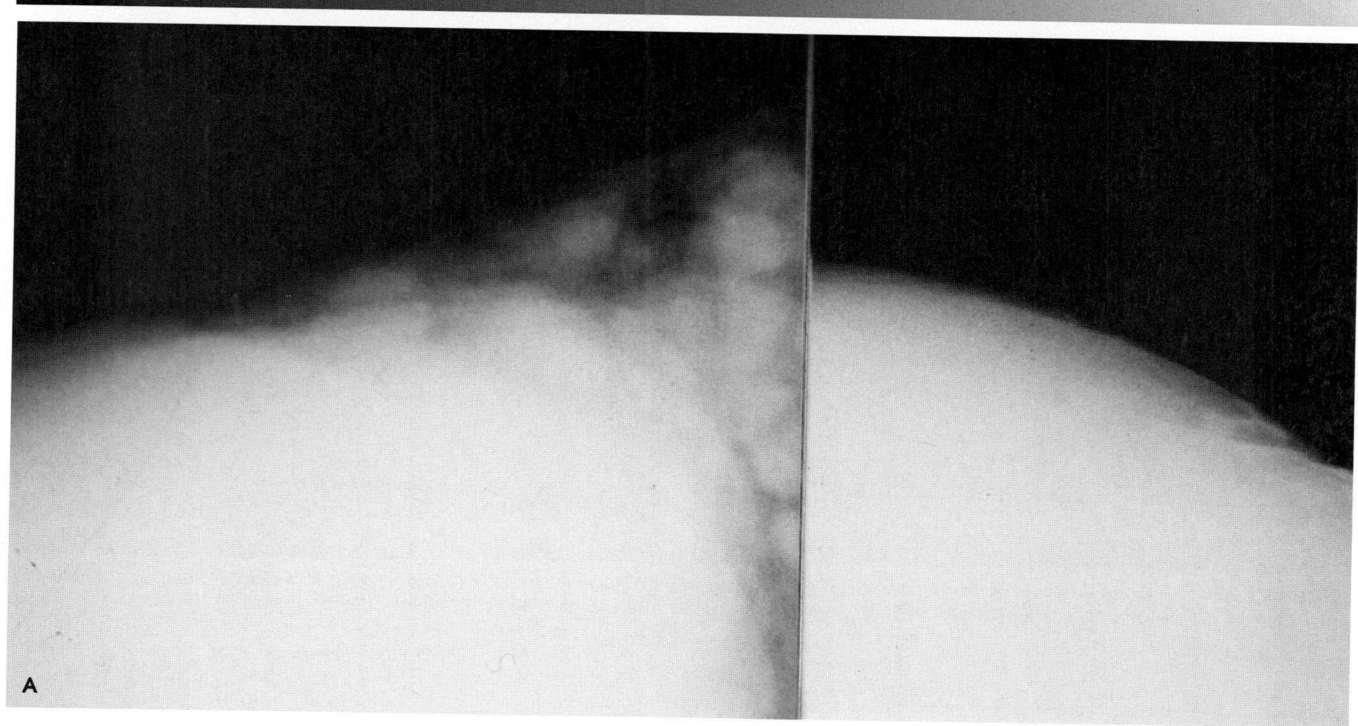

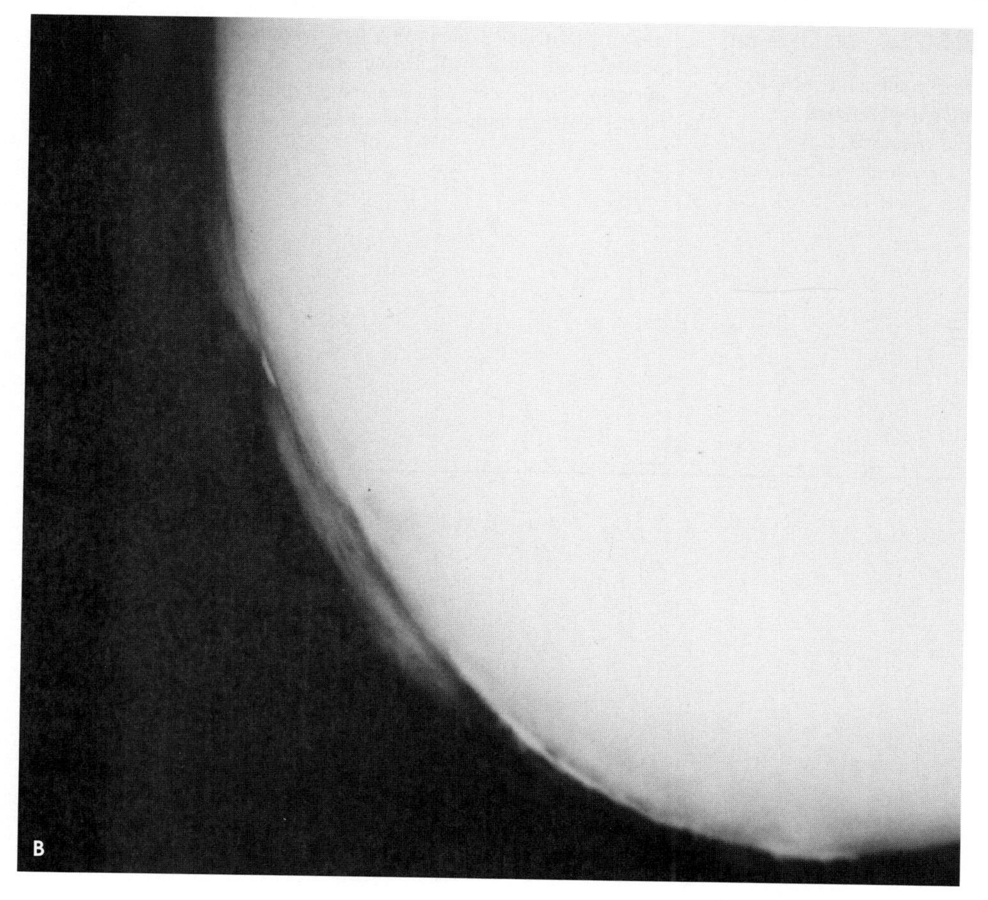

Figure 1.23. Diagnostic study, 57-year-old patient presenting with a "lump" in the upper outer quadrant of the right breast. Craniocaudal **(A)** views, photographically coned laterally. Craniocaudal **(B)** view, right breast, photographically coned medially.

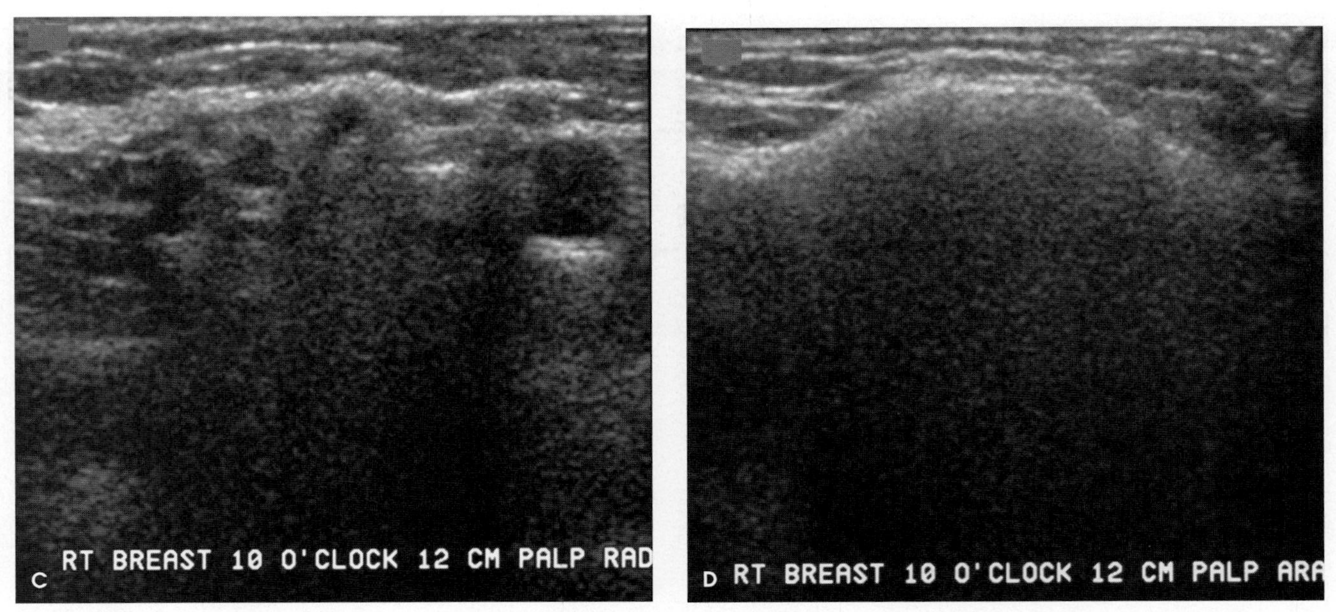

Figure 1.23. *(Continued)* Ultrasound image **(C)**, radial (RAD) projection at the site of the palpable (PALP) finding, 10 o'clock position, 12 cm from the right nipple. Ultrasound image **(D)**, antiradial (ARAD) projection at the site of the palpable (PALP) finding, 10 o'clock position, 12 cm from the right nipple.

How would you describe the imaging findings, and what is your diagnosis?

High-density globules adjacent to the right implant (arrows, Fig. 1.23E, F) are diagnostic of an extracapsular implant rupture. On ultrasound, round and irregular hypoechoic masses (arrows, Fig. 1.23G), some with angular margins and an echogenic halo, are imaged at the site of the palpable abnormality, 10 o'clock position, right breast, 12 cm from the nipple. The "snowstorm" appearance of extravasated silicone is also demonstrated in some of the images obtained during the ultrasound study (Fig. 1.23D); an irregular curvilinear echogenic focus is imaged, characterized by shadowing associated with high specular echoes.

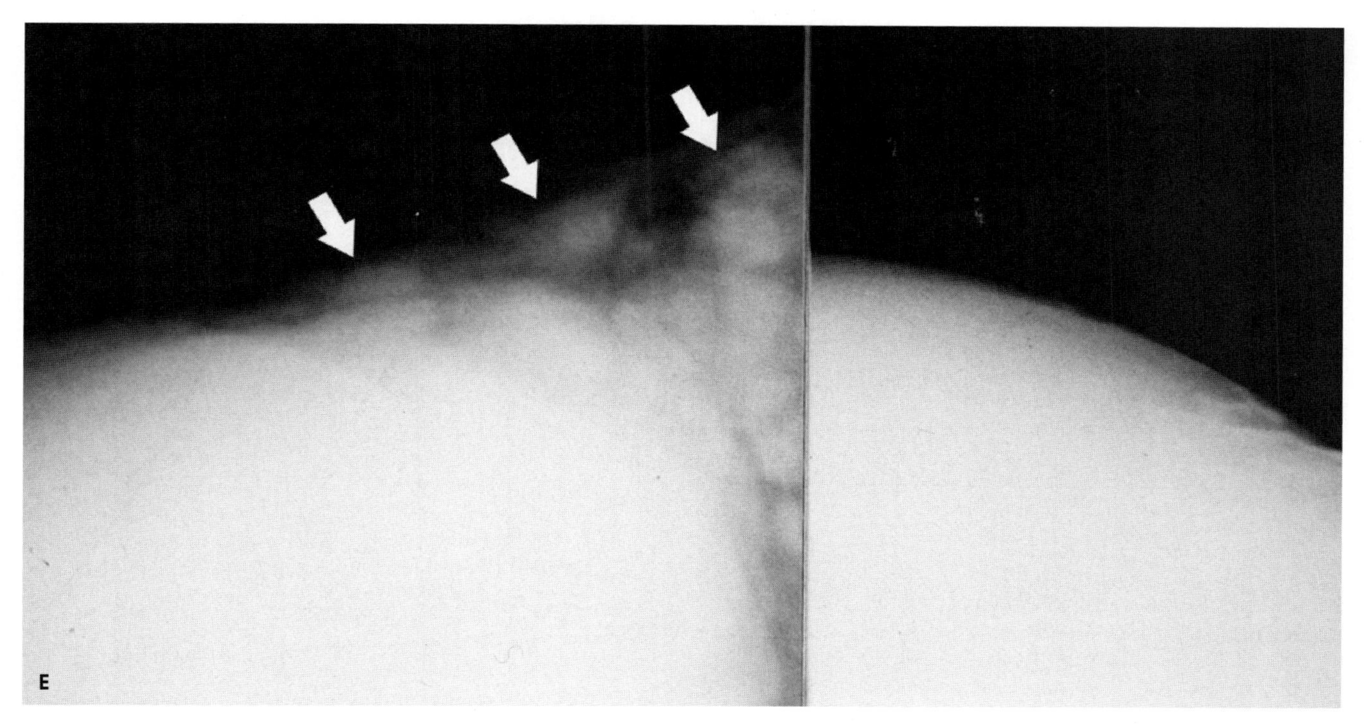

Figure 1.23. (*Continued*) Craniocaudal **(E)** views, photographically coned laterally. Extravasated silicone is present (*arrows*) closely apposed to the right implant posterolaterally.

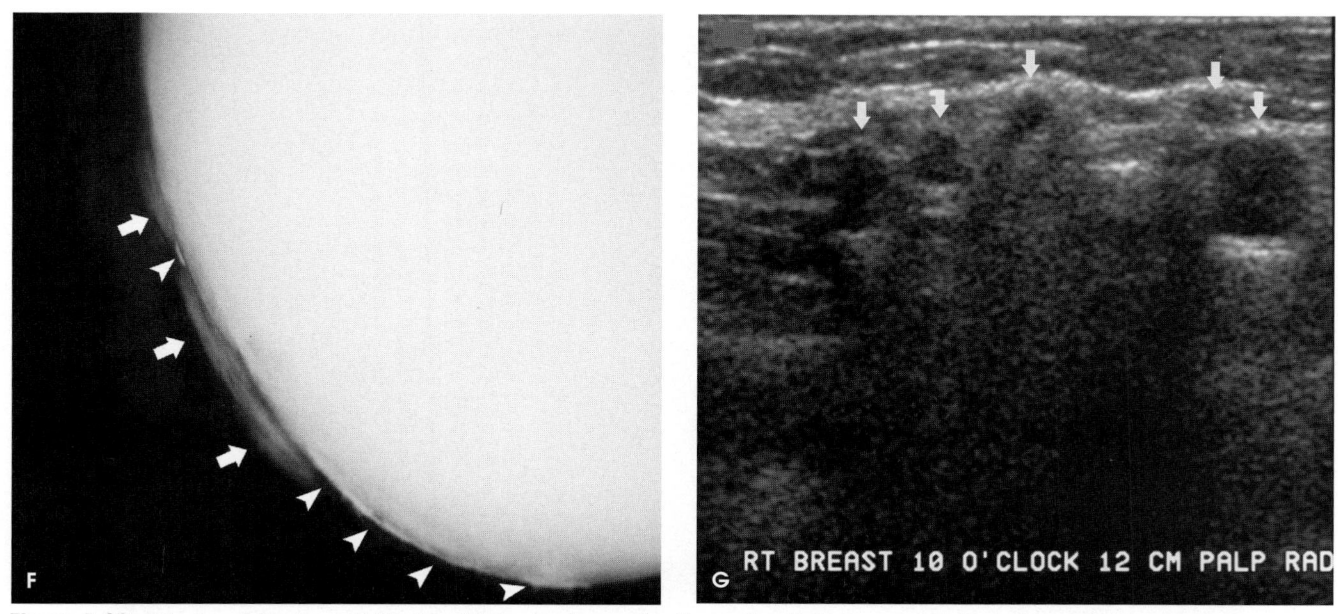

Figure 1.23. (*Continued*) Craniocaudal **(F)** view, right breast, photographically coned medially. Extravasated silicone is present (*arrows*) closely apposed to the right implant medially. Also noted is calcification of the capsule (*arrowheads*). Ultrasound image **(G),** radial (RAD) projection at the site of the palpable (PALP) finding, 10 o'clock position, 12 cm from the right nipple. The appearance of silicone on ultrasound is variable. In this image, extravasated silicone is imaged as a cluster of round and irregular hypoechoic masses.

PATIENT 24

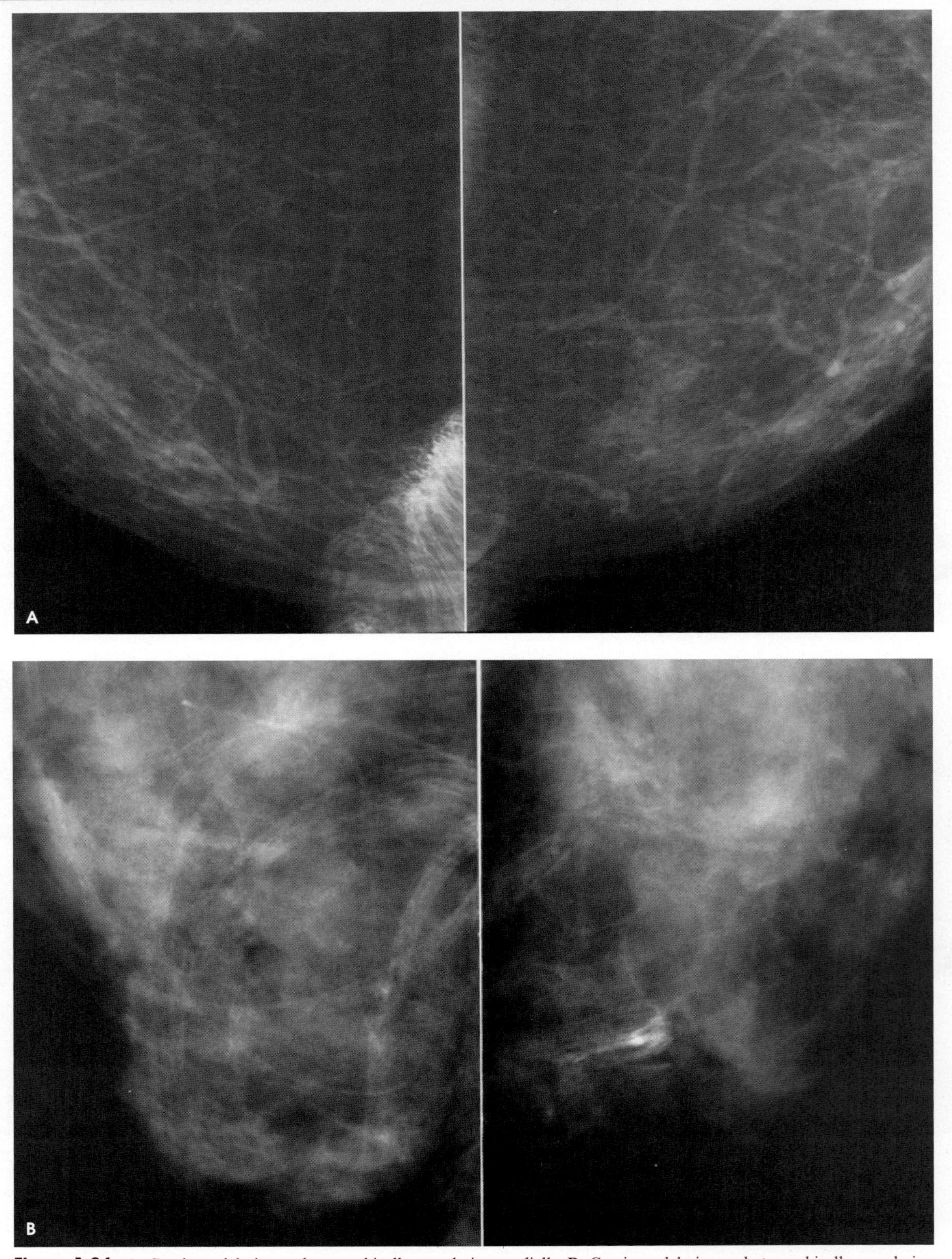

Figure 1.24. **A:** Craniocaudal views, photographically coned view medially. **B:** Craniocaudal views, photographically coned view medially.

What is the pertinent observation?

Swirls of hair are seen on one (Fig. 1.24A, *right*) and both (Fig. 1.24B) craniocaudal views posteromedially. As the patient is positioned for the craniocaudal view she is asked to turn her head away from the breast being imaged. As this is done, hair can come down along the neck and project on the breast. Because the hair is a distance from the cassette, the swirls are not sharp (geometric unsharpness). Although hair may be superimposed on any image and in any posterior location, it is most commonly seen posteromedially on craniocaudal views. The technologist needs to make sure that all the patient's hair is pulled back. Repeat views may be indicated if a potential lesion could be obscured. In the examples presented, the right craniocaudal (Fig. 1.24A) needs to be repeated because the density of the superimposed hair may obscure a cluster of calcifications or a small spiculated mass.

PATIENT 25

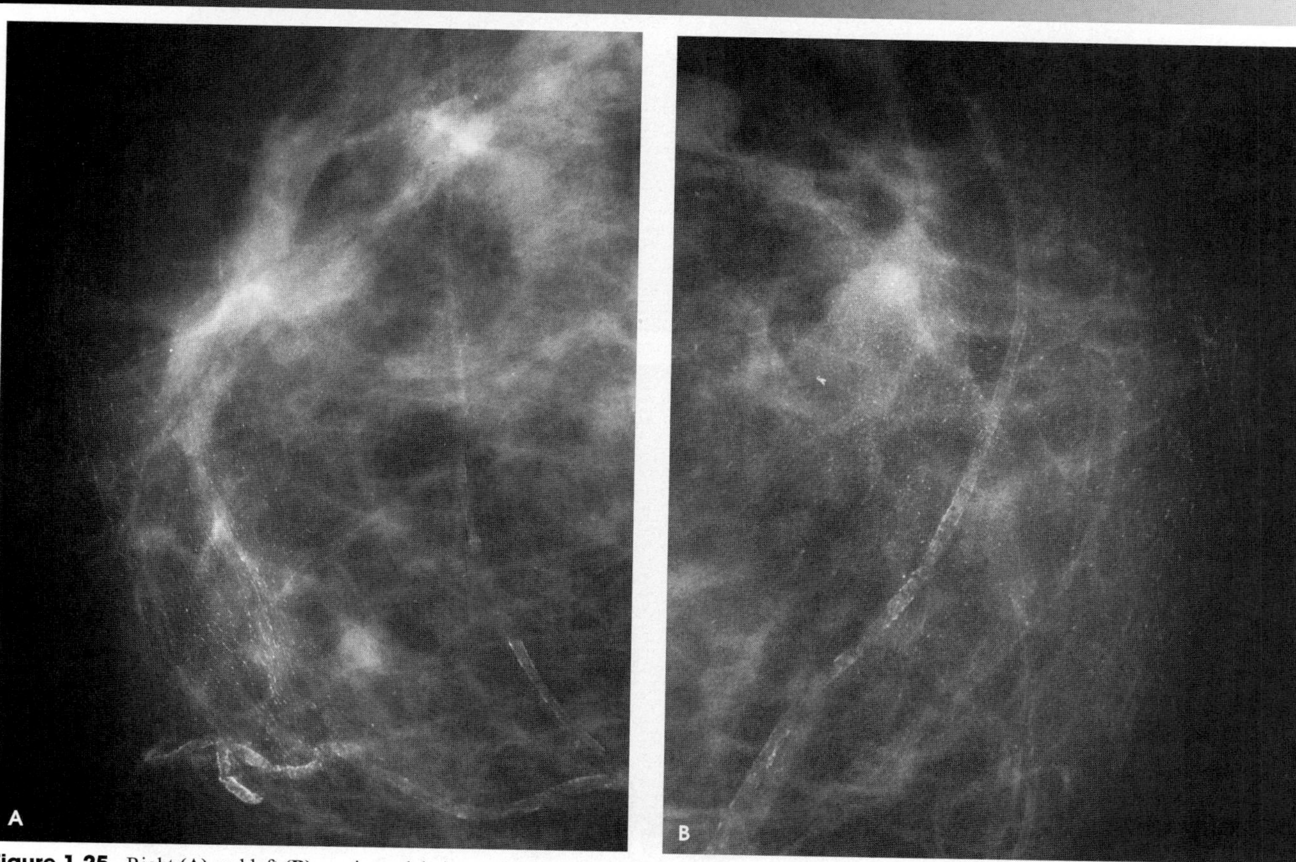

Figure 1.25. Right **(A)** and left **(B)** craniocaudal views, photographically coned anteriorly.

How would you describe the findings? What is your working hypothesis, and how can it be tested?

High-density material with linear (wavy) and punctate forms involving the anterior aspect of the breasts represents an artifact. This is zinc oxide ointment (Desitin) on the skin. If there is any question that this may represent calcifications, the patient is asked if she applied something to her skin; she can be examined and asked to wipe her breast clean before follow-up films are taken to confirm partial or complete removal of the artifact. Note the presence of bilateral arterial calcification.

PATIENT 26

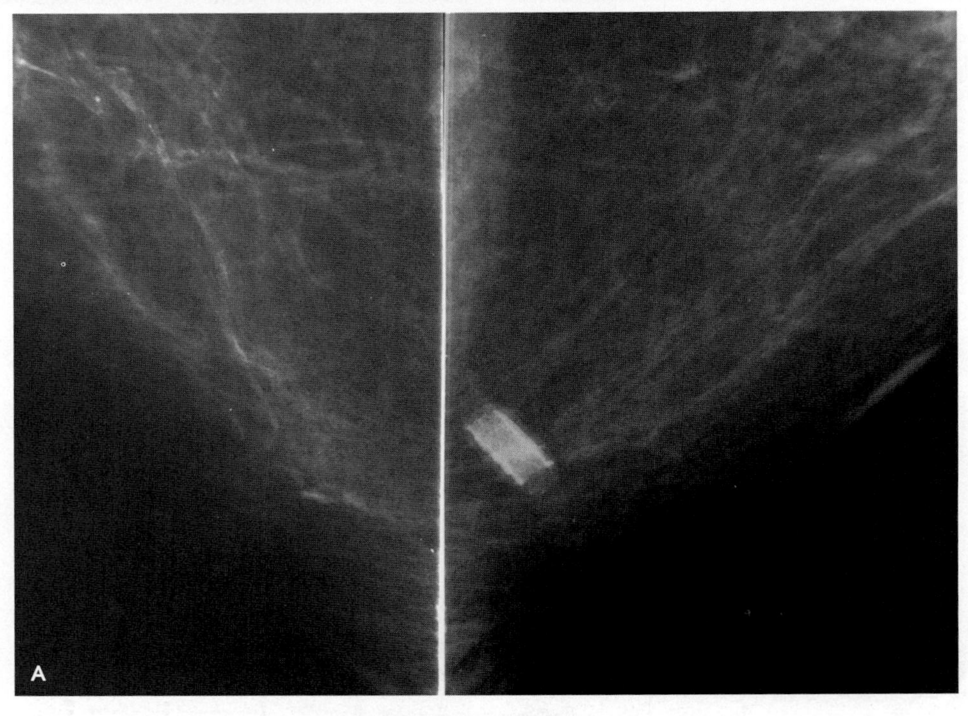

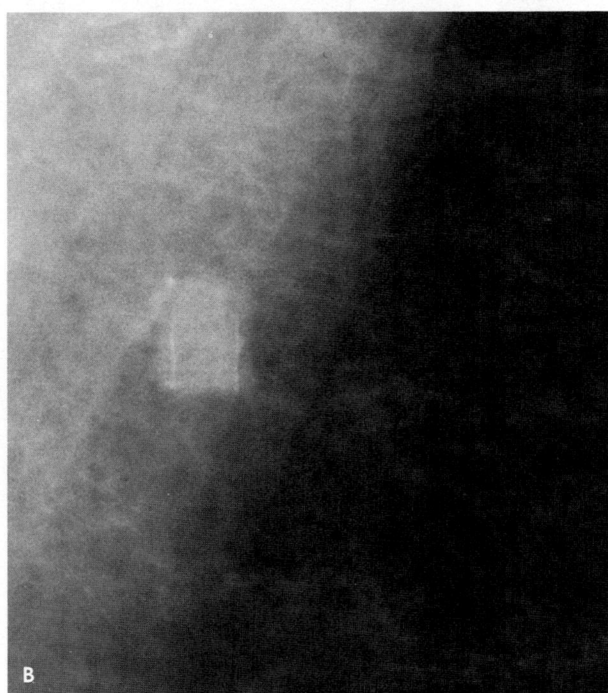

Figure 1.26. **A:** Craniocaudal views, photographically coned medially. **B:** Different patient. Mediolateral oblique view, photographically coned superiorly.

What is demonstrated in these two patients?

A high-density, tubular structure is imaged posteromedially in the left breast (Fig. 1.26A). Similarly, a tubular structure with dense edges is seen superimposed on the left pectoral muscle in a different patient (Fig. 1.26B). These are retained Dacron cuffs from Hickman central venous catheters. These are typically found in the upper inner quadrants of either the right or left breast. Although rare, abscess formation around the cuff has been reported and should be suspected if an irregular mass that may contain air is seen associated with the cuff.

PATIENT 27

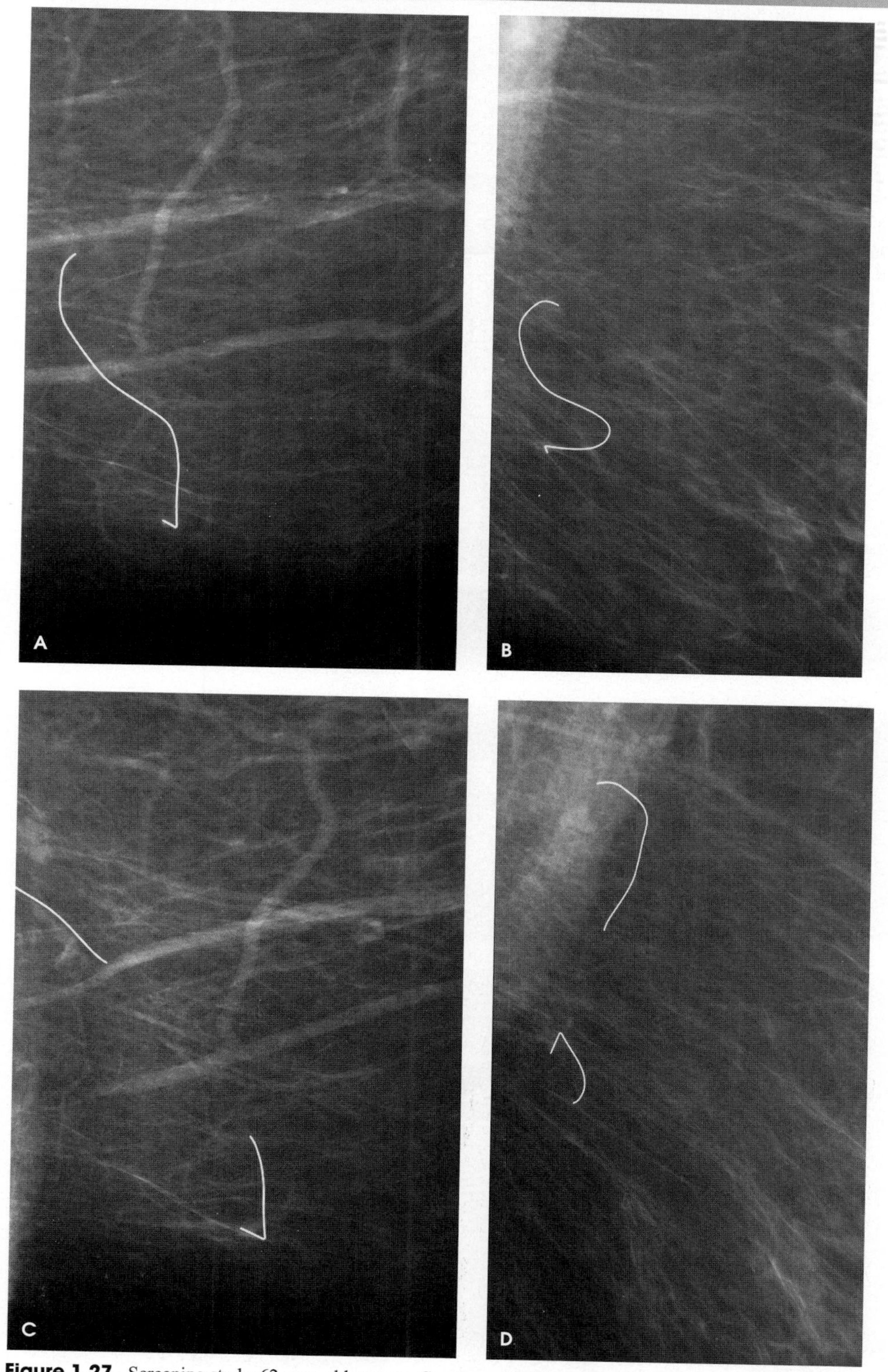

Figure 1.27. Screening study, 62-year-old woman. Craniocaudal **(A)** and mediolateral oblique **(B)** views, left breast, photographically coned. Craniocaudal **(C)** and mediolateral oblique **(D)** views, 1 year after **(A)** and **(B)**, photographically coned.

What is your impression?
What recommendation would you make based on the most recent set of images?

A retained wire fragment is imaged in the upper inner quadrant of the left breast, consistent with the history provided by the patient of a breast biopsy preceded by wire localization "many" years ago (Fig. 1.27A, B). The wire fragment is stable in appearance and position compared with several prior mammograms, and the patient is asymptomatic. On her next screening mammogram (Fig. 1.27C, D), the wire is fragmented and the larger of the two fragments has migrated such that it may be embedded in the pectoral muscle; however, this cannot be confirmed because the wire could not be imaged in its entirety on the craniocaudal view. Given the changes noted in the wire, excisional biopsy following preoperative wire localization of the fragments is recommended. A specimen radiograph obtained following the surgical procedure documents excision of the wire fragments, as well as the wire used for the current localization procedure.

Specimen radiography is indicated following all preoperative wire localizations for several reasons, including documentation that the localized lesion and localization wire have been excised. The radiograph is also used to mark the location of the lesion of interest for the pathologist. Rarely, additional unsuspected lesions may be identified on the specimen radiograph, and proximity of the lesion to the margins may be suggested. However, it is important to recognize that the radiograph is a two-dimensional representation of a three-dimensional structure and therefore the status of the margins requires histologic evaluation. The surgeon is contacted following a review of the specimen radiograph. If the localizing wire is not seen on the specimen radiograph, the surgeon is asked if it was pulled during the surgical procedure. If the surgeon is unable to provide reassurance about the location of the wire, a follow-up mammogram is obtained 6 to 8 weeks following the surgery.

PATIENT 28

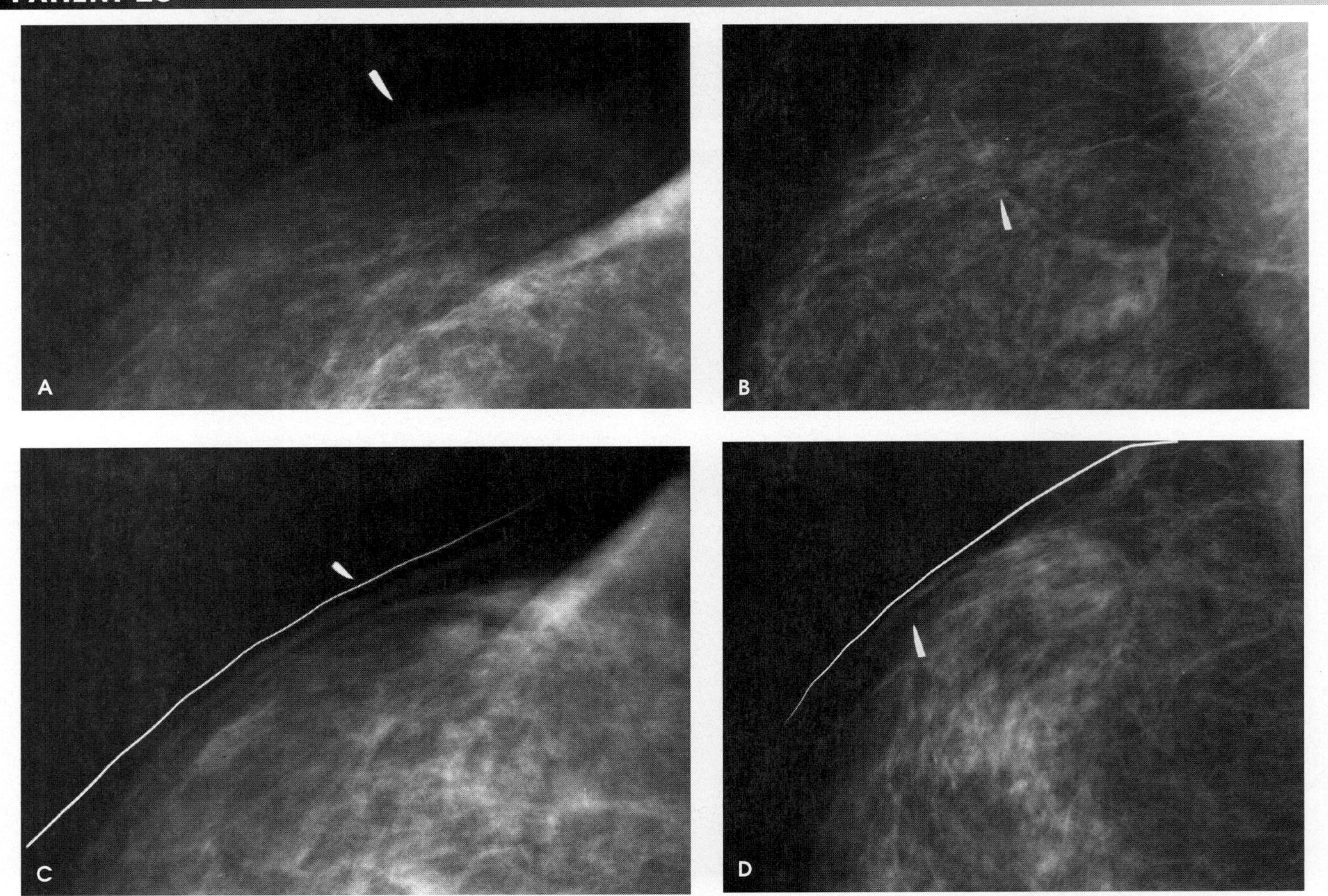

Figure 1.28. Screening study, 88-year-old woman. Craniocaudal **(A)** and mediolateral oblique **(B)** views, photographically coned views, right breast. Craniocaudal **(C)** and mediolateral oblique **(D)** views, photographically coned, right breast, screening study 8 years prior to **(A)** and **(B)**.

What do you think, and what are the possible explanations?

A needle tip is present in the subcutaneous tissue. A biopsy marker is seen at this site on films done 8 years ago; its association with the needle tip on both images suggests the possibility that the needle tip is retained from a breast surgical procedure the patient had 30 years previously. Alternatively, the location of the needle tip at a prior biopsy site may be coincidental and not related to the surgery. Foreign bodies that can be seen in the breast include, but are not limited to, needle tips, sewing needles, lead pencil tips, bullets, bullet fragments, and buckshot. Patients are usually asymptomatic and unaware of the presence of a foreign body in their breast. Iatrogenic sources of foreign bodies include acupuncture needles, surgical clips following lumpectomy and axillary dissection, retained wire fragments following preoperative wire localizations, metallic markers placed to mark the site of a prior percutaneous needle biopsy, port-a-catheters, pacemakers, and retained Dacron cuffs from a Hickman catheter.

PATIENT 29

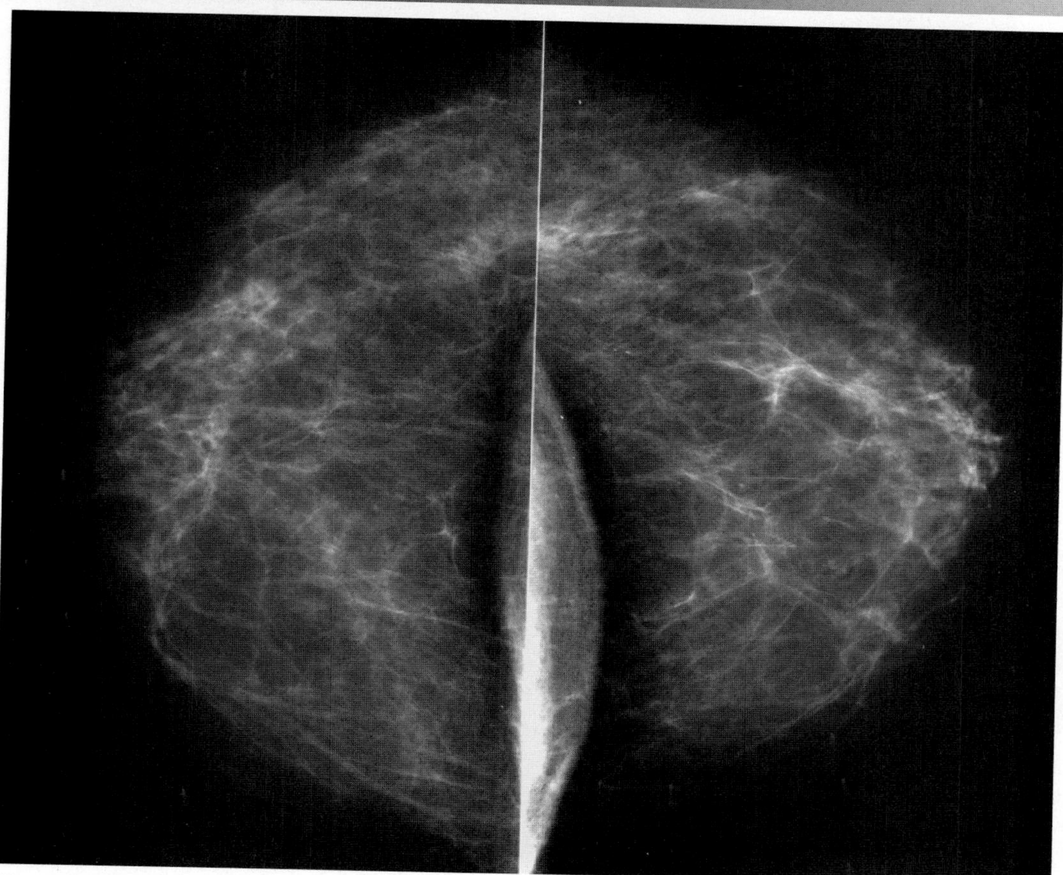

Figure 1.29. Screening study. Craniocaudal views.

What do you think of these images? Why are the pectoral muscles sharply outlined by radiolucency?

The images are of fairly good quality, in that exposure and contrast are optimal; however, there are large skin folds inferiorly (at inframammary fold (IMF)/abdomen) simulating pectoral muscles. Air outlining the skin folds accounts for the radiolucency noted at the anterior edge of the folds. The tissue surrounding the skin folds should be evaluated carefully for blurring, because the skin folds may limit compression.

In positioning the breast for the craniocaudal projection, the technologist should identify the inframammary fold at its neutral position and lift the breast up from the inframammary fold as much as the natural mobility of the breast will allow. After lifting the breast, it is important to pull the breast out away from the chest wall and to tug on the lateral aspect of the breast as much as the natural mobility of the breast allows. As the breast is lifted, a skin fold can be created inferiorly if a portion of abdominal wall skin is lifted with the breast. Since this fold develops inferiorly, the technologist is unable to see it as she inspects the breast superiorly before the exposure is made. As in this patient, when this skin fold develops, it can simulate the pectoral muscle. Unlike the pectoral muscle, a sharp radiolucency (air) is seen abutting the skin fold.

PATIENT 30

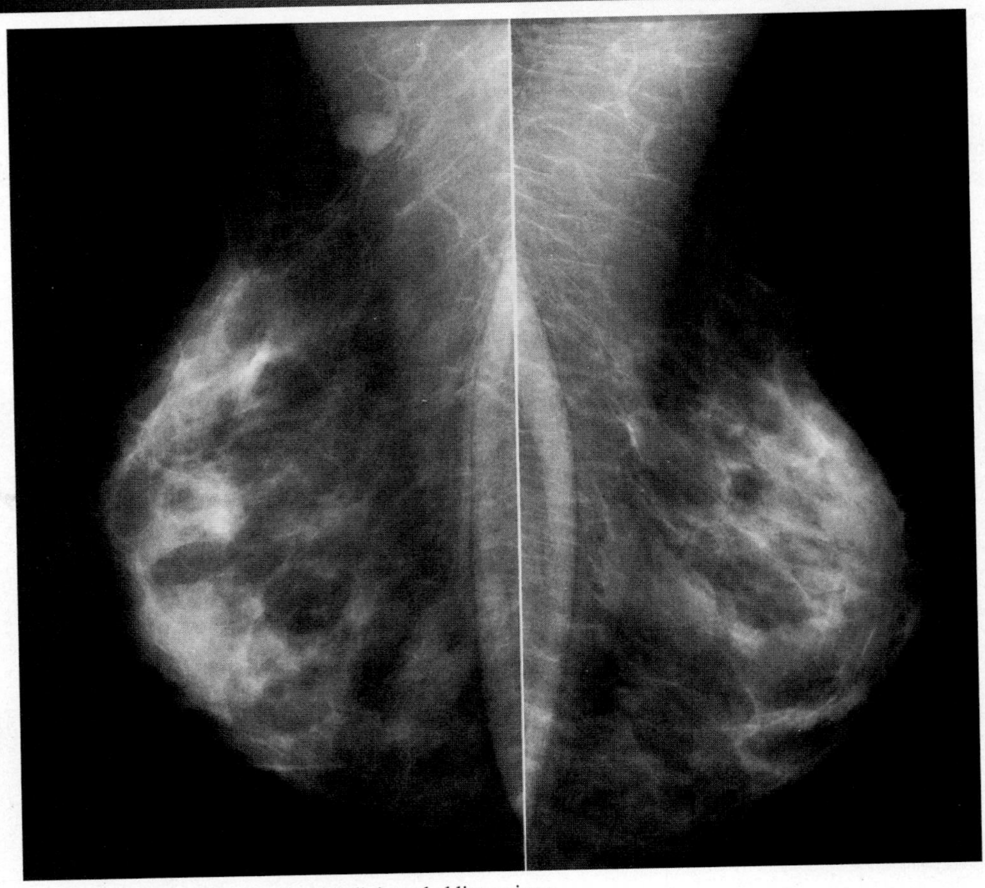

Figure 1.30. Screening studies. Mediolateral oblique views.

What do you think?
Are these optimally positioned mediolateral oblique views?

The pectoral muscles are wide at the axilla. The anterior margin is slightly concave, but the muscles reach the level of the nipples. There are, however, large skin folds superimposed on the pectoral muscles posteriorly.

In positioning the breast for the mediolateral oblique projection, the angle of obliquity is determined by the orientation of the pectoral muscle. The breast and underlying pectoral muscle are then mobilized medially as much as possible. If care is not taken, a skin fold can develop laterally as the breast is mobilized medially. If the technologist looks at the medial aspect of the breast after compression is applied, she is unable to see the skin fold because it is up against the bucky and therefore is not apparent. The edge of the fold is outlined by air so a thin radiolucency is noted abutting the skin fold. A lymph node is incidentally noted, superimposed on the right pectoral muscle.

PATIENT 31

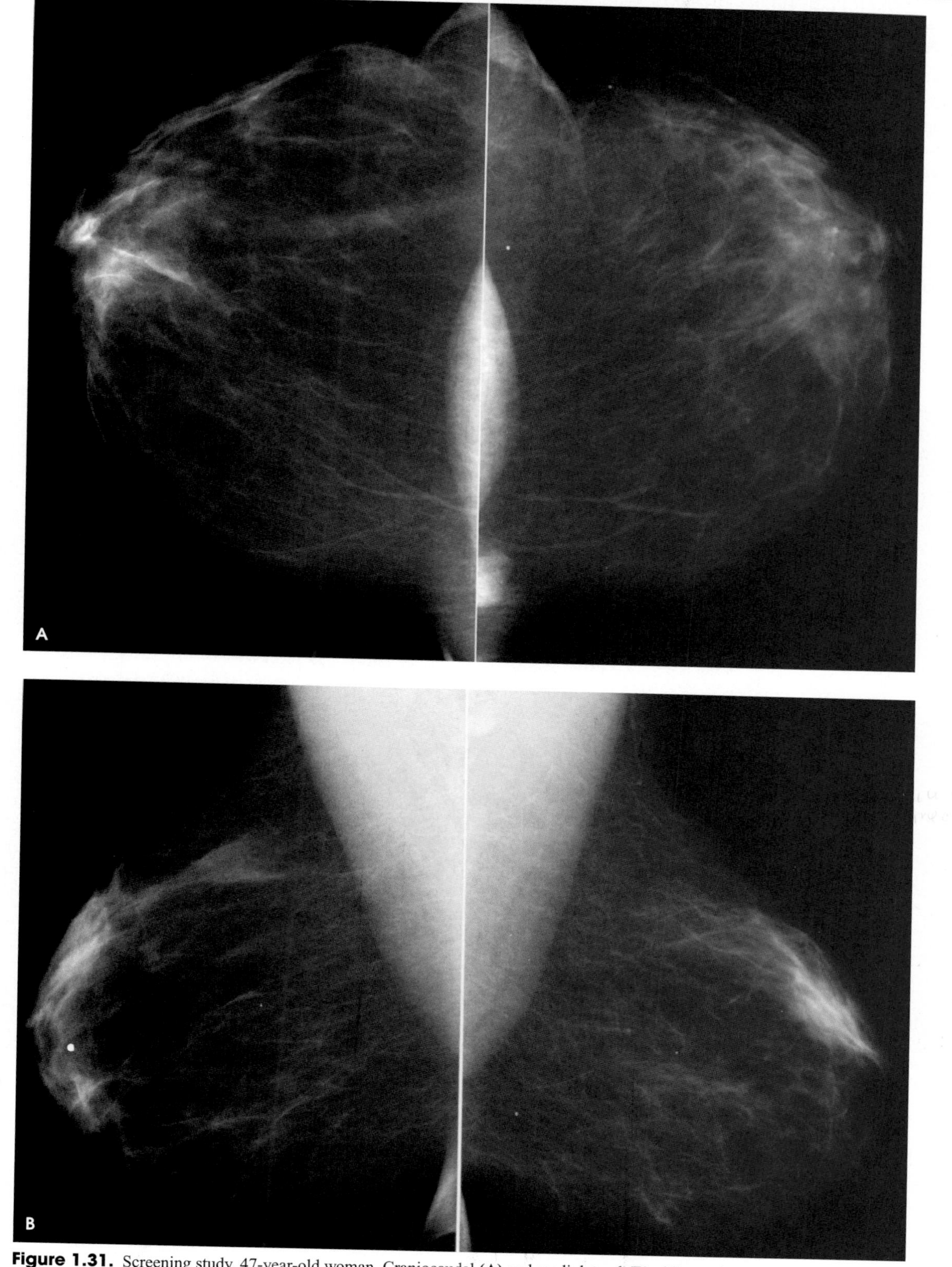

Figure 1.31. Screening study, 47-year-old woman. Craniocaudal **(A)** and mediolateral **(B)** oblique views.

Is this a normal mammogram, or do you think additional evaluation is indicated?
What BI-RADS® category would you use?

This is a normal mammogram. Skin folds are noted laterally on the craniocaudal (CC) views. These often develop as the technologist actively tugs on the lateral aspect of the breasts in an attempt to include as much lateral tissue as possible. Pectoral muscle can be seen posteriorly on the CC views. On the mediolateral oblique (MLO) views, the pectoral muscles are thick in the axillary region, extend to the level of the nipples, and have a convex anterior margin indicating excellent positioning technique.

Oh. . . you ask. . . what about the mass partially visualized at the posteromedial edge of the left breast on the CC view (Fig. 1.31C, *arrow*)? Where is this on the MLO view? This is the sternalis muscle, a normal variant. It is typically seen medially on craniocaudal views that include a maximum amount of posterior tissue (i.e., pectoral muscle is usually seen) and can have a variety of appearances. It is usually surrounded by fat and can be round in shape, as shown here, or it can be more triangular in shape. As in this patient, thin swirls of fatty tissue are seen in the "mass." The oblique view is normal, as are any lateral views that may be obtained. Although it has been reported in as many as 8% of the population, based on cadaveric studies, the sternalis muscle is an uncommon finding on mammographic studies. It is more commonly unilateral, but can occur bilaterally and typically runs parasternally, from the infraclavicular area to the caudal aspect, lying anterior to the medial margin of the pectoralis major muscle.

No additional evaluation is indicated. BI-RADS® category 1: negative. Next screening mammogram is recommended in 1 year.

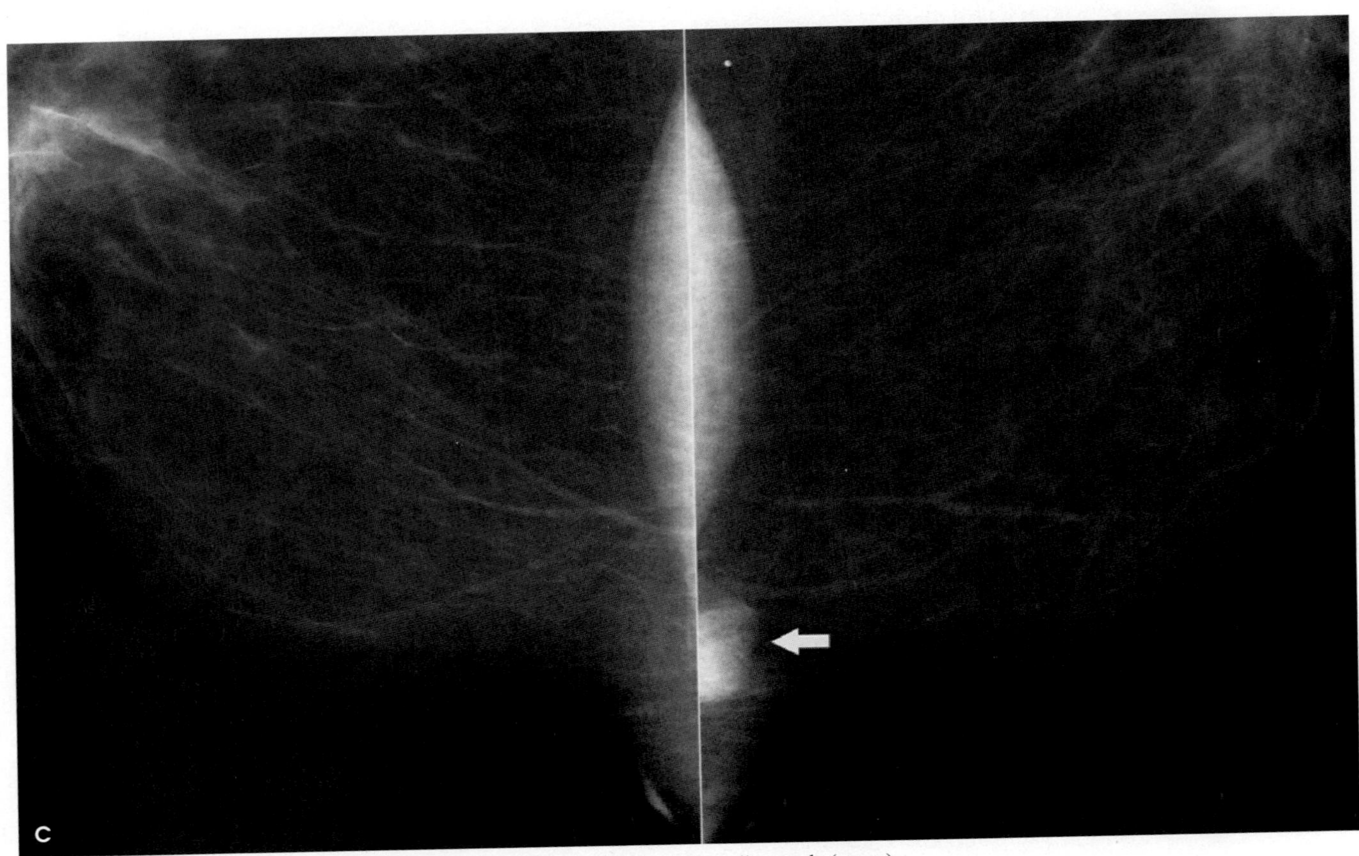

Figure 1.31. (*Continued*) Craniocaudal views (**C**) photographically coned. Sternalis muscle (arrow).

PATIENT 32

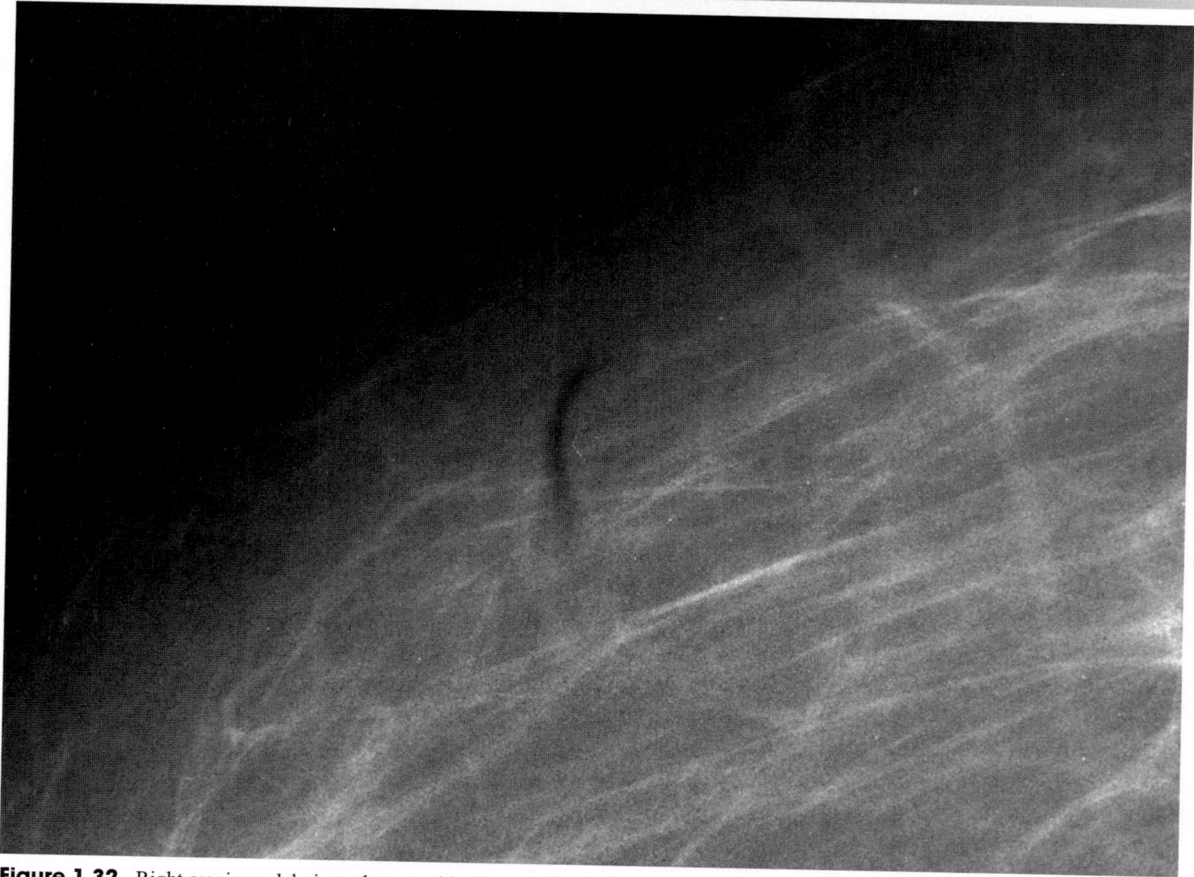

Figure 1.32. Right craniocaudal view, photographically coned laterally.

What is the observation? When did this occur, before or after the exposure was made?

A curvilinear, plus-density artifact from a nail is present, reflecting improper handling or pressure on the film, after the exposure was made but before processing. If the film is palpated at this site, a crimp will be found corresponding to the artifact.

PATIENT 33

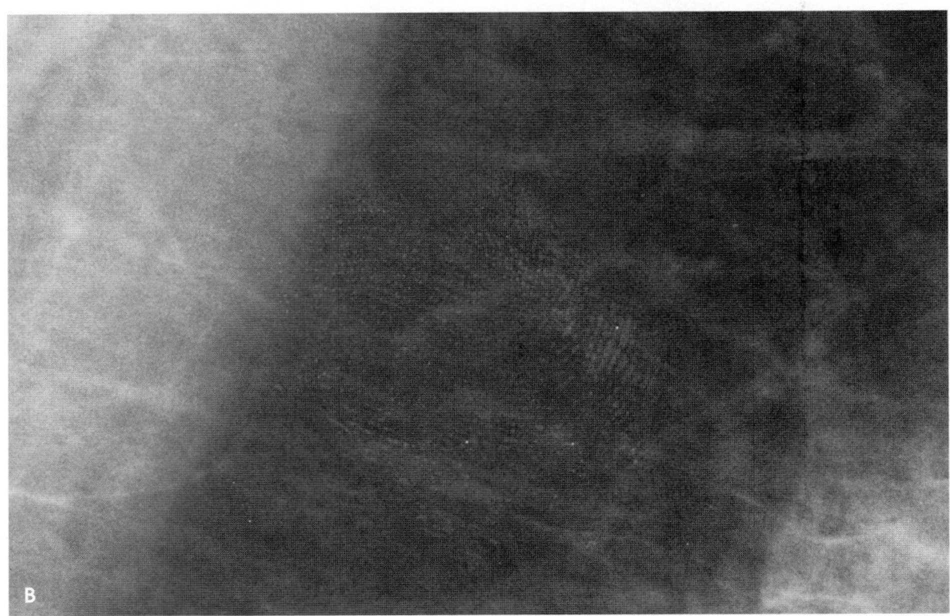

Figure 1.33. Craniocaudal **(A)** view, photographically coned. Mediolateral oblique **(B)** view, photographically coned.

What is the observation? When did this occur, before or after the exposure was made?

Curvilinear, negative-density artifacts, from fingerprints, reflect improper handling or pressure on the films before the exposure was made. Films should always be handled by the edges.

PATIENT 34

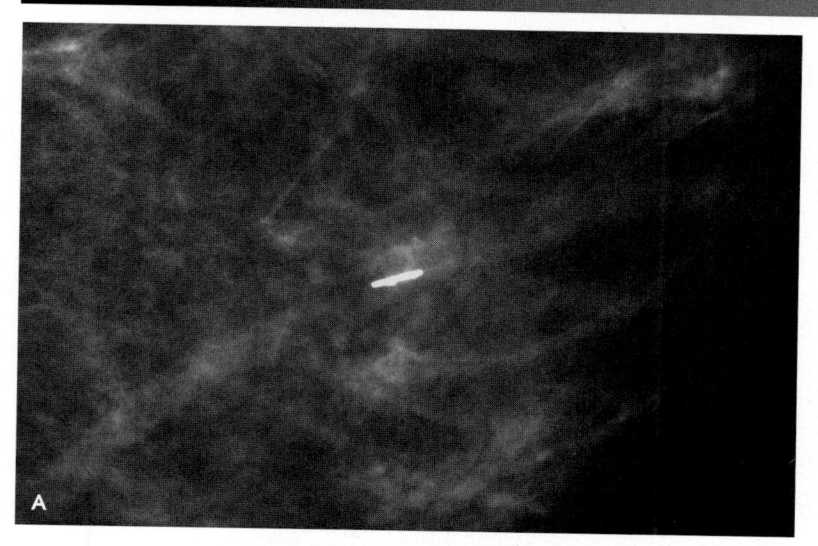

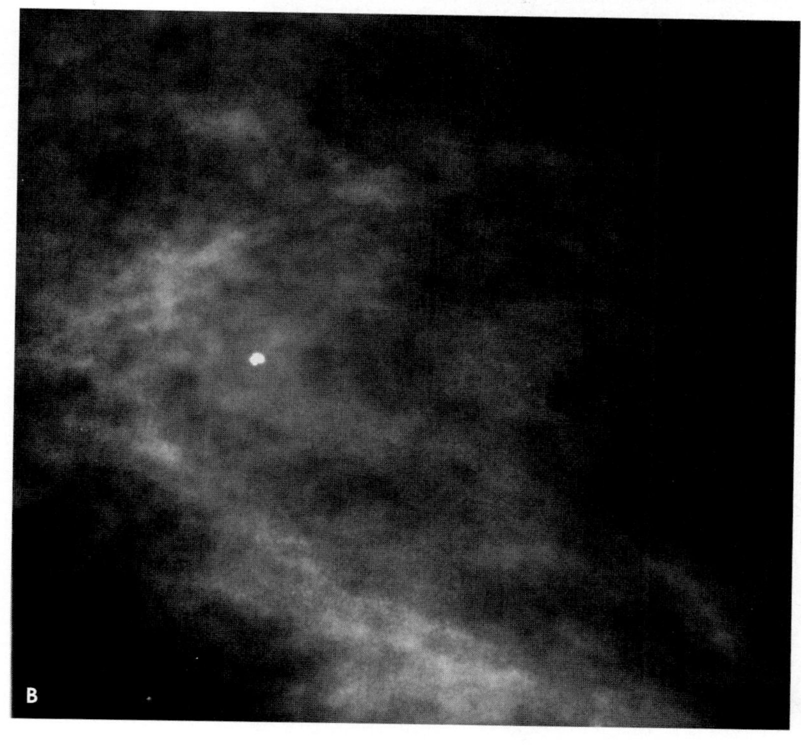

Figure 1.34. Craniocaudal **(A)** view, photographically coned. Craniocaudal **(B)** view, photographically coned.

What observations can you make? What happened?

On these images, a high-density artifact is present, surrounded by an area of blurring. This is consistent with poor film–screen contact. The artifact is on the screen and prevents the film from making direct contact with the screen. The blur surrounding the artifact reflects the lack of direct contact between film and screen. Depending on the size and shape of the artifact, the high-density material varies in size and shape and with it the surrounding area of blur. Unlike motion blur, this type of nonsharpness is more localized, symmetric, and the area of blur is more geometrically marginated.

What is the recommendation with respect to the amount of time that should elapse between loading cassettes with film and making an exposure, and why is this recommended? How often should screens be cleaned?

It is recommended that approximately 15 minutes be allowed to elapse between loading a cassette with film and making an exposure. This is so any entrapped air between film and screen can escape and good film–screen contact can develop. Screens should be cleaned at least weekly or immediately after dust artifacts are noted in an image by either the technologist or radiologist.

PATIENT 35

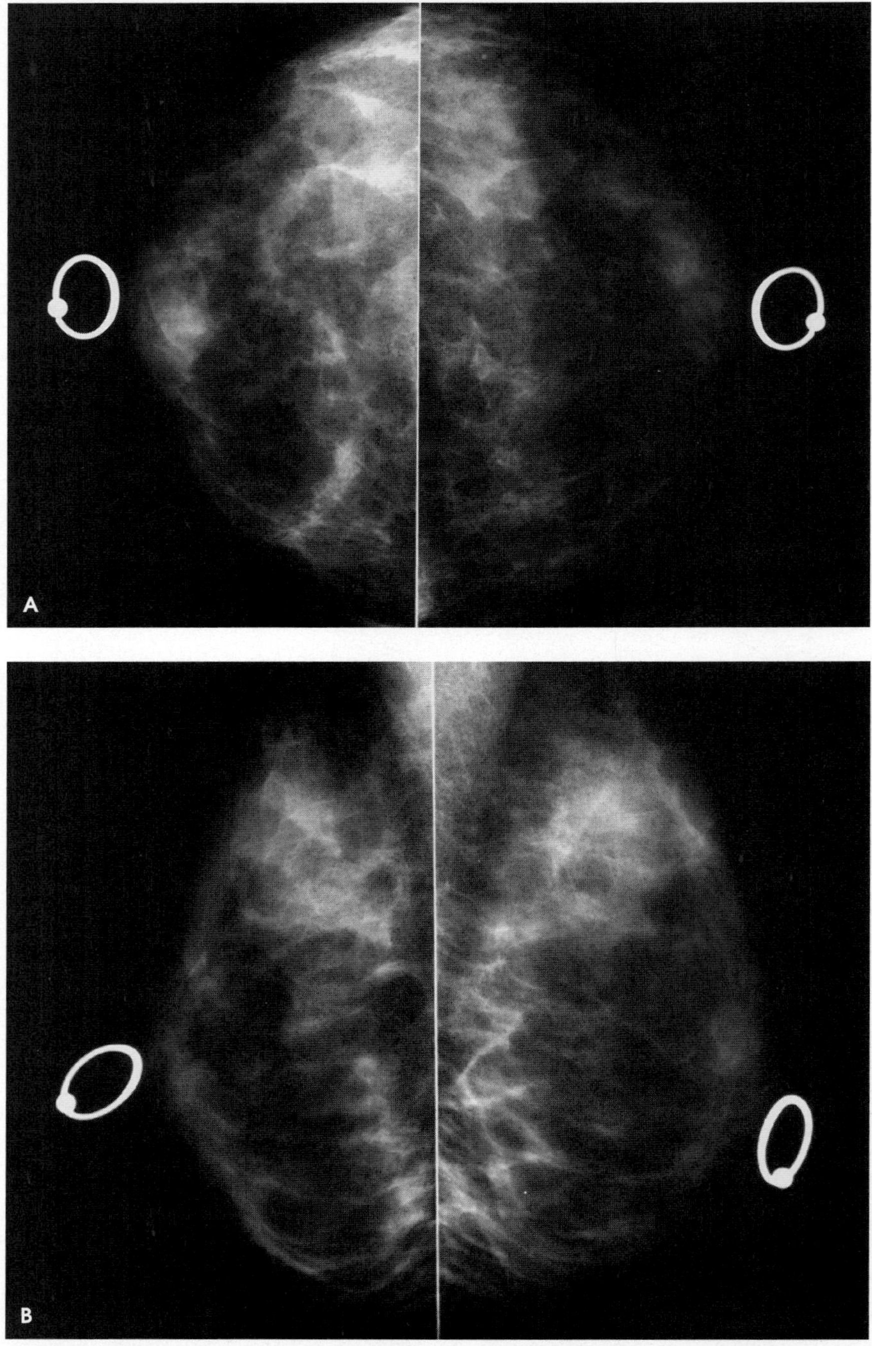

Figure 1.35. Screening study, 42-year-old woman. Craniocaudal **(A)** and mediolateral oblique **(B)** views.

What is your observation?

These are nipple rings: They are used uni- or bilaterally and are variable in shape.

PATIENT 36

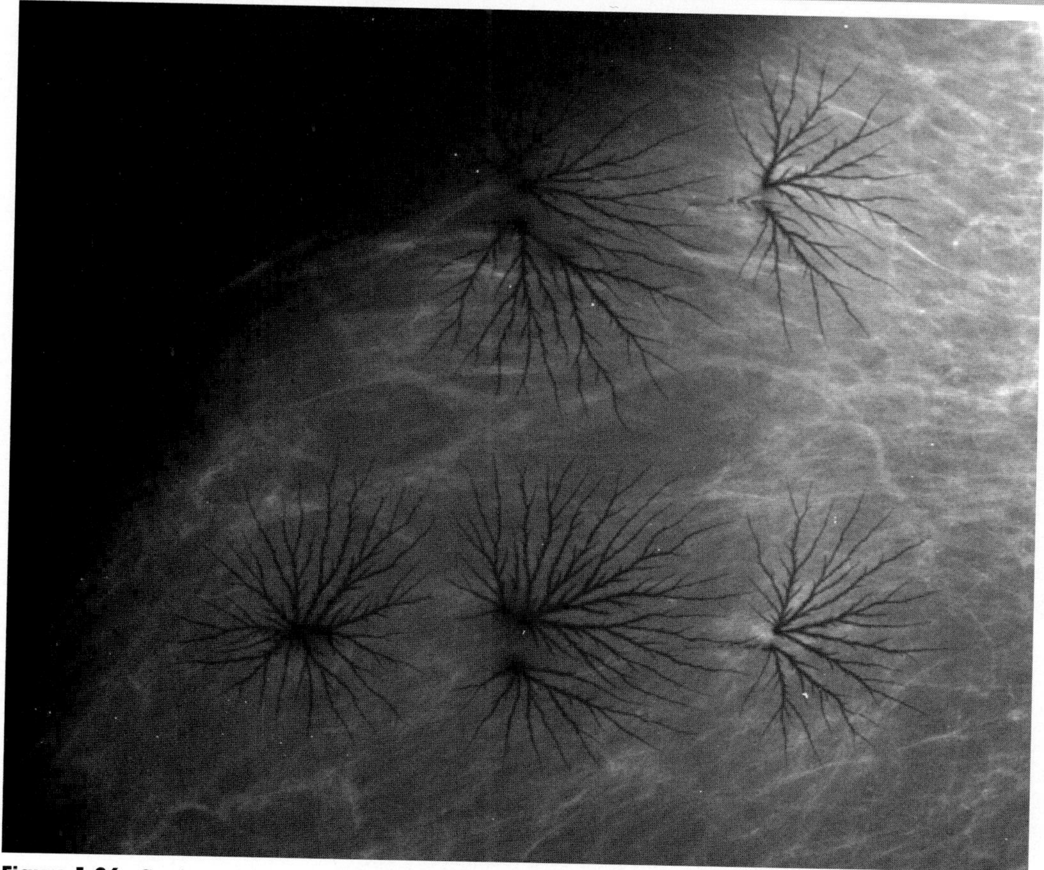

Figure 1.36. Craniocaudal view, right breast, photographically coned.

What is the observation?

Static results in fogging of the film in a fairly distinctive appearance and is related to the processor (as in this patient) or improper film handling.

PATIENT 37

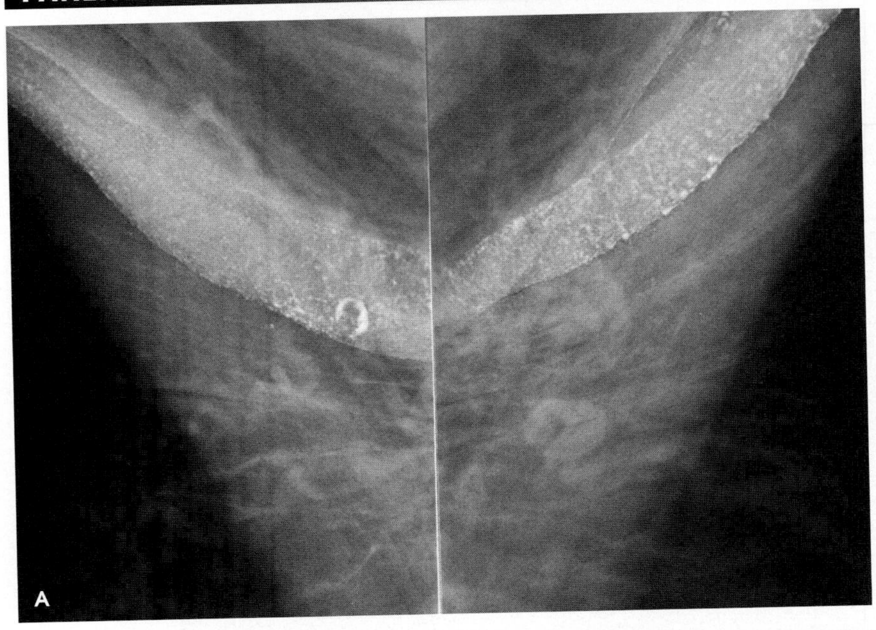

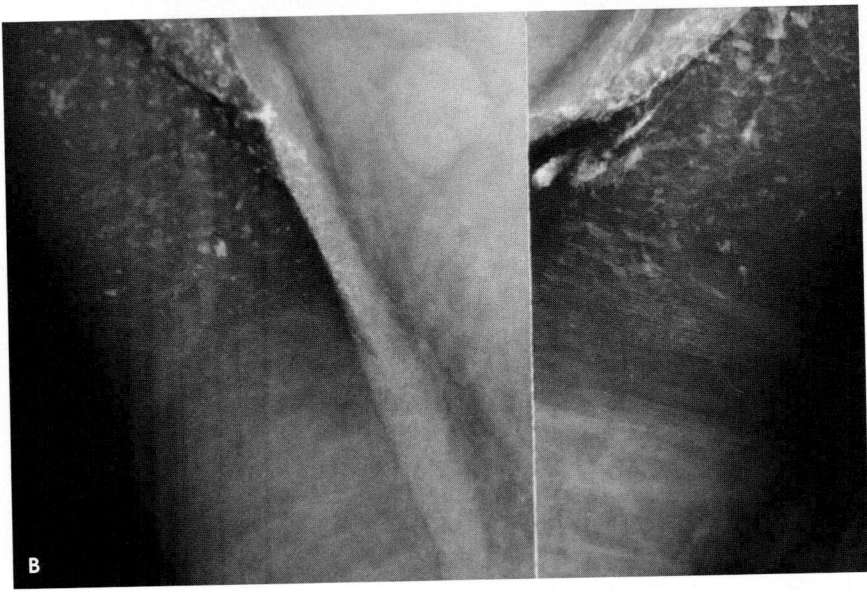

Figure 1.37. **A:** Mediolateral oblique views, photographically coned. **B:** Mediolateral oblique views, photographically coned.

What is the observation?

High-density material observed bilaterally in the axilla simulating calcifications reflects the presence of deodorant. A prominent skin fold and an axillary lymph node are present, superimposed on the right mediolateral oblique view (Fig. 1.37B).

When a mammogram is scheduled, what instructions may be helpful for the patient in preparation for her mammogram?

Patients are asked to not apply deodorant prior to their mammogram. They are also advised to consider wearing a two-piece outfit (e.g., skirt and blouse or pants and blouse) to facilitate changing for the exam. If at the time of the mammogram the patient states that she is wearing deodorant, an attempt is made to have her wipe it clean before any images are taken. We provide spray deodorant in the dressing rooms for patients to use following their mammogram.

PATIENT 38

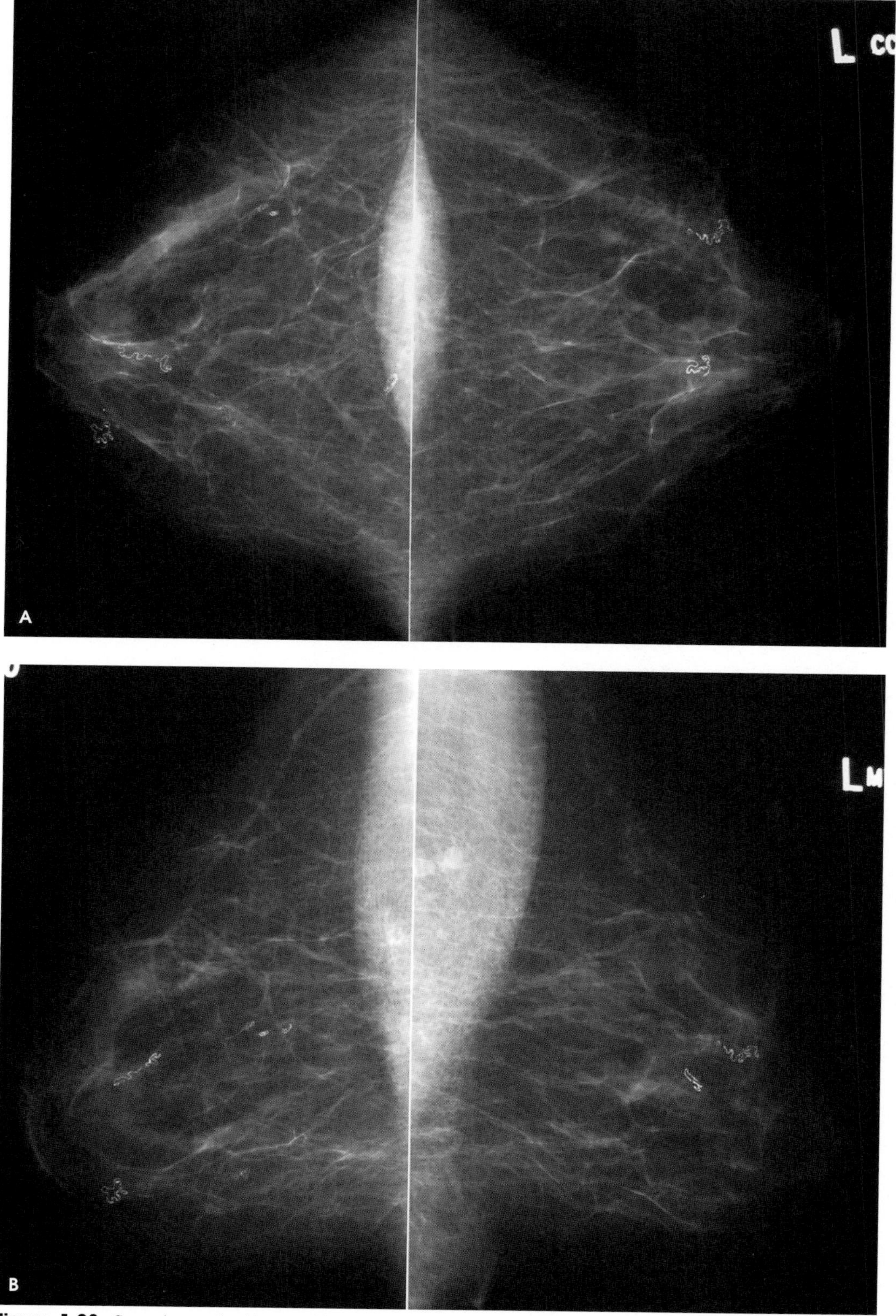

Figure 1.38. Screening study, 49-year-old woman. Craniocaudal **(A, B)** view. Screening study, 49-year-old woman. Mediolateral oblique **(B)** view.

How would you describe the findings, and what is the diagnosis?
What BI-RADS® category would you use?

Multiple clusters of coiled, serpiginous, linear and curvilinear calcifications are present bilaterally. These findings are consistent with calcified parasites. Several different parasites have been reported as occurring in the breast parenchyma or subcutaneous tissue (filariasis, loiasis, onchocerciasis, cysticercosis, dracunculosis, schistosomiasis, cutaneous myasis, etc). The dead parasites calcify, resulting in distinctive linear, curvilinear, coiled, lacelike, beadlike, or serpiginous calcifications scattered bilaterally. Sharply defined, round and punctate calcifications, limited to the pectoral muscles bilaterally, are seen in women with trichinosis.

BI-RADS® category 1: negative. Next screening mammogram is recommended in 1 year. BI-RADS® category 2: benign finding is used if the calcifications are described in the body of the report. Next screening mammogram is recommended in 1 year.

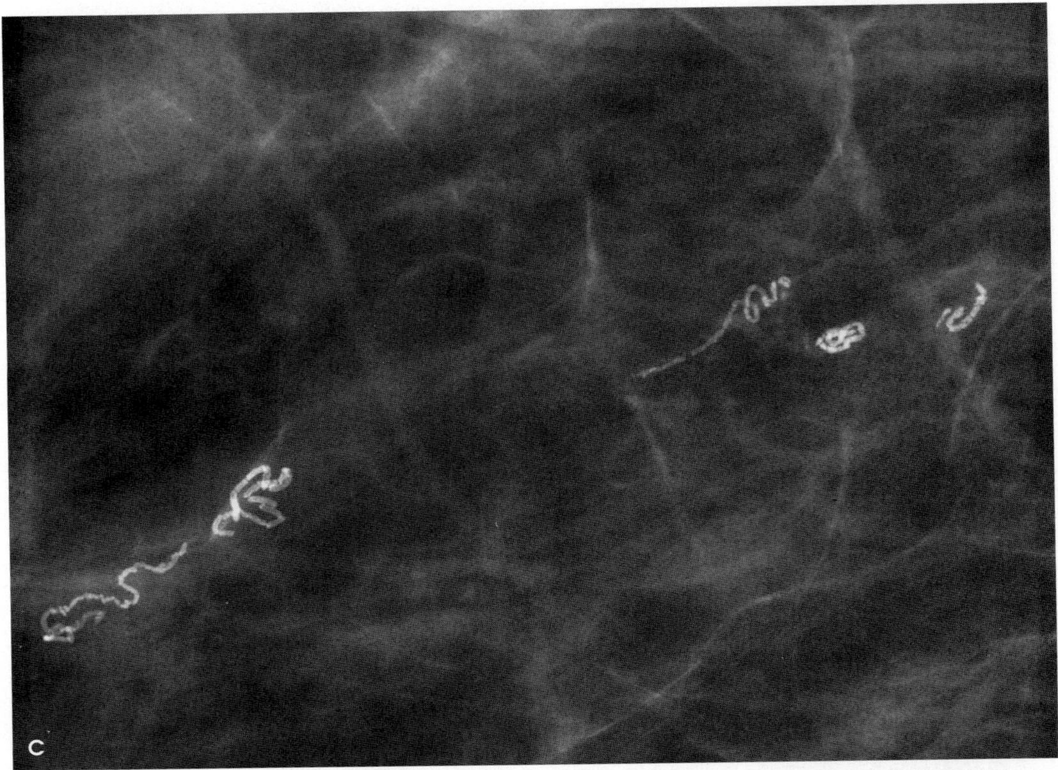

Figure 1.38. *(Continued)* Mediolateral oblique **(C)** view, right breast, photographically coned. Calcified parasites.

PATIENT 39

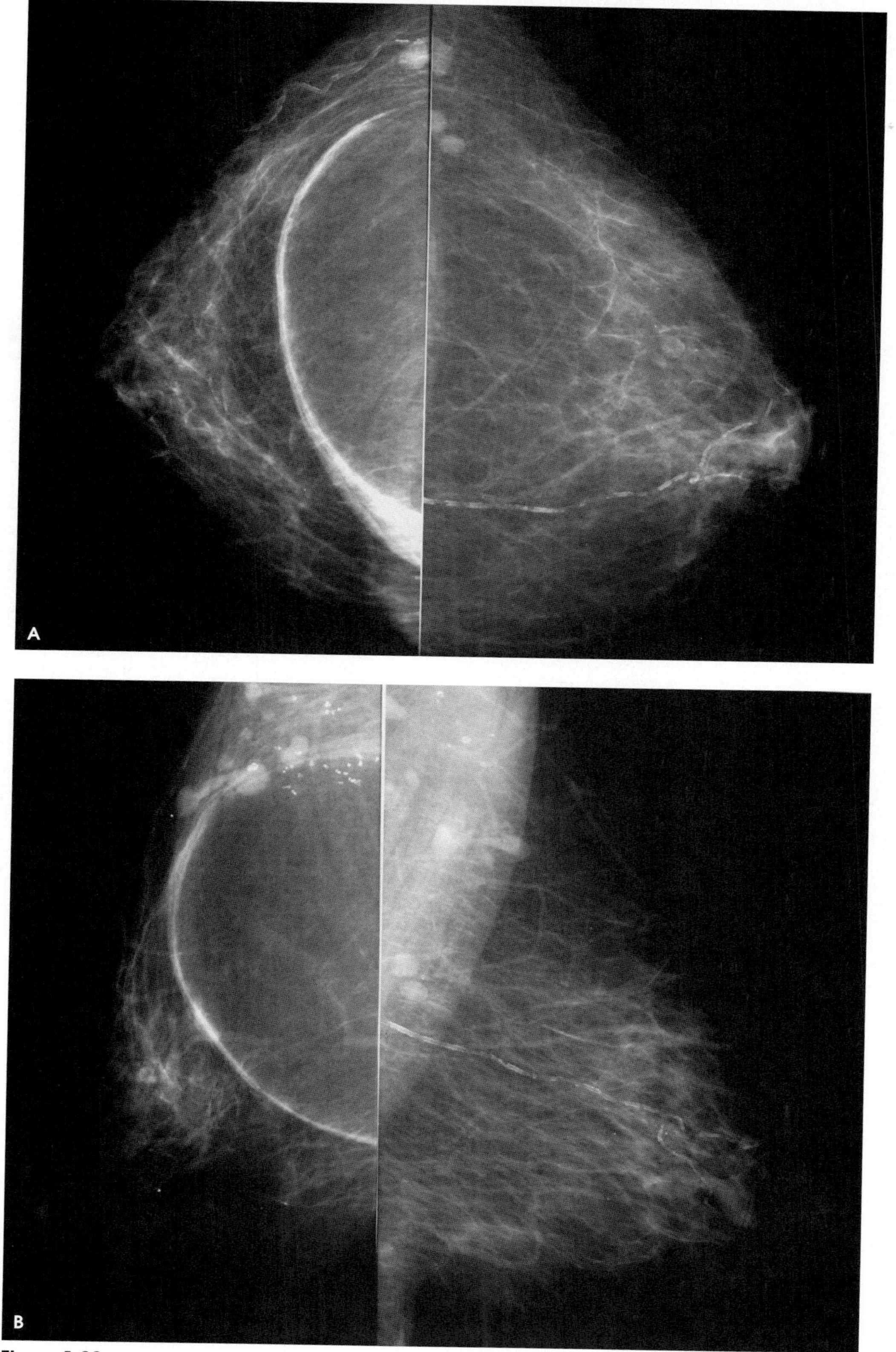

Figure 1.39. Screening study, 73-year-old woman. Craniocaudal **(A)** and mediolateral oblique **(B)** views.

What is your diagnosis?

Multiple axillary and intramammary lymph nodes are noted bilaterally, as are benign-type skin and vascular calcifications. A radiolucent mass is imaged in the right pectoral muscle consistent with a lipoma (Fig. 1.39C). The differential for radiolucent masses in the breast is limited and includes lipomas, oil cysts, and, rarely, galactoceles. Although ultrasound is not needed because the diagnosis is established mammographically, ultrasound is sometimes helpful in distinguishing between a lipoma and an oil cyst. Lipomas are often homogeneously iso- to slightly hyperechoic, well-circumscribed solid masses. Oil cysts have a variable appearance on ultrasound, ranging from cystic to complex cystic to solid masses, some with associated shadowing.

BI-RADS® category 1: negative. Next screening mammogram is recommended in 1 year. BI-RADS® category 2: benign finding is used if the lipoma is described in the body of the report. Next screening mammogram is recommended in 1 year.

Lipomas are slow-growing tumors presenting as soft, discrete, round, single or multiple masses, most commonly in the subcutaneous tissues; however, they can develop anywhere, including in breast tissue, muscles, and internal organs. Rarely, they can be associated with hereditary multiple lipomatosis, adiposis dolorosa (Dercum disease), and Gardner syndrome. They are composed of mature adipocytes that may be surrounded by a fibrous capsule. Although most do not require treatment, steroid injections, liposuction, or surgery are options that have been described for their management.

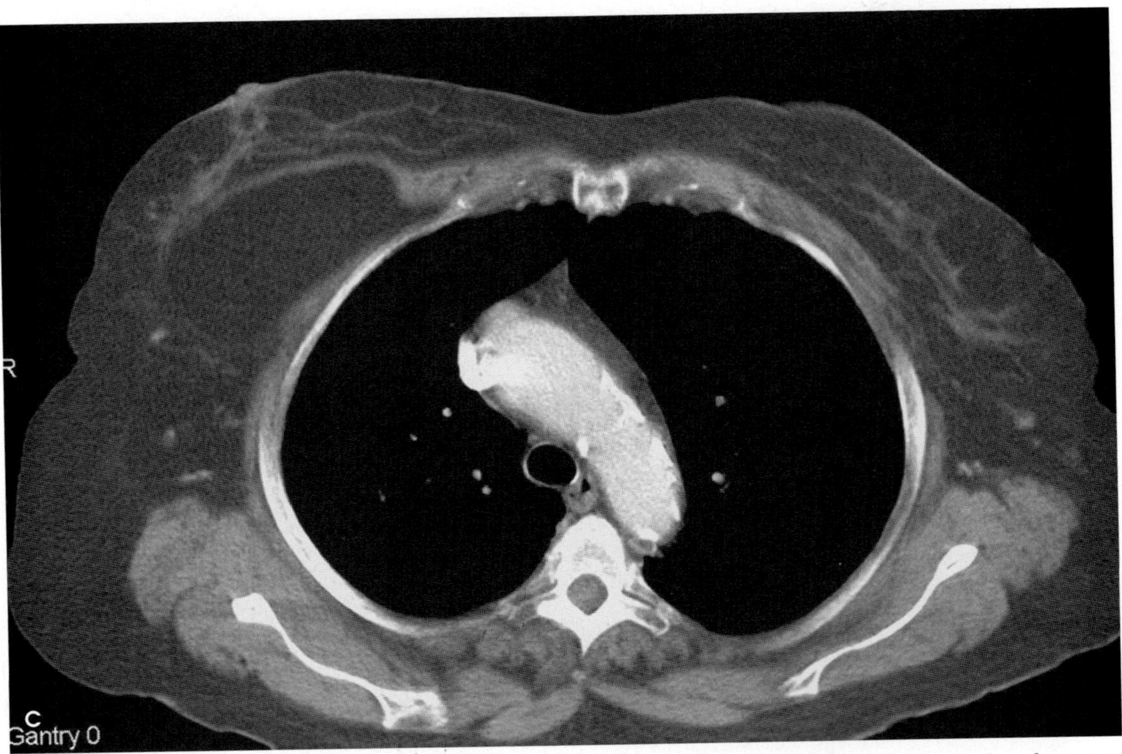

Figure 1.39. Chest CT scan **(C)** confirms the presence of a lipoma in the right pectoral muscle (CT scan was done for reasons other than the lipoma).

PATIENT 40

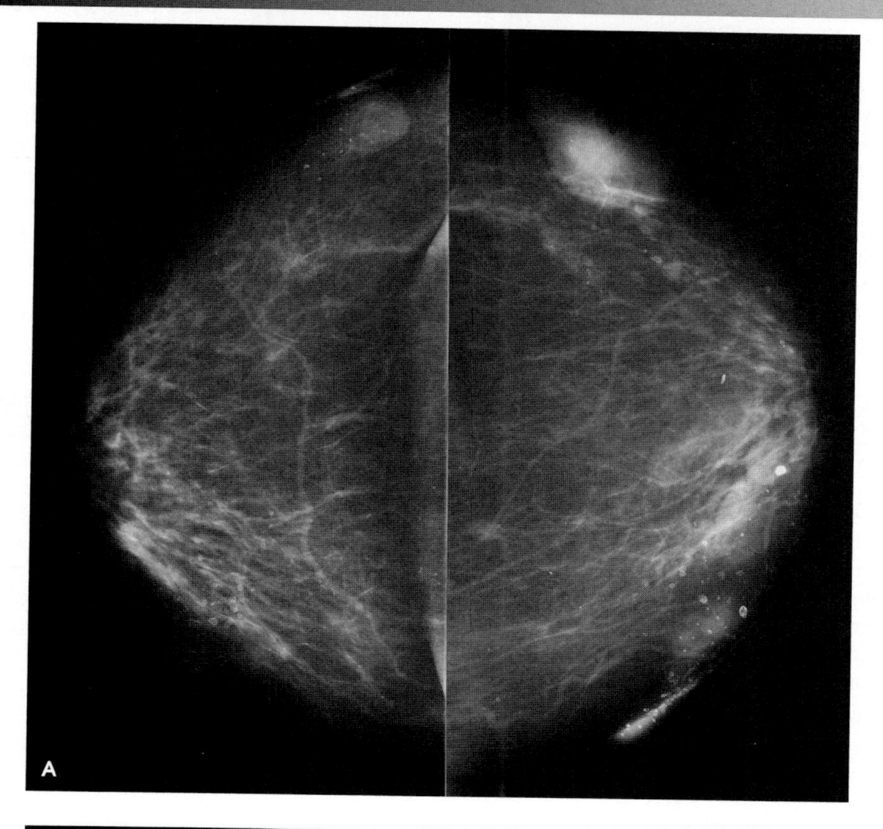

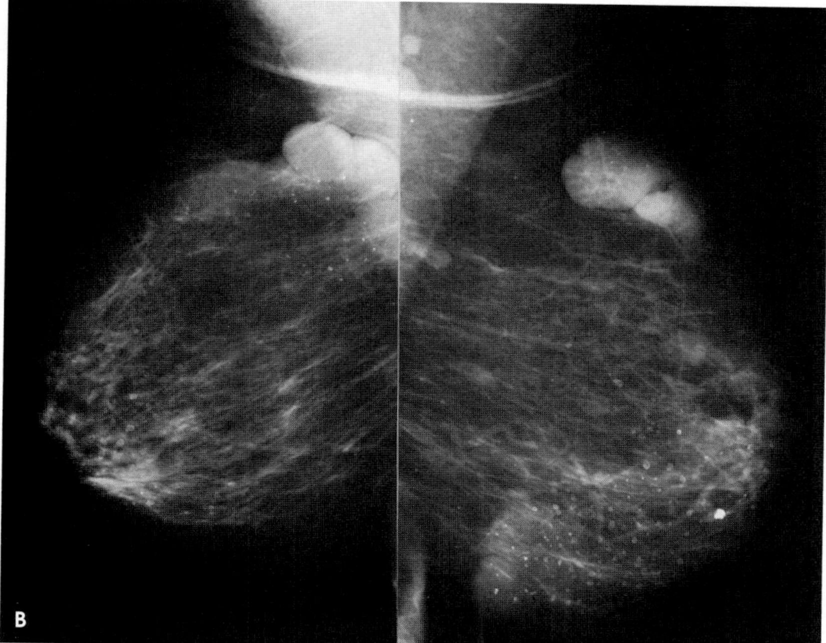

Figure 1.40. Screening study, 63-year-old woman. Craniocaudal **(A)** and mediolateral oblique **(B)** views.

What is your diagnosis? Does this patient require any additional evaluation?

Multiple densities of various sizes and shapes, some appearing tubular, are seen bilaterally. Associated round, lucent-centered calcifications consistent with skin calcifications are also present. The margins of some of these densities are partially or completely outlined by a sharp lucency consistent with air (Fig. 1.40C). The sharply defined margins in conjunction with the shapes of these structures and the associated skin calcifications suggest that these may represent keloids forming at prior sites of surgery. Review of prior mammograms with markers placed at the prior biopsy sites confirms this impression (Fig. 1.40D–G). No further evaluation is indicated.

BI-RADS® category 1: negative. Next screening mammogram is recommended in 1 year. BI-RADS® category 2: benign finding is used if the keloids are described in the body of the report. Next screening mammogram is recommended in 1 year.

Wound healing is a complex process controlled by soluble mediators characterized by a fine equilibrium between the deposition and removal of structural proteins and glycoproteins. Disruption in these normal anabolic and catabolic processes can lead to abnormal wound repair and scar formation, including hypertrophic scars and keloids. Hypertrophic scars are raised but typically confined to the borders of the original wound and increase in size by expanding the margins of the scar not by invading surrounding tissue. They arise in the first 4 weeks following injury and are characterized by rapid growth followed by regression. The collagen fibers in hypertrophic scars are oriented parallel to the skin surface. In contrast, keloids extend beyond the borders of the original wound and involve the adjacent normal dermis. These lesions typically appear later, gradually progress, and can proliferate indefinitely; they do not regress. The collagen fibers in keloids are larger, thicker, wavier, and randomly distributed as compared to those found in hypertrophic scars. Hypertrophic scars and keloids are often familial and are associated with a higher incidence of occurrence in black and Hispanic patients.

Various theories have been advanced into the causes of keloid formation. These include increases in growth-factor activity (e.g., transforming growth factor and platelet-derived growth factor), alterations in the extracellular matrix, abnormal regulation of collagen turnover, mechanical tension on the healing wound, genetic factors leading to abnormal immune responses to dermal injury, and an immune reaction to sebum. Various treatments including steroid (triamcinolone) injections, surgery, radiation therapy, topical application of silicone gel, pressure therapy, laser, intralesional 5-fluorouracil, interferon, retinoids, calcium channel blockers, cryosurgery, and antihistamines have been tried. Results, however, have been mixed, and the treatment and management of patients with keloids remains a challenge.

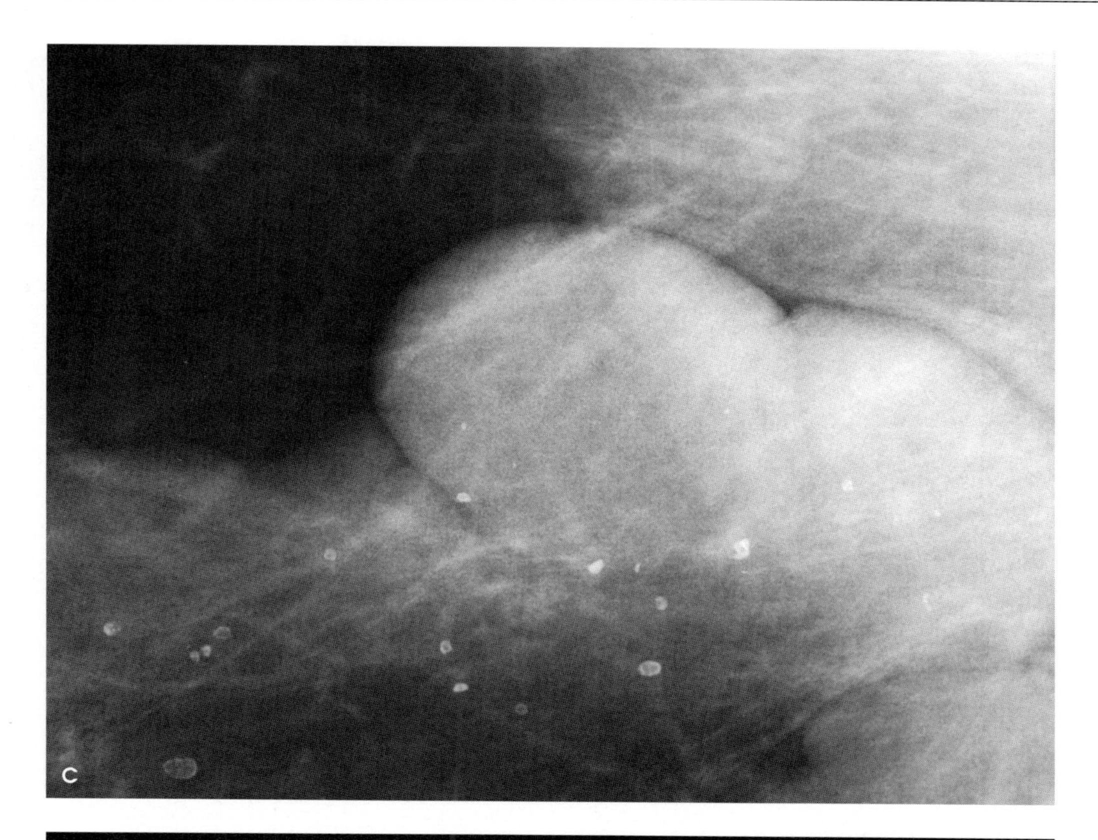

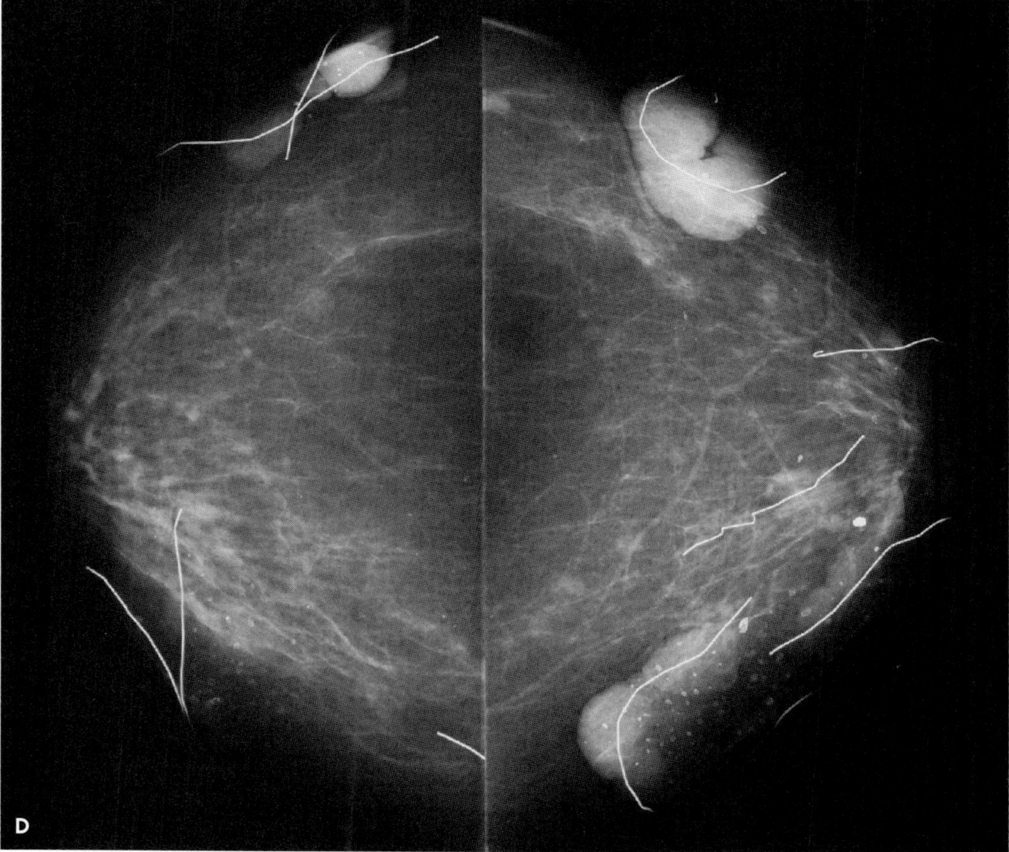

Figure 1.40. (*Continued*) Mediolateral oblique **(C)** view, right breast, photographically coned. Sharp lucency consistent with air partially outlines the lobulated mass. Adjacent lucent-centered calcifications consistent with skin calcifications are noted. Craniocaudal **(D)** and mediolateral oblique **(E)** views taken 1 year prior to **(A)** and **(B)** with metallic wires used to mark prior biopsy sites and keloids.

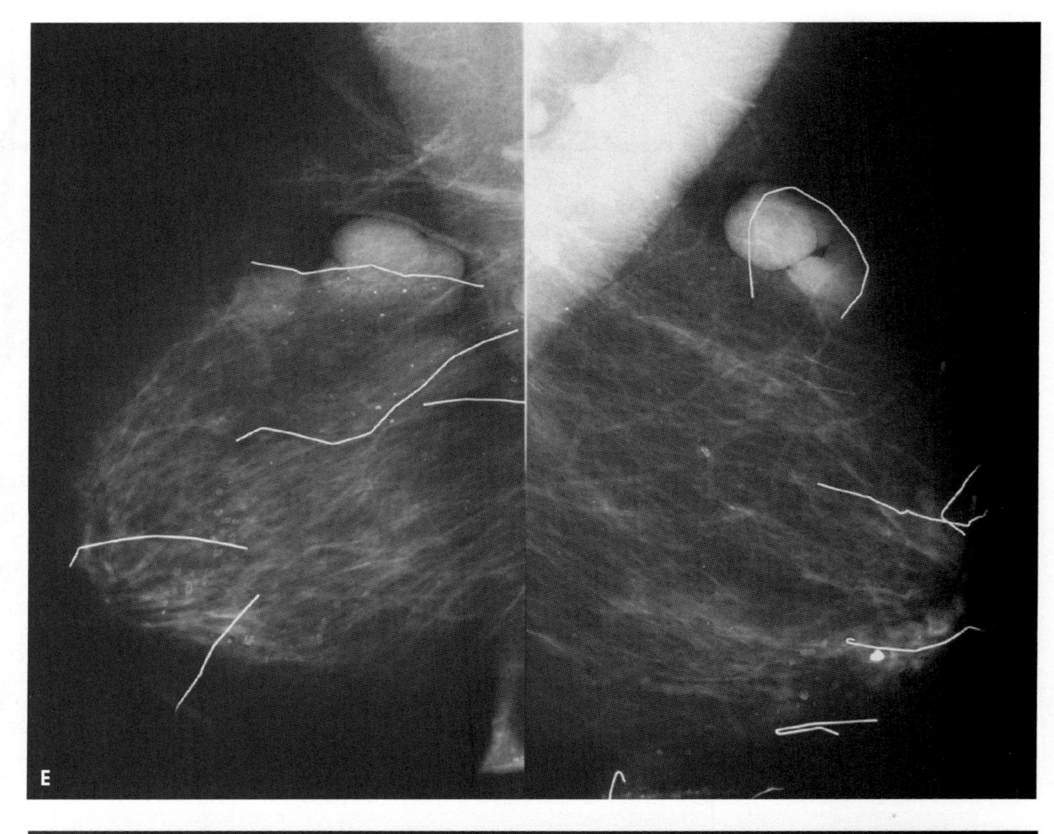

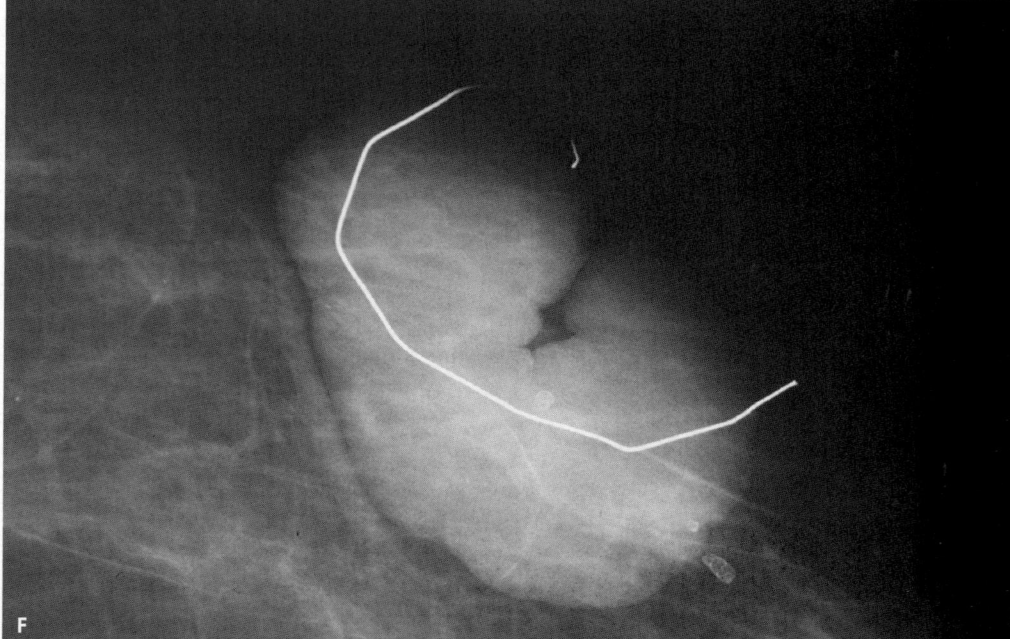

Figure 1.40. (*Continued*) Mediolateral oblique **(F)** view, left breast, and craniocaudal **(G)** view, right breast, photographically coned. Metallic wires used to mark prior biopsy sites and keloids. The linear and curvilinear shape and sharply defined margins resulting from air surrounding the protuberant portion of the keloids are diagnostic. Associated lucent-centered calcifications consistent with skin calcifications are also noted.

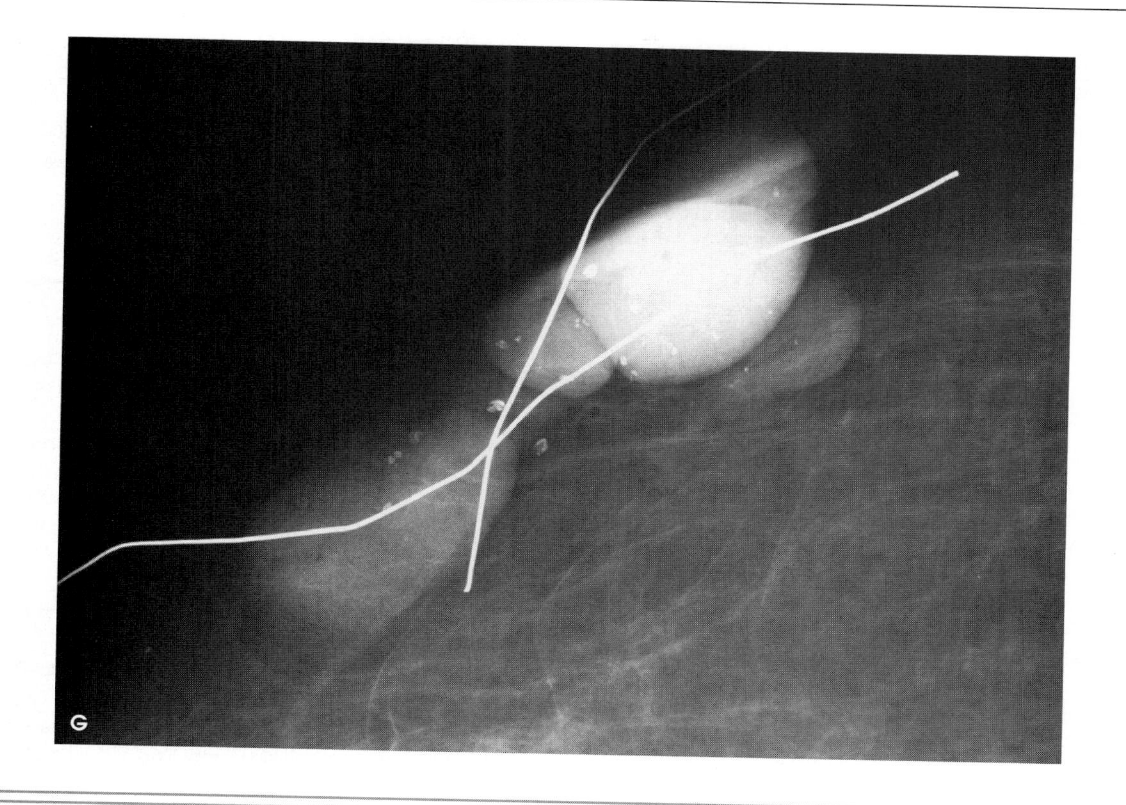

PATIENT 41

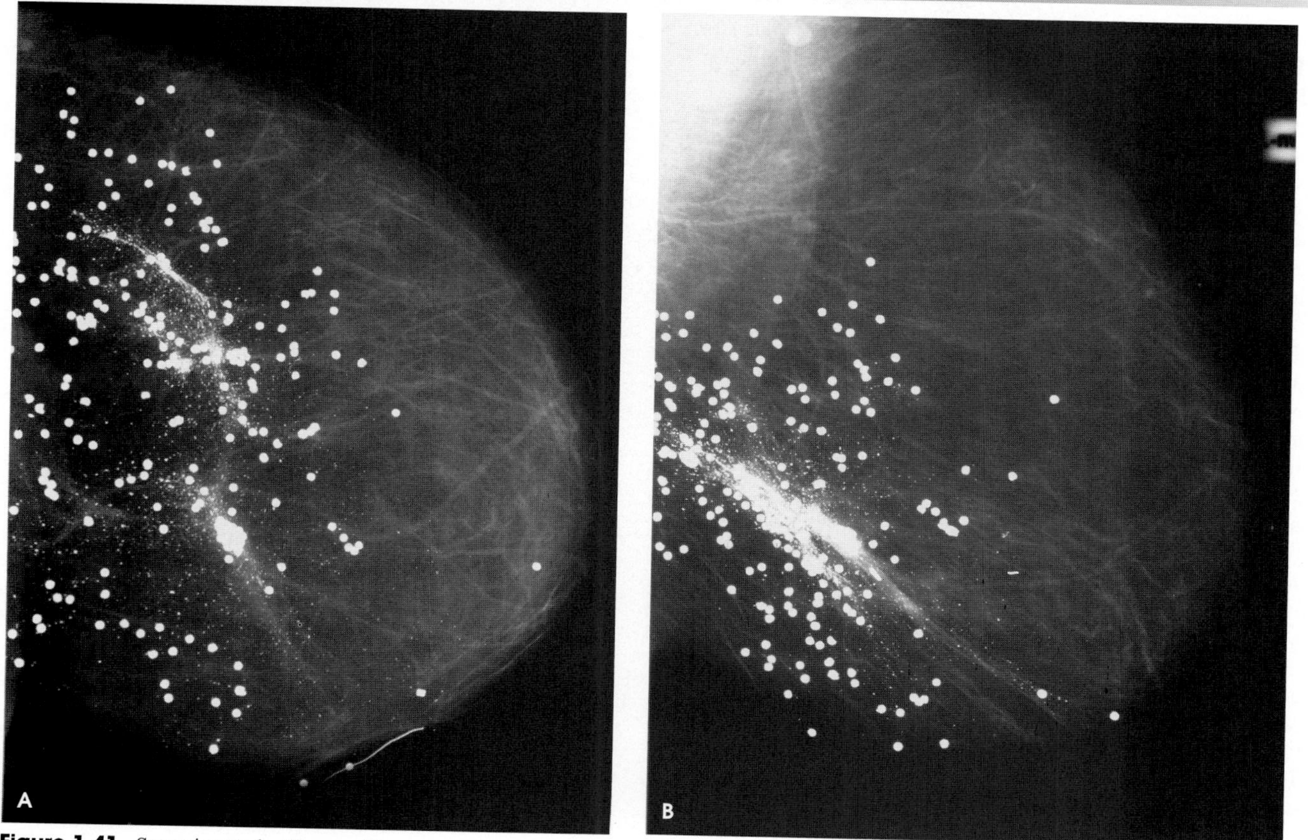

Figure 1.41. Screening study, 60-year-old woman. Craniocaudal **(A)** and mediolateral oblique **(B)** views, left breast.

What is your diagnosis?

Buck shot and bullet fragments with associated shrapnel are present in the left breast. Although the buck shot is distributed randomly, the bullet fragments and shrapnel demonstrate a more linear distribution, delineating the path of the bullets in the breast. No further intervention is warranted.

BI-RADS® category 1: negative. Next screening mammogram is recommended in 1 year. BI-RADS® category 2: benign finding is used if the metallic fragments are described in the body of the report. Next screening mammogram is recommended in 1 year.

BIBLIOGRAPHY

Al-Attar A, Mess S, Thomassen JM, et al. Keloid pathogenesis and treatment. *Plast Reconstr Surg.* 2006;117:286–300.

American College of Radiology (ACR). ACR BI-RADS®—Mammography. 4th ed. In: *ACR Breast Imaging Reporting and Data System, Breast Imaging Atlas.* Reston, VA: American College of Radiology; 2003.

American College of Radiology. *Mammography Quality Control Manual.* Reston, VA: American College of Radiology; 1999.

Apesteguia L, Mellado MT, Inchusta MI, Cordero JL. Mammographic demonstration of steatocystoma multiplex. *Eur Radiol.* 1998;8:647–648.

Apesteguia L, Murillo A, Biurrun J, et al. Calcified trichinosis of pectoral muscle: mammographic appearance. *Eur Radiol.* 1995; 5:414–416.

Asch T, Frey C. Radiographic appearance of mammary duct ectasia with calcification. *N Engl J Med.* 1962;266:86–87.

Atiyeh BS, Costagliola M, Hayek SN. Keloid or hypertrophic scar. The controversy: review of the literature. *Ann Plast Surg.* 2005; 54:676–680.

Bercovitch L, Schepps B, Koelliker S, et al. Mammographic findings in pseudoxanthoma elasticum. *J Am Acad Dermatol.* 2003; 48:359–366.

Beyer GA, Thorsen MK, Shaffer KA, et al. Mammographic appearance of the retained Dacron cuff of a Hickman catheter. *AJR Am J Roentgenol.* 1990;155:1204.

Bilgen IG, Ustun EE, Memis A. Fat necrosis of the breast: clinical, mammographic and sonographic features. *Eur J Radiol.* 2001; 39:92–99.

Bolognia JL, Jorizzo JL, Rapini RP, eds. *Dermatology.* Edinburgh: Mosby, 2003.

Borges da Silva B, Rodrigues JS, Borges US, et al. Large mammary hamartoma of axillary supernumerary breast tissue. *Breast.* 2005 Jun 27 (Epub).

Bradley FM, Hoover HC, Hulka CA, et al. The sternalis muscle: an unusual normal finding seen on mammography. *AJR Am J Roentgenol.* 1996;166:33–36.

Burd A, Huang L. Hypertrophic response and keloids diathesis: two very different forms of scar. *Plast Reconstr Surg.* 2005;116: 105e–157e.

Caskey CI, Berg WA, Anderson ND, et al. Breast implant rupture: diagnosis with US. *Radiology.* 1994;190:819–823.

Cetin M, Cetin R, Tamer N. Prevalence of breast arterial calcification in hypertensive patients. *Clin Radiol.* 2004;59:92–95.

Cetin M, Cetin R, Tamer N, Kelekci S. Breast arterial calcifications associated with diabetes and hypertension. *J Diabetes Complications.* 2004;18:363–366.

Chow CK, McCarthy JS, Neafie R, et al. Mammography of lymphatic filariasis. *AJR Am J Roentgenol.* 1996;167:1425–1426.

Cox J, Simpson W, Walshaw D. An interesting byproduct of screening: assessing the effect of HRT on arterial calcification in the female breast. *J Med Screen.* 2002;9:38–39.

de Barros N, D'Avila MS, Bauab SP, et al. Cutaneous myiasis of the breast: mammographic and US features—report of five cases. *Radiology.* 2001;218:518–520.

DeBruhl ND, Gorczyca DP, Ahn CY, et al. Silicone breast implants: US evaluation. *Radiology.* 1993;189:95–98.

Dershaw DD, Selland D, Tan LK, et al. Spiculated axillary adenopathy. *Radiology.* 1996;201:439–442.

Doeger KM, Whaley DH, Berger PB, et al. Breast arterial calcification detected on mammography is a risk factor for coronary artery disease. *Radiology.* 2002;225:552(abst).

Ellis RL, Dempsey PJ, Rubin E, et al. Mammography of breasts in which catheter cuffs have been retained: normal, infected and postoperative appearances. *AJR Am J Roentgenol.* 1997;169: 713–715.

Everson LI, Parentainen H, Detlie T, et al. Diagnosis of breast implant rupture: imaging findings and relative efficacies of imaging techniques. *AJR Am J Roentgenol.* 1994;163:57–60.

Fitzpatrick TB, Johnson RA, Wolff K, Suurmond D. *Color Atlas and Synopsis of Clinical Dermatology.* 4th ed. New York: McGraw-Hill; 2001.

Fornage BD, Tassin GB. Sonographic appearance of superficial soft tissue lipomas. *J Clin Ultrasound.* 1991;19:215–220.

Friedman PD, Kalisher L. Case 43: filariasis. *Radiology.* 2002; 515–517.

Fuster M, Saez JJ, Orozco D, et al. Breast arterial calcification: a new cardiovascular risk marker. *Radiology.* 2002;225:553–554 (abst).

Georgian-Smith D, Kricun B, McKee B, et al. The mammary hamartoma: appreciation of additional imaging characteristics. *J Ultrasound Med.* 2004;23:1267–1273.

Gravier A, Picquenot JM, Berry M. Invasive lobular carcinoma in a breast hamartoma. *Breast J.* 2003;9:246–248.

Harris KM, Ganott MA, Shestak KC, et al. Silicone implant rupture: detection with US. *Radiology.* 1993;187:761–768.

Harvey JA, Moran RE, Maurer EJ, DeAngelis GA. Sonographic features of mammary oil cysts. *J Ultrasound Med.* 1997; 16:719–724.

Haus AG, Jaskulski SM. *The Basics of Film Processing in Medical Imaging.* Madison, WI: Medical Physics Publishing; 1997.

Herbert M, Sandbank J, Liokumovich P, et al. Breast hamartomas: clinicopathological and immunohistochemical studies of 24 cases. *Histopathology.* 2002;41:30–34.

Hogge JP, Palmer CH, Muller CC, et al. Quality assurance in mammography: artifact analysis. *Radiographics.* 1999;19:503–522.

Hogge JP, Robinson RE, Magnant CM, et al. The mammographic spectrum of fat necrosis in the breast. *Radiographics*. 1995; 15:1347–1356.

Iribarren C, Go AS, Tolstykh I, et al. Breast vascular calcification and risk of coronary heart disease, stroke and heart failure. *J Womens Health (Larchmt)*. 2004;13:381–389.

Kim HS, Cha ES, Kim HH, Yoo JY. Spectrum of sonographic findings in superficial breast masses. *J Ultrasound Med*. 2005;24:663–680.

Kopans DB, Meyer JE, Homer MJ, et al. Dermal deposits mistaken for breast calcifications. *Radiology*. 1983;149:592–594.

Kuroda N, Sugimoto T, Numoto S, Enzan H. Microinvasive lobular carcinoma associated with intraductal spread in a mammary hamartoma. *J Clin Pathol*. 2002;55:76–77.

Lee CH, Giurescu ME, Philpotts LE, et al. Clinical importance of unilaterally enlarging lymph nodes on otherwise normal mammograms. *Radiology*. 1997;203:329–334.

Lee EH, Wylie EJ, Bourke AG, Bastiaan De Boer W. Invasive ductal carcinoma arising in a breast hamartoma: two case reports and a review of the literature. *Clin Radiol*. 2003;58:80–83.

Linden SS, Sickles EA. Sedimented calcium in benign cysts: the full spectrum of mammographic presentations. *AJR Am J Roentgenol*. 1989;152(5):967–971.

Mathers ME, Shrimankar J. Lobular neoplasia within a myxoid hamartoma of the breast. *Breast J*. 2004;10:58–59.

Mester J, Darwish M, Deshmukh SM. Steatocystoma multiplex of the breast: mammographic and sonography findings. *AJR Am J Roentgenol*. 1998;170:115–116.

Mester J, Simmons RM, Vasquez MF, et al. In situ and infiltrating ductal carcinoma arising in a breast hamartoma. *AJR Am J Roentgenol*. 2000;175:64–66.

Miller CL, Feig SA, Fox JW. Mammographic changes after reduction mammoplasty. *AJR Am J Roentgenol*. 1987; 149:35–38.

Montrey JS, Levy JA, Brenner RJ. Wire fragments after needle localization. *AJR Am J Roentgenol*. 1996;167:1267–1269.

Moshyedi AC, Puthawala AH, Kurland RJ, et al. Breast arterial calcifications: association with coronary artery disease. *Radiology*. 1995;194:181–183.

Park KY, Oh KK, Noh TW. Steatocystoma multiplex: mammographic and sonographic manifestations. *AJR Am J Roentgenol*. 2003;180:271–274.

Pollack AH, Kuerer HM. Steatocystoma multiplex: appearance at mammography. *Radiology*. 1991;181:836–838.

Pui MH, Movson IJ. Fatty tissue breast lesions. *Clin Imaging*. 2003;27:150–155.

Ravakhah K, Javadi N, Simms R. Hamartoma of the breast in man: first case report. *Breast J*. 2001;7:266–268.

Scott Soo M, Kornguth PJ, Hertzberg BS. Fat necrosis in the breast: sonographic features. *Radiology*. 1998;206:261–269.

Sickles EA. Breast calcifications: mammographic evaluation. *Radiology*. 1986;160:289–293.

Sickles EA. Breast masses: mammographic evaluation. *Radiology*. 1989;173:297–303.

Sickles EA, Abele JS. Milk of calcium within tiny benign breast cysts. *Radiology*. 1981;141:655.

Sickles EA, Galvin HB. Breast arterial calcification in association with diabetes mellitus: too weak a correlation to have clinical utility. *Radiology*. 1985;155:577–579.

Stigers KB, King JG, Davey DD, Stelling CB. Abnormalities of the breast caused by biopsy: spectrum of mammographic findings. *AJR Am J Roentgenol*. 1991;156:287–291.

Svane G, Franzen S. Radiologic appearance of nonpalpable intramammary lymph nodes. *Acta Radiol*. 1993; 34:577–580.

Takeuchi M, Kashiki Y, Shibuya C, et al. A case of muscular hamartoma of the breast. *Breast Cancer*. 2001;8:243–245.

Tse GM, Law BK, Ma TK, et al. Hamartoma of the breast: a clinicopathological review. *J Clin Pathol*. 2002;55:951–954.

Tse GM, Law BK, Pang LM, Cheung HS. Ductal carcinoma in situ arising in mammary harmartoma. *J Clin Pathol*. 2002;55: 541–542.

Venta LA, Salomon CG, Flisak ME, et al. Sonographic signs of breast implant rupture. *AJR Am J Roentgenol*. 1996;166: 1413–1419.

Wahner-Roedier DL, Sebo TJ, Gisvold JJ. Hamartomas of the breast: clinical, radiologic and pathologic manifestations. *Breast J*. 2001;7:101–105.

Walsh R, Kornguth PJ, Scott Soo M, et al. Axillary lymph nodes: mammographic, pathologic and clinical correlation. *AJR Am J Roentgenol*. 1997;168:33–38.

Chapter 2

Screening

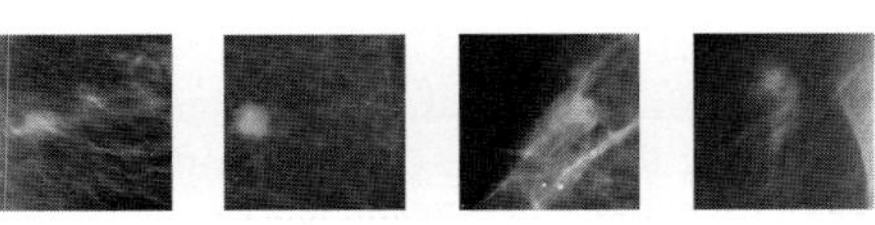

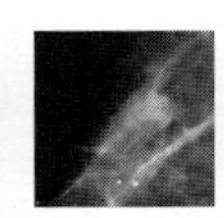
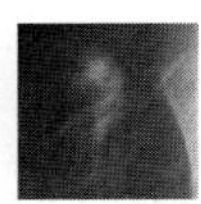

TERMS

Apocrine carcinomas
Artifacts
Axillary nodal metastasis
Batch interpretation
Biopsy changes
Breast cancer statistics
Call-back (recall) rates
Contrast
Craniocaudal views (CC)
Cysts
Diffuse changes
Distortion
Ductal carcinoma in situ (DCIS)
Exaggerated craniocaudal views laterally (XCCL)
Exposure
Fibroadenoma
Focal parenchymal asymmetry
Global parenchymal asymmetry
Invasive ductal carcinoma, not otherwise specified (NOS)
Invasive lobular carcinoma
Isolated tumor cells
Kilovoltage peak (kVp)
Lymphovascular space involvement
Mediolateral oblique views (MLO)
Micrometastasis
Milliamperage output (mAs)
Mondor disease
Ninety-degree lateromedial views (LM)
Ninety-degree mediolateral views (ML)
Poland syndrome
Posterior nipple line (PNL)
Reduction mammoplasty
Quantum mottle
Shrinking breast
Screening guidelines
Screening views
Sharpness
Triangulation

INTRODUCTION

Mammography can demonstrate clinically occult breast cancers. Is this significant? Does this make a difference? Does finding clinically occult cancers affect overall mortality from breast cancer? Yes, yes, and yes. Support for the routine use of screening mammography is provided by results from seven of eight randomized controlled trials in large populations of women, including 40- to 49-year-old women. These studies demonstrated a 20% to 32% reduction in breast cancer mortality among the women invited to undergo screening mammography. Updates from the two-county Swedish trial have reported 20-year survivals of 87.3% and 83.8% among women identified with tumors <0.9 cm and 1.0 to 1.4 cm in size, respectively. The goal of screening mammography (and our job), therefore, is to consistently identify breast cancers that are <1.4 cm (ideally, <0.9 cm). It is noteworthy that the most common method of breast cancer detection is now screening mammography (as opposed to breast self-examination), and that mortality rates from breast cancer continue to drop.

Based on the scientific evidence and expert opinion available, an independent panel of 42 medical and scientific experts developed new breast cancer screening guidelines that were adopted and published by the American Cancer Society (ACS) in 2003. The ACS recommends annual screening mammography starting at age 40 years and continuing for as long as a woman is in good health. Clinical breast exams should be part of a periodic health exam about every 3 years for women in their 20s and 30s and annually for women aged 40 years and older. Women should report any breast change they detect promptly to their health care provider. Beginning in their 20s, women should be told about the benefits and limitations of breast self-examination (BSE). It is acceptable for women to choose not to do BSE or to do it only occasionally. Women known to be at increased risk (e.g., personal or strong family history of breast cancer, a genetic tendency or prior mediastinal radiation therapy for Hodgkin lymphoma) may benefit from earlier initiation of early-detection testing, screening at shorter intervals, and/or the addition of breast ultrasound or magnetic resonance imaging (MRI). Indeed, since 2003, several reports have supported the use of MRI for the detection of small cancers in high-risk women.

It was estimated that 211,240 new cases of breast cancer would occur in 2005 among women in the United States. Among men, 1,690 new breast cancer cases were expected in 2005. The estimated numbers of deaths resulting from breast cancer in 2005 among women and men were 40,410 and 460, respectively. A decline in the mortality rate from breast cancer of 2.3% per year from 1990 to 2000 has been reported among all women, with larger decreases in women under age 50 years. The decline in the mortality rate is attributed to earlier detection and improved treatment.

SCREENING VIEWS

Craniocaudal (CC) and mediolateral oblique (MLO) views are the standard screening views. In addition to routine views, our technologists obtain anterior compression and exaggerated craniocaudal (XCCL) views, as needed, to tailor the screening study to the individual woman.

INTERPRETATION

Compared to online reading, batch interpretation of screening mammograms is cost-effective and efficient. With batch interpretation, the patient leaves the imaging facility after her routine views are done and reviewed by the technologist for technical adequacy. The mammograms are hung on high-luminance, dedicated mammography multiviewers for interpretation by the radiologist at a later time. At our facility, right and left CC and right and left MLO views are hung back to back. The two CC views are placed side by side with the two MLO views. If they are available, films from 2 years before are hung above the current study for comparison. Subtle changes may not be apparent from one year to the next, but may be more easily perceived if a study other than the one from 1 year ago is used for comparison. However, before calling a patient back for a diagnostic study, reviewing the mammogram from the year before is often helpful to make sure the current area of concern was not evaluated last year. Any additional studies done at our center are kept in jackets close to the multiviewer so that they can be reviewed as deemed necessary by the interpreting radiologist.

In evaluating screening mammograms, I recommend developing a viewing strategy that is systematic and is used consistently. I also think it is important to have a proactive and focused mindset when reviewing studies, rather than waiting passively for more subtle findings to become apparent. In other words, send your eyes out looking for potential lesions in specific locations; otherwise you may miss subtle findings or study limitations (e.g., blurring) that may preclude detection of possible abnormalities. Chance favors a prepared mind. Ideal viewing conditions are equally important. All extraneous light should be eliminated so that the only light in the room is coming through the films being reviewed. Paper work and interruptions should be minimized.

Whatever approach you use, it should begin with a review of the films for technical adequacy. Specifically, is positioning acceptable? Has any tissue, and possibly a lesion, been excluded from the films (e.g., do you see tissue at the edge of any of the films)? Is glandular tissue adequately compressed and penetrated (exposed)? Are the films high in contrast? Are there any artifacts that may preclude adequate interpretation? Is there any blurring?

Look for diffuse changes that may be difficult to perceive, particularly if you are focused on detecting smaller potential lesions. Is one breast larger or more dense than the other? Don't assume that the larger breast is the abnormal breast; the smaller breast may be progressively "shrinking." Are the technical factors needed for adequate exposure of one breast significantly different from those used to expose the contralateral side? Is compression limited (e.g., centimeters of compression or decanewtons used)? Is there prominence of the trabecular markings? Do you see trabecular markings superimposed on the pectoral muscles (e.g., reminiscent of "kerley" B lines)? Are there any findings in the axillary regions?

After evaluating the mammogram globally for technical adequacy and diffuse changes, look specifically both with and without a magnification lens for masses, areas of asymmetry, architectural distortion, and calcifications. Narrowing the search is helpful in focusing your review. On CC views, look at the lateral, middle, and medial thirds of the breasts (Fig. 2.1). On MLO views, evaluate the

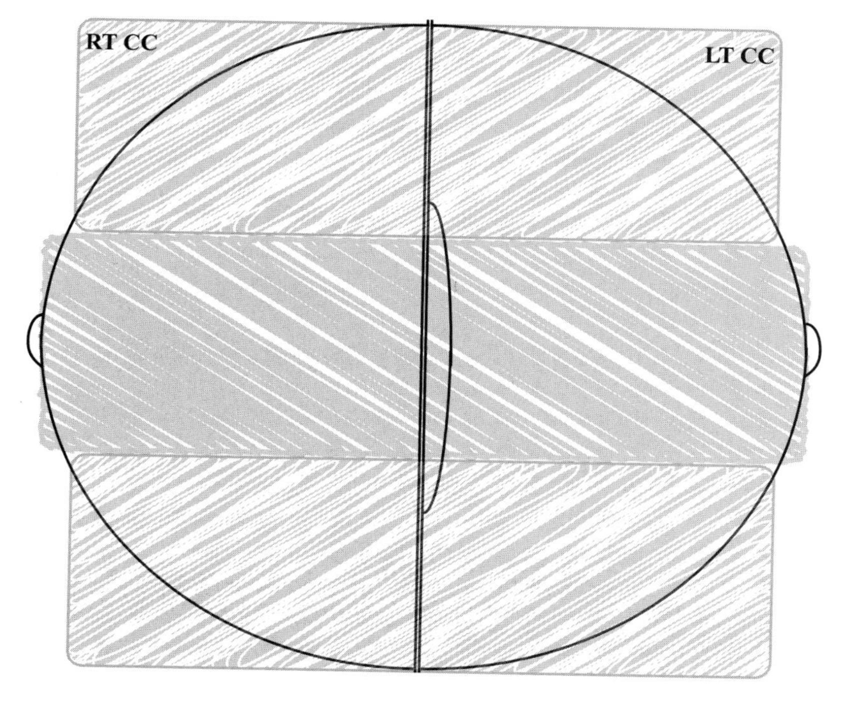

Figure 2.1. Image evaluation. On craniocaudal views, narrow the search for potential lesions by splitting the images in thirds. This will help you to focus attention on smaller amounts of tissue. Go back and forth between the right and left craniocaudal views, looking specifically for asymmetries, possible masses, distortion, or calcifications.

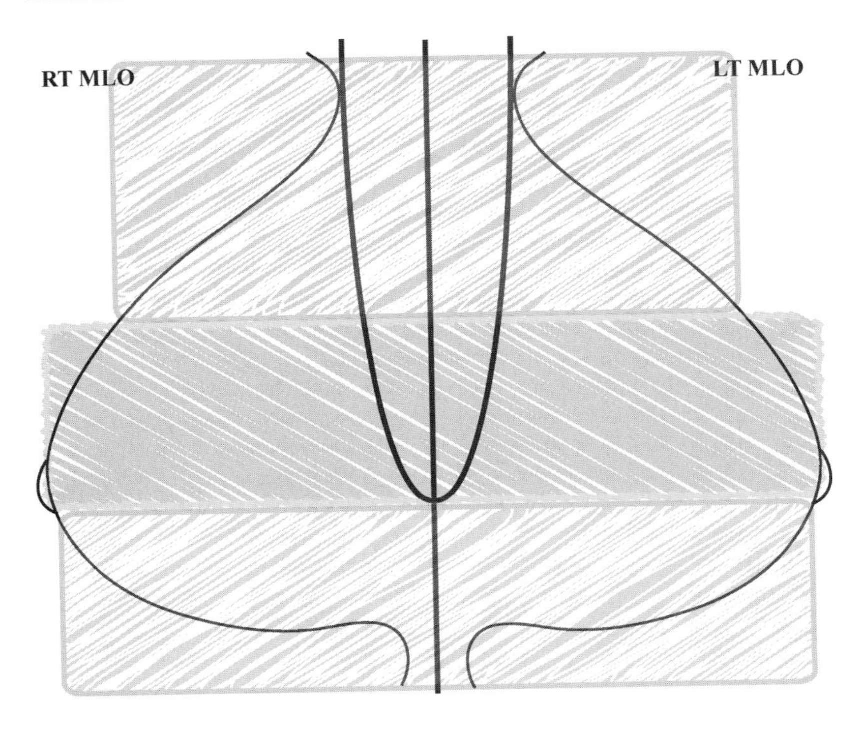

Figure 2.2. Image evaluation. On mediolateral oblique views, narrow the search for potential lesions by splitting the images in thirds. This will help you to focus attention on smaller amounts of tissue. Go back and forth between the right and left mediolateral oblique views, looking specifically for asymmetries, possible masses, distortion, or calcifications.

upper, middle, and lower thirds of the breasts (Fig. 2.2). Search out potentially abnormal areas as you go back and forth between the right and left breasts. Also, evaluate fat–glandular interfaces specifically for straight lines or convex tissue bulges, the fatty stripe of tissue between the pectoral muscle and glandular tissue on MLO views, the superior cone of tissue on MLO views, the subareolar areas, and the medial portions of the breasts on CC views (Fig. 2.3).

After formulating a working hypothesis on a given mammogram, compare it with prior studies and look at the history form for potentially relevant factors (hormone replacement therapy, prior breast surgery, family history of breast cancer, skin lesions etc.). Be careful not to let prior films influence decisions regarding the relevance of a finding on the current study. In some women, it is important to look at several comparison studies. If you perceive an area of spiculation or distortion that cannot be explained by a history of surgery, trauma, or mastitis at that specific site, the patient should be evaluated in spite of apparent stability. *Stability of a lesion does not assure that it is benign.*

Make no assumptions. If you assume something is benign or malignant, it becomes very difficult to think otherwise. Also, if there is an obvious finding, make a conscientious effort to look at the remainder of the mammogram first. Do not focus your attention on obvious findings to the exclusion of other subtle, and potentially more significant, findings.

On screening studies, my goal is to detect potential abnormalities. I make no particular effort to characterize potential or true lesions on screening studies. Over the years it has become apparent to me that sometimes what I think is a significant lesion on the screening mammogram turns out to be insignificant after additional evaluation and what I initially think is almost certainly benign is cancer. Similarly, in some patients, what is seen on the screening studies turns out to represent a more extensive lesion ("the tip of the iceberg"). Why make decisions with insufficient and potentially misleading information? Why work with low confidence? Additional evaluation increases certainty in making appropriate recommendations and narrows differential considerations to one or two options. Recommendations are more easily justified following complete and thorough evaluations. With the confidence generated by the additional evaluation, succinct, definitive, and directive reports can be generated.

MANAGEMENT OF PATIENTS NEEDING ADDITIONAL EVALUATION

For women with an obvious lesion on the screening study, additional evaluation helps characterize the extent of the lesion and sometimes establishes the presence of other, initially unsuspected, lesions. It provides an opportunity to communicate directly with the patient and undertake imaging-guided biopsies at the time of call-back. In essence, we expedite patient care. Consequently, the only BI-RADS® assessment categories I use on screening studies are category 1 (negative), category 2 (benign finding), and category 0 (needs additional imaging evaluation or needs prior mammograms for comparison).

Category 0 is used when additional studies are indicated or when prior studies are to be requested and comparison is needed to make a final assessment. For those women in whom a potential abnormality is detected, we categorize the call-back as level 1, 2, or 3. These levels are used internally to indicate the amount of time that should be allotted for the patient's diagnostic appointment. Fifteen, thirty, and sixty minutes are allowed for level 1, 2, and 3 call-backs, respectively. In general, level 1 designates those patients for whom physical examination, additional mammographic images, or an ultrasound are all that should be needed to resolve the question. If the interpreting radiologist expects that a patient will need additional mammographic images and an ultrasound, the call-back is designated as level 2. When the radiologist expects that the patient will need a biopsy, level 3 is used so that an adequate amount of time is

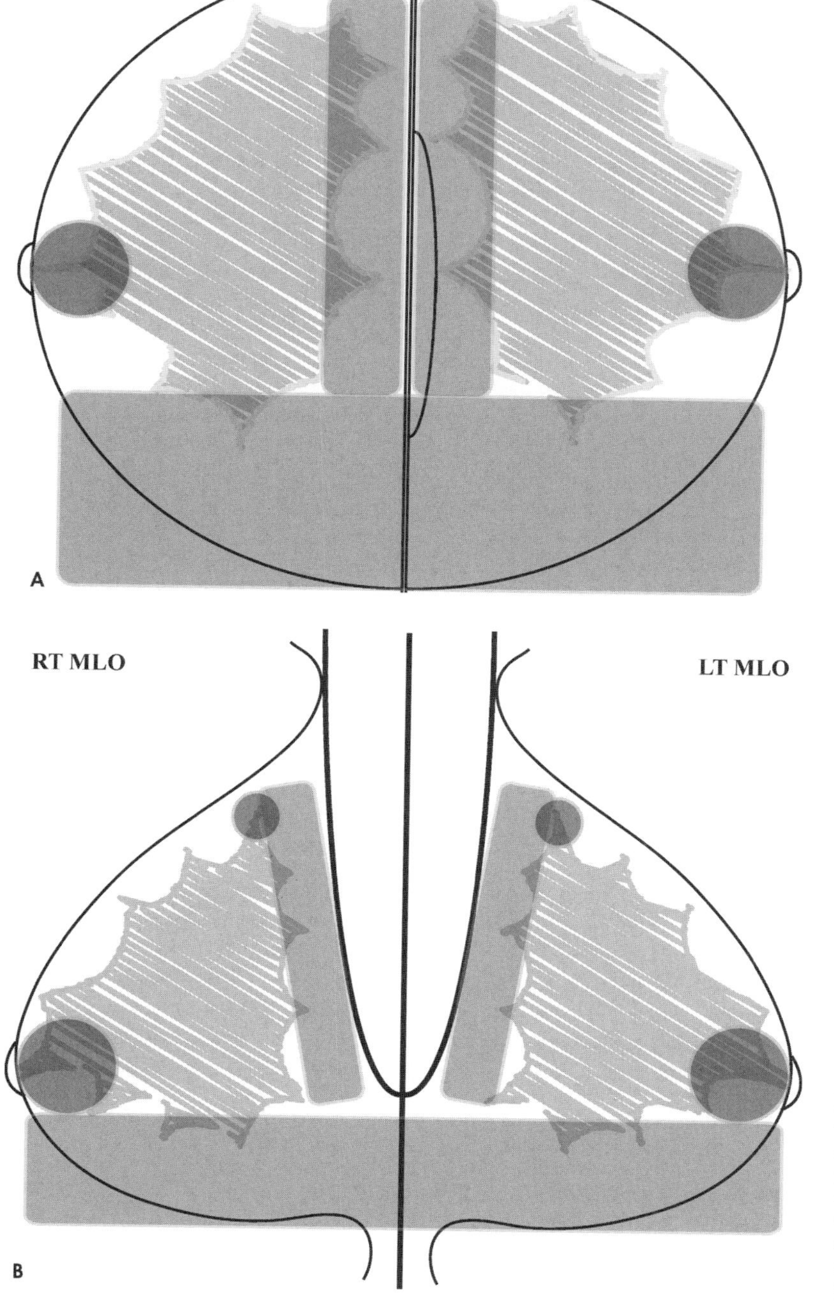

Figure 2.3. Image evaluation. **A:** On the craniocaudal views, evaluate areas where breast cancers are likely to develop—specifically, the medial quadrants, subareolar areas, fat–glandular interfaces, and the retroglandular areas posteriorly. **B:** On the mediolateral oblique views, evaluate areas where breast cancers are likely to develop—specifically, the fatty stripe of tissue between the pectoral muscle and glandular tissue, the superior cone of tissue, subareolar areas, and the inferior aspects of the breasts.

available to do a biopsy when the patient returns for additional evaluation. Although this is an arbitrary classification, characterized by times when, after completing the evaluation, a level 1 call-back patient requires a biopsy and a level 3 call-back patient does not, the system works well. It provides for more efficient use of the schedule and allows us to complete evaluations in one visit. It has enabled us to optimize patient care in a practical and cost-effective manner.

At the time of the screening study, the technologist informs the patient about the possibility of a call-back for further evaluation. In addition, each woman is given a written statement that describes the process for reviewing her mammogram, issuing a report to her doctor, sending her a letter with results, and the possibility of being called back for a diagnostic evaluation. *It is important for women to be informed of the process and to know that being called back does not necessarily mean they have cancer.* Our goal is to minimize some of the anxiety experienced by patients when they are called back for additional evaluation. It does not always work, but it does help some women.

All women who require additional evaluation are contacted directly by a member of our staff. By communicating with the patient directly, we can explain the reason for the call-back more appropriately than others might (e.g., as opposed to having a referring physician's office tell the patient that the first images taken were no good), and we reassure the patient regarding the need for additional studies. This method also expedites patient care by decreasing the amount of time needed to schedule the diagnostic evaluation. If we are unable to contact the woman by phone within 48 hours following her screening study, we send a letter via regular mail asking her to call us. If after a week from mailing the letter we still have not heard from the patient, a certified letter is mailed to her with a copy to the referring physician. All efforts to communicate with the patient are documented in her chart.

A report is generated for all studies in which a prior mammogram is requested and comparison is needed to make a final assessment. These reports are assigned to a category "0"; we do not keep undictated studies aside pending arrival of comparison films. By generating a report, the referring physician is informed that we are working on obtaining prior studies and a system to track the patient is set in motion that minimizes the likelihood of a patient "falling through the cracks." We allow a 2-week interval during which we make every effort to locate prior studies; this includes calling the facility indicated by the patient on her history form. If this action is unsuccessful, we contact the referring physician and request prior mammogram reports that will indicate the name of the facility and the date of the prior study. Lastly, we sometimes call the patient to verify the information she provided. If we are unable to obtain prior films after 2 weeks, an addendum to the initial report is issued and we dictate the findings as though there were no prior studies. Every effort we make to procure prior studies is documented in the patient's file.

CALL-BACK RATES

What is an appropriate call-back (recall) rate? This is an important question to consider and is something radiologists involved in screening mammography should monitor routinely. Calling a patient back for diagnostic evaluation is not innocuous and should never be trivialized. In some women, it is associated with significant morbidity that at times is (unfortunately) grossly underestimated. Regardless of how much you try to prepare a woman for the possibility of a call-back, it is guaranteed to provoke anxiety and stress in most women. High recall rates are also associated with increased costs and decreased efficiency of screening programs. Counter this with our goal of never missing an opportunity to diagnose an early breast cancer. Undoubtedly, to call back or not is a fine line that needs to be considered carefully. Depending on the availability of prior films, you can expect call-back rates to be higher among women with no prior studies compared to those women in whom prior films are available. In considering the call-back rate for individual radiologists, I think it is important not to consider this a static figure but rather a work in progress. Early in the career of a radiologist one should expect and accept higher call-back rates. However, the rate should decrease progressively with the number of screening mammograms evaluated over time. Although it is inconvenient and not usually easy to schedule, the ideal learning situation is for the radiologist recommending the call-back to be the one involved in the diagnostic workup. Under these circumstances, meaningful call-back rates can be generated and improvement shown over the years. It is also important to recognize that most call-backs for diagnostic evaluations do not lead to biopsies. Based on published reports, the American College of Radiology recommends that call-backs be maintained at a rate of 10% or less.

CONCLUSION

In this chapter, the screening mammogram is the starting point for all patients discussed. Focus your attention initially on systematically reviewing the images as described above. Determine if the mammogram is normal or potentially abnormal. Some differentials are included, and pathology results are provided for those patients for whom biopsy is appropriate. I also need to state the obvious at the onset of this chapter: What I present is an artificial situation. For didactic purposes, I have presented a significant number of patients with breast cancer in this chapter; in a true screening program, most of the mammograms you review are normal.

PATIENT 1

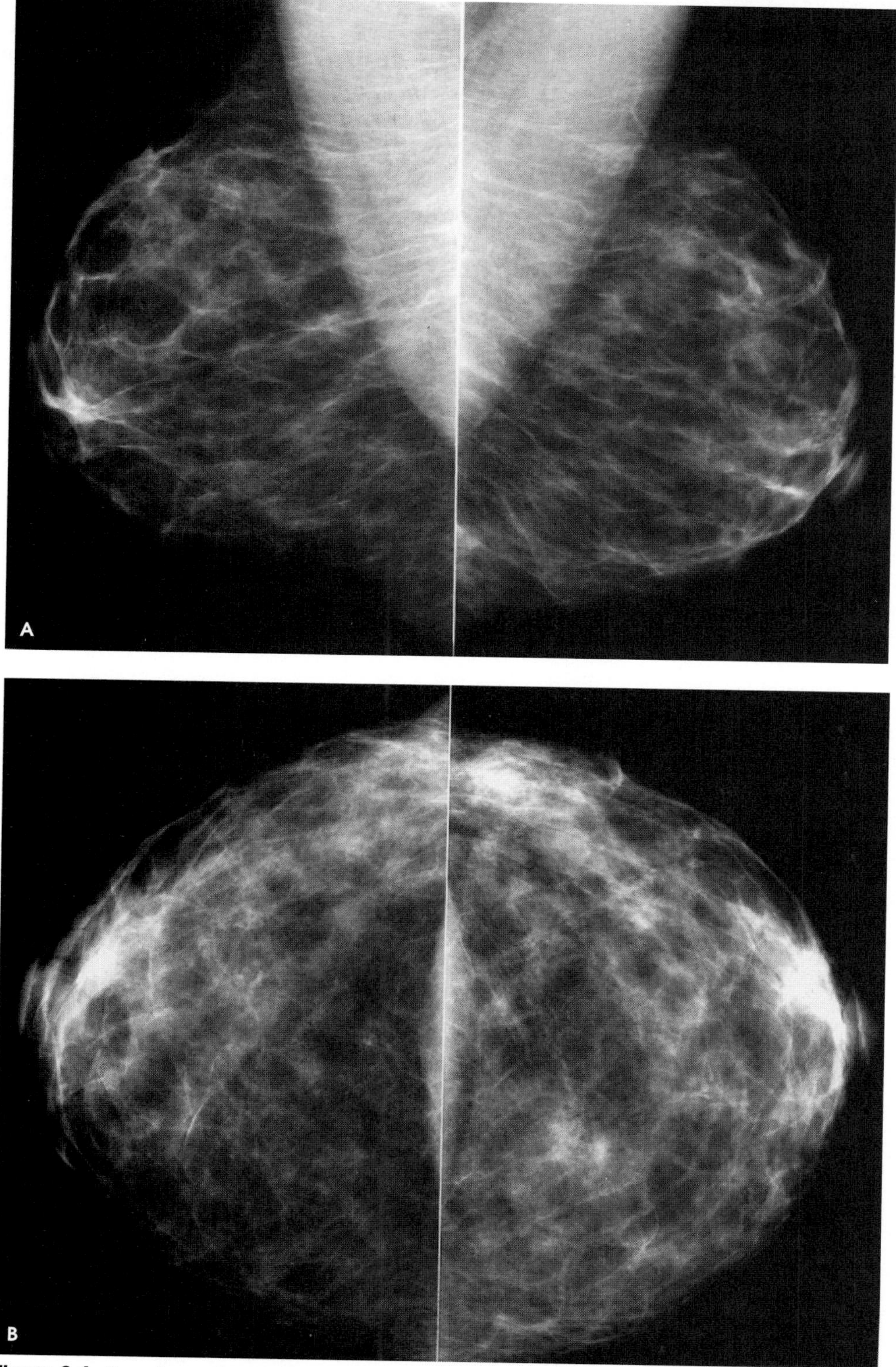

Figure 2.4. Screening studies. Mediolateral oblique **(A)** and craniocaudal **(B)** views.

In assessing images for technical adequacy, what factors should you evaluate?

The technical factors you should evaluate before focusing on potential abnormalities include positioning, compression, exposure, contrast, sharpness, noise, artifacts, and film labeling. *As an interpreting radiologist, you are the gatekeeper for image quality and overall patient care at your facility.* If you are willing to routinely interpret suboptimal studies without a good explanation that is well documented (a patient with Parkinson's disease, a frozen shoulder, history of stroke, etc.), you are basically willing to accept a potential delay in the diagnosis of breast cancer. The overall quality bar at your facility will be as high as you set it.

In evaluating positioning on mediolateral oblique (MLO) views, the pectoral muscles should be wide in the axillary regions, extend to the level of the nipples, and have convex margins anteriorly. The breast needs to be lifted (e.g., not sagging or drooping) so that the inframammary fold is open and a small amount of upper abdomen is included on the image (Fig. 2.4A). As the technologist positions the breast, she needs to establish the angle of obliquity of the patient's pectoral muscle; it is easier to mobilize tissue maximally away from the body if it is pulled parallel to underlying muscle fibers. Using the appropriate angle for the patient and having the patient lean in slightly to relax the muscle, the technologist needs to mobilize the breast and muscle medially as much as possible and maintain the medial mobilization of the breast as compression is applied and the breast is lifted up and pulled out. If an incorrect angle of obliquity is selected, the breast is not mobilized as much as possible medially, or if the patient moves out of the unit as compression is applied, the pectoral muscle may not be thick at the axilla, extend to the level of the nipple, or it may have a concave margin, a triangular shape, or be parallel to the edge of the film (Fig. 2.4C).

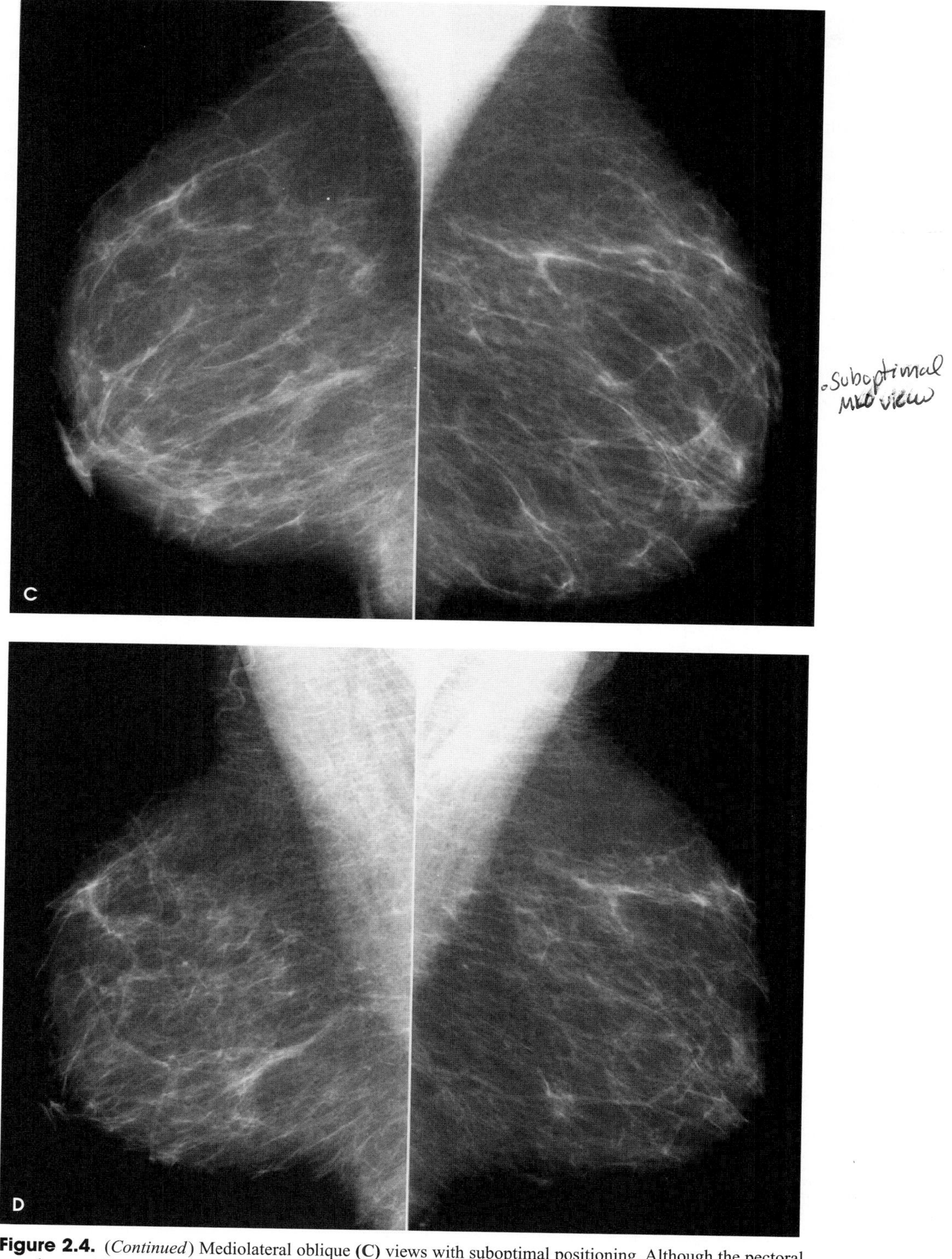

Figure 2.4. (*Continued*) Mediolateral oblique **(C)** views with suboptimal positioning. Although the pectoral muscles are thick at the axilla, the anterior margins are not convex and they do not extend to the level of the nipple. The shape of the muscles is triangular. Repeat mediolateral oblique **(D)** views, using optimal technique, show thick pectoral muscles at the axilla with convex anterior margins extending to the level of the nipples.

Positioning

In positioning patients for craniocaudal views, the technologist needs to identify the inframammary fold and lift the breast as much as the natural mobility of the breast permits. Next she needs to pull the breast tissue out and actively tug on the lateral aspect of the breast so as to include as much posterolateral tissue as possible. On craniocaudal (CC) views, you should expect to see pectoral muscle in 30% to 40% of patients. When you see pectoral muscles on the CC views, you can be assured that posterior tissue has been included on the images (Fig. 2.4B). If pectoral muscle is not seen on the CC view, look for cleavage as an indication that medial tissue has not been excluded from the image. If no pectoral muscle or cleavage is seen, measure the posterior nipple line (PNL) on the MLO view and compare it with the measurement on the CC view (Fig. 2.4E, F). The measurements should be within 1 cm of each other. Also, evaluate the lateral aspect of the images. If there is tissue extending to the edge of the film, the technologist did not pull lateral tissue in, or an exaggerated craniocaudal view laterally (XCCL) may need to be done to evaluate the patient adequately in the craniocaudal projection.

① pect. mm
② cleavage
③ PNL

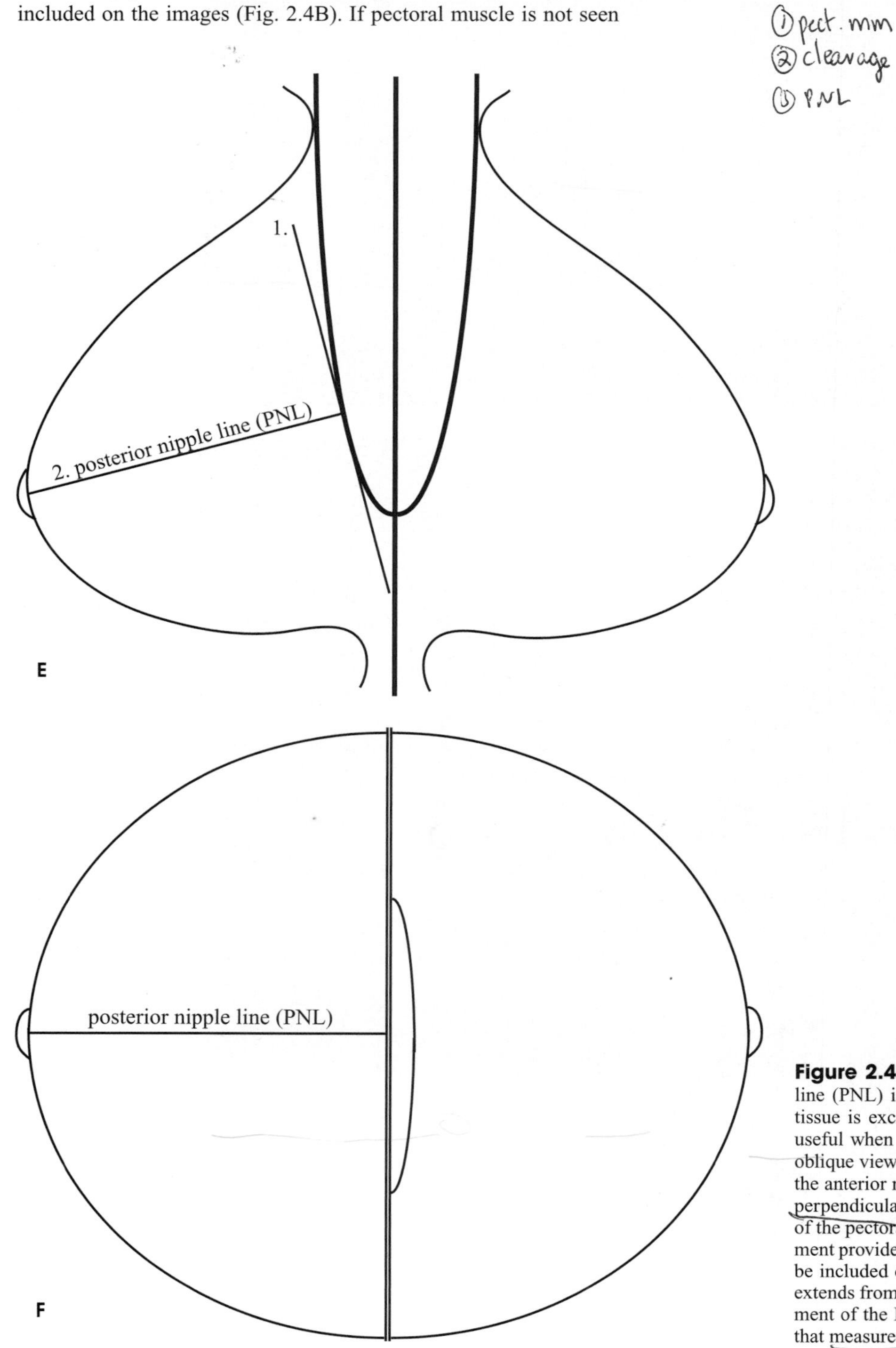

Figure 2.4. Posterior nipple line. **E:** The posterior nipple line (PNL) is measured when it is suspected that posterior tissue is excluded on a craniocaudal (CC) view. It is most useful when positioning on the corresponding mediolateral oblique view is optimal. A line (1) can be drawn to delineate the anterior margin of the pectoral muscle. The PNL (2) is a perpendicular line drawn from the nipple to the anterior edge of the pectoral muscle. The PNL is measured. This measurement provides an estimate of the amount of tissue that should be included on the CC views. **F:** On the CC view, the PNL extends from the nipple to the edge of the film. The measurement of the PNL on the CC view should be within 1 cm of that measured on the MLO view.

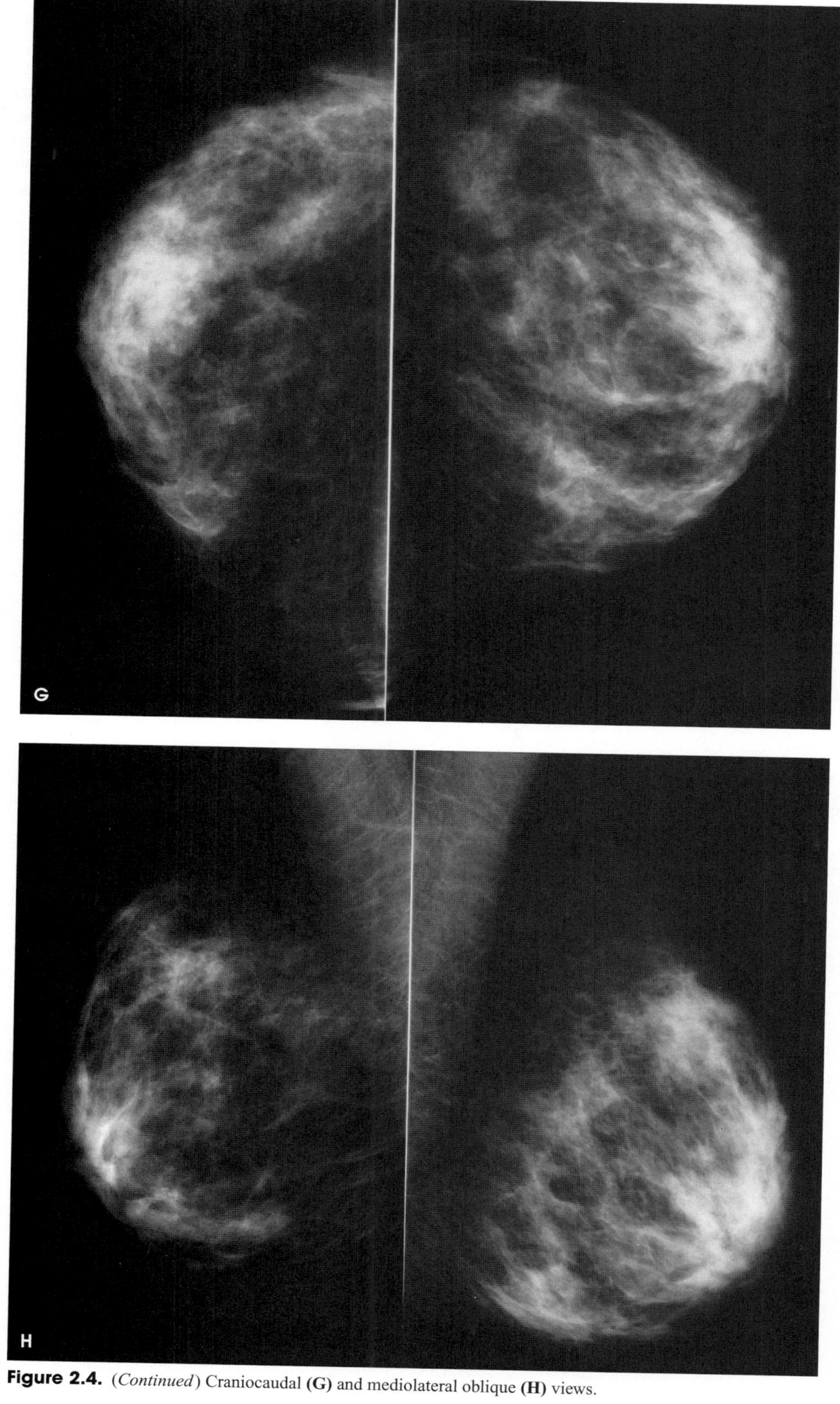

Figure 2.4. (*Continued*) Craniocaudal **(G)** and mediolateral oblique **(H)** views.

What are your observations concerning the positioning on this patient's mammogram?

Retroglandular fat is seen laterally on the left craniocaudal view. Tissue is seen extending to the edge of the film on the right craniocaudal view, and although the right breast is smaller than the left, is there an adequate amount of posterior tissue on the right craniocaudal view? How can you determine this? Measuring the PNL is helpful in assessing if the amount of tissue imaged on the craniocaudal view is adequate (Fig. 2.4I, J). In this patient, the PNL measurement on the right MLO view is 10 cm, compared to 7.2 cm on the right CC view. A significant amount of posterior tissue is excluded from the right CC view and therefore it needs to be repeated. Focusing on technique, a repeat CC view (Fig. 2.4K) is obtained and demonstrates a significantly greater amount of tissue. There is now fat at the edge of the film and the PNL measurement on this second CC view (Fig. 2.4L) is 10 cm, which is equal to what is measured on the MLO view. If images that are missing 2.8 cm of posterior tissue (as on the original right CC view in this patient) are accepted and interpreted, our goal of finding cancers that are less than 1 cm in size is compromised significantly.

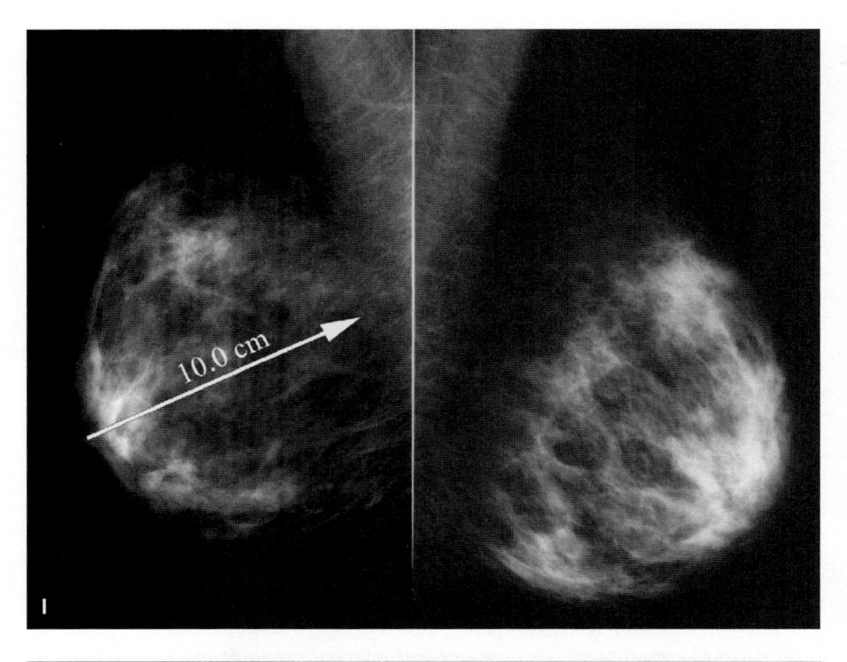

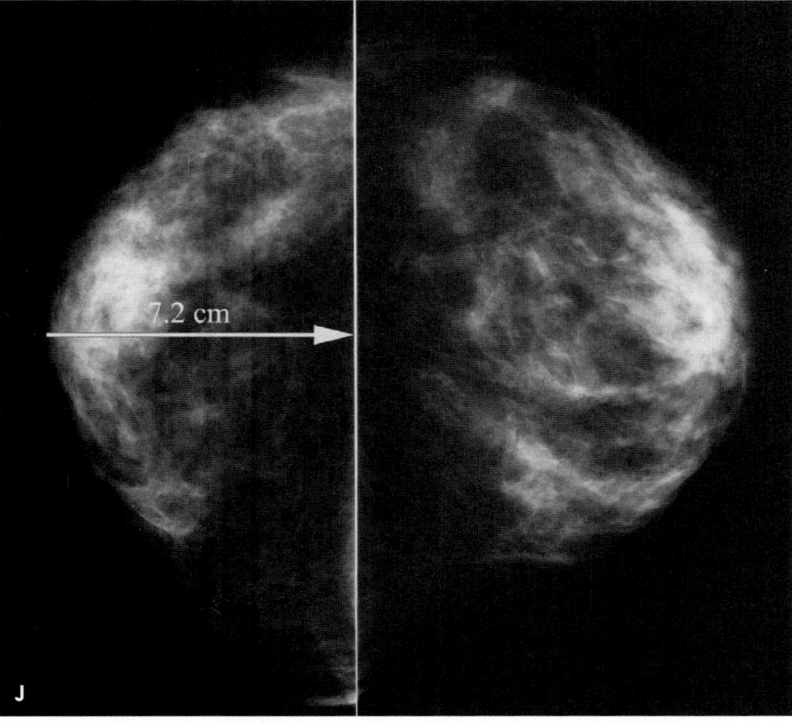

Figure 2.4. *(Continued)* Mediolateral oblique **(I)** and craniocaudal **(J)** views showing the posterior nipple line measurements. An inadequate amount of tissue is included on the right craniocaudal view.

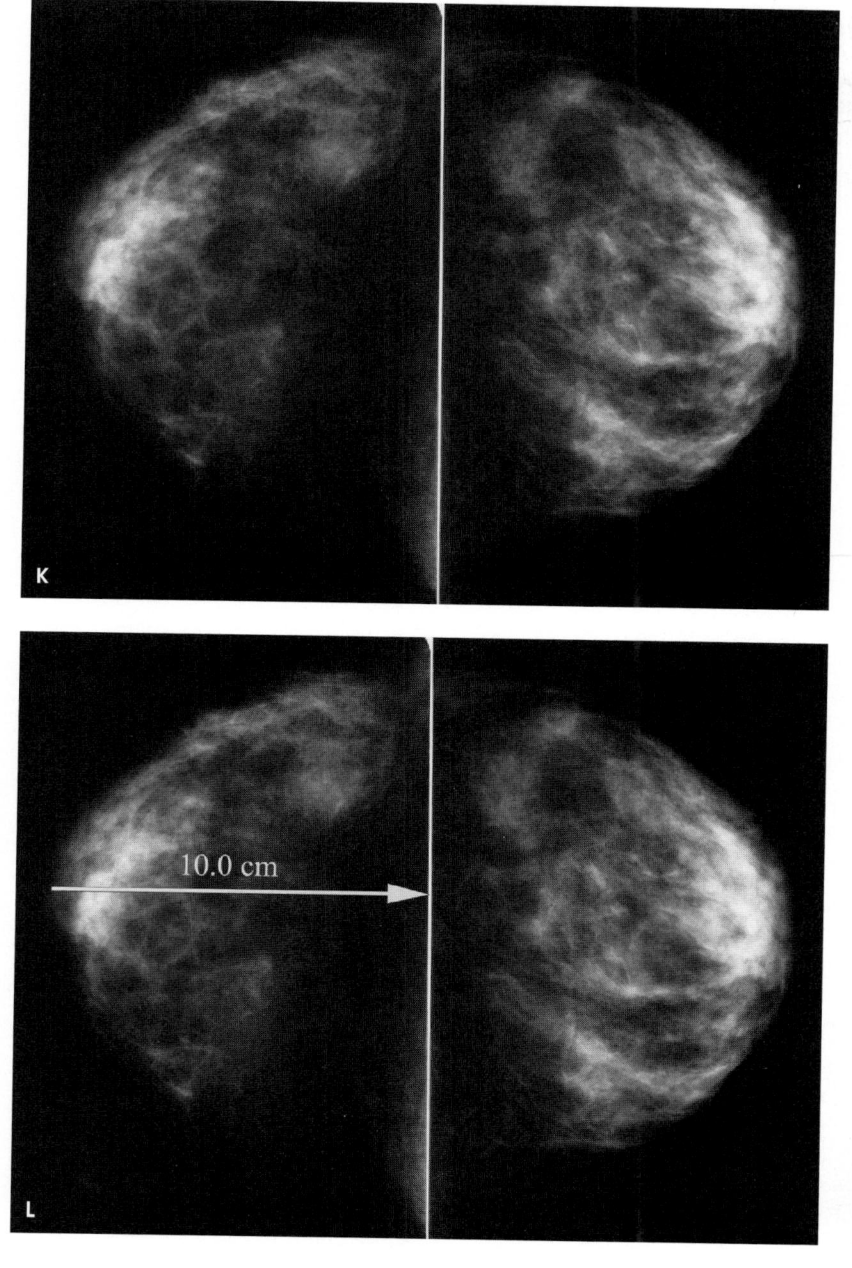

Figure 2.4. (*Continued*) Repeat right craniocaudal **(K)** view. Fat is now seen at the edge of the film. Repeat right craniocaudal **(L)** view with the posterior nipple line measuring 10 cm, which is comparable to that measured on the original mediolateral oblique view.

In addition to positioning, compression needs to be assessed by specifically evaluating the images for uneven or inadequate exposure, motion blur, and poor separation of parenchymal densities.

Additional Technical Factors to Assess

Glandular tissue needs to be adequately exposed so that there is visualization of trabecula, small tubular structures, and vessels. In many women, adequate penetration of the glandular tissue overexposes the skin and subcutaneous tissue. Image contrast is also important. Ideally, contrast is maximized so that subtle density differences in glandular tissue can be appreciated. Subcutaneous and retroglandular fat is dark gray or nearly black in high-contrast images. Poor-contrast images are characterized by dull gray retroglandular and subcutaneous fat, and the skin is readily apparent.

Sharpness needs to be evaluated by looking specifically for blurring (i.e., unsharpness). The most common cause of blur is patient motion. This is why adequate breast compression is critical. Short exposures (ideally, <2 s) are also helpful in minimizing motion blur. Motion blur does not always involve the entire image. It can be localized to one area on the mammogram, where it is commonly caused by lack of uniformity in breast compression. Poor film screen contact can also be a cause of localized unsharpness. Sharpness is also affected by focal spot size, object-to-image distance, and source-to-image distance. Increases in focal spot size and object-to-image distance as well as decreases in source-to-image distance contribute to geometric unsharpness.

The ability to detect small structures such as calcifications is decreased by noise (e.g., radiographic mottle). Quantum mottle is the major cause of noise in mammography. Noise can be identified on an image by a background density that is not homogeneous and results in loss of sharpness and visualization of low-contrast structures.

Artifacts can result from x-ray equipment (filter, compression paddle, image receptor holder, grid, etc.), patient factors (deodorant, hair, jewelry, tattoos, etc.), and cassette, film, and screen factors (upside-down cassette in bucky, film scratches, dents, fingerprints, pick-off, moisture, incorrect film loading so that the emulsion side is away from the screen, fog, static, foreign objects on the screen, etc.). Ideally, most images are artifact free. Depending on the overall effect on image quality, films with artifacts may need to be repeated.

With respect to film labeling, the following information is required on all films: patient name, unique patient identification number, date of study, radiopaque laterality and projection markers placed closest to the axilla, facility name, facility location (city, state, and Zip code), technologist identification, cassette/screen identification number, and mammography unit identification number if there is more than one unit in the facility.

PATIENT 2

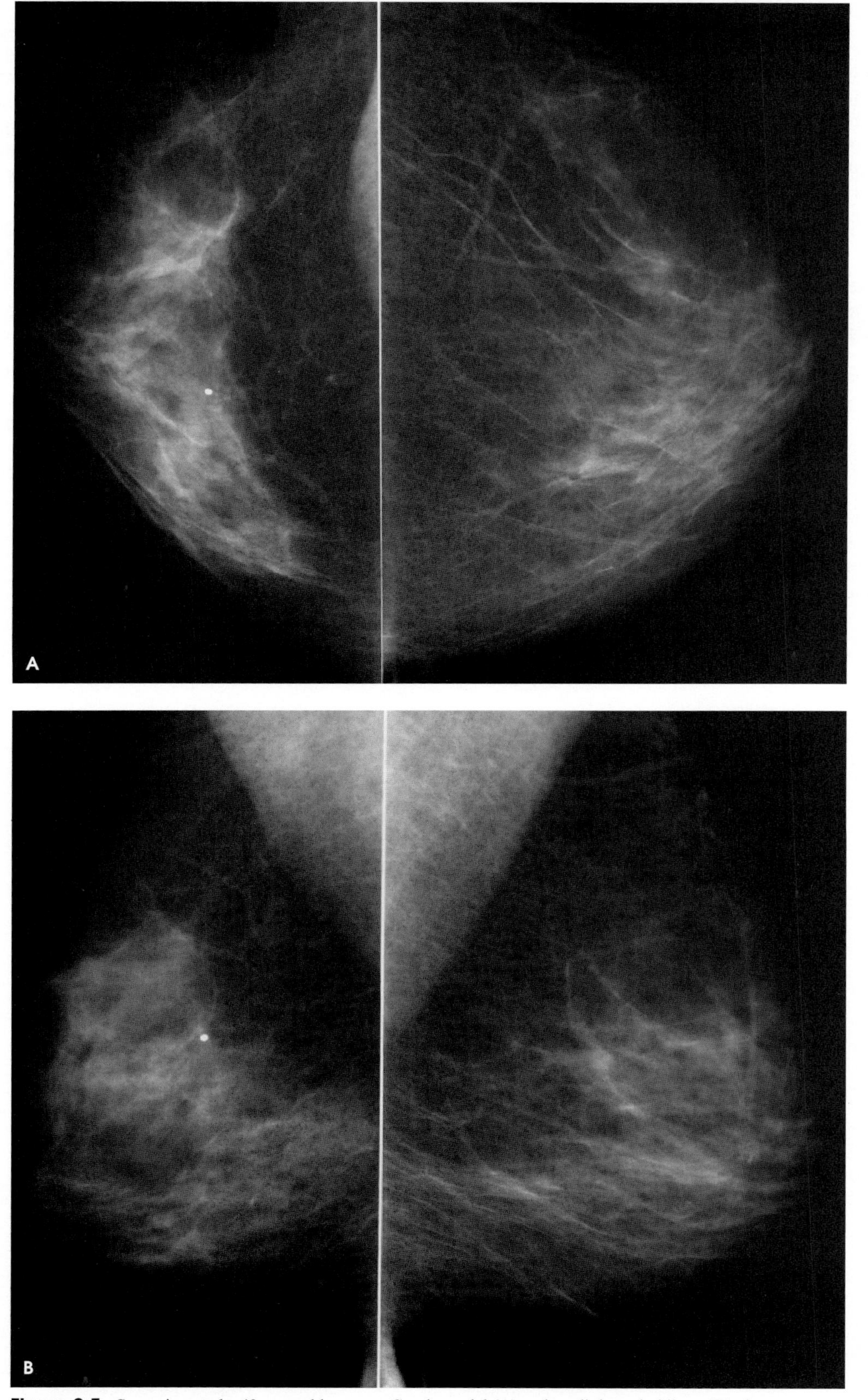

Figure 2.5. Screening study, 43-year-old woman. Craniocaudal **(A)** and mediolateral oblique **(B)** views.

How would you describe the findings on this mammogram?

Compared to the left breast, the right breast is smaller, with dense, asymmetrically distributed tissue (i.e., global parenchymal asymmetry). Although breast size and tissue are commonly symmetric, asymmetries in breast size and tissue distribution can be seen in numerous women as a normal variant. No mass or distortion is noted in the area of increased tissue on the right. The tissue in the right breast is scalloped and contains areas of fatty lobulation. A solitary dense dystrophic calcification is present in the right breast.

What two pieces of information are critical in this patient?

In this woman, it is important to determine that there is no palpable abnormality in the right breast and that the asymmetry in size (either a decrease in size on the right or an increase in size on the left) is not a new or developing change. If they are available, comparison with multiple prior studies is critical, as is a history of prior right breast surgery or trauma. If there is any question about a corresponding palpable abnormality or a progressive change in breast size, the patient can be asked to return for correlative physical examination and, if needed, additional mammographic views, ultrasound, or, occasionally, magnetic resonance imaging. When they are abnormal, asymmetric changes may be the result of chest wall trauma (e.g., burns), congenital abnormalities (e.g., Poland syndrome), or surgery. Invasive ductal carcinomas can present with global areas of parenchymal asymmetry, but these are usually clinically apparent and readily palpable. Invasive lobular carcinoma can also present with global areas of parenchymal asymmetry and progressive changes in breast size (either increases or decreases); palpable findings may be present, but they are often more subtle in patients with invasive lobular carcinomas. Rarely, lymphoma can present with diffuse, asymmetric involvement of one breast.

What do you think about the amount of posterior tissue imaged on the right craniocaudal view?
What BI-RADS® category would you assign?
Are you sure?

Pectoral muscle and retroglandular fat are imaged on the right craniocaudal view and there is no tissue extending to the edge of the film, so it is unlikely that posterior tissue has been excluded from the image.

No change is noted in comparing with multiple prior studies (not shown).

This is categorized as BI-RADS® category 1: negative. BI-RADS® category 2: benign finding can be used if the observations are described in the report. Annual screening mammography is recommended.

PATIENT 3

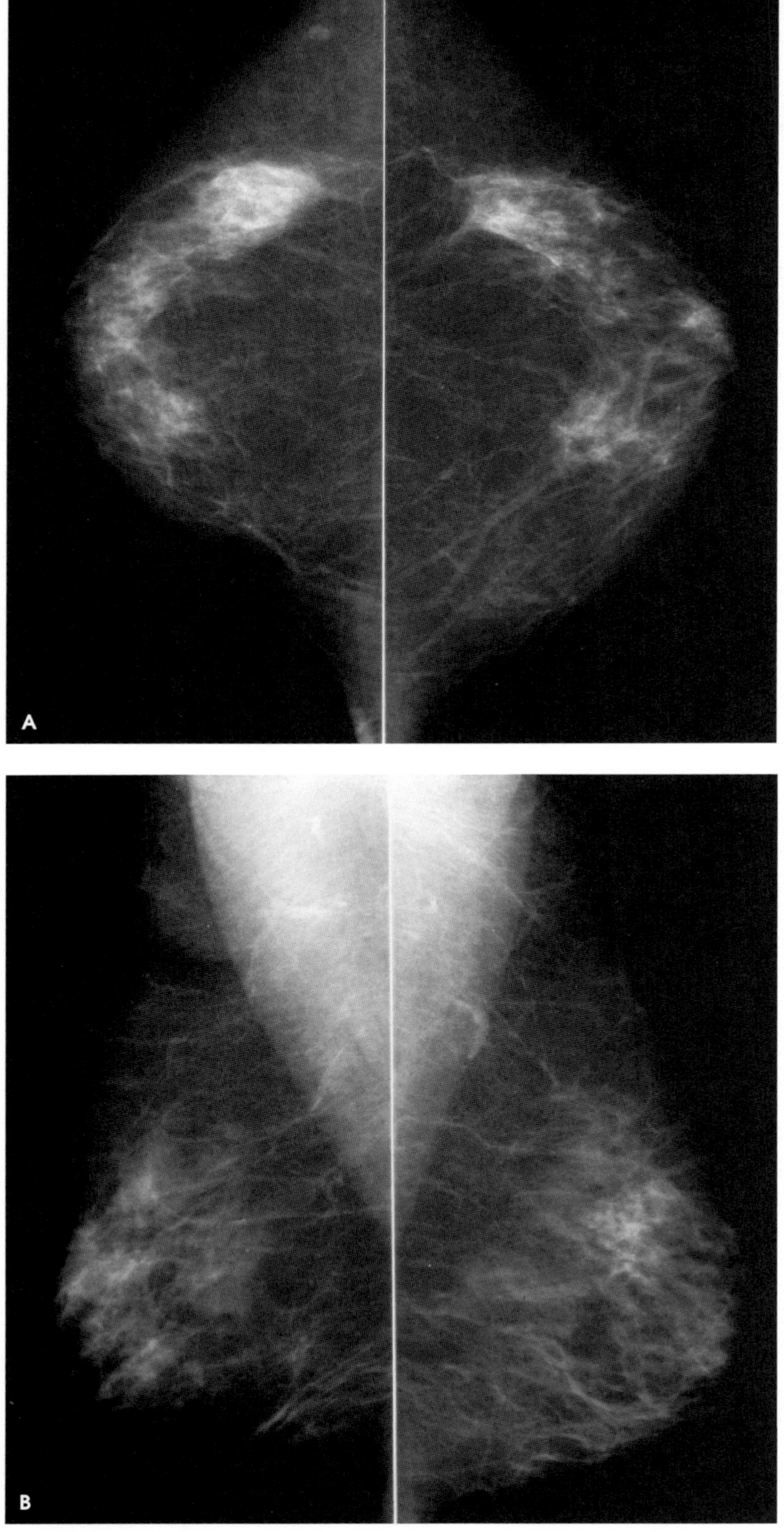

Figure 2.6. Screening study, 81-year-old woman. Craniocaudal **(A)** and mediolateral oblique **(B)** views.

What do you think of the positioning on the craniocaudal (CC) views?
What BI-RADS® category would you assign, and what is your recommendation?

Patient positioning in this study is acceptable. Although no pectoral muscle is seen on the craniocaudal views, cleavage is seen medially and there is retroglandular fat bilaterally (i.e., no tissue is seen at the edge of the films). A lymph node is noted superimposed on the left pectoral muscle, and one is seen laterally on the right craniocaudal view.

What do you think of the rounded area of asymmetric tissue laterally in the right breast?

Do you see a potential abnormality of comparable size, shape, and density when you evaluate the mediolateral oblique (MLO) view? Based on the location of this area on the CC view, look specifically at where you would expect to find the corresponding area on the MLO view. Using the distance of this area from the nipple on the CC view (Fig. 2.6C), generate an arc on the MLO view (Fig. 2.6D) to help you approximate the expected location of this area on the MLO view.

With the exception of some invasive lobular carcinomas, most breast cancers are three-dimensional structures with comparably sized and shaped abnormalities on any view of the breast. In this woman, there is no comparable area in size, shape, or density on the MLO view. For potential lesions >1 cm in size noted on one view, a comparable abnormality should be identified on the other projection at approximately the same distance from the nipple.

BI-RADS® category1: negative. Annual screening mammography is recommended.

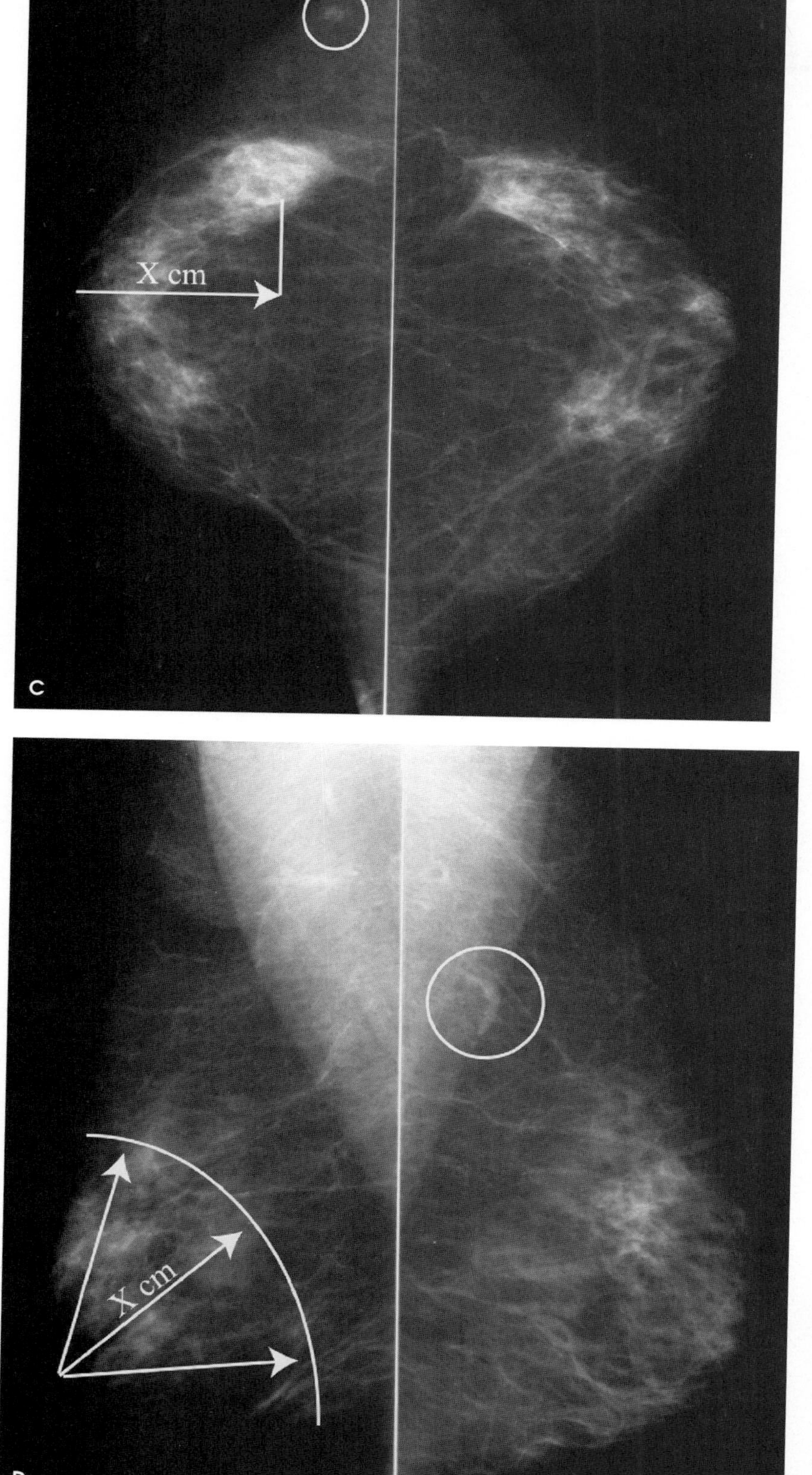

Figure 2.6. (*Continued*) Craniocaudal **(C)** and mediolateral oblique **(D)** views. The distance to the possible lesion is measured from the nipple as "X" cm on the craniocaudal (CC) view. As "X" cm is measured back from the nipple on the mediolateral oblique (MLO) view, an arc can be created that describes the approximate location for the possible lesion noted in the right CC view. No comparably sized area is identified in the MLO view. Intramammary lymph nodes described above are within the circles on the images.

PATIENT 4

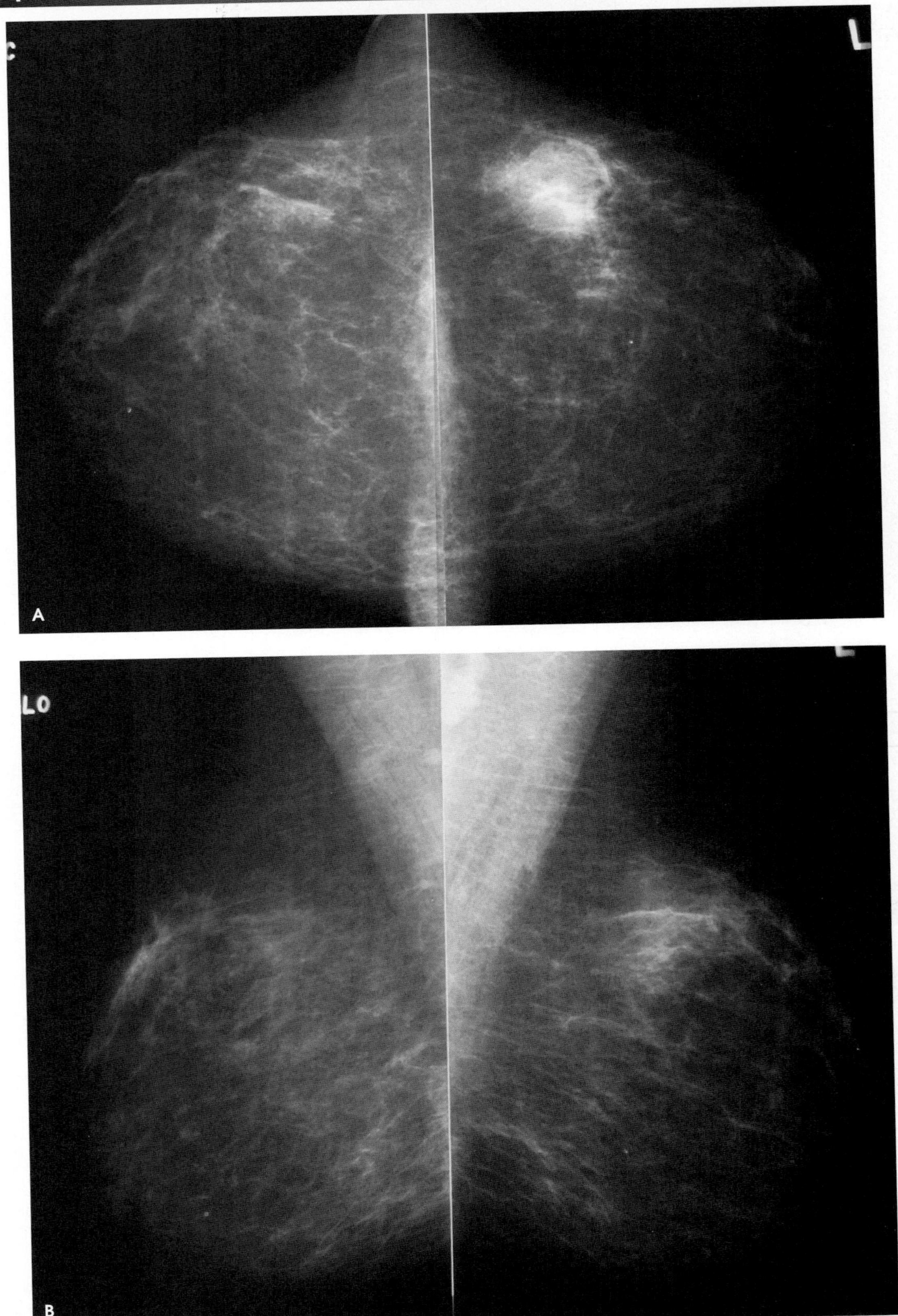

Figure 2.7. Screening study, 45-year-old woman. Craniocaudal **(A)** and mediolateral oblique **(B)** views.

What do you think?
What BI-RADS® category would you assign, and what is your recommendation?

A rounded, asymmetric island of tissue is noted laterally in the left breast. However, in evaluating the mediolateral oblique view, no comparably sized or shaped area is identified that would correspond to the approximate location of this area on the craniocaudal view. Relatively low-density tissue is seen superiorly, characterized by scalloping, interposed fat, and a gradual transition in density. As illustrated here, asymmetric tissue is often planar (i.e., best seen in one projection and changes significantly in appearance on other views), scalloped, heterogeneous in density because of interspersed fat, and characterized by a gradual change in density at the margins. Masses are three-dimensional, with an abrupt change in density and a bulging (convex) margin. True lesions, particularly when >1 cm, are of comparable size, shape and density on the two standard projections and are at approximately the same distance from the nipple on the two views.

BI-RADS® category 1: negative. Annual screening mammography is recommended.

PATIENT 5

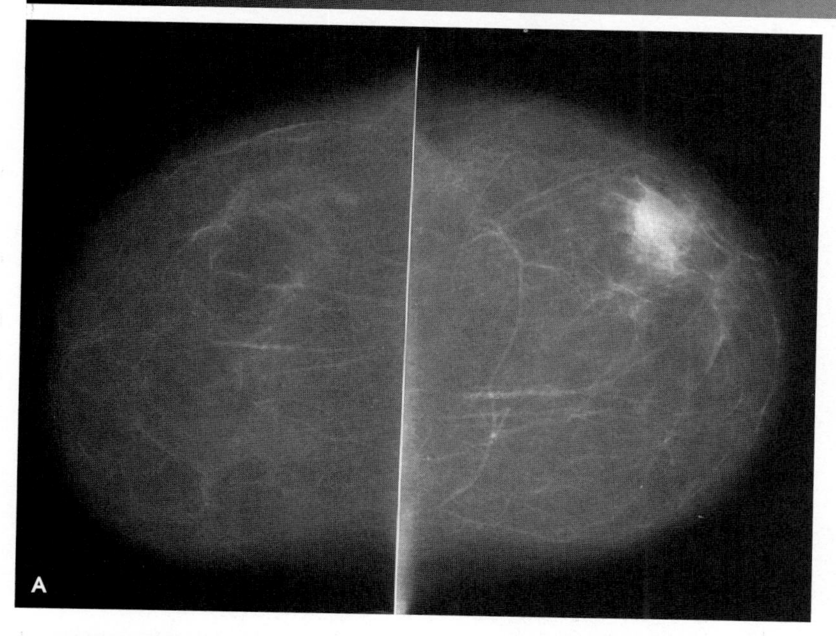

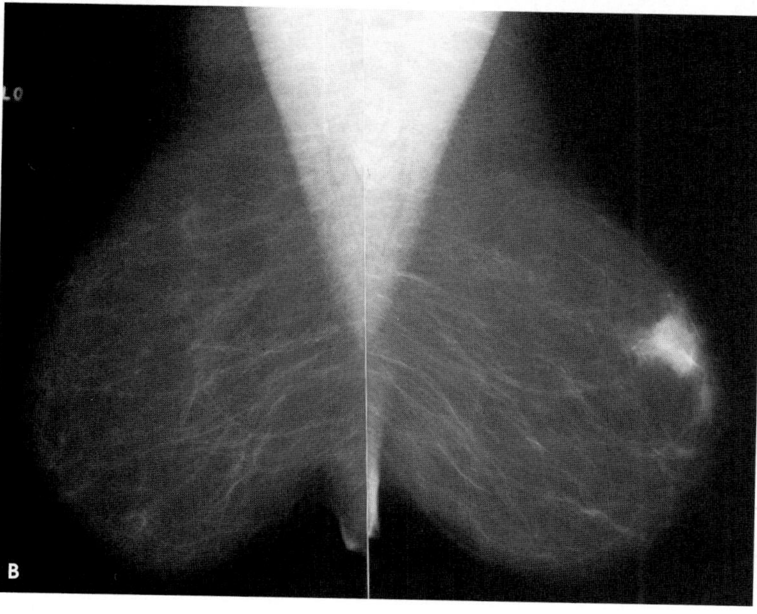

Figure 2.8. Initial screening study, 41-year-old woman. Craniocaudal **(A)** and mediolateral oblique **(B)** views.

What do you think?
What BI-RADS® category would you assign, and what is your recommendation?

A focal area of parenchymal asymmetry is present in the upper outer quadrant of the left breast. It is of comparable size and density and is at the same approximate distance from the nipple on the two projections. Differential considerations include normal variant, hormone replacement therapy effect, asymmetry secondary to prior surgical excision of the corresponding tissue in the right breast, focal fibrosis, pseudoangiomatous stromal hyperplasia (PASH), posttraumatic changes (evolving hematoma, fat necrosis), mastitis, fibroadenolipoma (hamartoma), invasive ductal carcinoma not otherwise specified, invasive lobular carcinoma, and lymphoma.

If, as in this woman, no prior studies are available for comparison, spot compression views and possibly ultrasound with correlative physical examination can be undertaken to exclude an underlying malignancy.

BI-RADS® category 0: need additional imaging evaluation.

What do you think of this predominantly fatty pattern in a 41-year-old woman?

Although it is routinely suggested that mammography in young women is not very good because dense tissue precludes the detection of breast cancer, it is clear that age alone cannot be used to establish the density of the parenchymal pattern in an individual woman. Regardless of childbearing, young women can have completely fatty tissue and older, postmenopausal women can have dense tissue. It is also important to recognize that there is large intra- and interobserver variability in the application of arbitrarily defined parenchymal patterns. Additionally, the perceived density of a tissue pattern is dependent on technical factors. Some "extremely dense" tissue is inadequately exposed fibroglandular tissue.

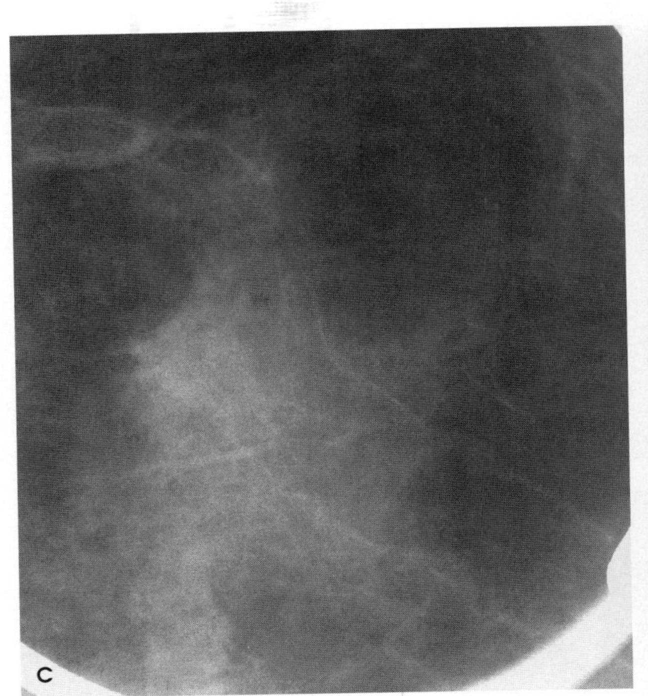

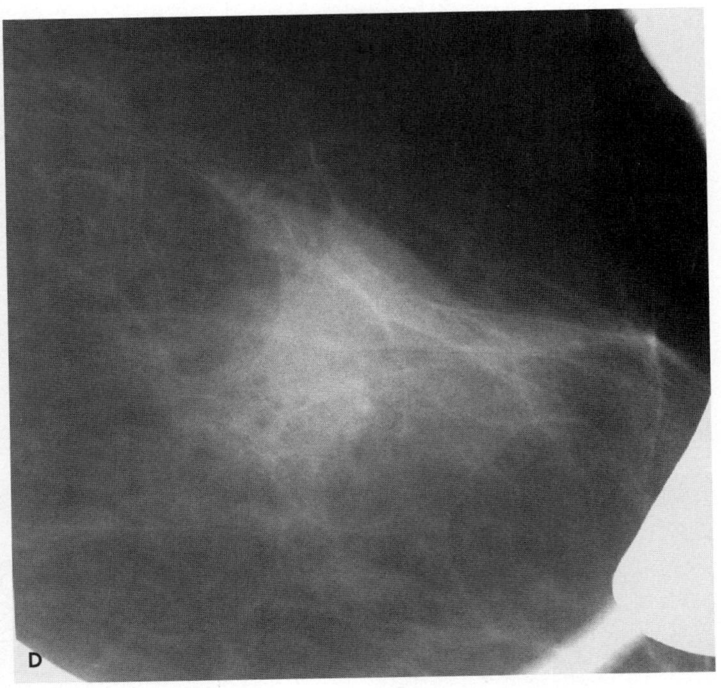

Figure 2.8. (*Continued*) Craniocaudal **(C)** and mediolateral oblique **(D)** spot compression views.

What do you think now?
What BI-RADS® category would you assign at this point, and what is your recommendation?

Normal tissue is imaged on the spot compression views. The overall appearance and density of this tissue is different in the two projections; there is scalloping and fatty tissue is interspersed with the glandular tissue. There is a gradual change in density at the margins. In contrast, masses are three-dimensional with comparable size and density regardless of projection. They are also characterized by an abrupt change in density at the margins. The patient has no history of breast surgery and recalls no trauma to the left breast. Physical examination of this area is normal and symmetric with the comparable site on the contralateral breast. No tenderness is elicited. Ultrasound demonstrates normal tissue throughout the upper outer quadrant of the left breast. This is benign focal parenchymal asymmetry, a normal variant.

BI-RADS® category 2: benign finding. Annual screening mammography is recommended.

PATIENT 6

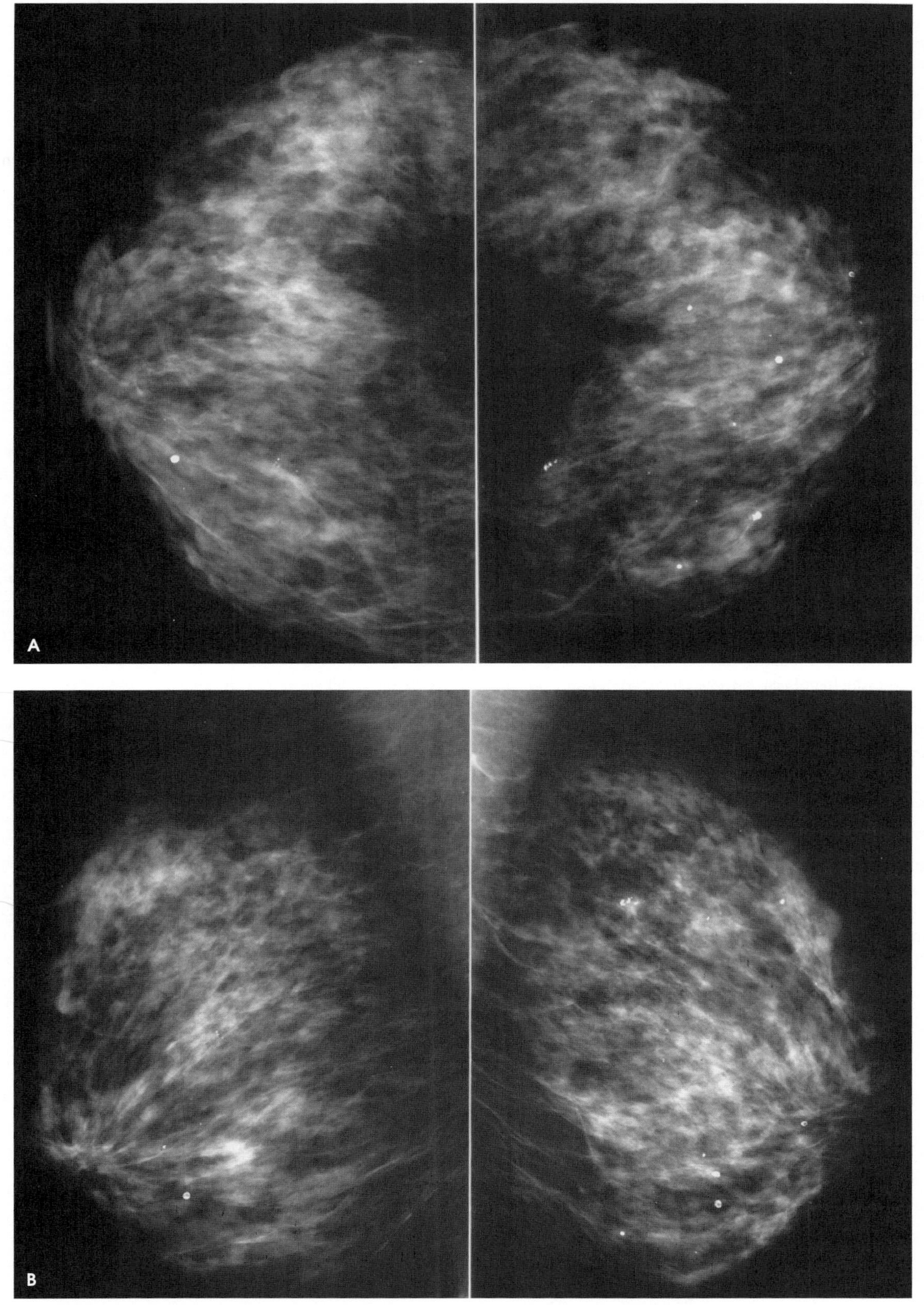

Figure 2.9. Screening study, 68-year-old woman. Craniocaudal **(A)** and mediolateral oblique **(B)** views.

How do you evaluate a screening mammogram?

The evaluation of screening mammograms can be approached in different ways. Develop a strategy that is systematic and use it consistently. Take a proactive approach, and actively send your eyes and brain looking for particular abnormalities in specific locations (subareolar area, medially on craniocaudal views, etc.). This helps you stay focused and minimizes the likelihood that you will miss significant findings. Whatever approach you settle on, it should include a review of the films for technical adequacy. Specifically, is the positioning acceptable? Has tissue and possibly a lesion been excluded (e.g., do you see tissue to the edge of any of the films)? Is glandular tissue adequately compressed and penetrated? Are the films high in contrast? Are there any artifacts that may preclude adequate interpretation of the films? Is there any blurring? Before focusing on perceiving localized findings, look for global or diffuse changes. These may be difficult to appreciate once you focus your attention on more subtle findings.

After evaluating the mammogram at a distance for technical adequacy and diffuse changes, look specifically (with and without a magnification lens) for masses, focal areas of asymmetry, architectural distortion, and calcifications. It is helpful to narrow your search, so on craniocaudal (CC) views, focus on the lateral, middle, and medial thirds of the breasts (Fig. 2.1). On the mediolateral oblique (MLO) views, focus on the upper, middle, and lower thirds of the breasts (Fig. 2.2). Search out potentially abnormal areas as you go back and forth between the right and the left breasts. Specifically, evaluate fat/glandular interfaces, the fatty stripe of tissue between pectoral muscle and glandular tissue on MLO views, the superior cone of tissue on the MLO views, subareolar areas, and the usually fatty tissue medially on CC views (Fig. 2.3). After developing a working hypothesis on a given mammogram, compare with prior studies and look at the history form for any pertinent information (family history of breast cancer or ovarian cancer, estrogen use, prior trauma or surgery, etc.).

What do you think?

In this patient, scattered dystrophic calcifications are present bilaterally. Did you find a potential abnormality? If you did not, look specifically for architectural distortion and move to the subareolar areas. Architectural distortion is present in the right subareolar area, best seen on the MLO view (Fig. 2.9C); it is not readily apparent on the CC view (Fig. 2.9D). Is it safe to assume that this is cancer? No! Benign-appearing lesions can turn out to be cancer, malignant-appearing lesions can reflect benign changes. Make no assumptions, or you will pigeonhole yourself and limit your ability to think through the possibilities. Most findings in the breast have benign and malignant etiologies in the differential. Our job is to sort through the possibilities accurately and efficiently.

What is your differential for architectural distortion?

Among the benign possibilities, consider fat necrosis related to trauma or prior surgery, mastitis, complex sclerosing lesions (sclerosing adenosis), papilloma, and focal fibrosis (rare). Invasive ductal carcinoma not otherwise specified (NOS), tubular carcinoma, ductal carcinoma in situ (rare), and invasive lobular carcinoma are among the invasive lesions that may present with architectural distortion. Armed with differential considerations, you can sort through them by integrating the imaging features of the lesion in question with the patient's age, pertinent history, and physical examination. If you develop and routinely follow a simple, logical, and systematic approach, the next appropriate step becomes readily apparent and is justifiable. This approach is rarely misleading.

What, if any, history would keep you from calling this patient back?
What BI-RADS® assessment category would you assign, and what is your recommendation?

In this patient, the overall characteristics of the lesion include long spicules, no significant central density, and a more pronounced appearance in one of the two routine views. It is critical to establish if the patient has had a biopsy (or significant trauma) in the right subareolar area. If there is a history of prior surgery, the location of the surgical procedure has to correspond directly to the area of distortion. Don't hesitate to examine the patient to establish the presence of a subtle periareolar scar even when the patient does not recall a prior breast biopsy. A complex sclerosing lesion is a good possibility in a woman with this type of lesion and no history of surgery or apparent scar on physical examination. Complex sclerosing lesions are often seen better in one projection and, given their size, usually have no corresponding palpable abnormality on physical examination. In considering mastitis, the breast is usually tender; there may be associated erythema and warmth as well as a history of prior inflammatory changes in the subareolar area.

In thinking about the malignant possibilities, an invasive ductal carcinoma (NOS) of this size and in this location will almost certainly have physical findings, including a palpable abnormality, dimpling, and possibly nipple retraction. Tubular carcinomas are usually fairly small and are more commonly identified in younger women (in their 40s). Invasive lobular carcinomas are more common in older patients, and physical findings are often subtle.

This patient has had surgery in the right subareolar area corresponding to the site of distortion. The findings reflect fat necrosis related to the prior biopsy. Architectural distortion related to prior surgery is often planar and therefore better seen in one projection, as in this patient. No additional evaluation is indicated.

BI-RADS® category 2: benign finding. Annual screening mammography is recommended.

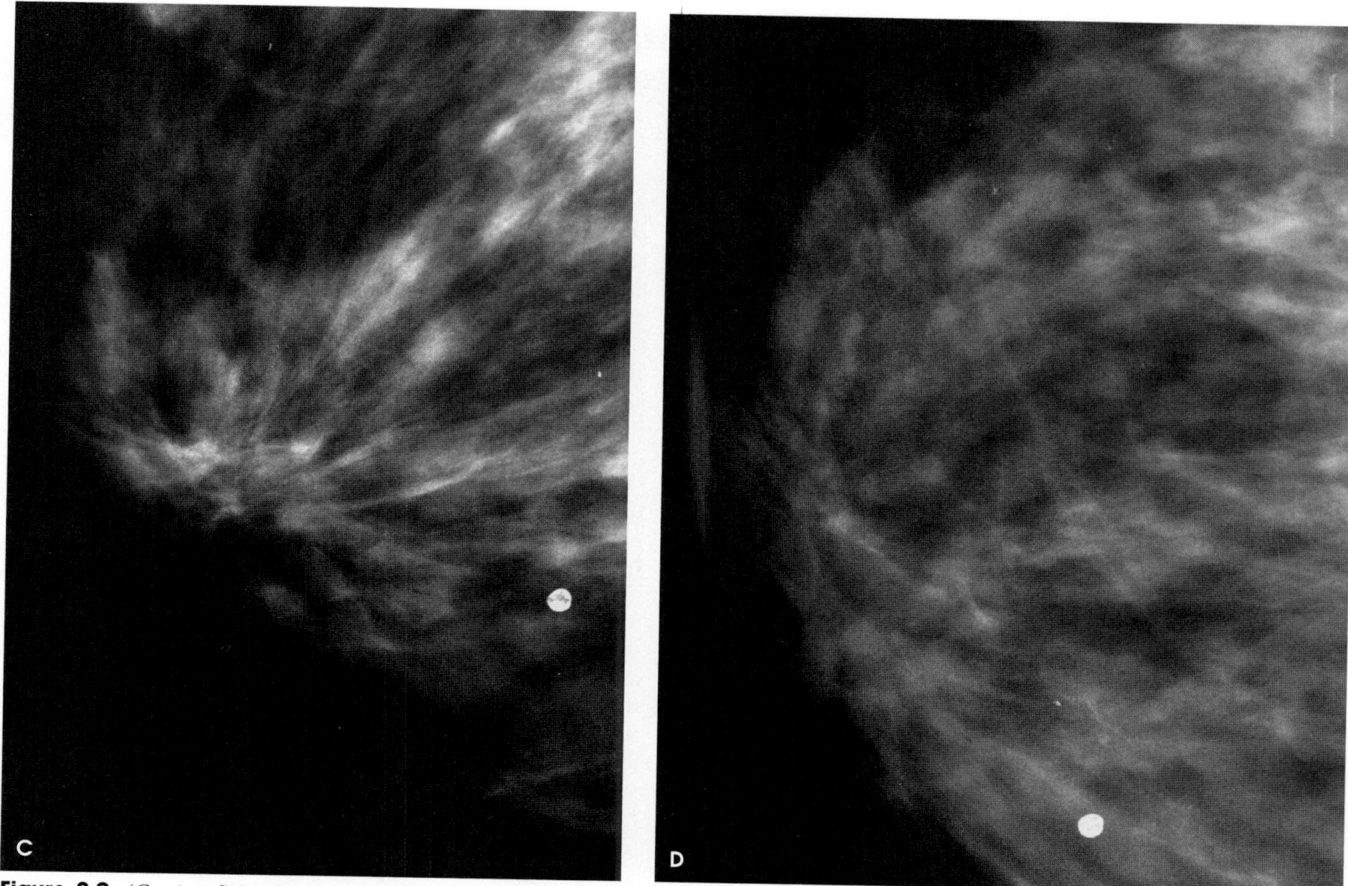

Figure 2.9. (*Continued*) Mediolateral oblique **(C)** and craniocaudal **(D)** photographically coned views. Architectural distortion readily apparent on the mediolateral oblique view, more subtle on the craniocaudal view.

PATIENT 7

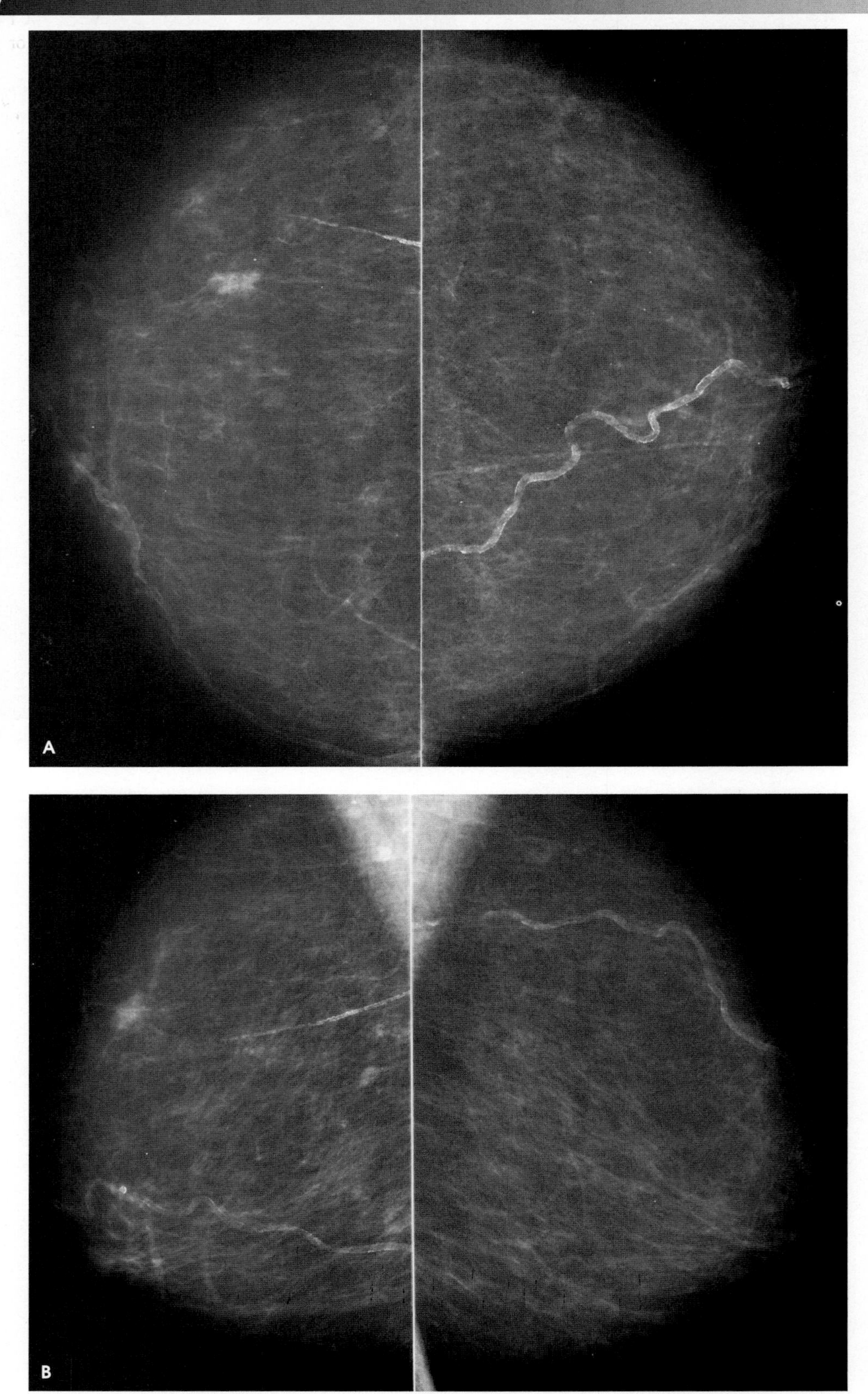

Figure 2.10. Screening study, 68-year-old woman. Craniocaudal **(A)** and mediolateral oblique **(B)** views.

What do you think?
What BI-RADS® assessment category would you assign, and what is your recommendation?

There are arterial calcifications bilaterally. Did you notice a mass in the right breast? This is new compared with prior studies (not shown). Additional evaluation is recommended. BI-RADS® category 0: need additional imaging evaluation.

Do you have any additional observations? Technically, are you happy with this study? Be specific in describing the problem.

Positioning on this study is not optimal. There is insufficient pectoral muscle on the mediolateral oblique (MLO) views. Ideally, pectoral muscle should be seen to the level of the nipple; it should be thick in the axilla and have a convex anterior margin. Given the triangular shape of the muscle in this patient, several things went wrong during positioning. It is likely that an incorrect angle of obliquity was selected, the muscles were not relaxed, and the breasts were not adequately mobilized medially (or if they were, the patient pulled out during positioning).

On the craniocaudal (CC) views, a significant amount of posterior tissue is excluded from the images. In determining if an adequate amount of tissue has been included on the CC views, look for pectoral muscle posteriorly or for cleavage medially. If neither of these is seen, measure the posterior nipple line (PNL) on the MLO views (and remember that in this patient, positioning on the MLO views is not optimal, so the PNL measurement is not an optimal measure of the amount of tissue this patient has) and compare it to that measured on the CC views (Fig. 2.4E, F). The PNL measurement on the CC view should be within 1 cm of that measured on the MLO view. It is not in this patient. Additionally, if you look at the length of the calcified artery laterally on the right CC and the relationship of the lesion to the edge of the film between CC and MLO views, it is clear that posterior tissue has been excluded on the CC views.

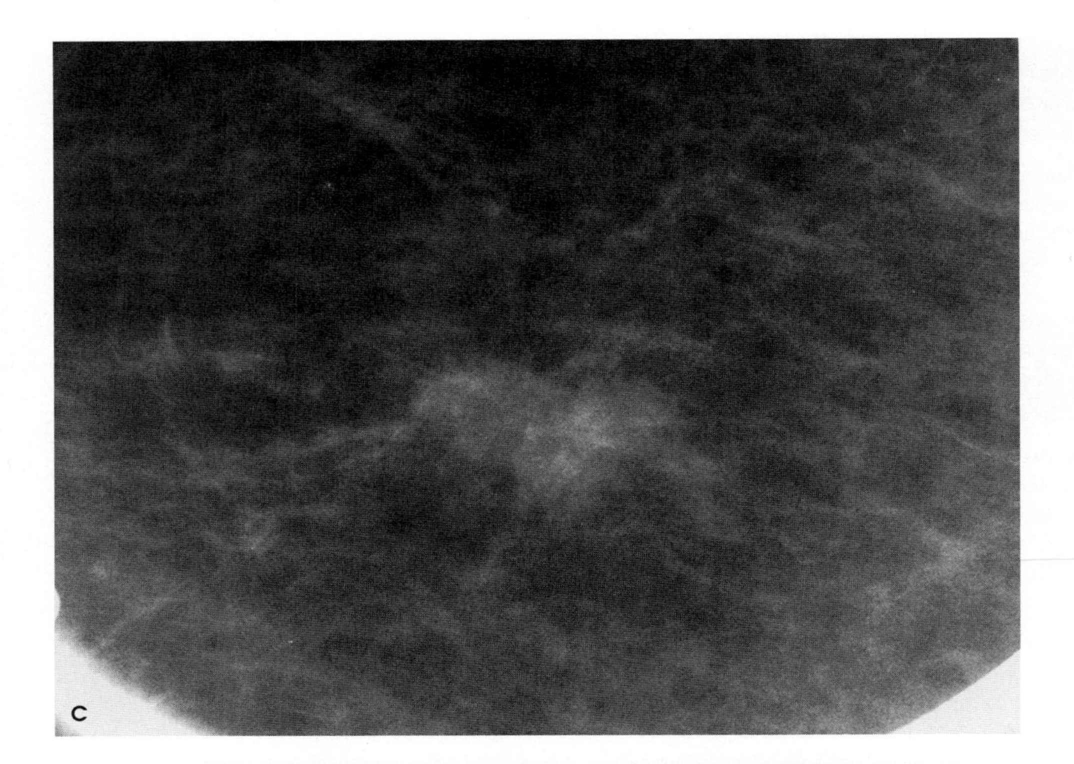

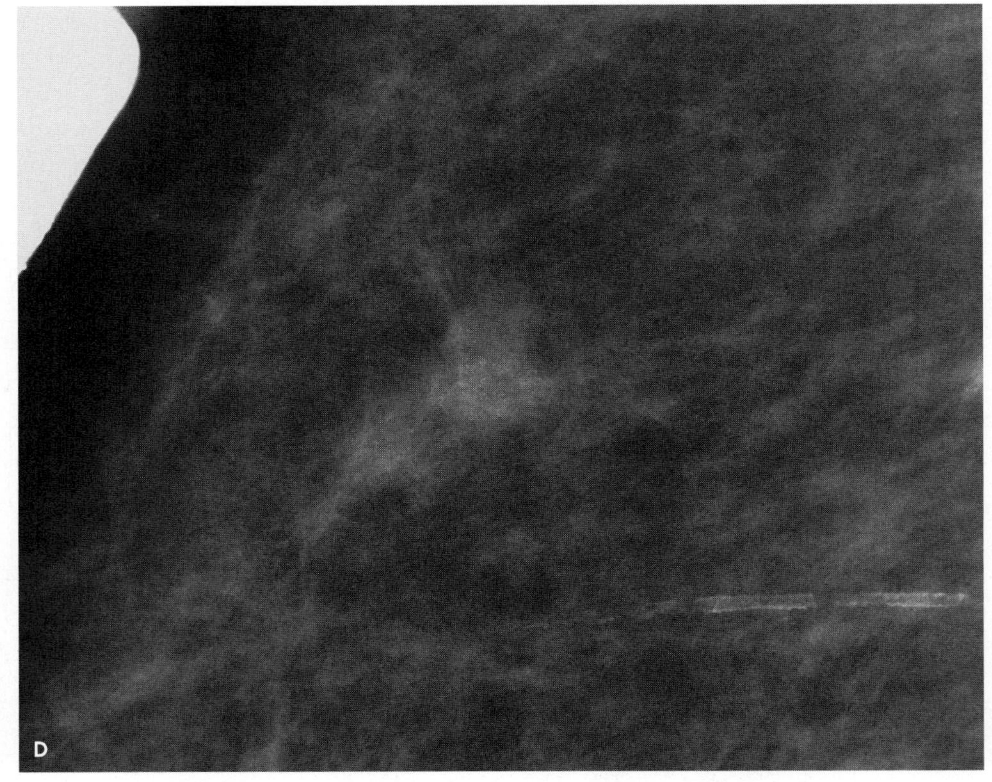

Figure 2.10. (*Continued*) Craniocaudal **(C)** and mediolateral oblique **(D)** spot compression views, right breast.

What do you think?
How would you describe the finding, and at what clock position would you expect to find this lesion?

The spot compression views confirm the presence of a 1-cm irregular mass with spiculated margins. A biopsy is indicated based on the mammographic findings.

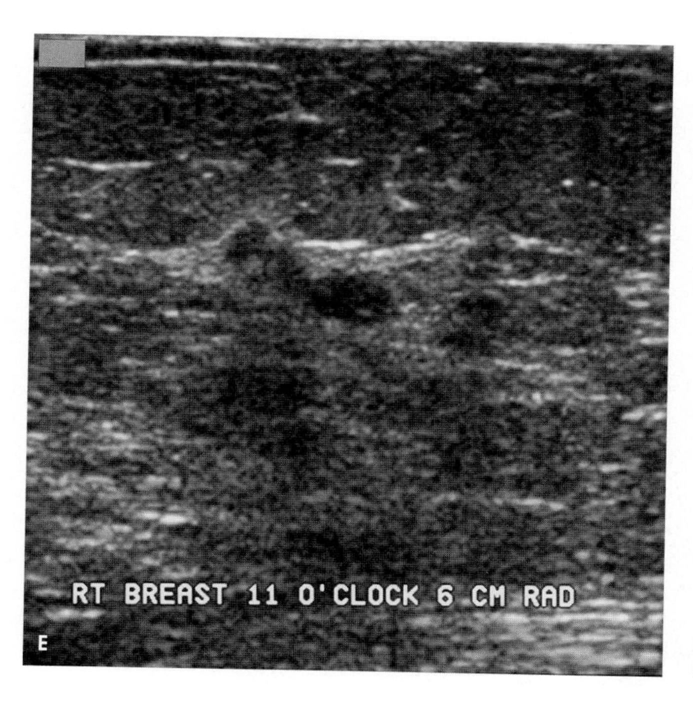

Figure 2.10. (*Continued*) Ultrasound image **(E)**, radial (RAD) projection of the lesion.

An irregular, hypoechoic mass with angular margins is imaged at the 11 o'clock position, 6 cm from the right nipple, corresponding to the expected location of the lesion seen mammographically.

BI-RADS® category 4: suspicious abnormality, biopsy should be considered. An ultrasound-guided core biopsy is done at the time of the diagnostic evaluation.

A poorly differentiated, invasive ductal carcinoma is reported histologically following the ultrasound guided core biopsy. A 1.2-cm, grade III, invasive ductal carcinoma is reported on the lumpectomy specimen. No metastatic disease is identified in four excised sentinel lymph nodes; [pT1c, pN0(sn)(i−), pMX; Stage I].

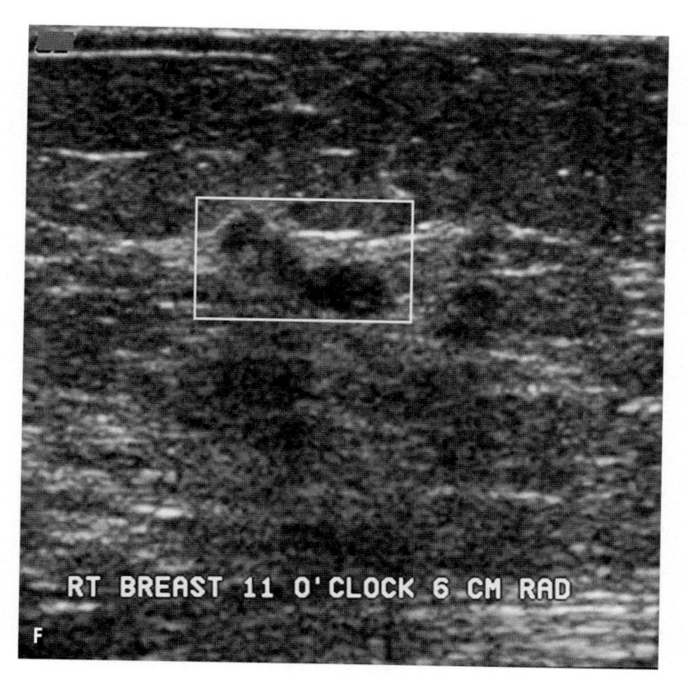

Figure 2.10. (*Continued*) Ultrasound image **(F)**, radial (RAD) projection. The lesion is contained in the box.

PATIENT 8

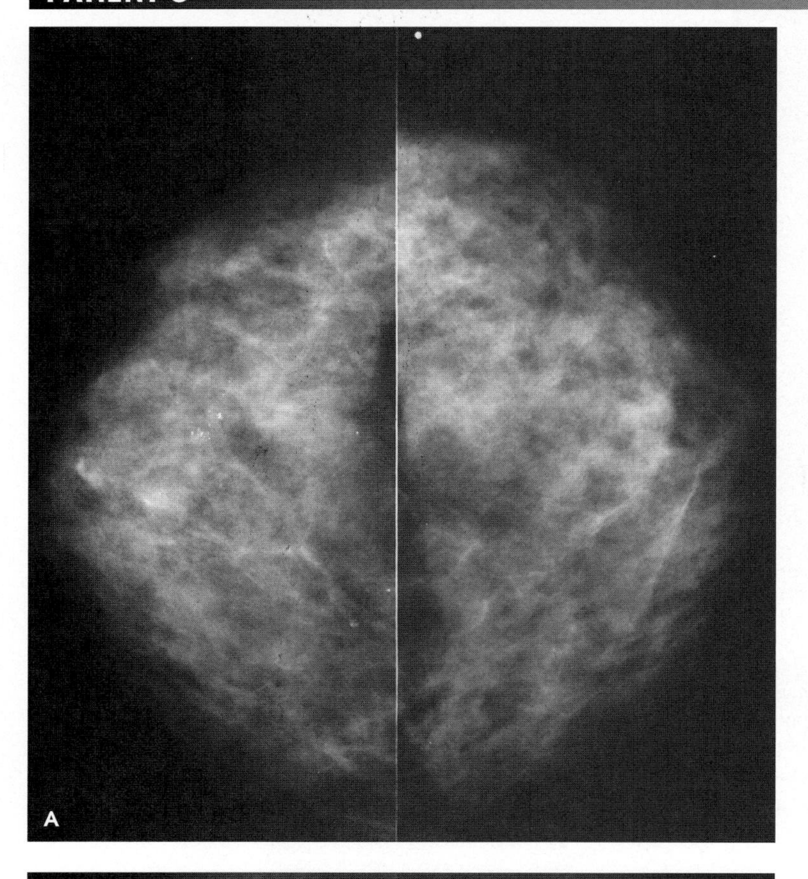

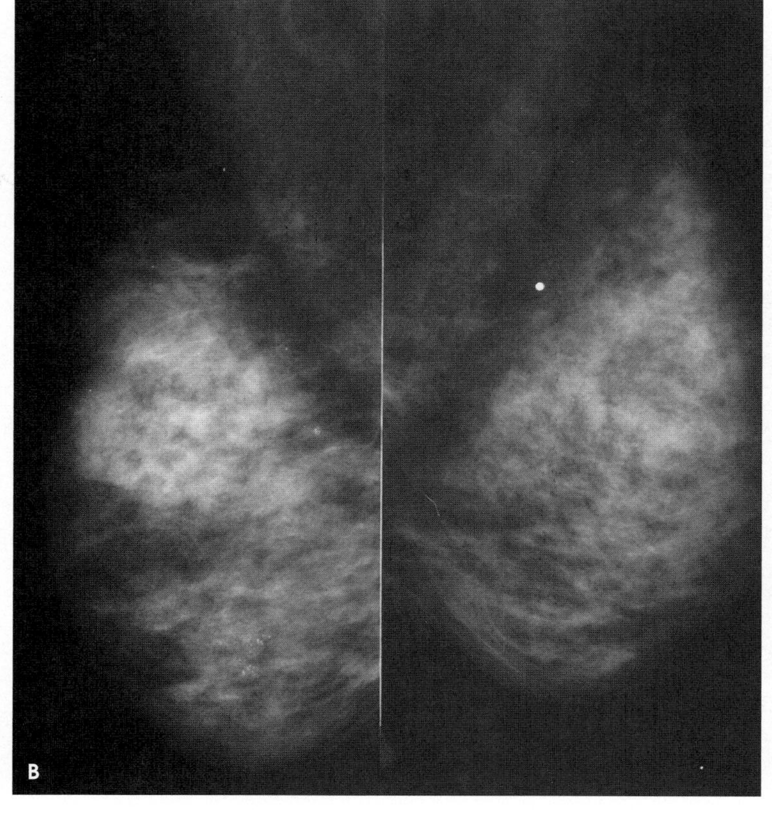

Figure 2.11. Screening study, 51-year-old woman. Craniocaudal **(A)** and mediolateral oblique **(B)** views. The metallic BB on the left is on a skin lesion. No history of breast surgery or significant trauma.

Any observations?
What BI-RADS® assessment category would you assign, and what is your recommendation?

Systematically review the images and actively look for potential lesions. In addition to splitting the craniocaudal (CC) and mediolateral oblique (MLO) views into thirds and evaluating the locations where cancers are likely to develop, look specifically for diffuse changes, masses, distortion, asymmetry, and calcifications. If you focus down with a magnification lens and look specifically for calcifications on every screening mammogram you review, you are unlikely to miss the relevant finding in this patient. Did you see the cluster of calcifications anteriorly at approximately the 6 o'clock position in the right breast? With what degree of confidence can you characterize these, and how definitive can you be with respect to their significance? Why not get more information in the form of double spot compression magnification views? There are other calcifications posteriorly (close to the edge of the film medially) in the lower inner quadrant on the right, but these contain lucent centers and are benign.

BI-RADS® category 0: need additional imaging evaluation.

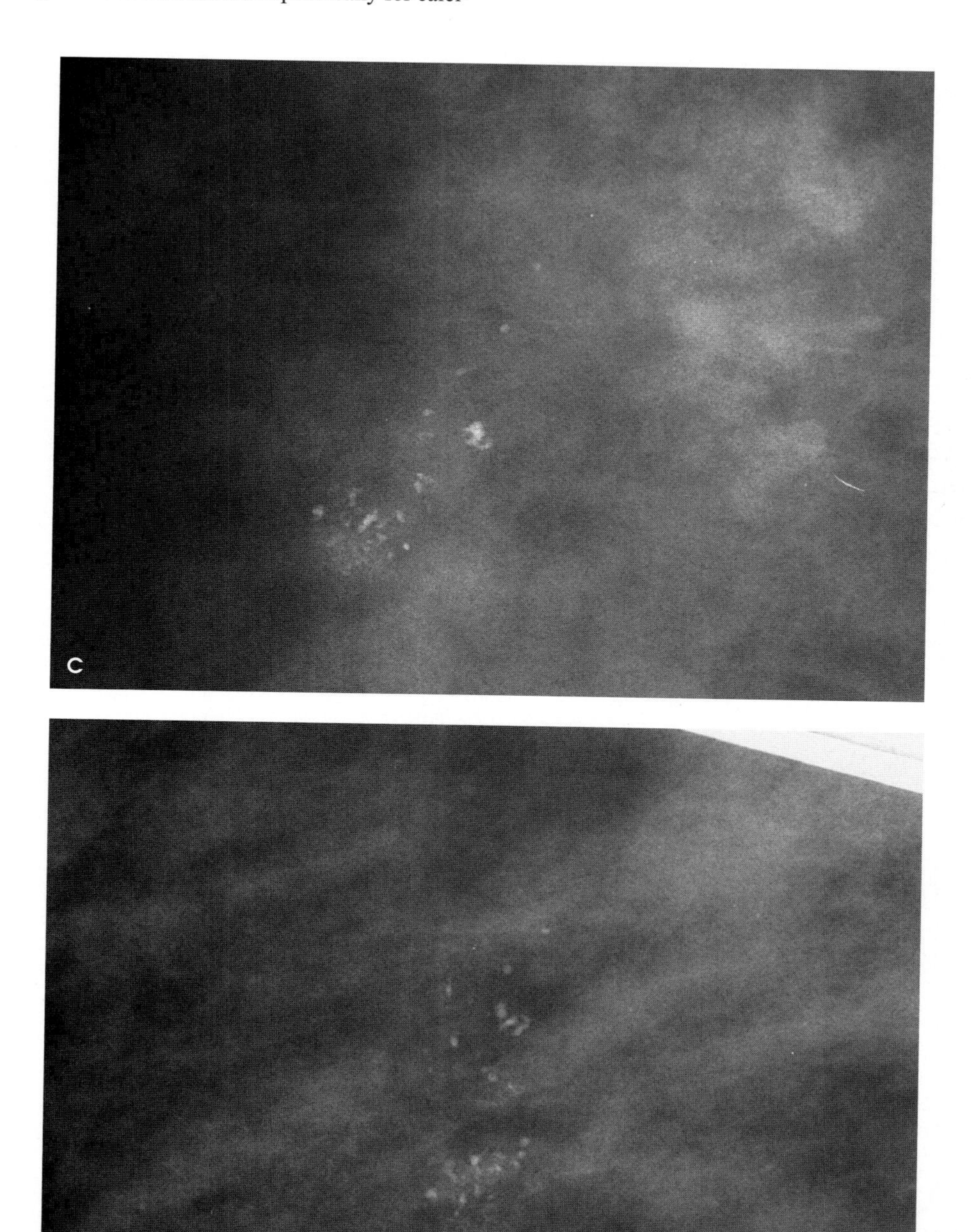

Figure 2.11. (*Continued*) Craniocaudal **(C)** and mediolateral oblique **(D)**, double spot compression magnification views.

pleomorphic calcs

What do you think?
What BI-RADS® assessment category would you assign, and what is your recommendation?

On the double spot compression magnification views, the morphology of the calcifications is much better demonstrated, as is the extent of the lesion. The calcifications in this cluster are pleomorphic, and there are linear forms. Armed with high-quality magnification views, our confidence in the likely diagnosis of ductal carcinoma in situ is increased significantly, and the need for a biopsy is easily justified.

BI-RADS® category 4: Suspicious abnormality; biopsy should be considered. A stereotactically guided needle biopsy is done on the same day as the magnification views. A high-nuclear-grade ductal carcinoma in situ with central necrosis is diagnosed on the core biopsy. A 1-cm area of high-nuclear-grade ductal carcinoma in situ with central necrosis and no associated invasion is described histologically on the lumpectomy specimen. No sentinel lymph node biopsy is done [pTis(DCIS), pNX, pMX; Stage 0].

PATIENT 9

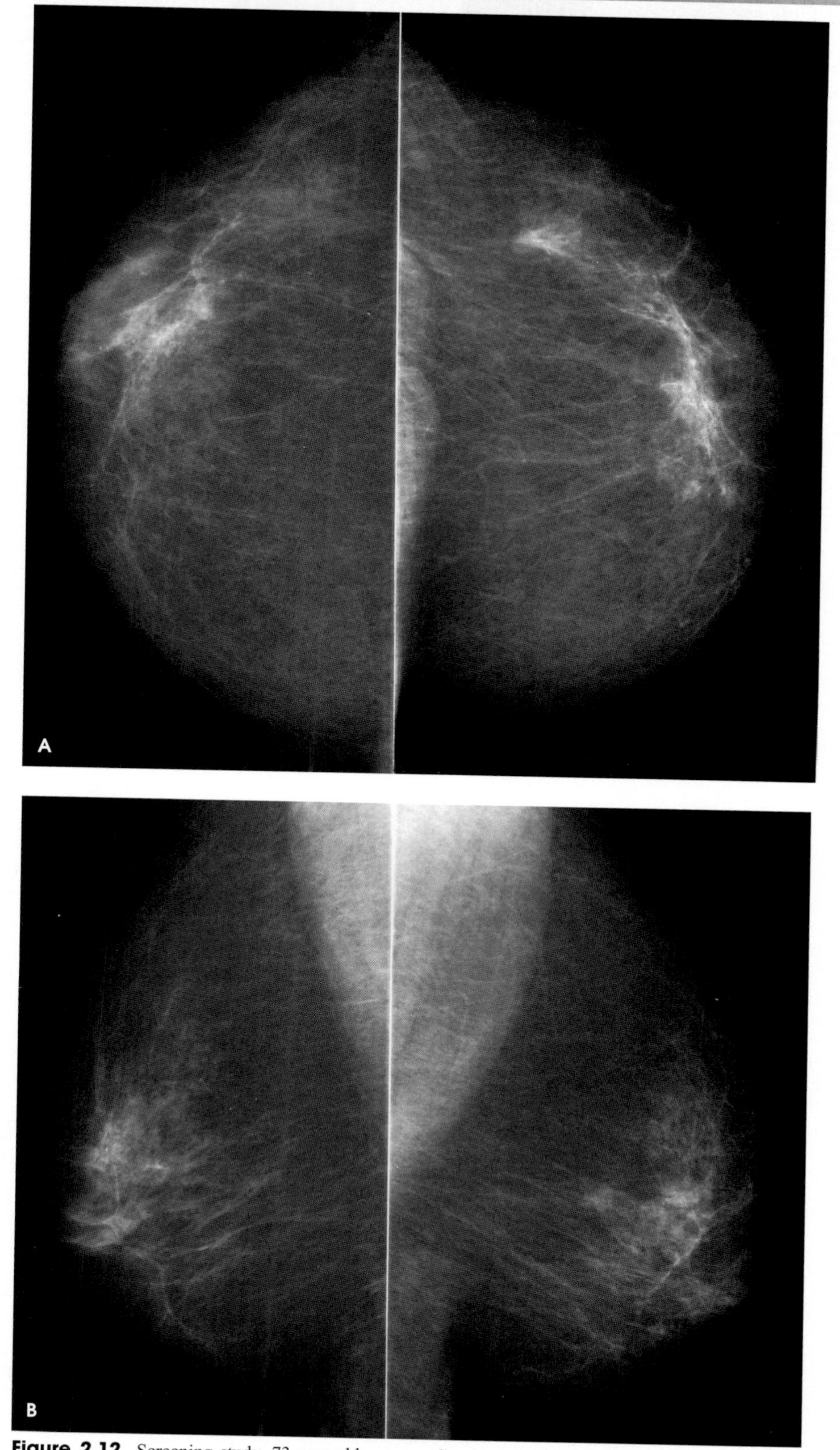

Figure 2.12. Screening study, 73-year-old woman. Craniocaudal **(A)** and mediolateral oblique **(B)** views, left breast. No prior films available for comparison.

Would you agree with a BI-RADS® assessment category 2: benign finding?

There is a mass in the left breast at approximately the 3 o'clock position, 4 cm from the left nipple. Did you see it (Fig. 2.12G, H)? What did you think? Good for you, if you are not willing to accept this as an intramammary lymph node. Although it may be that a fatty hilum and well-circumscribed margins are demonstrated with spot compression views, on these screening views no fatty hilum is apparent and the margins are not well defined. Remember: Make no assumptions. With what degree of certainty can you say this is a lymph node? If you are not sure, call the patient back for additional evaluation.

BI-RADS® category 0: need additional imaging evaluation.

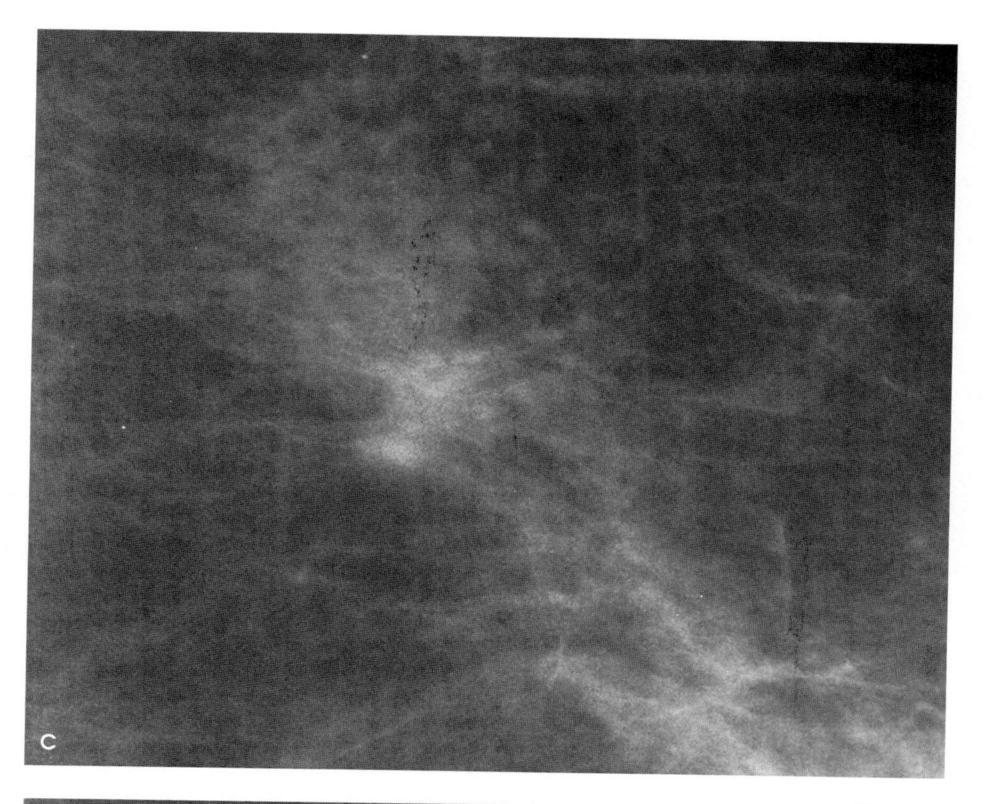

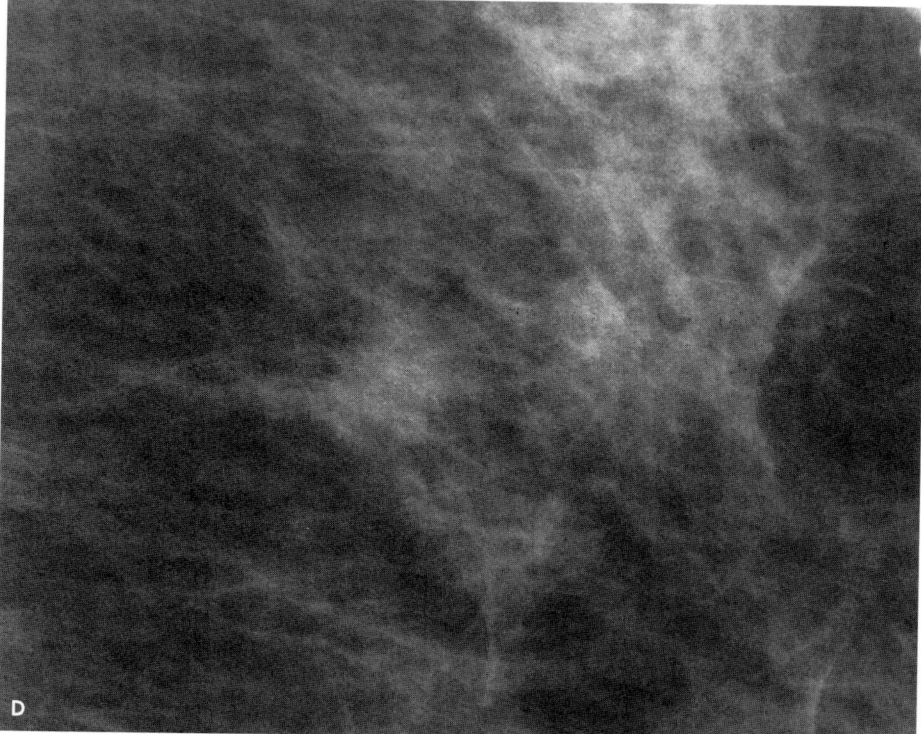

Figure 2.12. (*Continued*) Craniocaudal **(C)** and mediolateral oblique **(D)** spot compression views, left breast.

What do you think now?

A 1-cm spiculated mass is confirmed on the spot compression views. A biopsy is indicated. An ultrasound is done to determine whether the lesion is identified on ultrasound; if it is, ultrasound guidance can be used for the core biopsy.

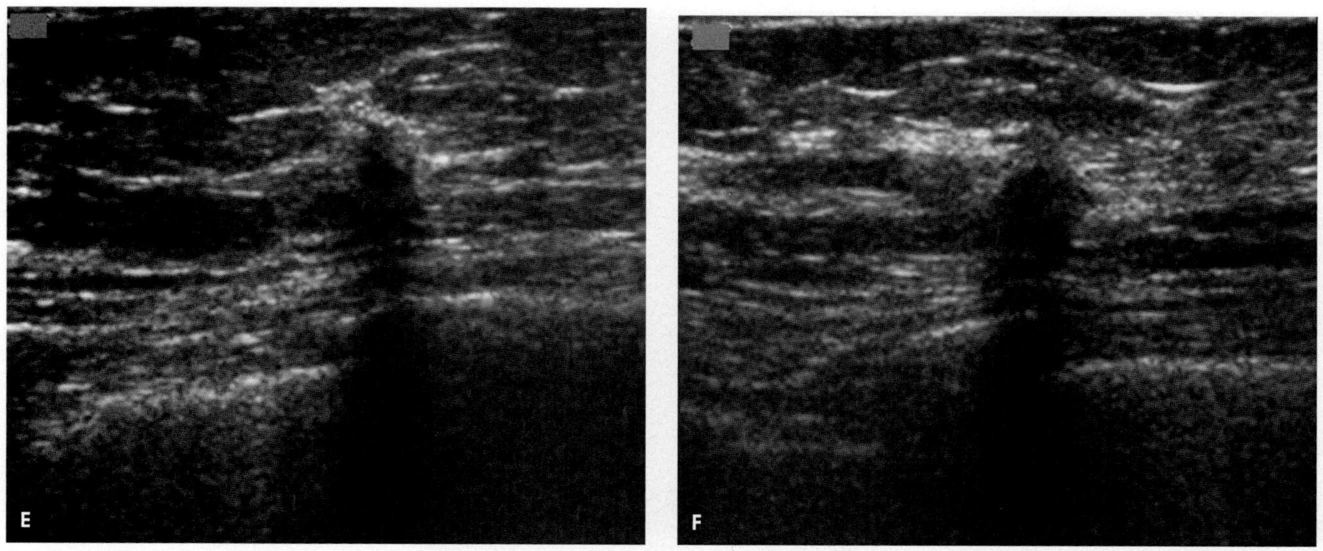

Figure 2.12. (*Continued*) Ultrasound images in radial (RAD) **(E)** and antiradial (ARAD) **(F)** projections, left breast.

How would you describe the ultrasound findings?

A vertically oriented, irregular hypoechoic mass with indistinct and angular margins, shadowing, and associated distortion of the surrounding tissue is imaged at the 3 o'clock position, 4 cm from the left nipple, correlating to the expected location of the lesion seen mammographically. With the additional views and the ultrasound we can issue a succinct, definitive report on the finding, the likely significance, and our recommendations. Would you now agree with the assignment of BI-RADS® category 4: suspicious abnormality; biopsy should be considered.

An invasive ductal carcinoma is diagnosed following an ultrasound-guided core biopsy. A 0.7-cm invasive ductal carcinoma with tubular features (grade I) is diagnosed on the lumpectomy specimen. No metastatic disease is diagnosed in two excised sentinel lymph nodes [pT1b, pN0(sn)(i−), pMX; Stage I].

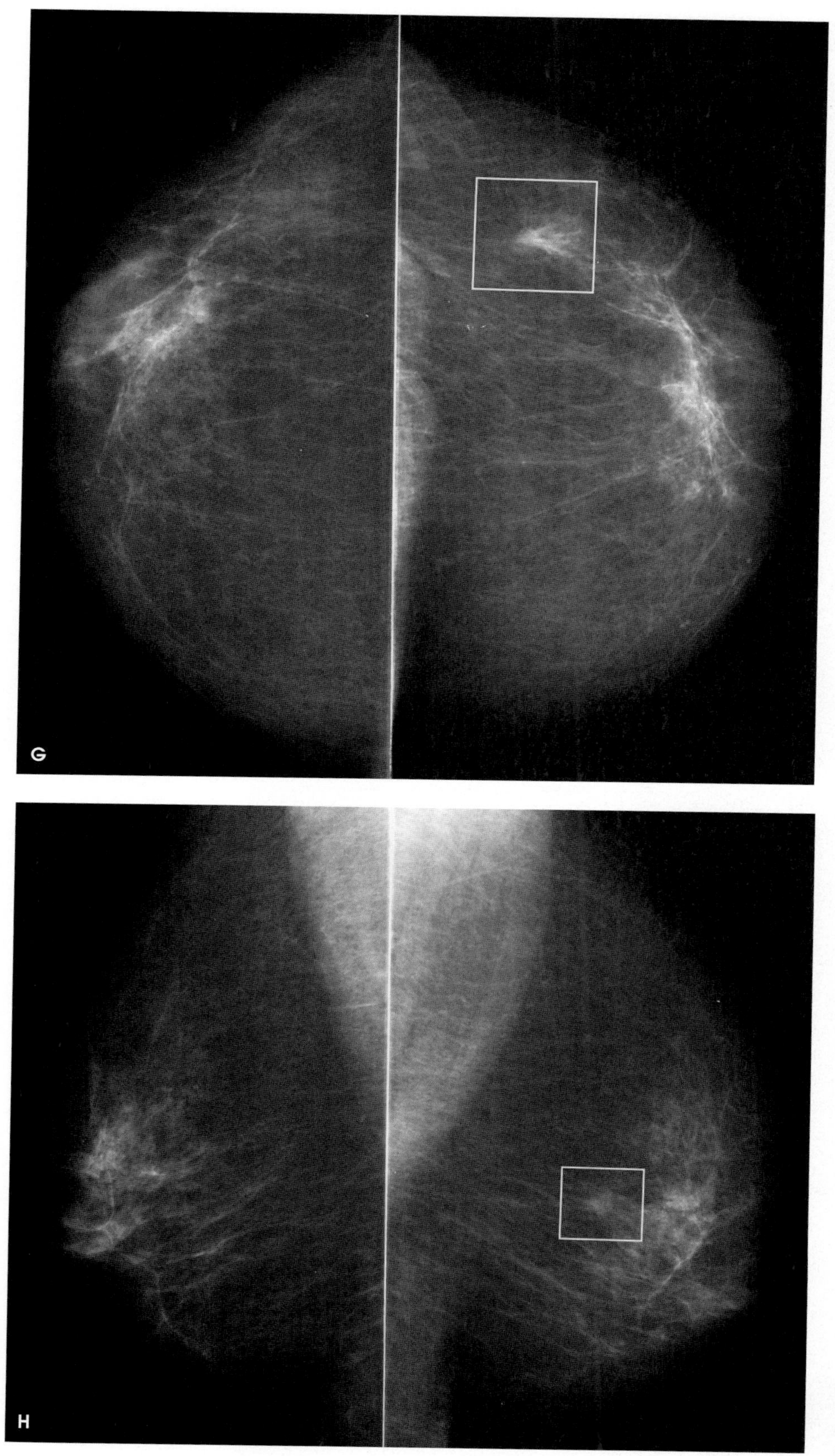

Figure 2.12. (*Continued*) Craniocaudal **(G)** and mediolateral oblique **(H)** views. Box indicating location of potential mammographic abnormality.

PATIENT 10

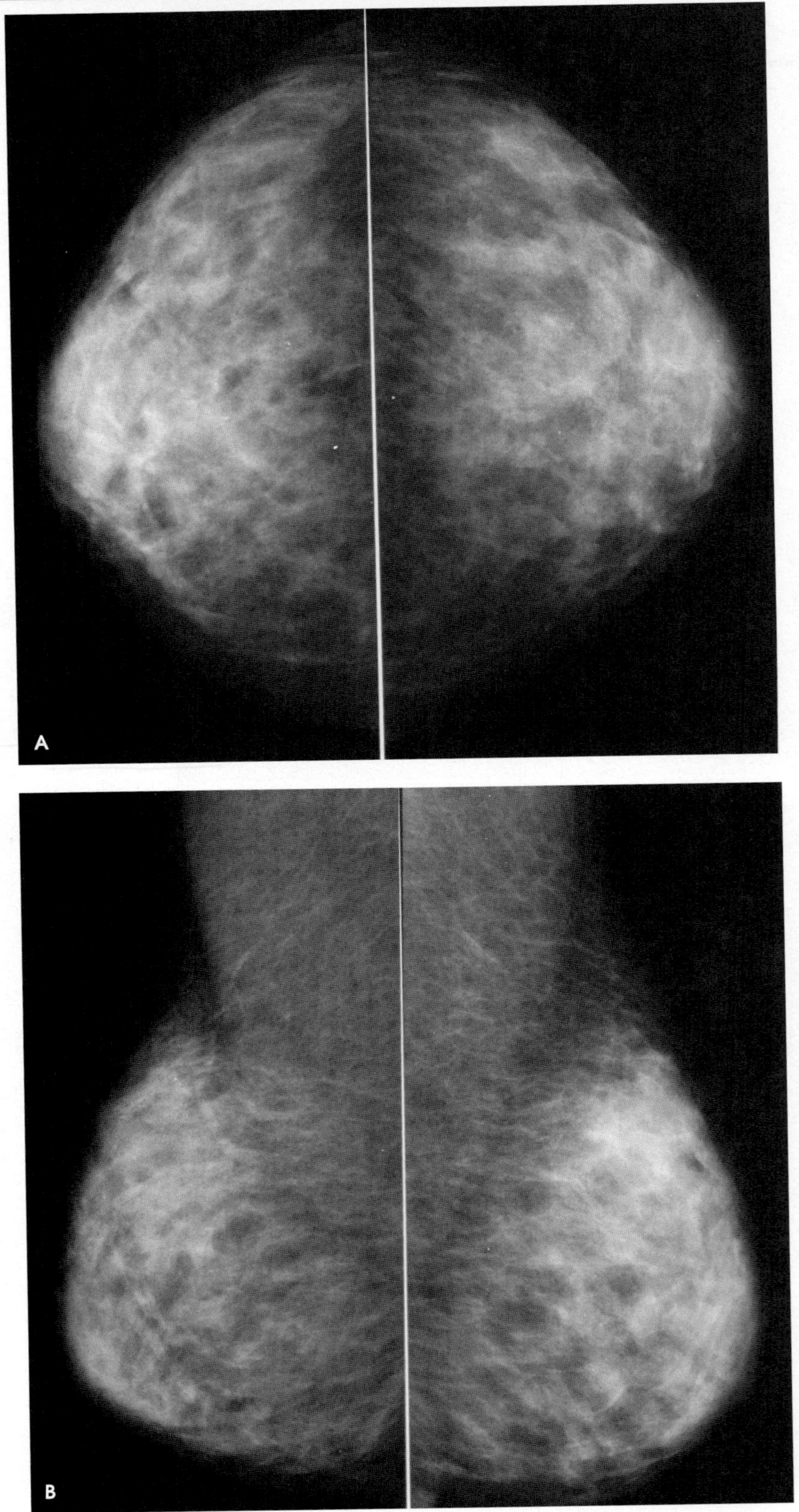

Figure 2.13. Screening study, 38-year-old woman. Craniocaudal **(A)** and mediolateral oblique **(B)** views.

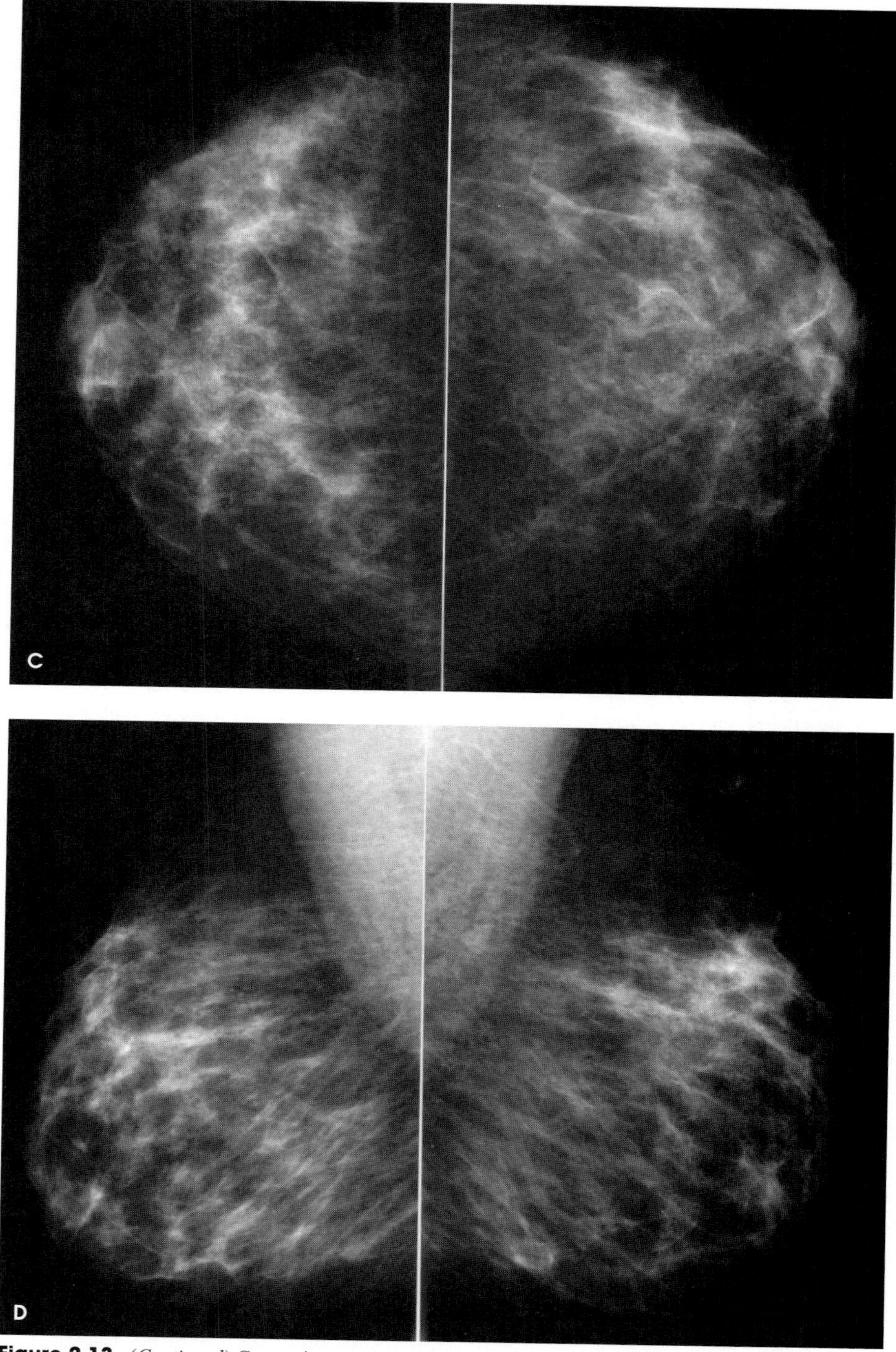

Figure 2.13. (*Continued*) Comparison study, craniocaudal **(C)** and mediolateral oblique **(D)** views.

Technical factors used for exposures:

Factor	RCC (A)	RCC (C)	LCC (A)	LCC (C)	RMLO (B)	RMLO (D)	LMLO (B)	LMLO (D)
kV	26	26	26	26	26	27	26	27
mAs	36	294	41	334	47	363	43	352
Comp(mm)	22	67	24	71	24	74	24	72
Target/filter	mo/mo	mo/rh	mo/mo	mo/rh	mo/mo	mo/rh	mo/mo	mo/rh

What do you think?
Are these mammograms from two different women?
If they are from the same woman, what is your working hypothesis?
Are there any significant findings in either mammogram?

These mammograms are normal and from the same woman, taken 20 months apart. In the interval, she lost 150 pounds. On the current study (Fig. 2.13A, B), breast size is decreased and parenchymal density is increased, with a concomitant decrease in fat compared with the study from 20 months before (Fig. 2.13C, D). The changes are bilateral and symmetric. There is no skin or trabecular thickening. The breasts are significantly thinner, as evidenced by the millimeters of compression used for exposure on the current study compared with 20 months before. Given similar kilovoltage peaks on both studies, the resulting milliamperage output is consistently lower on the current images. Also, note that rhodium kicked in for all of the films done on the comparison study.

Given the milliamperage output on the current study, what could the technologist have done to improve image quality?

Image contrast is partially related to the voltage used for exposure. As you increase voltage, you decrease image contrast. Optimally, you want to use a high enough voltage to penetrate the tissue adequately, but not much more than that. At a given voltage, the resulting amperage also needs to be considered, because this indirectly reflects the length of the exposure. As the amperage is increased, exposure time is increased, and as exposure time increases, motion blur may become an issue if the patient is unable to hold her breath. If, at a given voltage, the resulting amperage is high (>400 mAs) and the tissue is not adequately exposed, either voltage or compression (or both) need to be increased. As voltage is increased, the resulting amperage (and exposure time) decreases; as voltage is decreased, the resulting amperage (and exposure time) increases. In this woman, the resulting amperages on the current study are well below 400 mAs, so the voltage can be lowered without sacrificing adequate exposure of the tissue. As voltage is lowered, contrast is increased, improving overall image quality. Did you notice the low image contrast on the current images? Overall, the images (and particularly the fat) look gray, reflecting the poor contrast.

What is your differential for diffuse breast changes?

Differential considerations for diffuse changes that are usually unilateral, although rarely can be bilateral, include radiation therapy effect, inflammatory changes (e.g., mastitis), trauma, ipsilateral axillary adenopathy with lymphatic obstruction, dialysis shunt in the ipsilateral arm with fluid overload, invasive ductal carcinoma not otherwise specified, inflammatory carcinoma, invasive lobular carcinoma, or lymphoma. Invasive lobular carcinoma can lead to increases in breast density and size, or a decrease in breast size (the shrinking breast). Differential considerations for diffuse changes that are usually bilateral, although they can be unilateral, include hormone replacement therapy (e.g., estrogen), weight changes, congestive heart failure, renal failure with fluid overload, and superior vena cava syndrome. Additional rare benign causes include granulomatous mastitis, coumadin necrosis, arteritis, and autoimmune disorders (e.g., scleroderma). Obtaining a thorough history, examining the patient, and obtaining an ultrasound are often helpful in sorting through the differential considerations.

BI-RADS® category 1: negative. Next screening mammogram is recommended at age 40.

PATIENT 11

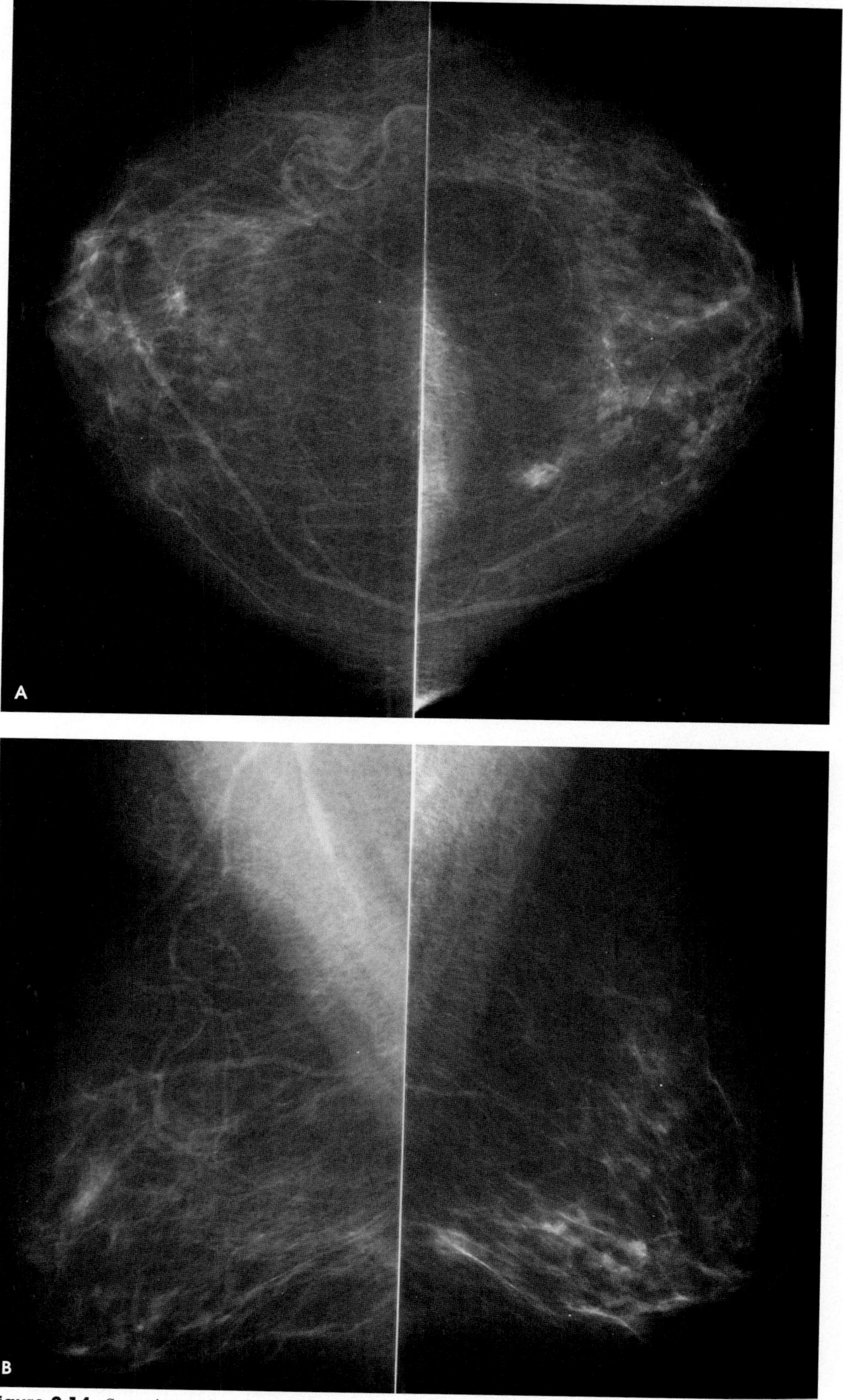

Figure 2.14. Screening study, 74-year-old woman. Craniocaudal **(A)** and mediolateral oblique **(B)** views.

What do you think?
Is this a normal mammogram, or do you think additional evaluation is indicated?

In this patient, by splitting the images (Fig. 2.14C, D) in thirds and focusing your attention to the medial portions of the breasts on the craniocaudal (CC) views, a mass is detected medially in the left breast. On the mediolateral oblique (MLO) views, the corresponding mass is imaged in tissue projecting on the lower third of the left breast. If they are available, previous films will be helpful in assessing a change and should be requested before calling the patient back for a diagnostic evaluation. In the absence of comparison films, or if this represents a change when comparison is made to several sequential mammograms, additional evaluation is indicated.

BI-RADS® category 0: need additional imaging evaluation.

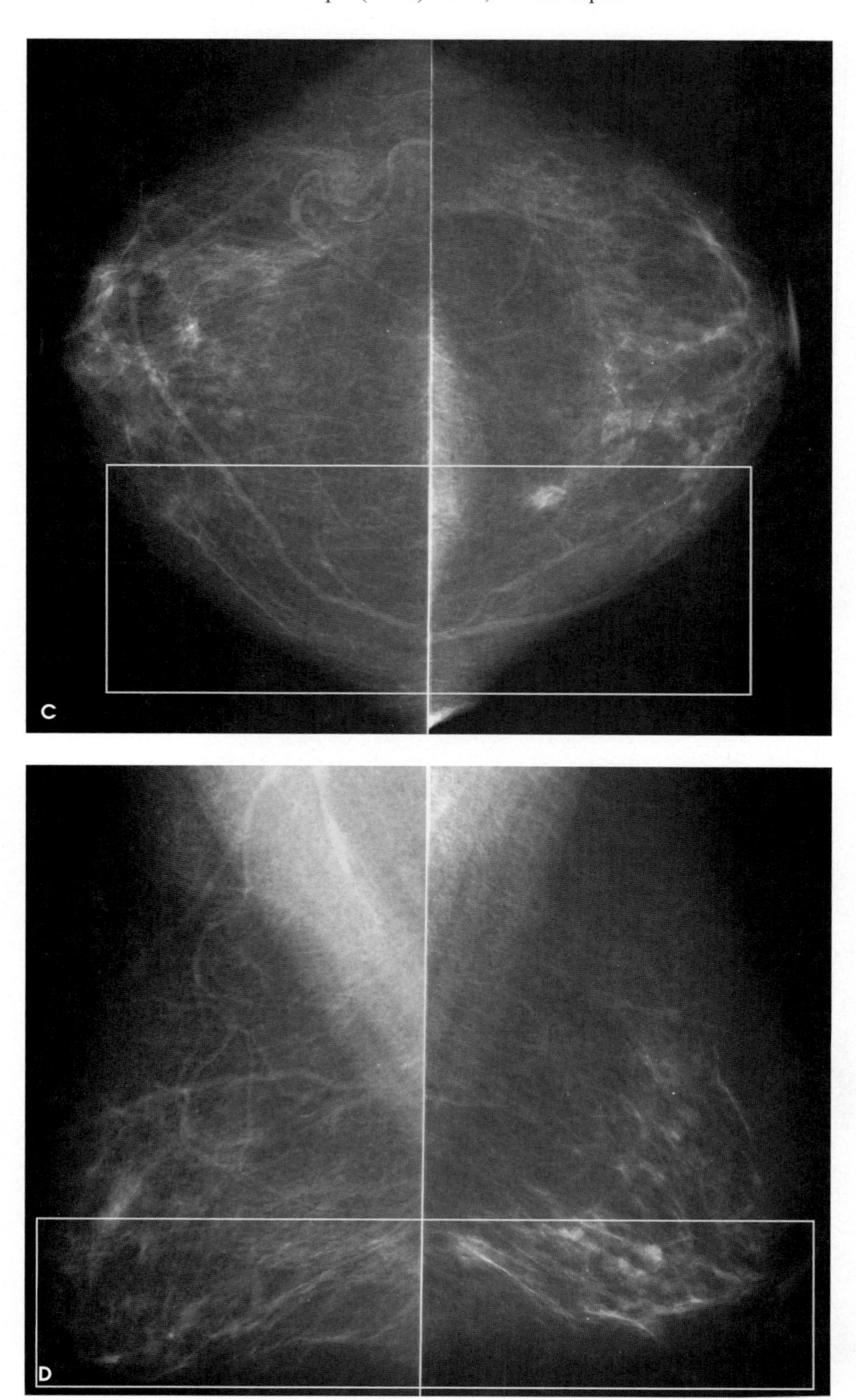

Figure 2.14. (*Continued*) Craniocaudal **(C)** and mediolateral oblique **(D)** views with boxes on the medial and lower thirds of the breasts, respectively.

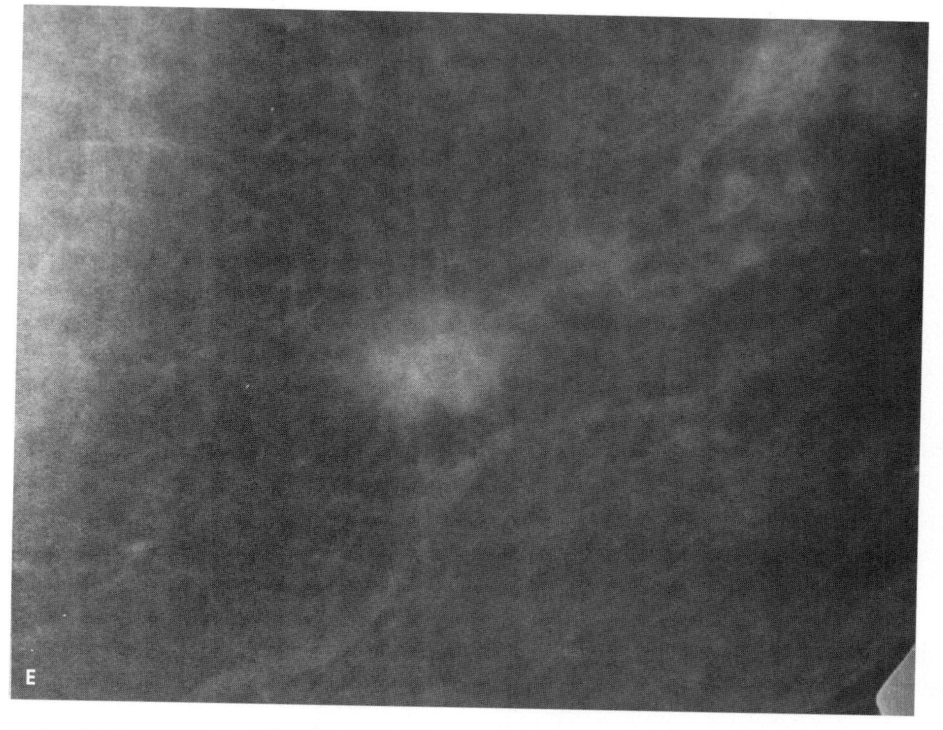

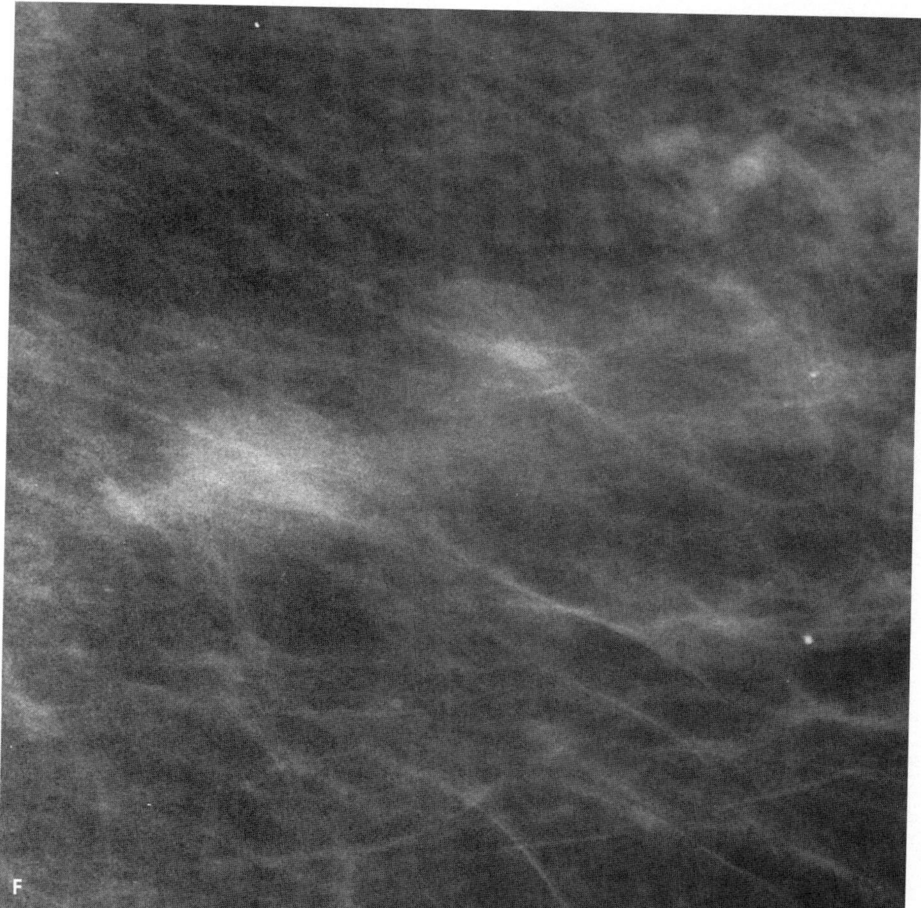

Figure 2.14. Craniocaudal **(E)** and mediolateral oblique **(F)** spot compression views, left breast.

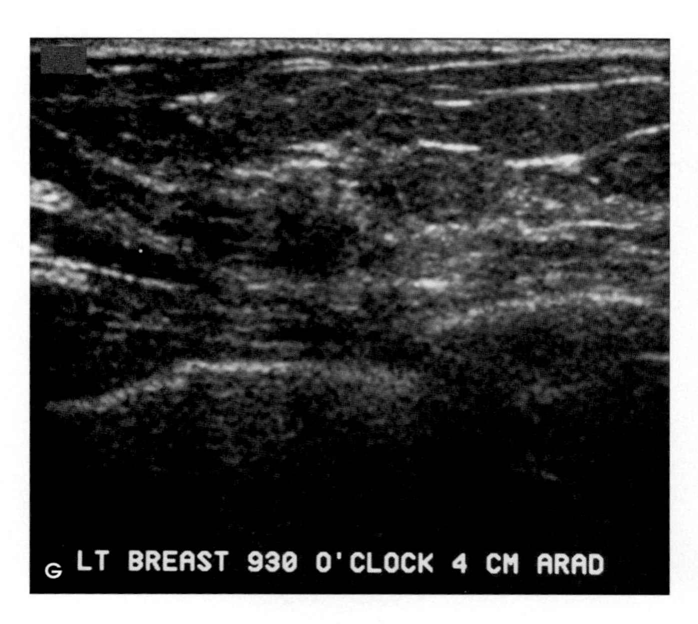

Figure 2.14. (*Continued*) Ultrasound image **(G),** antiradial (ARAD) projection, left breast.

Where would you place the ultrasound transducer? Be precise. (What clock position? How far back from the nipple?)
How would you describe the imaging findings?

Spot compression views confirm the presence of a 1-cm mass with indistinct margins. An irregular, hypoechoic mass with indistinct and spiculated margins and a partial echogenic halo is imaged on ultrasound (Fig. 2.14G, H). Although the lesion projects below the level of the nipple on the MLO view, be careful in assuming that this lesion is in the lower inner quadrant of the left breast. Some lesions that project below the level of the nipple on the mediolateral oblique (MLO) view are actually above the level of the nipple. In this patient, the lesion is in the lower aspect of the upper inner quadrant of the breast at the 9:30 o'clock position (see Fig. 3.6F–I), 4 cm from the left nipple.

BI-RADS® category 4: suspicious abnormality, biopsy should be considered. Rather than just consider it, a biopsy is done.

An invasive ductal carcinoma is diagnosed following the ultrasound-guided core biopsy. A grade II invasive ductal carcinoma measuring 1 cm is confirmed at the time of the lumpectomy, and the sentinel lymph node is negative for metastatic disease [pT1b, pN0(sn)(i−), pMX; Stage I].

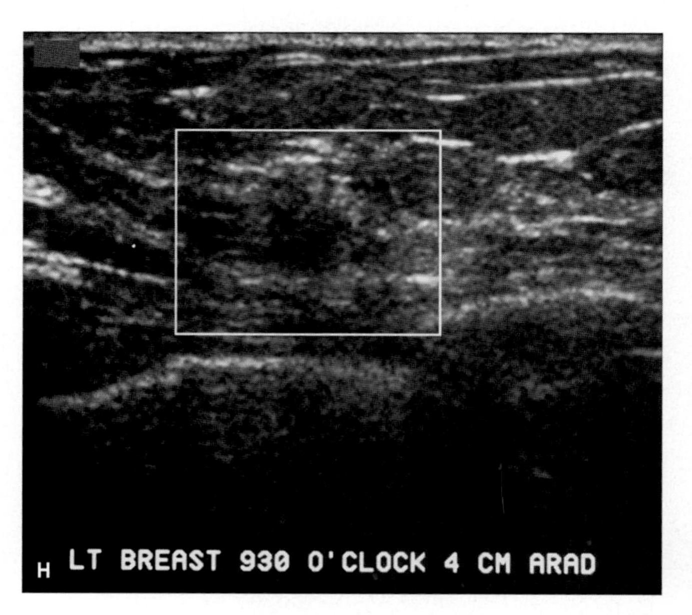

Figure 2.14. (*Continued*) Ultrasound image **(H),** antiradial (ARAD) projection, left breast at the 9:30 o'clock position, 4 cm from the left nipple. A box delineates the mass.

PATIENT 12

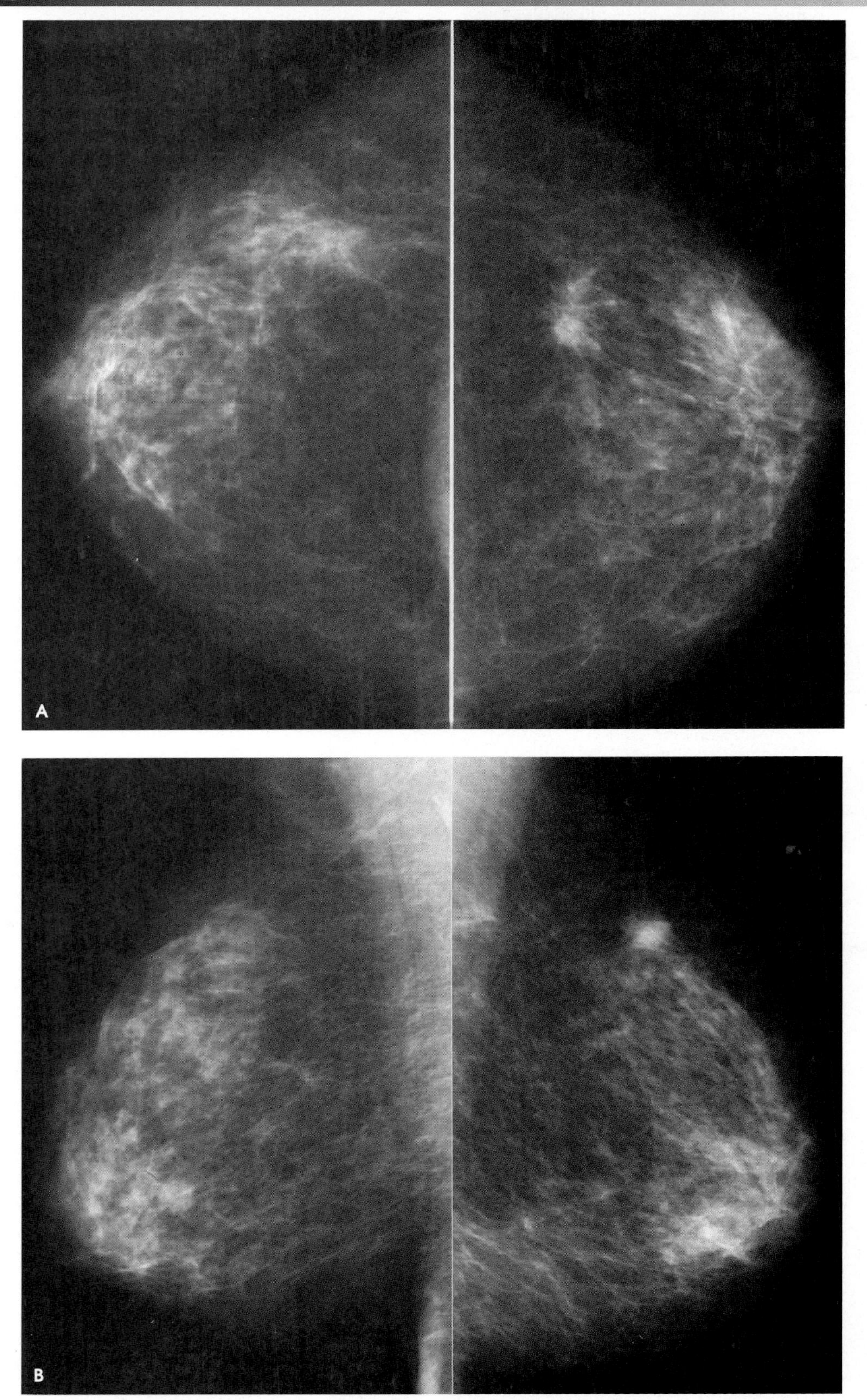

Figure 2.15. Screening study, 87-year-old woman. Craniocaudal **(A)** and mediolateral oblique **(B)** views.

**What do you think?
Is this a normal mammogram, or do you think additional evaluation is indicated?**

A mass is present in the upper cone of tissue on the mediolateral oblique (MLO) view. In many women, this area of tissue on the MLO is scalloped. If the tissue in this area rounds off asymmetrically, it should raise concerns about a developing lesion. A spiculated mass is seen laterally in the left craniocaudal view.

BI-RADS® category 0: need additional imaging evaluation.

How would you describe the imaging findings, and what is indicated?

Spot compression views (not shown) confirm the presence of a 1.5-cm spiculated mass at this site. A biopsy is indicated. Ultrasound-guided core biopsy is done at the time of the diagnostic study. An invasive mammary carcinoma is reported histologically. A 1.6-cm grade I invasive ductal carcinoma with associated low-nuclear-grade ductal carcinoma with central necrosis is reported on the lumpectomy specimen. No metastatic disease is diagnosed in two excised sentinel lymph nodes [pT1c, pN0(sn)(i−), pMX; Stage I].

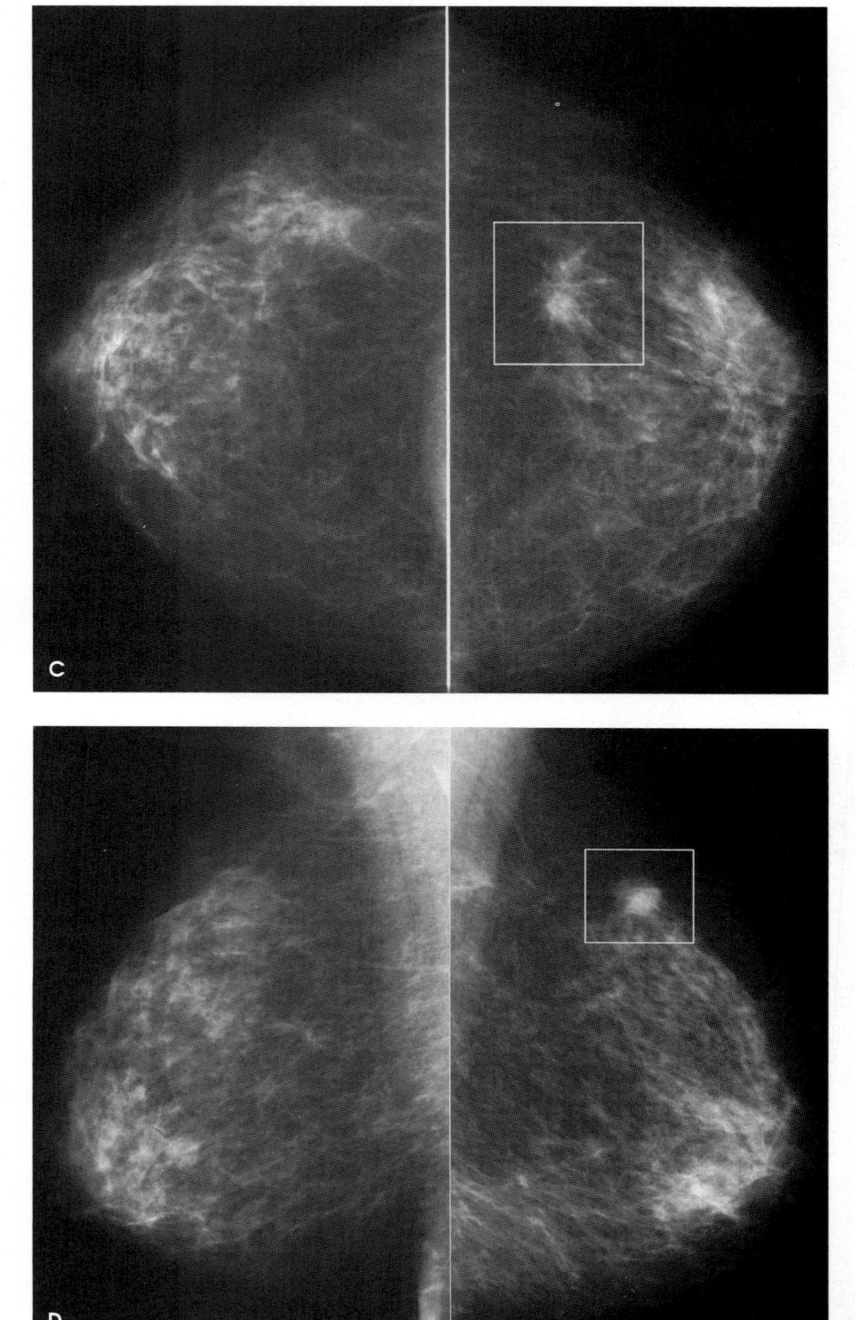

Figure 2.15. *(Continued)* Screening images with a box indicating the location of the lesion on the left craniocaudal **(C)** and mediolateral oblique **(D)** views.

PATIENT 13

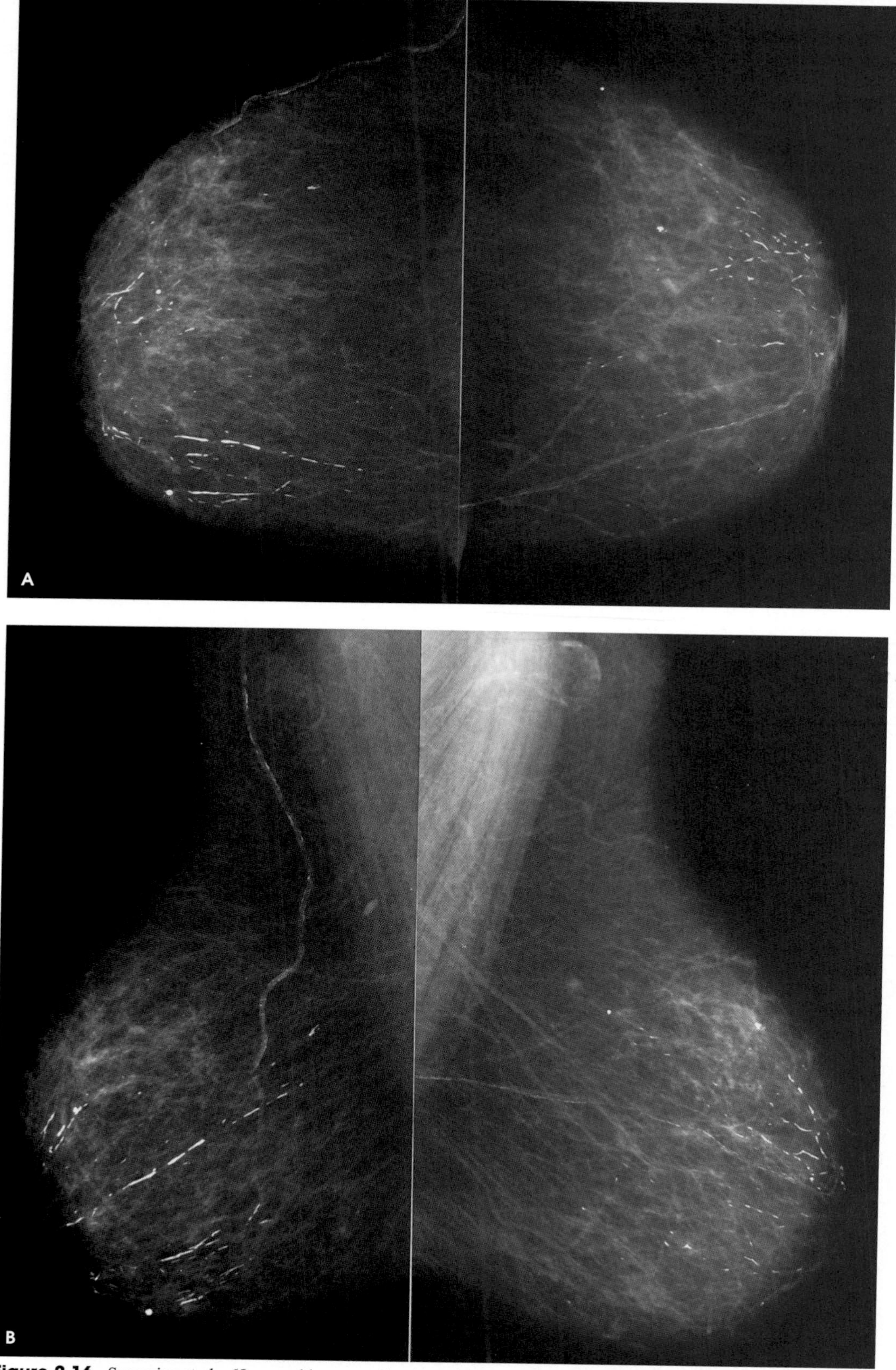

Figure 2.16. Screening study, 68-year-old woman. Craniocaudal **(A)** and mediolateral oblique **(B)** views.

What do you think?
Is this a normal mammogram, or do you think additional evaluation is indicated?

Arterial calcifications are present bilaterally. The artery, coursing inferiorly at the anterior edge of the right pectoral muscle on the mediolateral oblique (MLO) view, is the lateral thoracic artery. It is always seen coursing in the subcutaneous tissue laterally on the craniocaudal (CC) view. The calcified artery, entering the breast just inferior to the left pectoral muscle on the MLO view and extending toward the nipple, is likely a perforating branch of the internal mammary artery. On the CC views, these are more commonly medial in location but can also be seen laterally. Additionally, large rodlike calcifications, oriented toward the nipple, are noted scattered bilaterally, and a lymph node with a prominent fatty hilum is seen at the edge of the left pectoral muscle superiorly on the left MLO. Following a systematic review of the films, no significant finding is perceived. No additional views are indicated.

BI-RADS® category 1: negative. Annual screening mammography is recommended (or BI-RADS® category 2: benign finding can be used if you describe the arterial or secretory calcifications in your report).

PATIENT 14

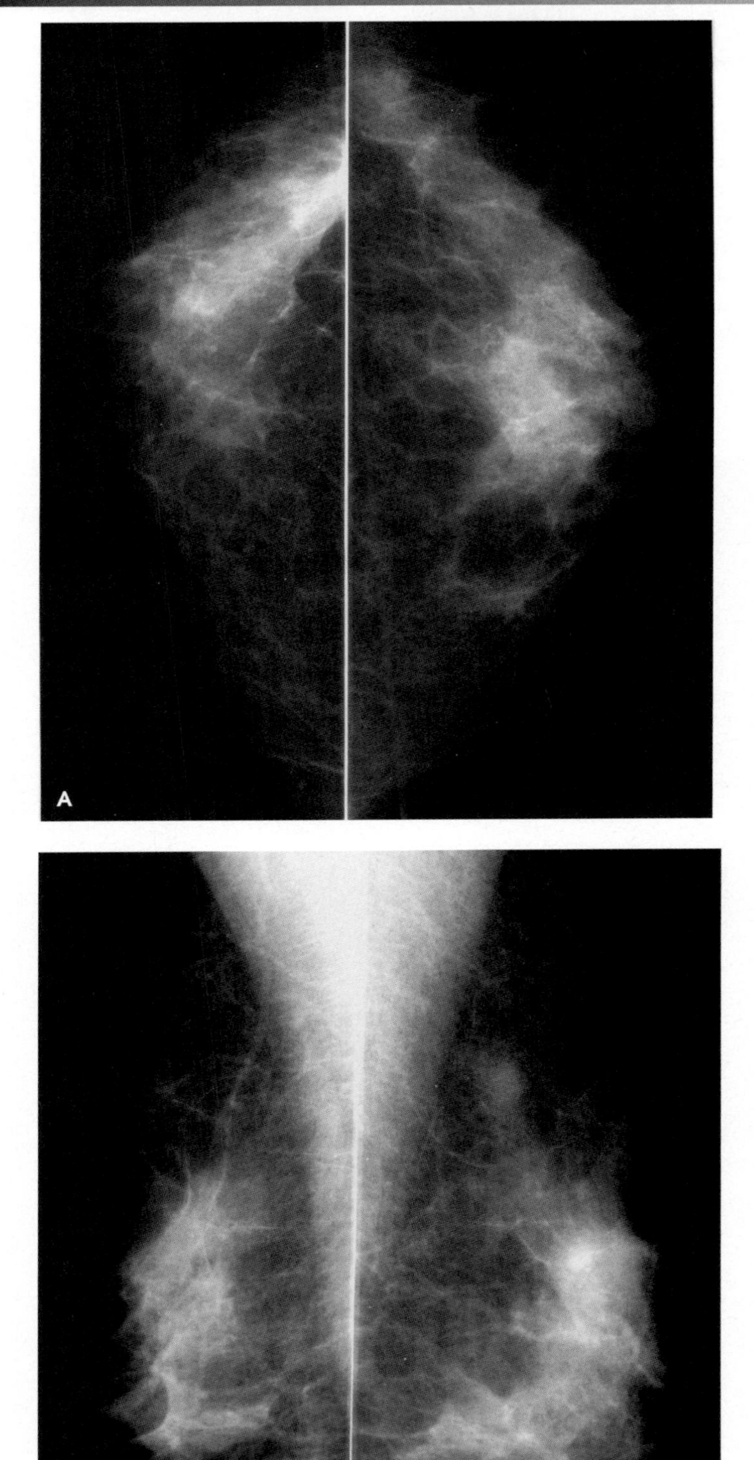

Figure 2.17. Screening study, 55-year-old woman. Craniocaudal **(A)** and mediolateral oblique **(B)** views.

What do you think?
Is this a normal mammogram, or do you think additional evaluation is indicated?

Review the images systematically. Focus your attention on smaller amounts of tissue by splitting the craniocaudal (CC) and mediolateral (MLO) views into thirds (Figs. 2.1 and 2.2). Look for specific findings, including diffuse changes, masses, distortion, asymmetry, and calcifications. Review areas on the mammograms where breast cancers are likely to develop, specifically, the fatty stripe of tissue between pectoral muscle and glandular tissue on MLO views, the superior cone of tissue on MLO views, medial tissue on CC views, fat–glandular interfaces, and subareolar areas (Fig. 2.3). Focus down with a magnification lens, particularly when looking for small masses, distortion, and clusters of calcifications.

Is there a potential mass in this patient?

Did you notice the possible mass in the fatty stripe of tissue between pectoral muscle and glandular tissue on the left MLO? No definite abnormality is identified on the CC view, but it may be partially imaged at the edge of the film in the far posterolateral aspect of the left breast. With what degree of confidence can you characterize this potential finding, and how definitive can you be about what the next step should be? How about prior films? If prior films are not available, or this represents an interval change, additional imaging may be helpful in determining the significance of this finding.

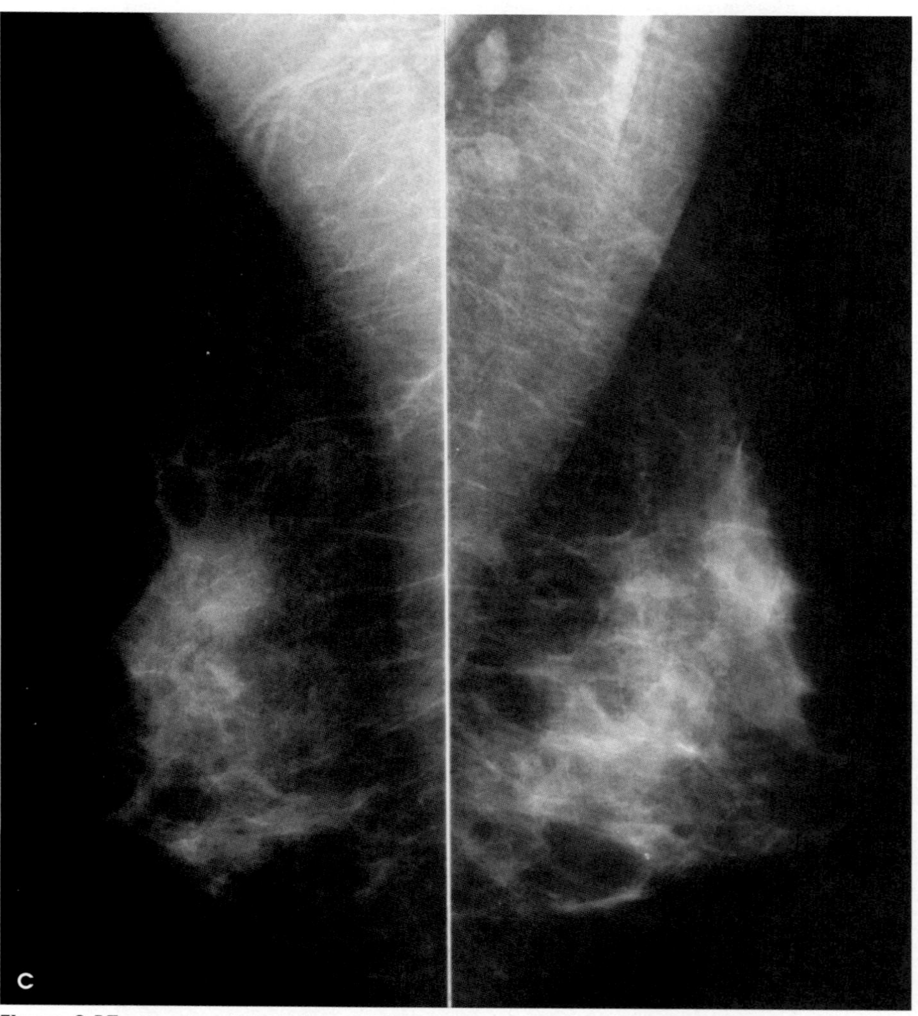

Figure 2.17. (*Continued*) Mediolateral oblique **(C)** views, 2 years prior to **(B)**.

The potential abnormality perceived on the current study is not seen on the prior film. Additional evaluation is indicated.

BI-RADS® category 0: need additional imaging evaluation.

What additional views will you request? Be specific.

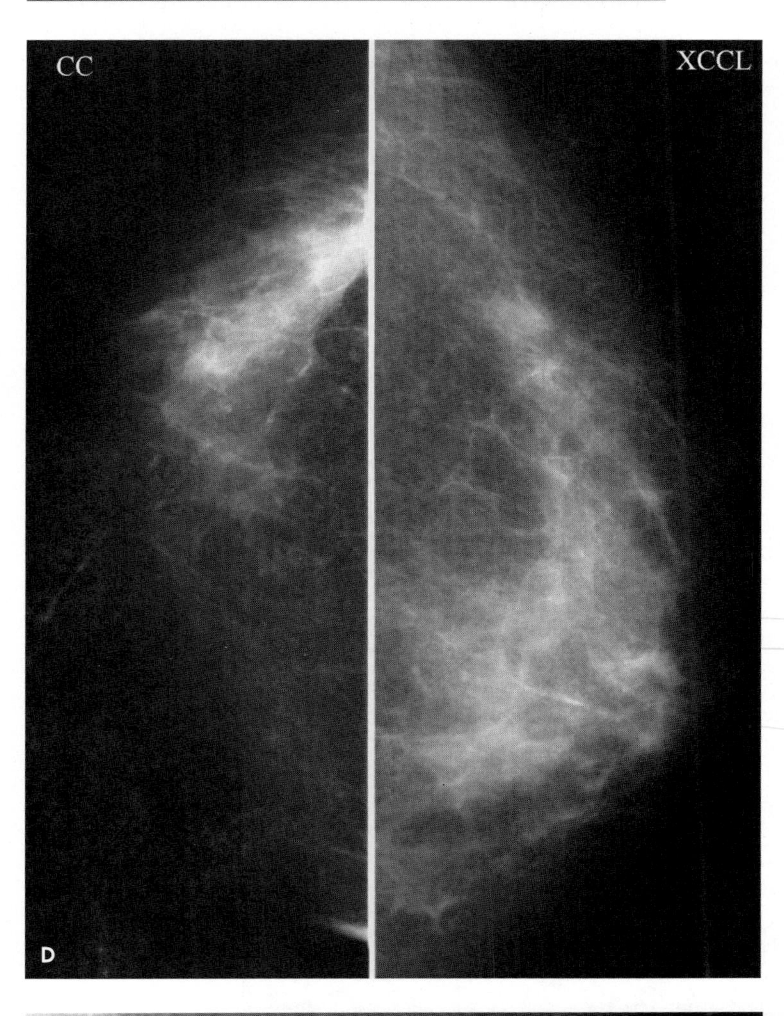

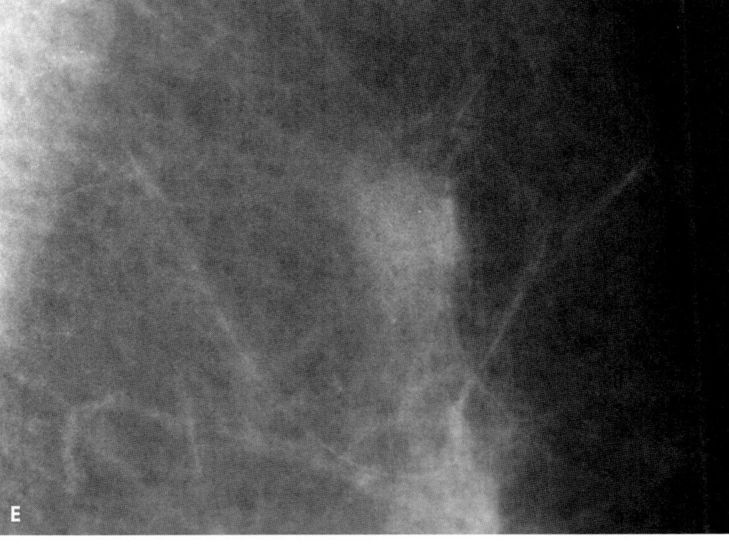

Figure 2.17. (*Continued*) Right craniocaudal and left craniocaudal exaggerated laterally views **(D)** and spot compression view, mediolateral oblique **(E)** projection.

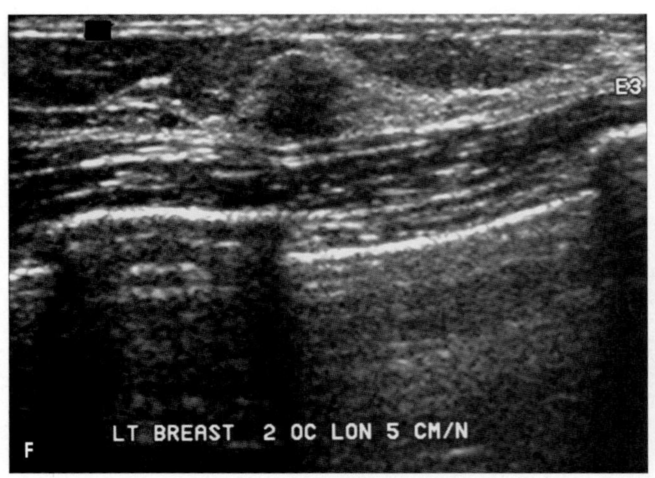

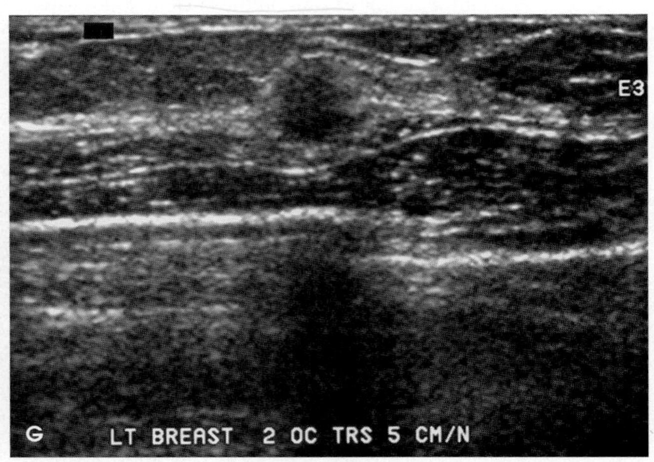

Figure 2.17. (*Continued*) Ultrasound images in longitudinal (LON) **(F)** and transverse (TRS) **(G)** projections of a mass at the 2 o'clock position, 5 cm from the left nipple.

How would you describe the imaging findings? What is your recommendation?

A 1-cm mass is confirmed laterally on the exaggerated craniocaudal views laterally (XCCL). The margins of the mass are indistinct and partially obscured on the mediolateral oblique (MLO) spot compression view. On ultrasound, a vertically oriented, irregular mass with indistinct, spiculated margins and an echogenic rim is imaged, corresponding to the area of mammographic concern. Associated disruption of Cooper ligaments is noted. With the patient supine, this mass is directly on the pectoral fascia and muscle. A developing solid mass with the described imaging features on a post- or perimenopausal woman requires biopsy.

BI-RADS® category 4: suspicious abnormality; biopsy should be considered. Rather than just consider it, a biopsy is done.

An invasive mammary carcinoma is reported on the ultrasound-guided core biopsy. A 0.9-cm, grade II invasive mammary carcinoma, apocrine type with associated intermediate-grade ductal carcinoma in situ, is diagnosed on the lumpectomy specimen. No metastatic disease is diagnosed in three excised sentinel lymph nodes [pT1b, pN0(sn)(i−), pMX; Stage I].

Apocrine carcinomas represent less than 1% of all breast cancers and usually present as a mass that is detected mammographically or clinically. The lesions are characterized by the presence of apocrine cells. Some of these cells are characterized by the presence of an eosinophilic granular cytoplasm, often localized to the apical portion of cells, and cells with foamy cytoplasm filled with small vacuoles. The presence of gross cystic disease fluid protein, GCDFP-15, characterizes both benign and malignant apocrine differentiation.

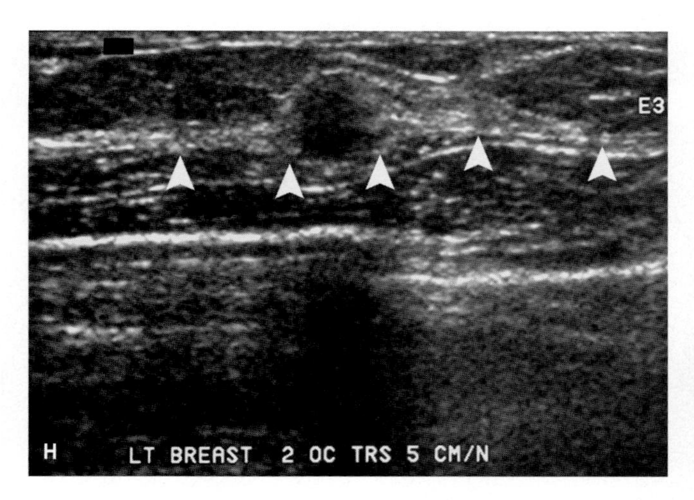

Figure 2.17. (*Continued*) Ultrasound image **(H)** in transverse (TRS) projection of a mass at the 2 o'clock position, 5 cm from the left nipple. With the patient in the supine position the mass is closely apposed to the deep pectoral fascia (*arrowheads*). As the patient is imaged and the mass is compressed, mass effect is noted on the deep pectoral fascia.

PATIENT 15

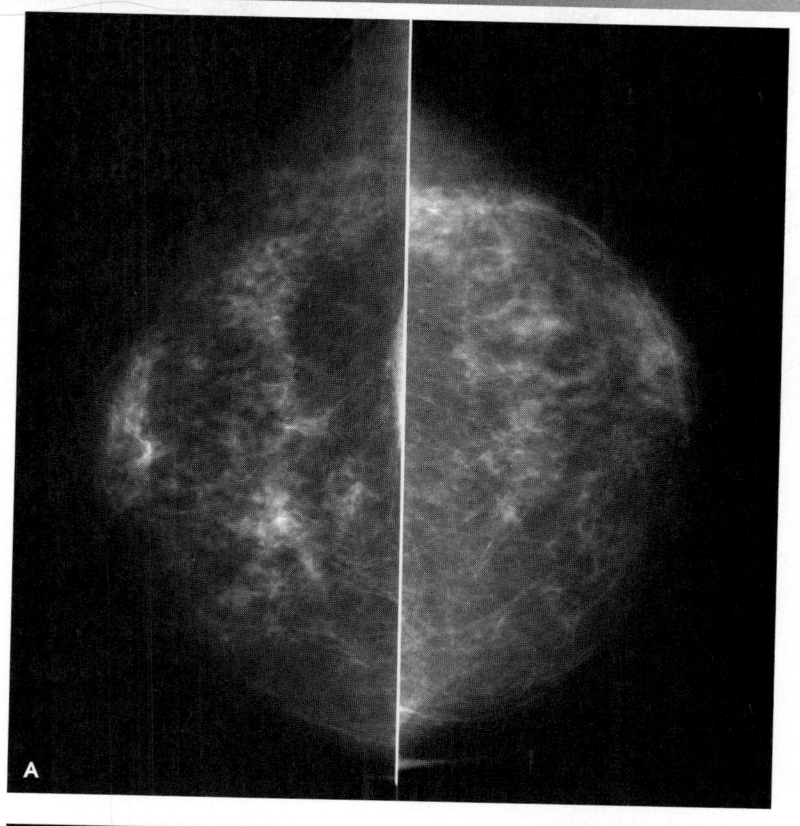

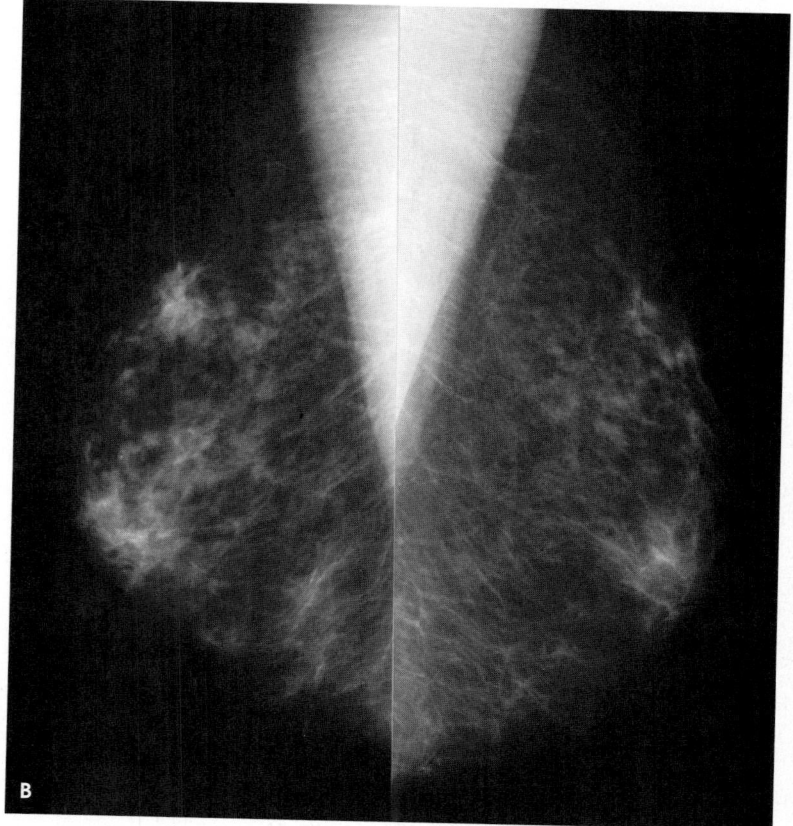

Figure 2.18. Screening study, 54-year-old woman. Craniocaudal **(A)** and mediolateral oblique **(B)** views.

What do you think?
Is this mammogram normal, possibly abnormal or definitely abnormal?

Review the images systematically. Do you see a potential mass? Split the craniocaudal (CC) and mediolateral (MLO) views into thirds and go back and forth between the right and left breasts (Fig. 2.18C, D). Does something catch your eye medially and superiorly in the CC and MLO views of the right breast, respectively? Although this is of concern, and it is in a comparable location on the two projections, it appears more spread out and less dense on the CC view (Fig. 2D). With what degree of certainty can you say this is normal or abnormal? How would you dictate the report? Prior films may be helpful. If these are not available, or this represents a change, why commit yourself when you can obtain spot compression views and, if needed, correlative physical examination and sonography? Depending on the workup, a biopsy may be indicated.

BI-RADS® category 0: need additional imaging evaluation.

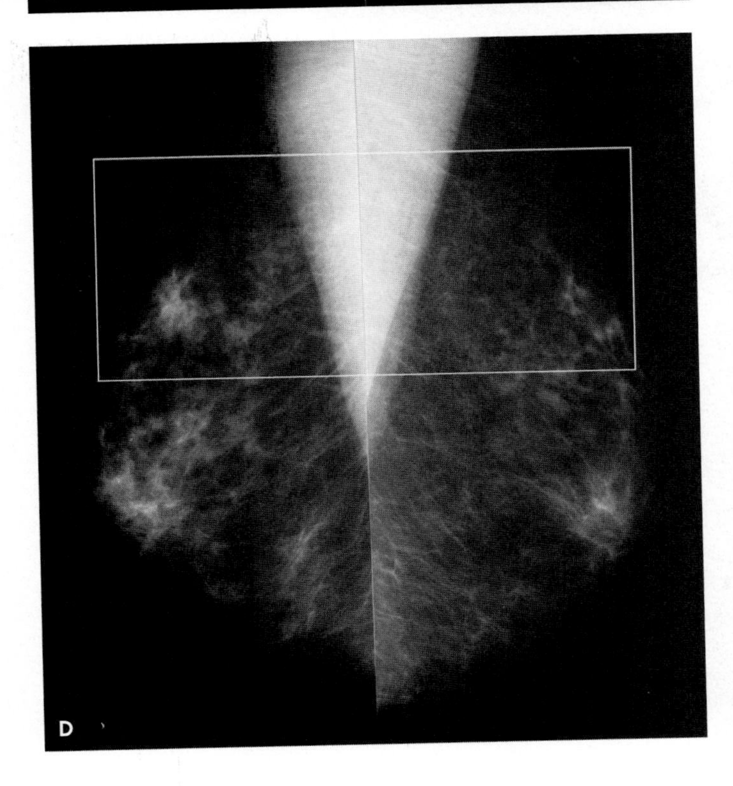

Figure 2.18. (*Continued*) Craniocaudal **(C)** and mediolateral oblique **(D)** views with boxes on the medial and upper thirds of the breasts respectively.

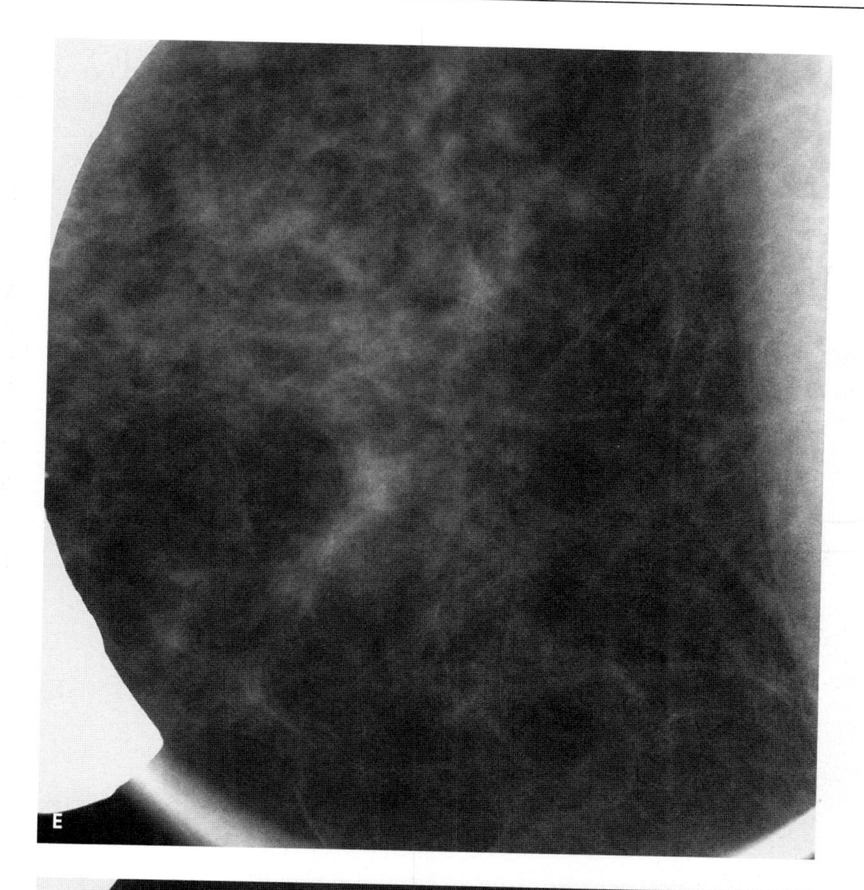

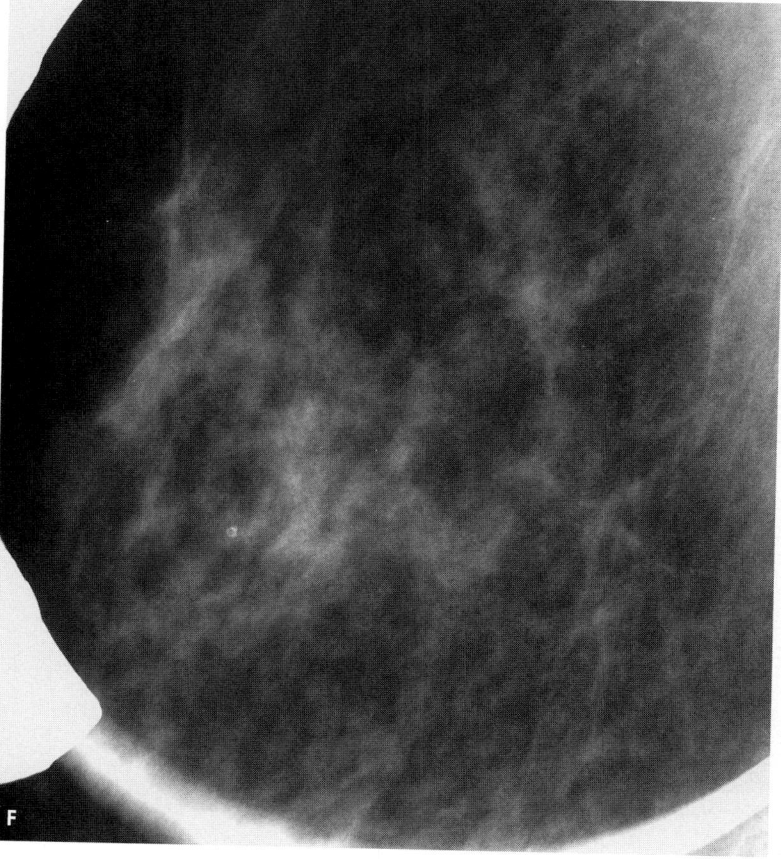

Figure 2.18. (*Continued*) Craniocaudal **(E)** and mediolateral oblique **(F)** spot compression views, right breast.

What do you think now?

Puff goes the magic dragon! Normal glandular tissue is imaged when focal spot compression is applied in the areas of initial concern. Although the additional mammographic images are definitive, correlative physical examination and sonography can be done in the medial quadrants of the right breast for added reassurance.

BI-RADS® category 1: negative. Annual screening mammography is recommended.

PATIENT 16

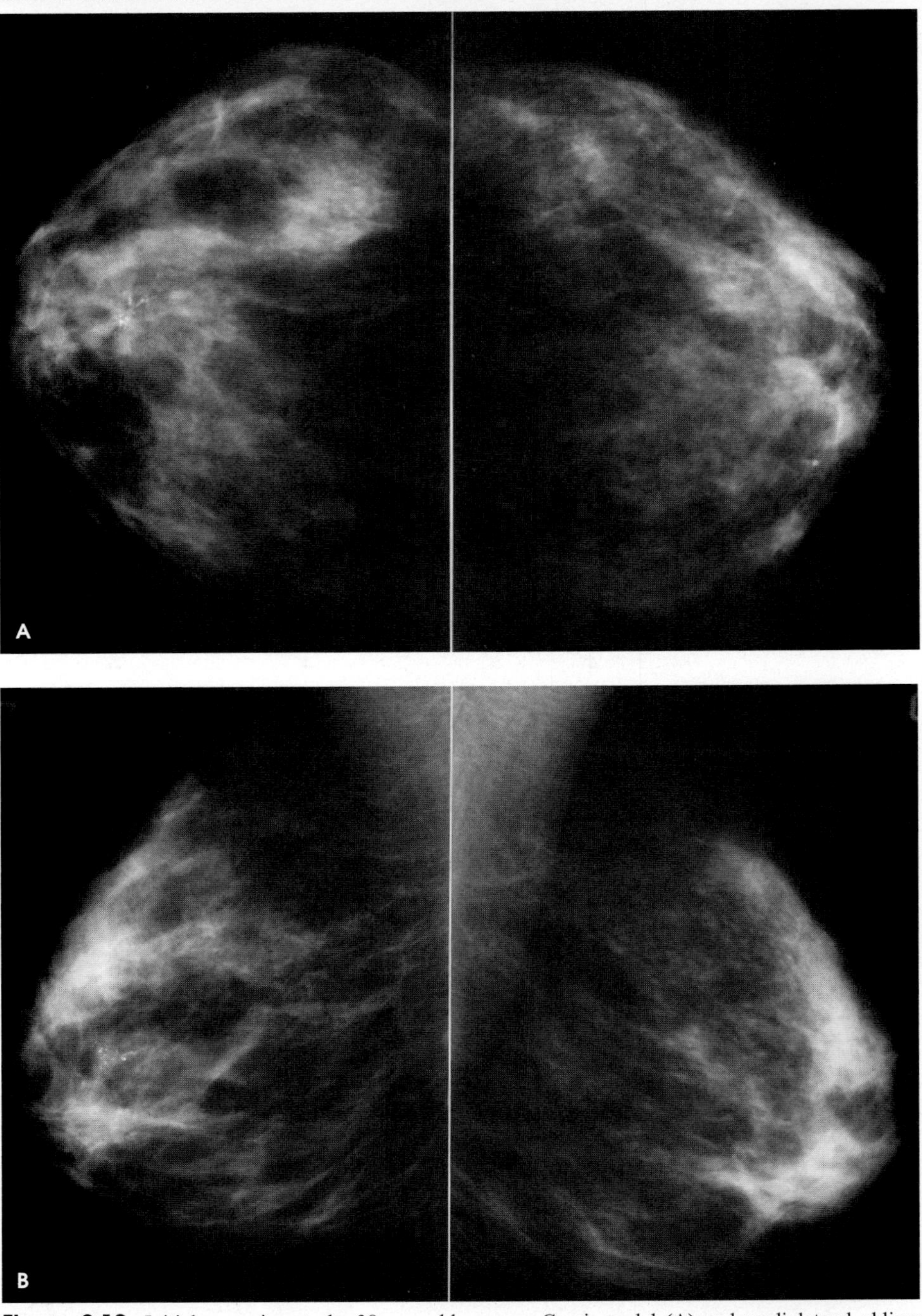

Figure 2.19. Initial screening study, 38-year-old woman. Craniocaudal **(A)** and mediolateral oblique **(B)** views.

Any observations?
What BI-RADS® assessment category would you assign?

Review the images systematically, looking actively for potential lesions. In addition to splitting the craniocaudal (CC) and mediolateral oblique (MLO) views into thirds and evaluating the locations where cancers often develop, look specifically for diffuse changes, masses, distortion, asymmetry, and calcifications. If you focus down with a magnification lens and look specifically for calcifications on every screening mammogram you review, you are unlikely to miss the relevant finding in this patient. Did you see the cluster of calcifications in the right subareolar area? Although the appearance of the calcifications is of concern, with what degree of confidence can you characterize these and their extent? Why not get more information in the form of double spot compression magnification views? If needed, and the patient consents, a biopsy can be done at the time of the magnification views.

BI-RADS® category 0: need additional imaging evaluation.

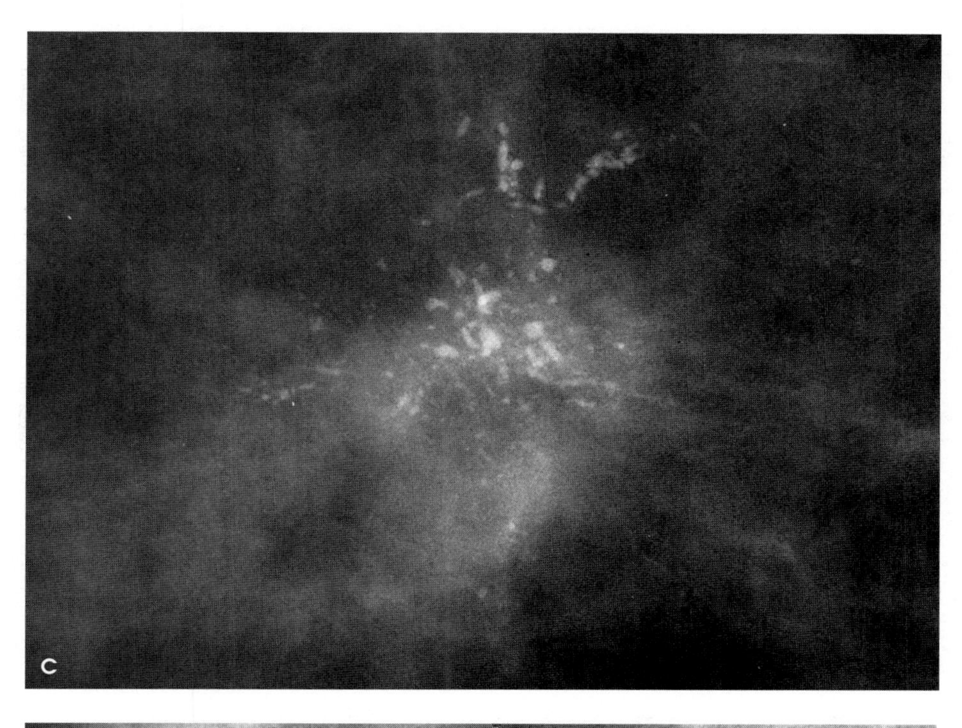

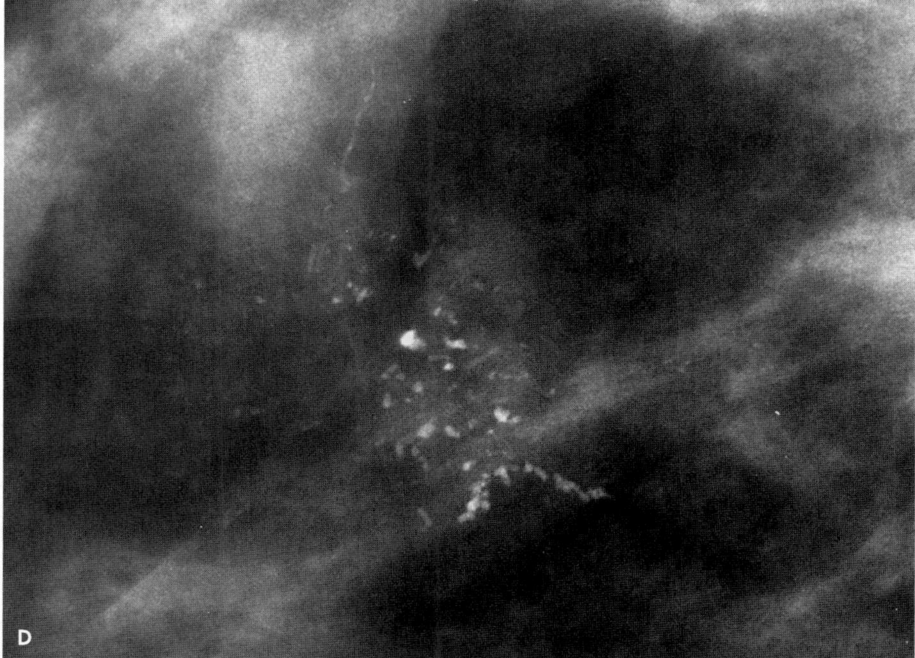

Figure 2.19. Craniocaudal **(C)** and mediolateral oblique **(D)** double spot compression magnification views, right breast.

How would you describe the imaging findings?

On the double spot compression magnification views, the morphology of the calcifications is much better demonstrated, as is the extent of the lesion. The calcifications in this cluster are pleomorphic and variable in density. In addition to some of the calcifications demonstrating linear orientation, others are linear. The borders of some of the linear calcifications are irregular and there are associated clefts. This is likely to represent ductal carcinoma in situ with central necrosis. There is an associated density such that gross or microscopic invasive ductal carcinoma may be present. Armed with high-quality magnification views, our confidence in the diagnosis and the appropriate recommendation is greatly enhanced. A succinct, definitive report can be generated.

BI-RADS® category 5: Highly suggestive of malignancy; appropriate action should be taken. Appropriate action, in the form of an imaging guided biopsy, is undertaken following completion of the magnification views.

A high-nuclear-grade ductal carcinoma in situ with central necrosis is diagnosed on the core samples. This diagnosis is confirmed at the time of the lumpectomy, and no invasion is identified. No sentinel lymph node biopsy is done [pTis(DCIS), pNX, pMX; Stage 0].

PATIENT 17

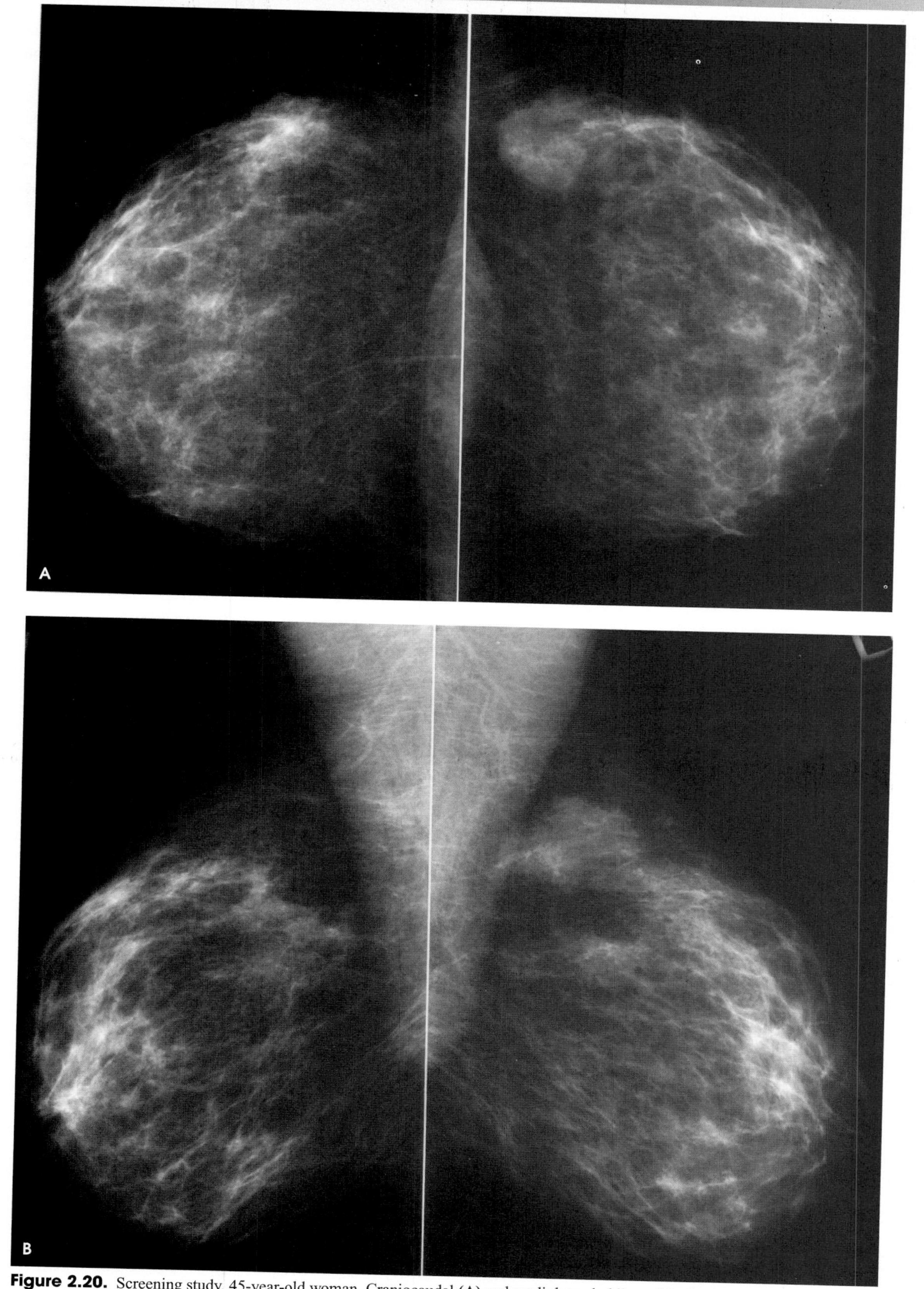

Figure 2.20. Screening study, 45-year-old woman. Craniocaudal **(A)** and mediolateral oblique **(B)** views.

What is the primary observation?

A focal area of parenchymal asymmetry is present in the upper outer quadrant of the left breast. It is of comparable size and density and in the same approximate distance from the nipple on the two projections, but there is fat interspersed in the glandular tissue. In most patients, focal parenchymal asymmetry is a normal variant. Progressive development of focal parenchymal asymmetry can be benign, presumably related to hormonal variations.

What additional information would you like?

A good history is important. Has the patient had any breast surgery (e.g., a comparable area of tissue excised from the right breast, or does this finding reflect fat necrosis postsurgery)? Is there any history of trauma to this site (e.g., hematoma)? Estrogen use? Presumably, if the patient had any focal tenderness, erythema, skin dimpling, or discoloration limited to this site, she would have been scheduled for a diagnostic evaluation or your technologist would have indicated this on the woman's history sheet.

Comparison with prior studies is critical. If the area of focal parenchymal asymmetry represents a change, or if no prior studies are available for comparison, spot compression views and ultrasound with correlative physical examination are recommended to exclude an underlying malignancy. If normal tissue is imaged on spot compression views and ultrasound, and there is no corresponding palpable abnormality on physical examination, no further intervention is recommended. Magnetic resonance imaging may also provide helpful information, particularly in high-risk patients. If concerns remain following the diagnostic evaluation, an imaging-guided biopsy can be undertaken. Fibrosis or pseudoangiomatous stromal hyperplasia (PASH) is often the diagnosis on core biopsies done through these areas.

What is your differential at this point?

Differential considerations include normal variant, hormone replacement therapy effect, asymmetry secondary to prior surgical excision of the corresponding tissue in the right breast, focal fibrosis, pseudoangiomatous stromal hyperplasia (PASH), posttraumatic changes (evolving hematoma; fat necrosis), mastitis, fibroadenolipoma (hamartoma), invasive ductal carcinoma not otherwise specified, invasive lobular carcinoma, and lymphoma.

In this patient, the area is unchanged from prior studies (not shown).

This mammogram can be categorized as BI-RADS® category 1: negative. BI-RADS® category 2: benign finding is used if the observation is described in the report. Annual screening mammography is recommended.

PATIENT 18

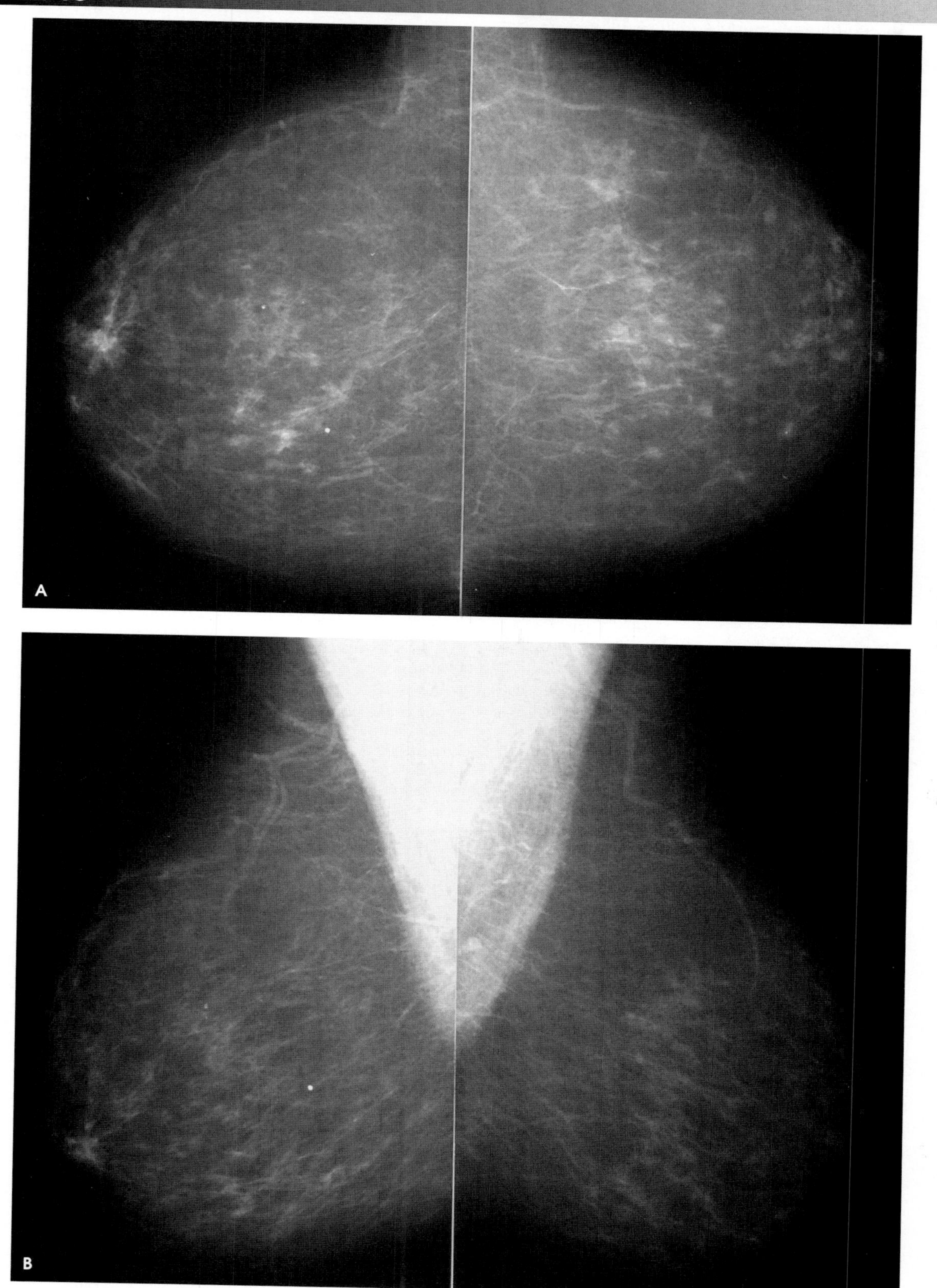

Figure 2.21. Screening study, 65-year-old woman. Craniocaudal **(A)** and mediolateral oblique **(B)** views.

What do you think?
Is this a normal mammogram, or do you think additional evaluation is indicated?

Review the images systematically. Look for specific findings, including diffuse changes, masses, distortion, asymmetry, and calcifications. Focus your attention on smaller amounts of tissue by splitting the craniocaudal (CC) and mediolateral oblique (MLO) views into thirds (Figs. 2.1 and 2.2). Review those areas where breast cancers commonly develop, specifically the fatty stripe of tissue between pectoral muscle and glandular tissue on MLO views, the superior cone of tissue on MLO views, medial tissue on CC views, the fat–glandular interfaces, and the subareolar areas (Fig. 2.3). Focus down with a magnification lens, particularly when looking for small masses, distortion, and clusters of calcifications. Is there a potential mass in this patient? Did you notice the right subareolar area? With what degree of confidence can you characterize this potential finding, and how definitive can you be in determining its significance? Prior films will be helpful, as will a surgical history. If prior films are not available (and the patient has no history of surgery), additional imaging is needed to determine the significance of this finding.

BI-RADS® category 0: need additional imaging evaluation.

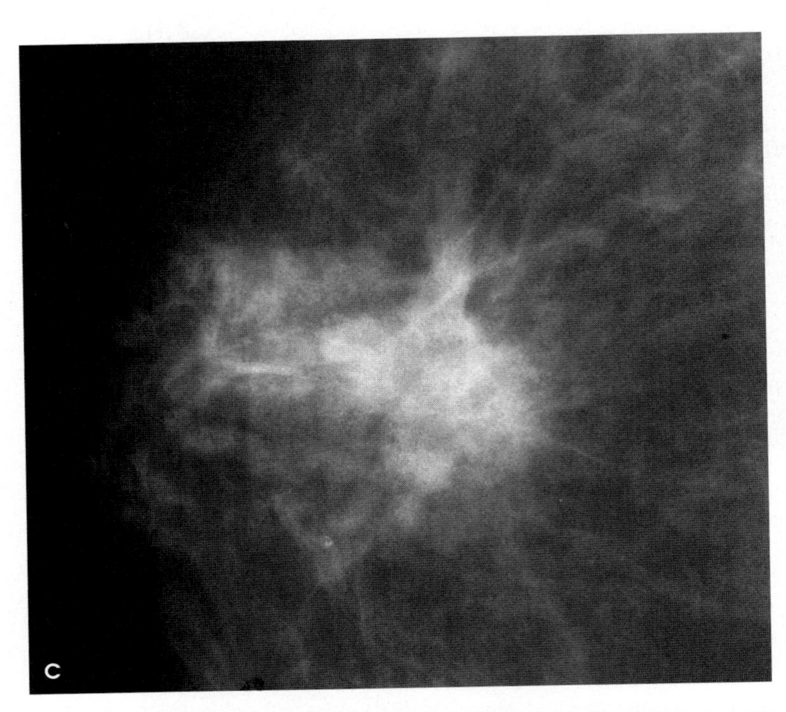

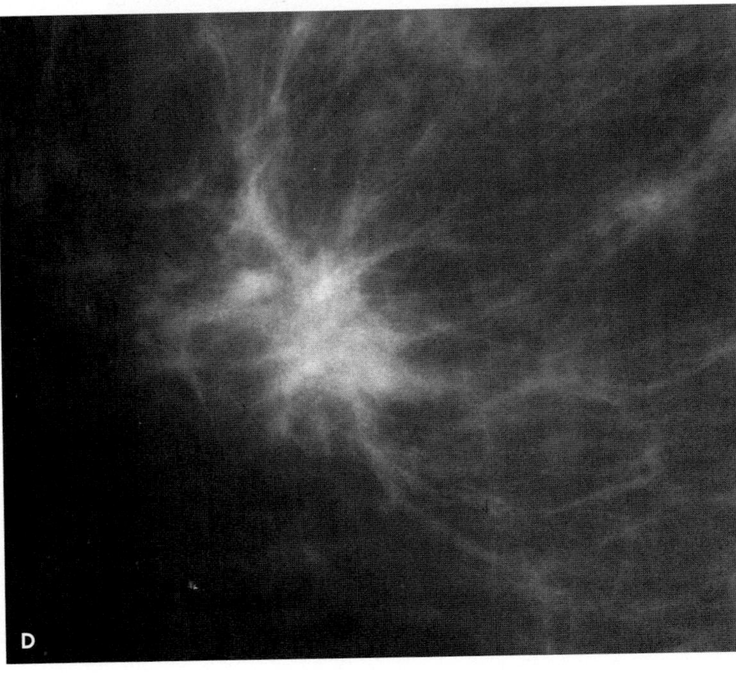

Figure 2.21. (*Continued*) Craniocaudal **(C)** and mediolateral oblique **(D)** spot compression views, right subareolar area.

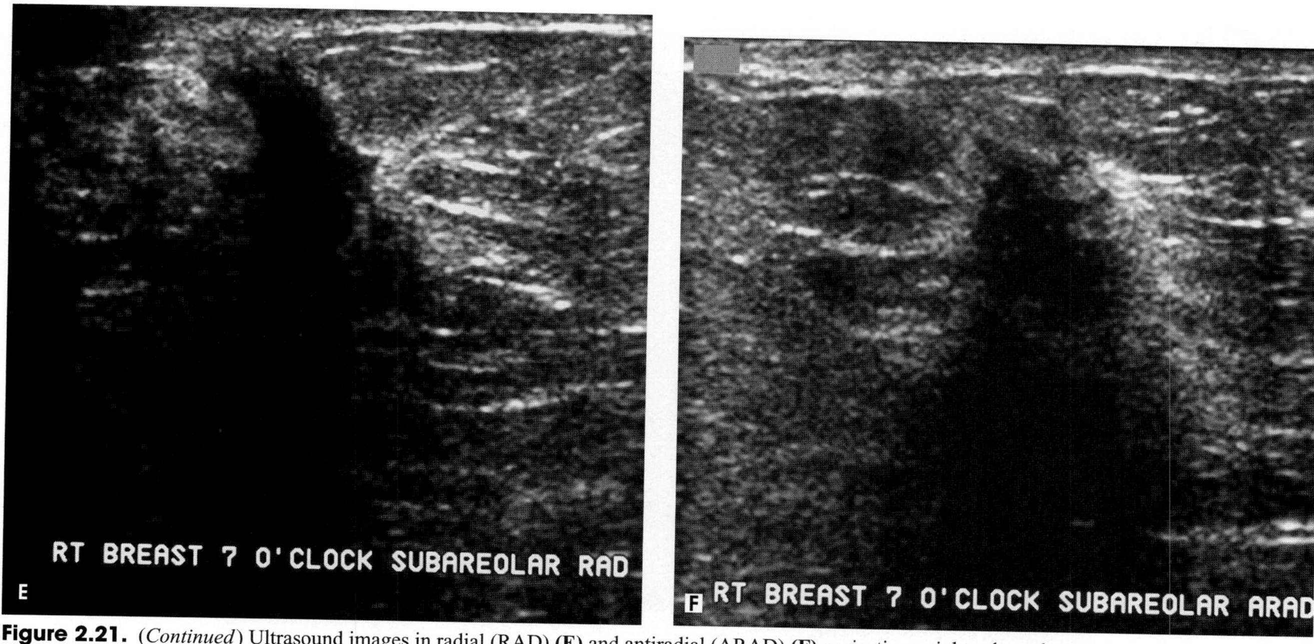

Figure 2.21. (*Continued*) Ultrasound images in radial (RAD) **(E)** and antiradial (ARAD) **(F)** projections, right subareolar area.

How would you describe the findings, and what is your recommendation?

Spot compression views of the right subareolar area confirm the presence of a 2-cm mass. The patient has no history of previous breast surgery. An irregular, vertically oriented, hypoechoic mass with spiculated and angular margins and associated shadowing is imaged in the right subareolar area on ultrasound. These findings, in a 65-year-old woman with no history of surgery at this site, require biopsy. The additional views are helpful in establishing the presence of a lesion and demonstrating the morphologic features of the lesion.

BI-RADS® category 4: Suspicious abnormality; biopsy should be considered.

Rather than just consider it, a biopsy is done. An invasive lobular carcinoma is diagnosed, following ultrasound-guided core biopsies. A 2.2-cm invasive lobular carcinoma is confirmed at the time of the lumpectomy. Lymphovascular space involvement is present and metastatic disease is found in the sentinel lymph node, so an axillary dissection is undertaken. Three of 12 lymph nodes have metastatic disease with extracapsular extension in one of the three positive lymph nodes (pT2, pN1a, pMX; Stage IIB).

What is the significance of lymphovascular space involvement?

Lymphovascular space involvement is described in approximately 15% of patients with invasive ductal carcinoma. It has been described as an unfavorable prognostic finding, particularly in node-negative patients treated with either mastectomy or lumpectomy. The significance in patients with positive axillary lymph nodes (as in our current patient) is not clear. Extracapsular extension has also been described as an unfavorable prognostic factor.

What is the single most important prognostic factor in women with an invasive breast cancer diagnosis?

The presence of metastatic disease in axillary lymph nodes is the single most important prognostic factor, and there is a direct correlation between the number of positive lymph nodes and disease-free survival, as well as mortality. In patients with tumors <2 cm in size, Carter et al. reported overall 5-year survival rates of 96.3% in patients with negative lymph nodes, 87.4% for patients with one to three positive axillary lymph nodes, and 66% for patients with four or more positive axillary lymph nodes. In the sixth edition of the American Joint Committee on Cancer (AJCC) Staging Manual, the pathologic status of node-positive patients has been revised to reflect the prognostic significance of the number of positive lymph nodes: pN1a for patients with one to three positive axillary lymph nodes; pN2a for patients with four to nine positive axillary lymph nodes, and pN3a for patients with 10 or more positive axillary lymph nodes.

PATIENT 19

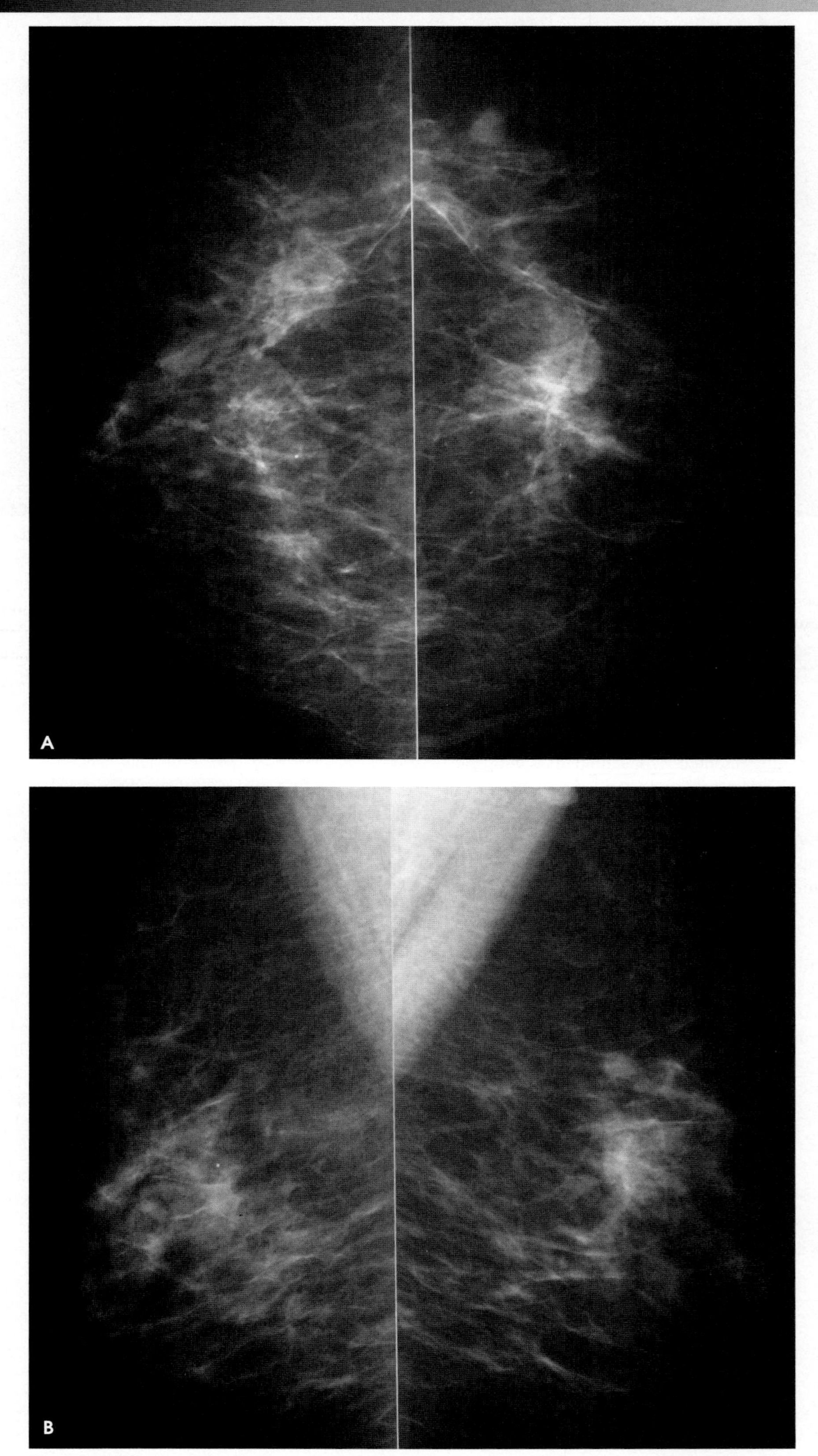

Figure 2.22. Screening study, 40-year-old woman. Craniocaudal **(A)** and mediolateral oblique **(B)** views.

What do you think?
Would you agree with a BI-RADS® assessment category 1 or 2 for this mammogram?

Did you review this study for technical adequacy as your starting point? Positioning and compression are not optimal. There is insufficient pectoral muscle on the mediolateral oblique (MLO) views. Although it is thick in the axillary region, pectoral muscle should be seen to the level of the nipple and it should have a convex anterior margin. Given the triangular shape of the muscle in this patient, several things went wrong during positioning. It is likely that an incorrect angle of obliquity was selected, the muscles were not relaxed, and the breasts were not adequately mobilized medially (or if they were, the patient pulled out during positioning).

On the craniocaudal (CC) views, a significant amount of posterior tissue is excluded from the images. In determining whether an adequate amount of tissue has been included on the CC views, look for pectoral muscle posteriorly or for cleavage medially. If neither of these is seen, measure the posterior nipple line (PNL) on the MLO (and remember, in this patient, positioning on the MLO views is not optimal, so the PNL measurement is not an optimal measure of the amount of tissue this patient has) and compare it to that measured on the CC views (Fig. 2.4E, F). The PNL measurement on the CC view should be within 1 cm of that measured on the MLO view. It is not in this patient. Also, notice the relationship of the mass to the edge of the film on the MLO view and compare it to that seen on the CC view.

There is inadequate separation of tissue, particularly on the MLO views, consistent with suboptimal compression. Additionally, if you evaluate the left MLO and specifically send your eyes looking for motion, you will notice blurring of tissue anteriorly; an additional sign of suboptimal compression. Blurring can tomogram small spiculated masses and clusters of calcification off the image; however, it often goes undetected because we do not specifically assess and insist on high image quality. As with subtle findings of breast cancer, blurring will go undetected unless you recognize how much it can limit your ability to perceive important lesions and you focus your attention on looking for it before attempting to look for potential lesions.

Did you notice anything else, and what would you like to do next?

How about the mass in the lateral aspect of the left breast? On the MLO view, it is likely to be on the upper cone of tissue. As a further indication of how much tissue is missing on the CC view, notice the relationship of this lesion to the edge of the film on the CC and the MLO view. Momentarily you might think that what you see on the CC view is not what you see on the MLO view; however, if you measure back from the nipple, the lesion is at approximately the same distance from the nipple. Based on the technical limitations of the study alone, the patient needs to be called back. With respect to the mass noted in the left breast, comparison studies may be helpful. If the mass is decreasing in size, or has been previously evaluated, it may not require additional evaluation at this time. If there are no prior studies, or these are unavailable, or if this represents an interval change, additional evaluation is indicated.

BI-RADS® category 0: need additional imaging evaluation.

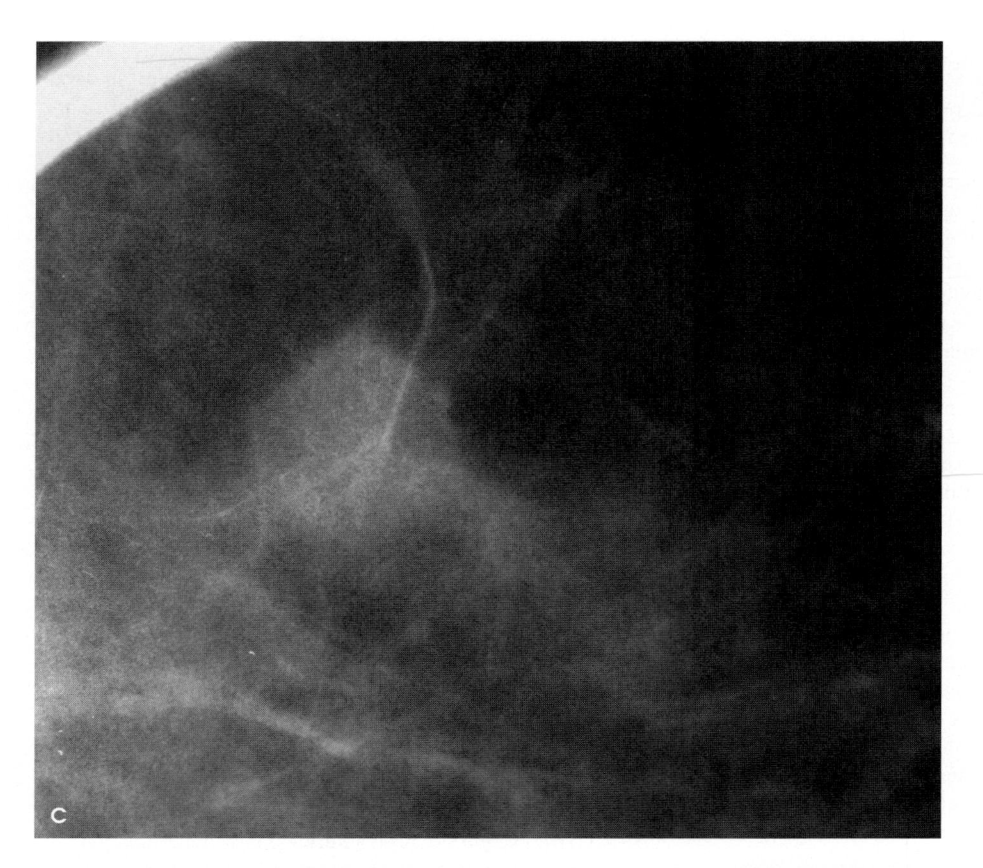

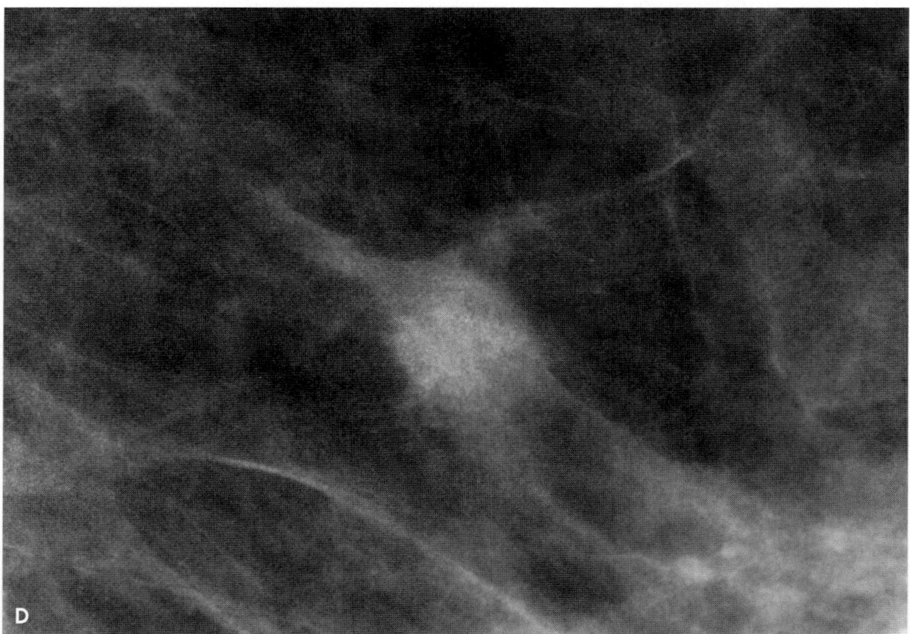

Figure 2.22. *(Continued)* Craniocaudal **(C)** and mediolateral oblique **(D)** spot compression views, left breast. Additional views to address described technical limitations are not shown.

What do you think now?
In a 40-year-old woman, what differential would you consider based on the mammographic findings alone?

A 1-cm mass with indistinct margins is confirmed on the spot compression views. At this point, in a 40-year-old woman, benign differential considerations are extensive and include an intramammary lymph node, cyst, fibroadenoma (complex fibroadenoma, tubular adenoma), papilloma, focal fibrosis, pseudoangiomatous stromal hyperplasia (PASH), sclerosing adenosis, phyllodes tumor, or a granular cell tumor. In the malignant category, one would consider an invasive ductal carcinoma not otherwise specified, medullary carcinoma, although possible mucinous and papillary carcinomas are usually diagnosed in postmenopausal women, a metastatic lesion (in patients with a known malignancy), and adenoid cystic carcinoma. Invasive lobular carcinomas do not typically present as a round-oval mass.

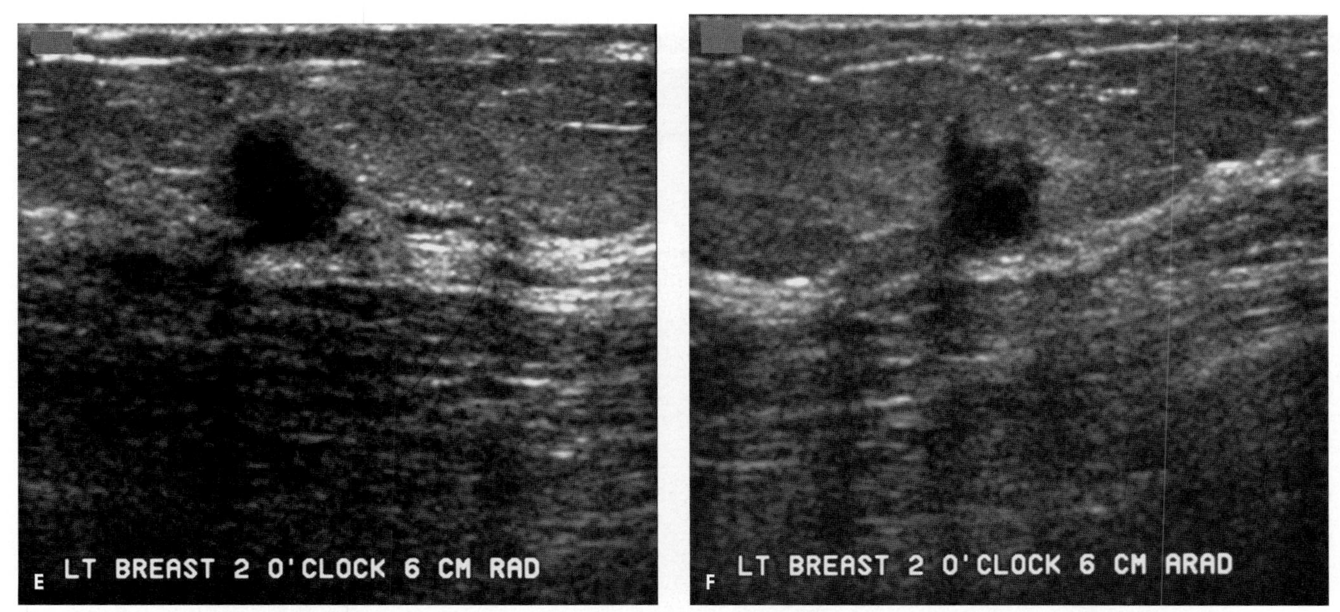

Figure 2.22. (*Continued*) Ultrasound images in radial (RAD) **(E)** and antiradial (ARAD) **(F)** projections, upper outer quadrant, left breast.

How would you describe the ultrasound finding? What is your recommendation?

An irregular, vertically oriented, hypoechoic mass with angular and spiculated margins is imaged at the 2 o'clock position, 6 cm from the left nipple. Given the indistinct margins mammographically, and the sonographic appearance of this lesion, a biopsy is indicated.

BI-RADS® category 4: Suspicious abnormality; biopsy should be considered.

A biopsy is done. An invasive ductal carcinoma is diagnosed, following an ultrasound-guided core biopsy. A 0.8-cm grade III invasive ductal carcinoma is diagnosed following the lumpectomy, and two excised sentinel lymph nodes are negative for metastatic disease [pT1b, pN0(sn)(i−), pMX; Stage I].

PATIENT 20

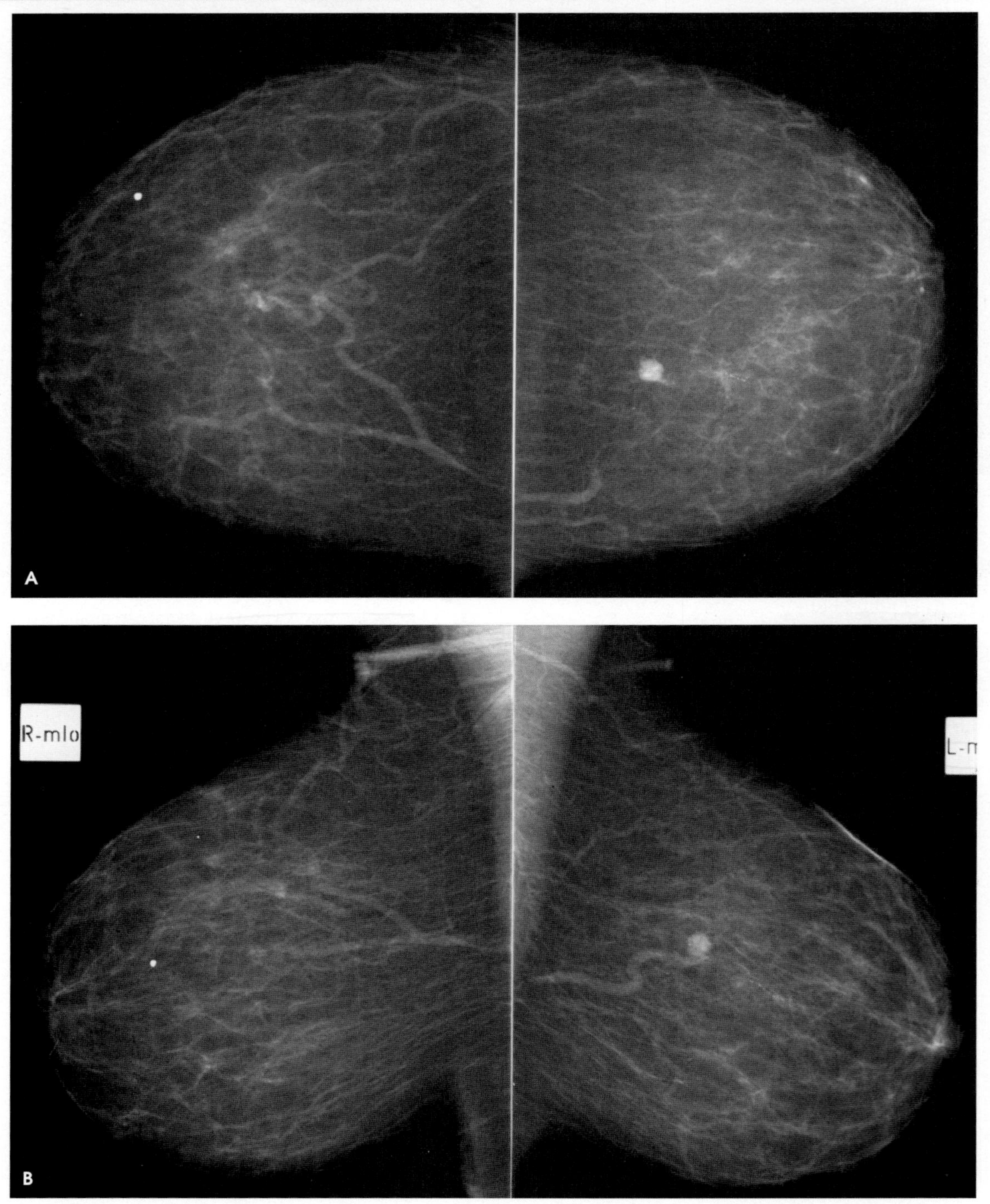

Figure 2.23. Screening study, 58-year-old woman. Craniocaudal **(A)** and mediolateral oblique **(B)** views.

What do you think, and what BI-RADS® assessment category would you assign?

A round mass with an adjacent area of calcifications is identified in the left breast. Although a malignancy is suspected, additional evaluation is beneficial in better characterizing the extent of the lesion and the morphology of the calcifications.

BI-RADS® category 0: need additional imaging evaluation.

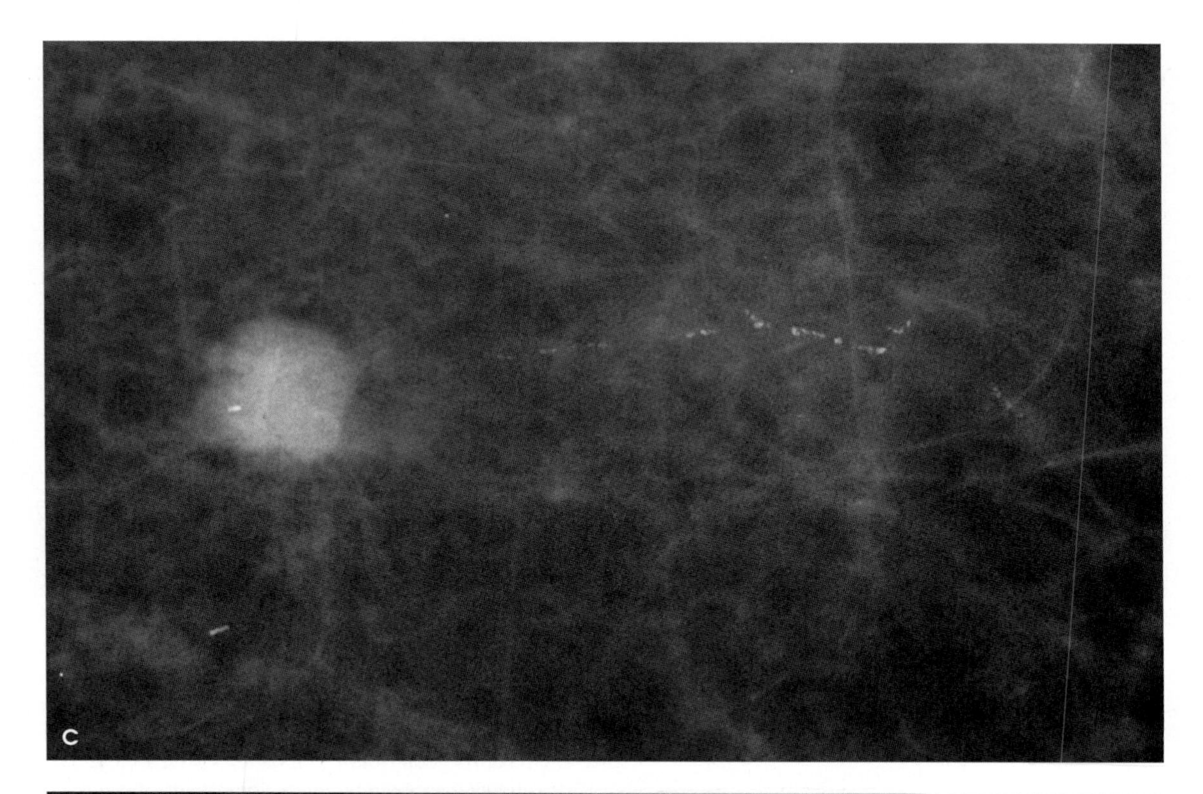

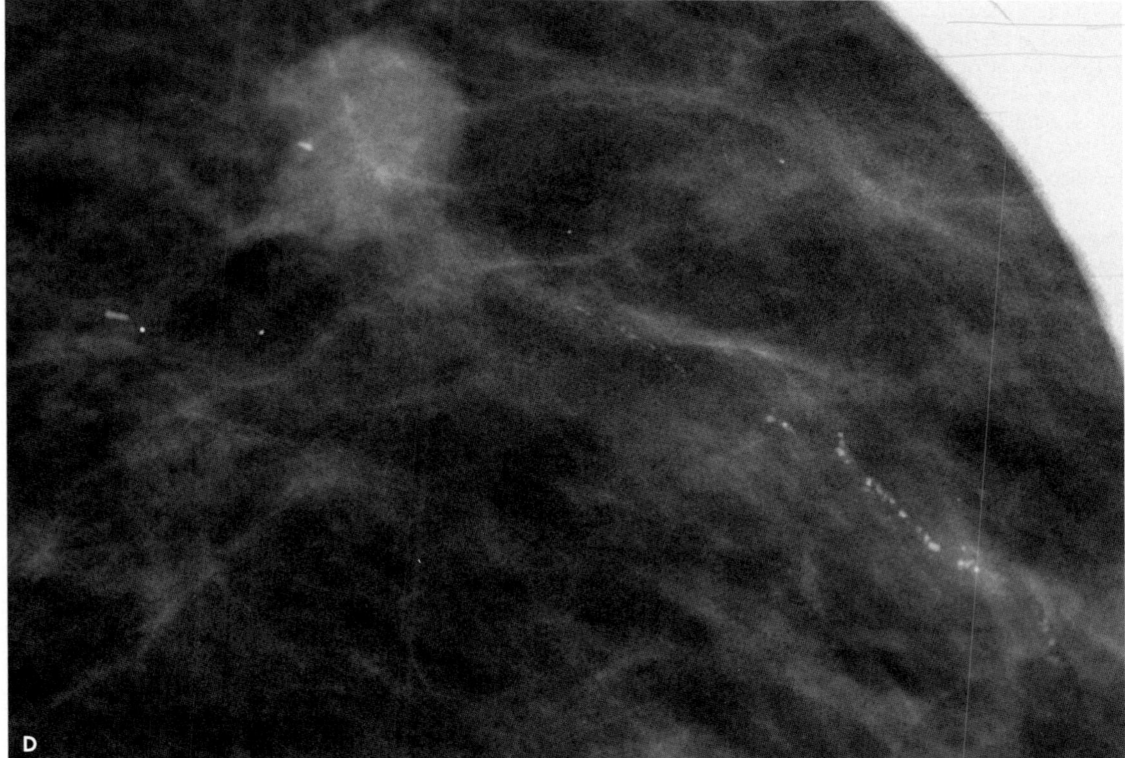

Figure 2.23. (*Continued*) Craniocaudal **(C)** and mediolateral oblique **(D)** double spot compression magnification views, left breast.

How would you describe the findings?

Double spot compression views demonstrate a 1-cm round mass with microlobulated, indistinct and spiculated margins. Predominantly round calcifications demonstrating a linear (branching) orientation extend for approximately 3 cm anterior to the mass.

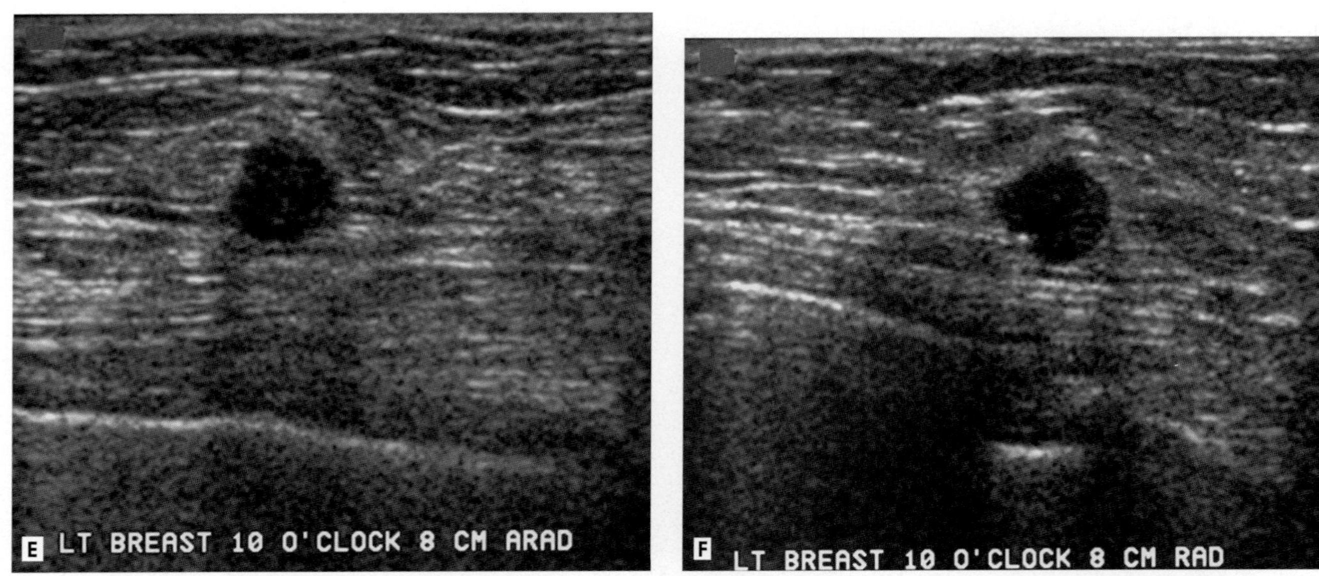

Figure 2.23. (*Continued*) Ultrasound images in radial (RAD) **(E)** and antiradial (ARAD) **(F)** projections in the upper inner quadrant of the left breast.

How would you describe the findings?

On ultrasound, a round mass with indistinct margins, an echogenic halo, minimal posterior enhancement, and disruption of Cooper ligaments is imaged at the 10 o'clock position, 8 cm from the left nipple. Did you notice the calcification in the mass mammographically and on ultrasound? The calcification noted in the mass mammographically on both projections is also identified on the ultrasound (Fig. 2.23G). However, the linearly oriented calcifications cannot be identified with certainty on ultrasound.

Based on the imaging finding, what is your diagnosis (don't just say "cancer"; be specific)?

The mass, in conjunction with the calcifications, is almost pathognomonic for an invasive ductal carcinoma (mass) with an associated ductal carcinoma in situ (calcifications). An invasive mammary carcinoma is diagnosed following an ultrasound-guided core biopsy of the mass. As is our routine on patients with a breast cancer diagnosis following an imaging-guided biopsy, magnetic resonance imaging is obtained. This further assesses the ipsilateral breast for unsuspected multifocal or multicentric disease, as well as the status of the contralateral breast.

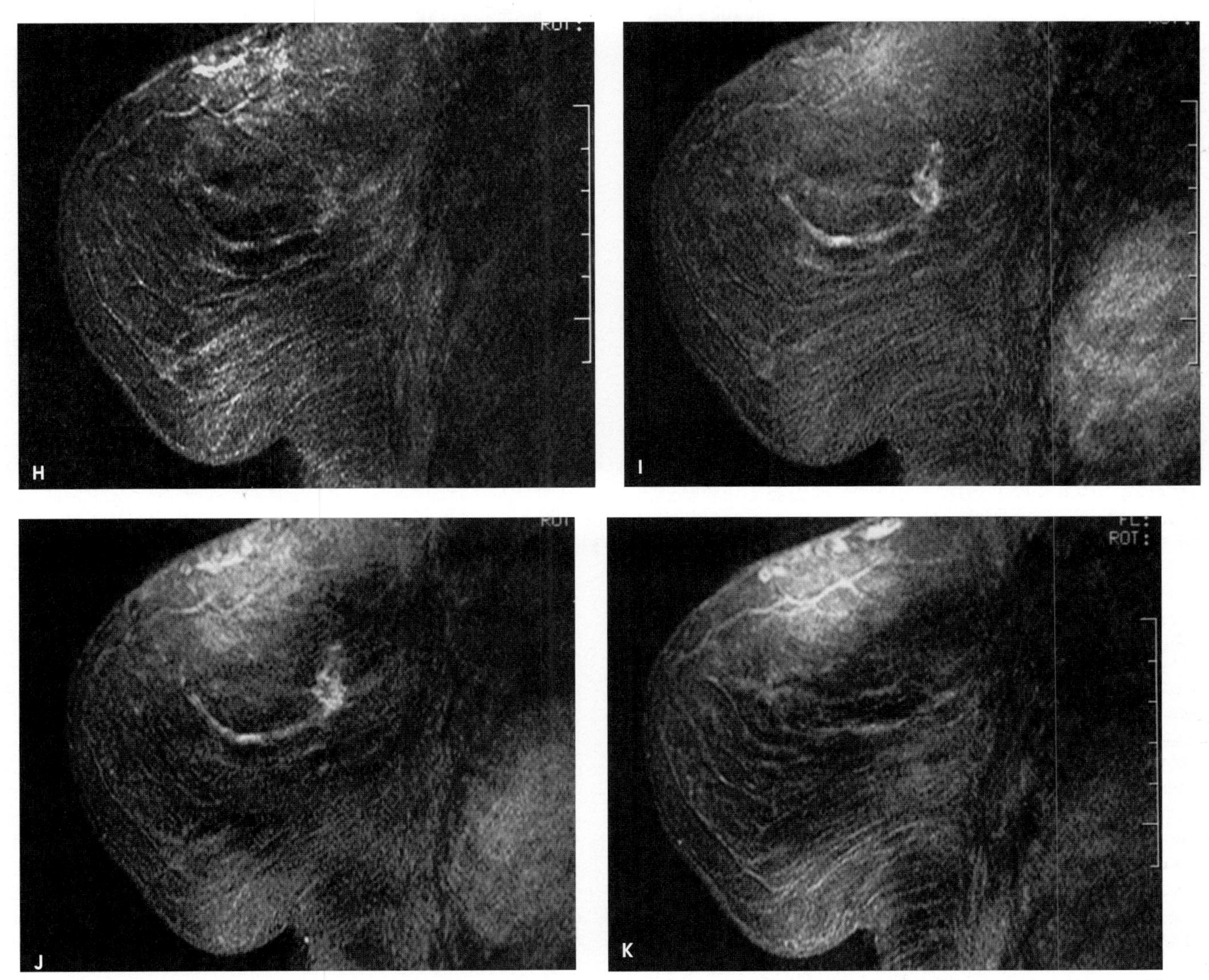

Figure 2.23. *(Continued)* T1-weighted, sagittal image **(H)** left breast, precontrast. T1-weighted, sagittal image **(I)**, left breast, same tabletop position as shown in **(H)**, 1 minute following contrast administration. T1-weighted, sagittal image **(J)**, left breast, same tabletop position as shown in **(H)**, 2 minutes following contrast administration. T1-weighted, sagittal image **(K)**, left breast, same tabletop position as shown in **(H)**, 10 minutes following contrast administration.

How would you describe the findings?

The dynamic sequence demonstrates a mass with rapid wash-in and wash-out of contrast, characteristic of malignant lesions. Morphologically, this is an irregular mass with irregular margins and heterogeneous enhancement. Ductal enhancement is present, corresponding to the area of calcifications seen mammographically. No additional lesions are noted in the left breast, and no masses or other abnormal areas of enhancement are seen in the right breast (images not shown).

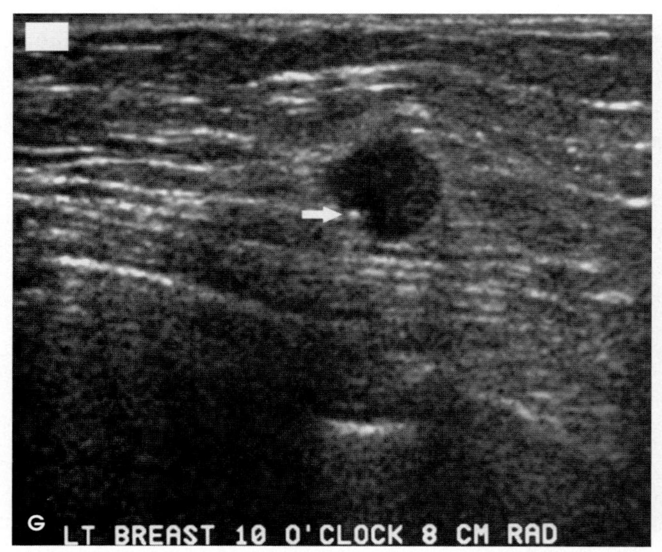

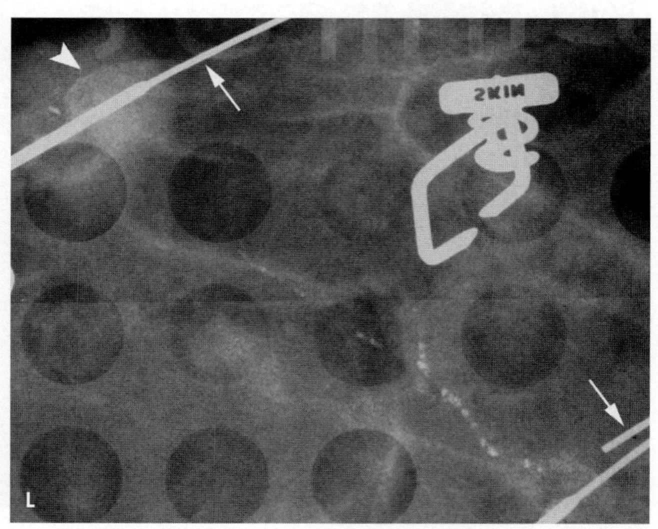

Figure 2.23. (*Continued*) Magnetic resonance image in radial (RAD) projection **(G)** demonstrating the calcification seen mammographically in the mass. Specimen radiograph **(L),** 3× magnification obtained on a dedicated specimen radiography unit.

At the time of the preoperative wire localization, the lesion is bracketed with two wires to assure complete excision of the lesion (i.e., the mass and all calcifications). One of the wires is used to skewer the mass and a second is placed anteriorly through the leading edge of the calcifications. The excised tissue is placed in a plastic container (a Dubin device) and an alphanumeric grid is used to compress the tissue. A radiograph of the specimen is taken to assure excision of the localized lesion(s). In this patient, the mass is seen at the edge of the image (Fig. 2.23L, arrowhead) and the calcifications extending away from the mass are also present. The apparent proximity of the mass to one of the margins on the radiograph is discussed with the surgeon so that additional tissue may be taken.

The Dubin device provides an alphanumeric grid (letters partially seen) with corresponding "holes" so that pins can be placed through the specimen to mark the location of the lesion(s) for the pathologist. Portions of the localizing wires are seen on the radiograph (arrows). Also noted is one of several markers placed by the surgeon intraoperatively to indicate the different margins, thereby orienting the specimen for the pathologist. The marker seen here is the skin marker; additional markers include caudal, cranial, medial, and lateral markers. In addition to these markers used by the surgeon, the pathologist inks the margins so that extension of tumor to the margins can be assessed at the time of histologic evaluation. If tumor is seen extending to the margins, re-excision is usually indicated.

A 1.2-cm invasive mammary carcinoma with apocrine features is reported histologically. Associated high-nuclear-grade ductal carcinoma in situ with central necrosis is present. The sentinel lymph node is normal [pT1c, pN0(sn)(i−), pMX; Stage I].

PATIENT 21

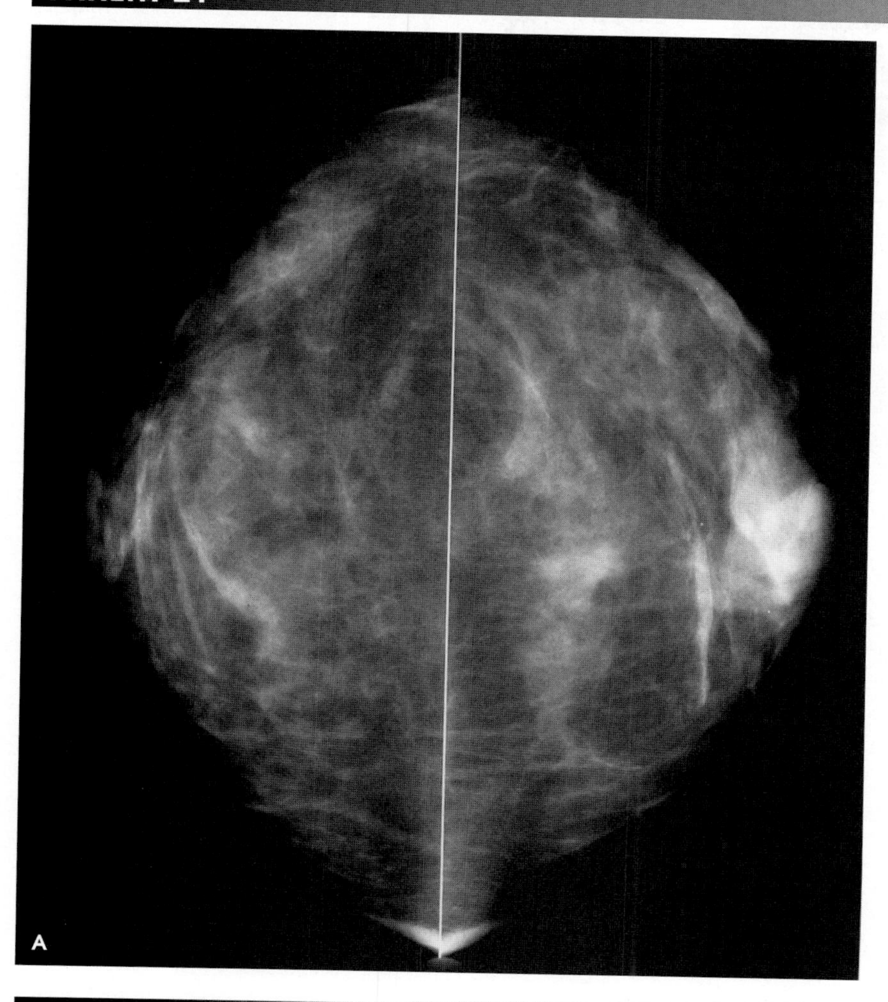

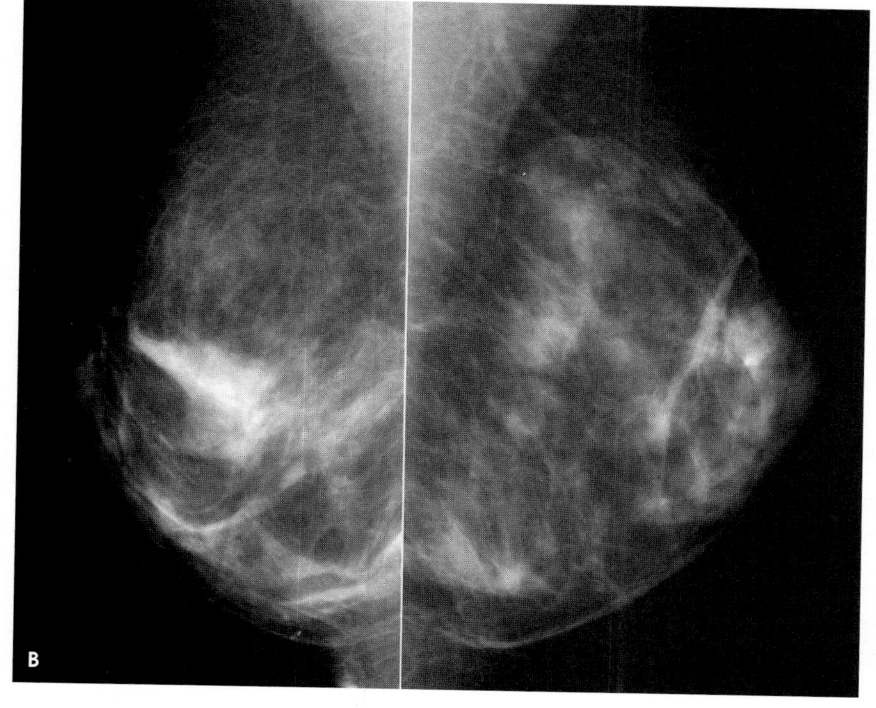

Figure 2.24. Screening study, 44-year-old woman. Craniocaudal **(A)** and mediolateral oblique **(B)** views.

What observations can you make on this patient's mammogram, and what conclusion can you draw? What recommendation would you make?

Pertinent observations include fibrotic bands in the subareolar areas on the craniocaudal views, islands of nonanatomically distributed tissue bilaterally, inferior displacement of tissue with a swirling pattern on the right mediolateral oblique (MLO) view, and skin thickening inferiorly on the left MLO. These findings are common in women following reduction mammoplasty. From a review of her history form, she has had a reduction mammoplasty. No masses or malignant type calcifications are present.

BI-RADS® category 1: negative. Annual screening mammography is recommended.

PATIENT 22

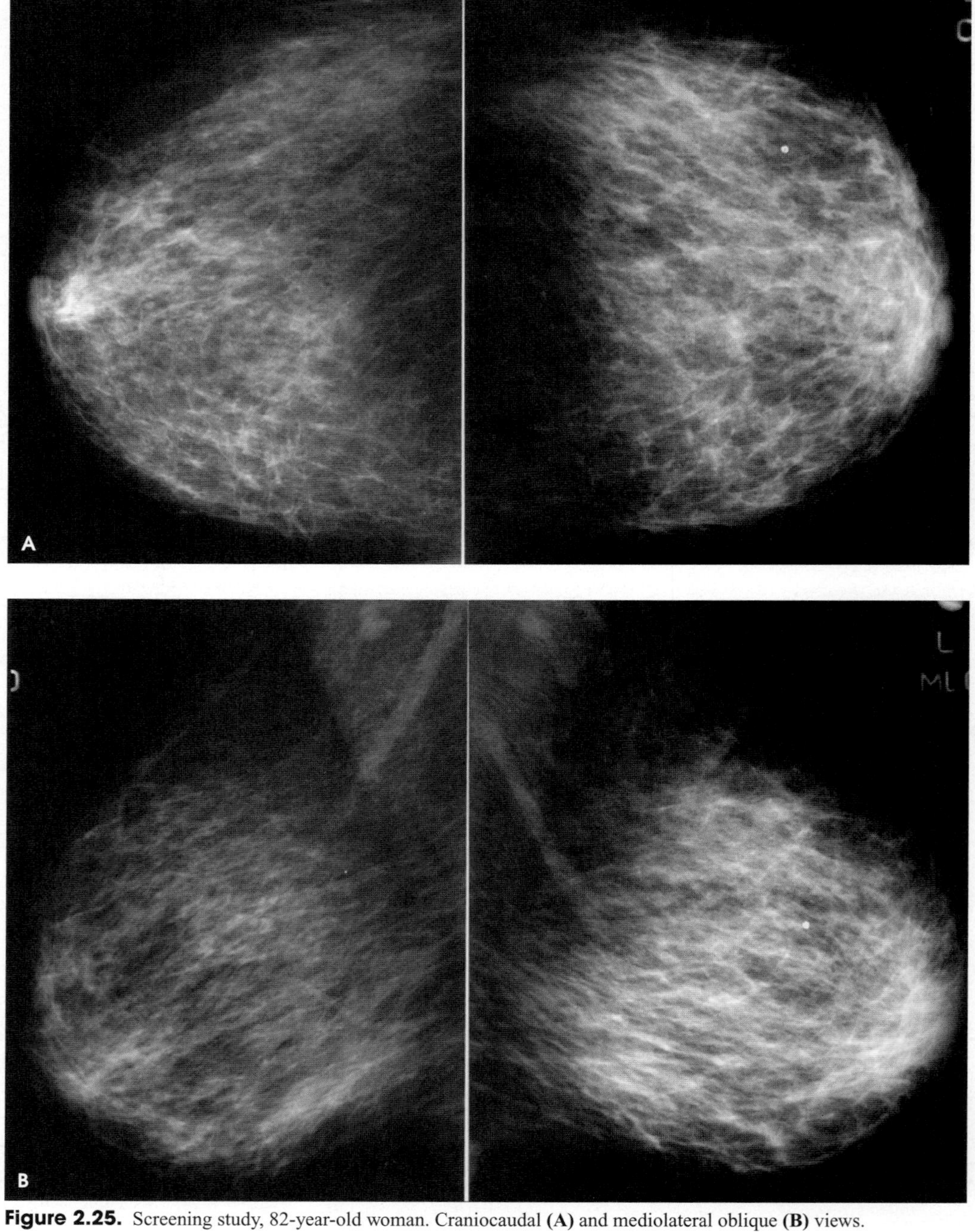

Figure 2.25. Screening study, 82-year-old woman. Craniocaudal **(A)** and mediolateral oblique **(B)** views.

What do you think and what would you like to do next?

In reviewing this mammogram, did you consider the possibility of a diffuse abnormality? *Remember to initially sit back and look at the study from a distance.* Assess technical adequacy and the possible presence of diffuse changes. The trabecular markings are increased diffusely, thickened, and extend close to the chest wall. For diffuse changes to be appreciated, particularly when they are bilateral, you need to consider them specifically as a possibility; otherwise they may go undetected.

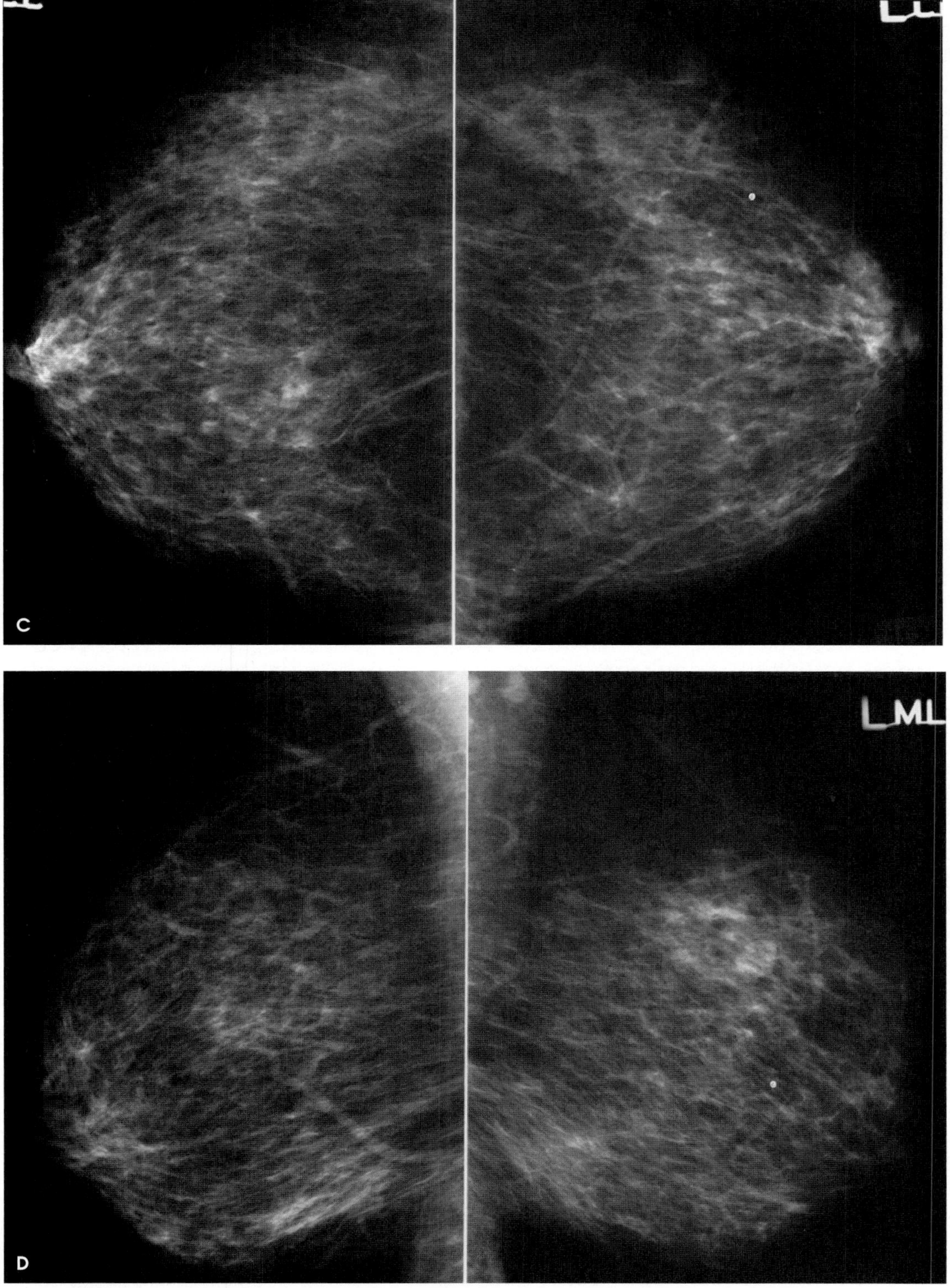

Figure 2.25. Craniocaudal **(C)** and mediolateral oblique **(D)** views, 3 years before those shown above.

What do you think a comparison of technical factors would show?
In addition to the comparison studies, what else might help you with the differential?

The initial perception of a diffuse abnormality can be confirmed by comparing present to prior mammograms (Fig. 2.25C, D). In comparing the two studies, consider the overall density of the breast parenchyma and the prominence of the trabecular pattern. As you would expect, peak kilovoltages and milliamperage output are higher and the breasts are less compressible on the current study compared with the study from 3 years earlier. Reviewing the patient's history form should be helpful as you consider the differential: The patient is short of breath (as detailed by the technologist), is on diuretics, and has a history of congestive heart failure (CHF). In this patient, the described findings are related to CHF and, as the CHF is treated, you can expect significant improvements in the mammographic findings.

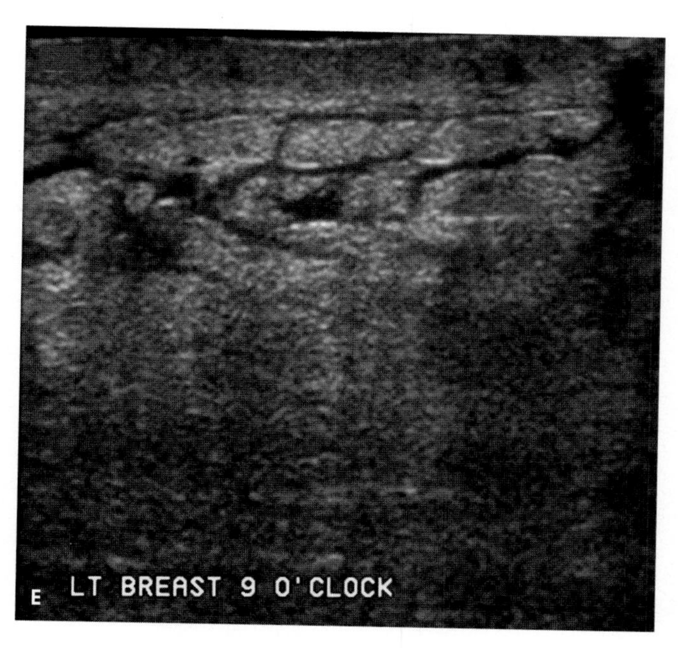

Figure 2.25. (*Continued*) Ultrasound image **(E)** of the left breast at the 9 o'clock position.

Although an ultrasound is not indicated in this patient, you can expect to see skin thickening, increased echogenicity of the tissue, and reticulation consistent with edema.

What is your differential for diffuse breast changes?

Differential considerations for diffuse changes that are usually unilateral, although rarely can be bilateral, include radiation therapy effect, inflammatory changes (e.g., mastitis), trauma, ipsilateral axillary adenopathy with lymphatic obstruction, dialysis shunt in the ipsilateral arm with fluid overload, invasive ductal carcinoma not otherwise specified, inflammatory carcinoma, invasive lobular carcinoma, or lymphoma. Invasive lobular carcinoma can lead to increases in breast density and size, or a decrease in breast size (the shrinking breast). Differential considerations for diffuse changes that are usually bilateral, although they can be unilateral, include hormone replacement therapy (e.g., estrogen), weight changes, congestive heart failure, renal failure with fluid overload, and superior vena cava syndrome. Additional rare benign causes include granulomatous mastitis, coumadin necrosis, arteritis, and autoimmune disorders (e.g., scleroderma). Obtaining a thorough history, examining the patient, and obtaining an ultrasound are often helpful in sorting through the differential considerations.

BI-RADS® category 2: benign finding. Annual screening mammography is recommended.

unil
radiation
inflammatory CA
mastitis
lymphatic obstruction
lymphoma
trauma

PATIENT 23

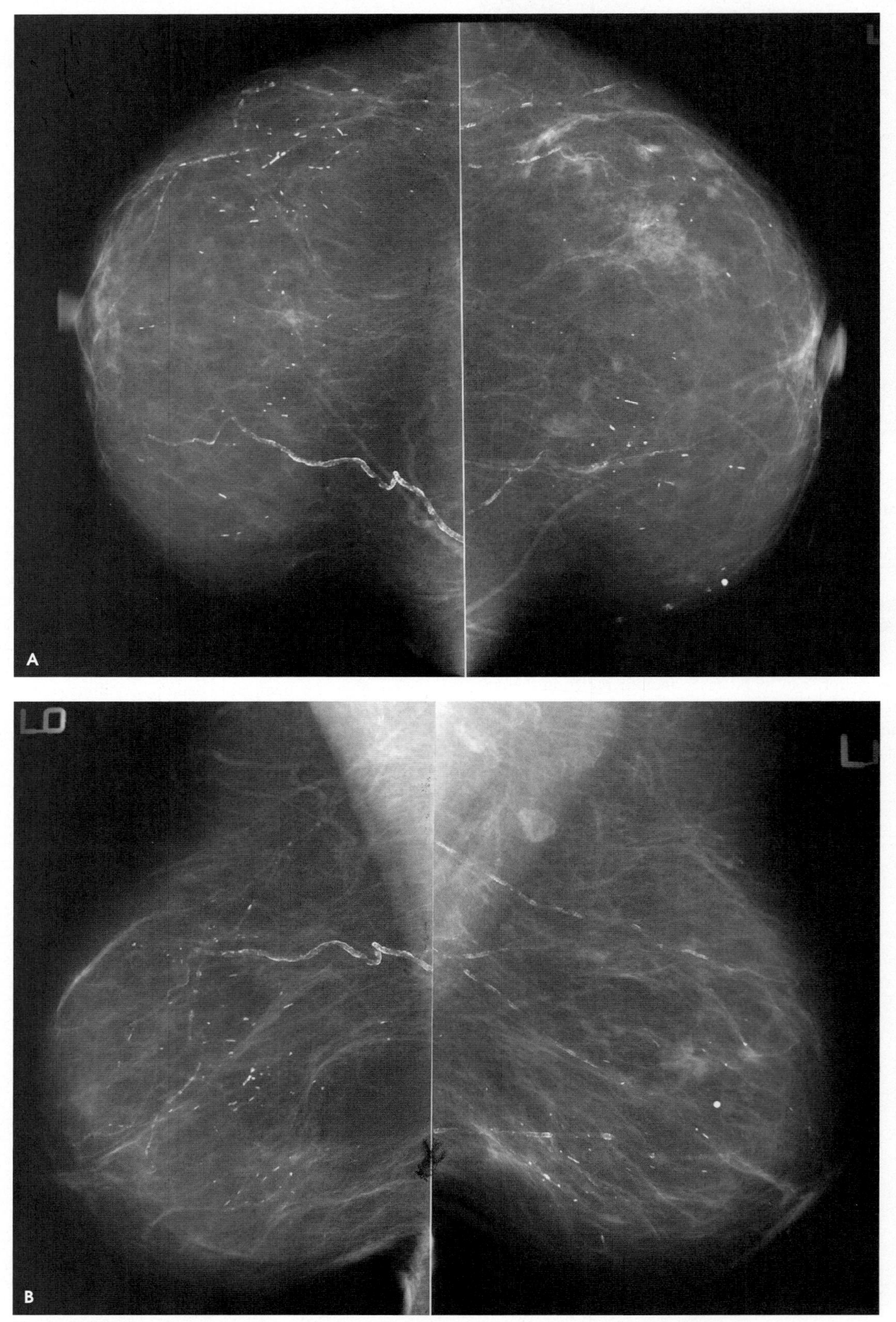

Figure 2.26. Screening study, 77-year-old woman. Craniocaudal **(A)** and mediolateral oblique **(B)** views.

What do you think, and would you like to do anything else?

There are scattered densities in an otherwise predominantly fatty pattern. Is it possible that any one of these densities represents an early malignancy? This is what makes what we do a challenge, particularly because it would not be ideal to call back all women with this mammographic appearance. Comparison with prior studies dating back several years is indicated in women with this type of parenchymal pattern. If any of these areas represents a change, additional evaluation is indicated; however, if the findings are stable, annual mammography is recommended. Arterial calcifications, noted bilaterally, are most likely perforating branches from the internal mammary artery. There are also large rodlike calcifications present bilaterally; these are benign and require no additional evaluation. Lymph nodes are seen projecting superimposed on the left pectoral muscle.

Did you notice the uneven exposure on the craniocaudal views posteromedially (more prominent on the right)? What does this reflect?

This usually reflects suboptimal compression with an associated air pocket. Consequently, evaluate the tissue in these areas carefully for blur, because the compression of the tissue in these areas is probably not optimal.

BI-RADS® category 2: benign finding. Annual screening mammography is recommended.

PATIENT 24

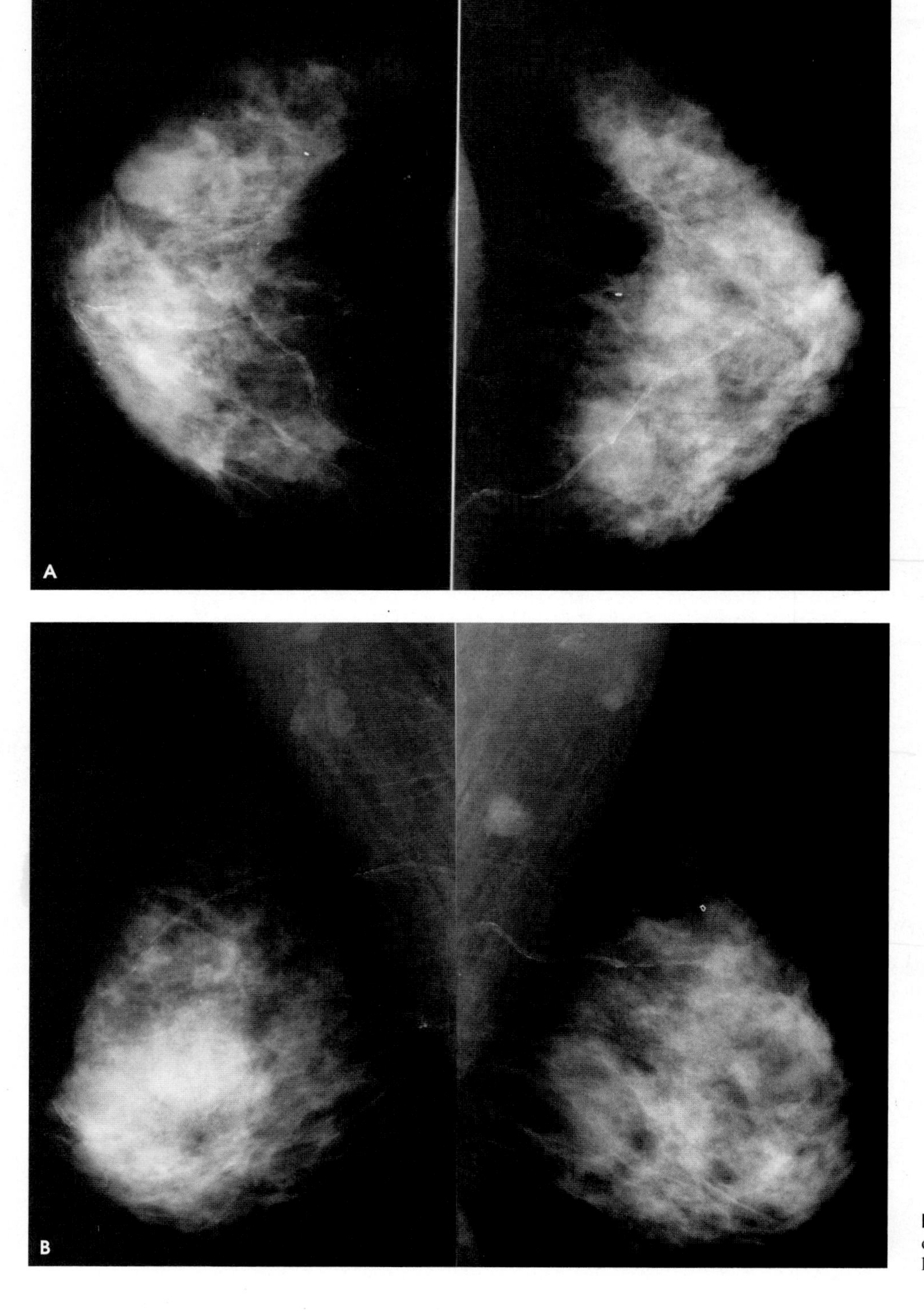

Figure 2.27. Screening study, 59-year-old woman. Craniocaudal **(A)** and mediolateral oblique **(B)** views.

What do you think?
Is the tissue too dense for a 59-year-old woman?
What is your working hypothesis, and what would you like to do next? How about prior films for comparison?

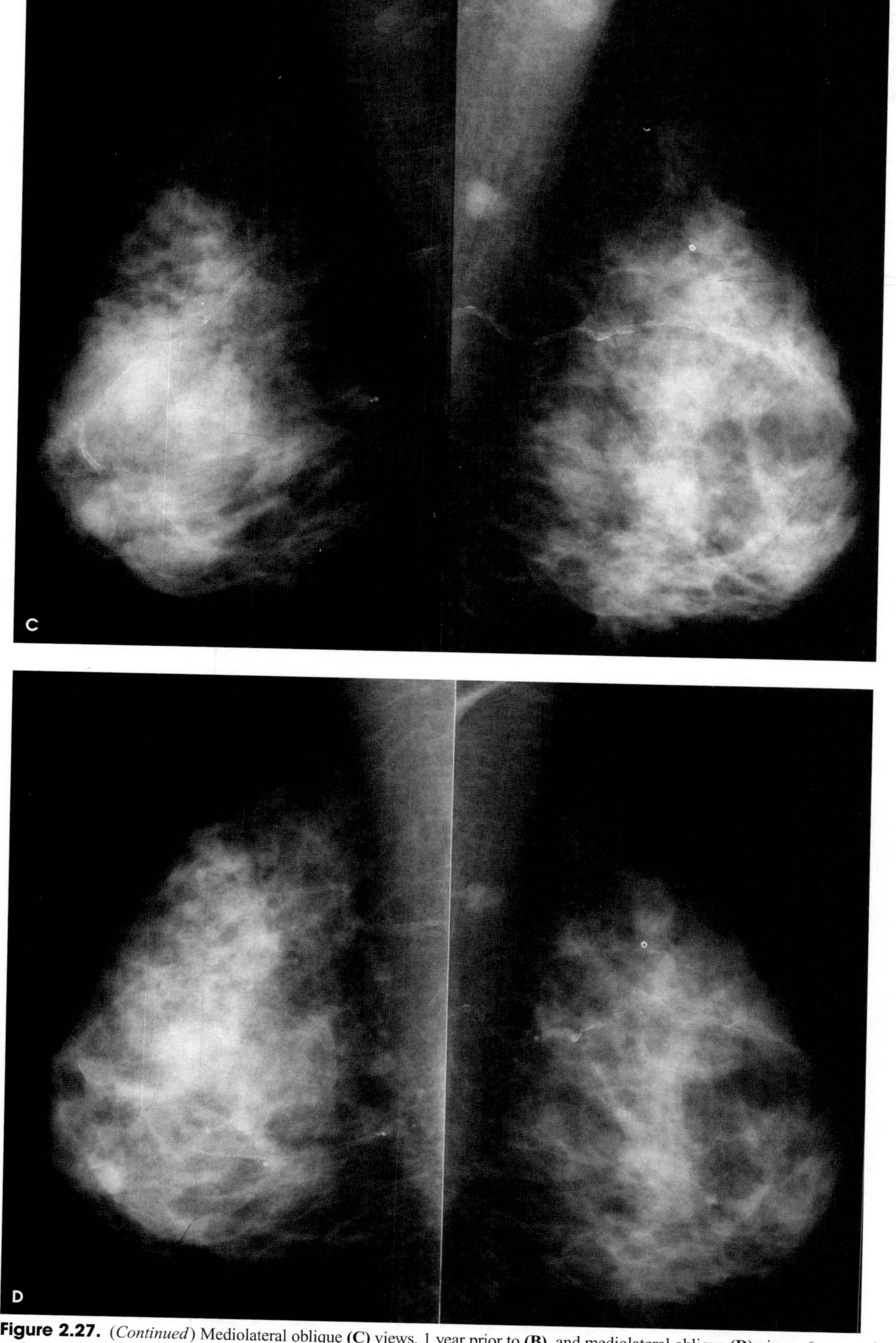

Figure 2.27. (*Continued*) Mediolateral oblique **(C)** views, 1 year prior to **(B)**, and mediolateral oblique **(D)** views, 6 years prior to those of **(B)**.

What do you think now? When screening studies are hung on the multiviewer, what is the routine for which comparison films to hang?

A micromark clip is present in the upper outer quadrant of the left breast, consistent with the history of a prior stereotactially guided biopsy (Fig. 2.27E). Arterial calcifications are noted bilaterally, as are several benign-appearing lymph nodes superimposed on the pectoral muscles. However, with careful evaluation, the mass superimposed on the lower aspect of the left pectoral muscle does not have an identifiable fatty hilum (Fig. 2.27E). When compared with prior studies, this mass has increased in size and the change in size is best appreciated when comparison is made to the earliest study available (Fig. 2.27D). Subtle changes are more difficult to appreciate from one year to the next, but may be readily apparent when an earlier study is used. Consequently, when the screening board is hung, we use the study from 2 years previous to the current study. If the patient has other studies, these are also immediately available in the patient's jacket for our review. It is common for us to review several prior studies, including the earliest study available in the patient's jacket, particularly before calling a patient back.

On the craniocaudal (CC) view, where would you expect to find this lesion and what views do you want your technologist to do to image this lesion in the CC projection?

Obviously, this will depend on the location of the lesion; however, this is not known because the lesion is not seen on the CC view. Did you assume this lesion is in the lateral aspect of the left breast? *Remember: make no assumptions.* When you make assumptions, you pigeonhole yourself. Logically, how can we establish if this lesion is medial, central, or lateral in location? A 90-degree lateral view can help us determine the location of this lesion. If the lesion moves up in going from mediolateral oblique (MLO) to lateral view, the lesion is in the medial aspect of the breast. If the lesion moves down in going from MLO to lateral view, the lesion is in the lateral aspect of the breast; and if the lesion does not shift in position, it is central in location. Alternatively, line up lateral, MLO, and CC views with the nipple on the same horizontal plane for the three views and draw a line connecting the lesion on the lateral and MLO views and extend it into the CC view. On the CC view, the lesion can be found somewhere along the course of the resulting line. You can localize the lesion more precisely by measuring how far posteriorly the lesion is in the breast with respect to the nipple (Fig. 2.27F).

As you can see from the ultrasound (Fig. 2.27G), this lesion is in the upper, inner quadrant of the left breast at the 11 o'clock position, posteriorly (Z3) sitting on the pectoral muscle. An oval, nearly isoechoic mass with parallel orientation, indistinct margins, and some shadowing as well as straightening and thickening of Cooper ligaments is imaged on ultrasound.

BI-RADS® category 4: suspicious abnormality; biopsy should be considered.

An invasive ductal carcinoma is diagnosed following the ultrasound-guided core biopsy. A 1.2-cm tubular carcinoma is diagnosed on the lumpectomy specimen. No metastatic disease is diagnosed in four excised sentinel lymph nodes [pT1c, pN0(sn)(i−), pMX; Stage I]. The well-differentiated nature of this lesion could have been suggested based on the relatively slow growth of the mass compared with 1 and 6 years previously.

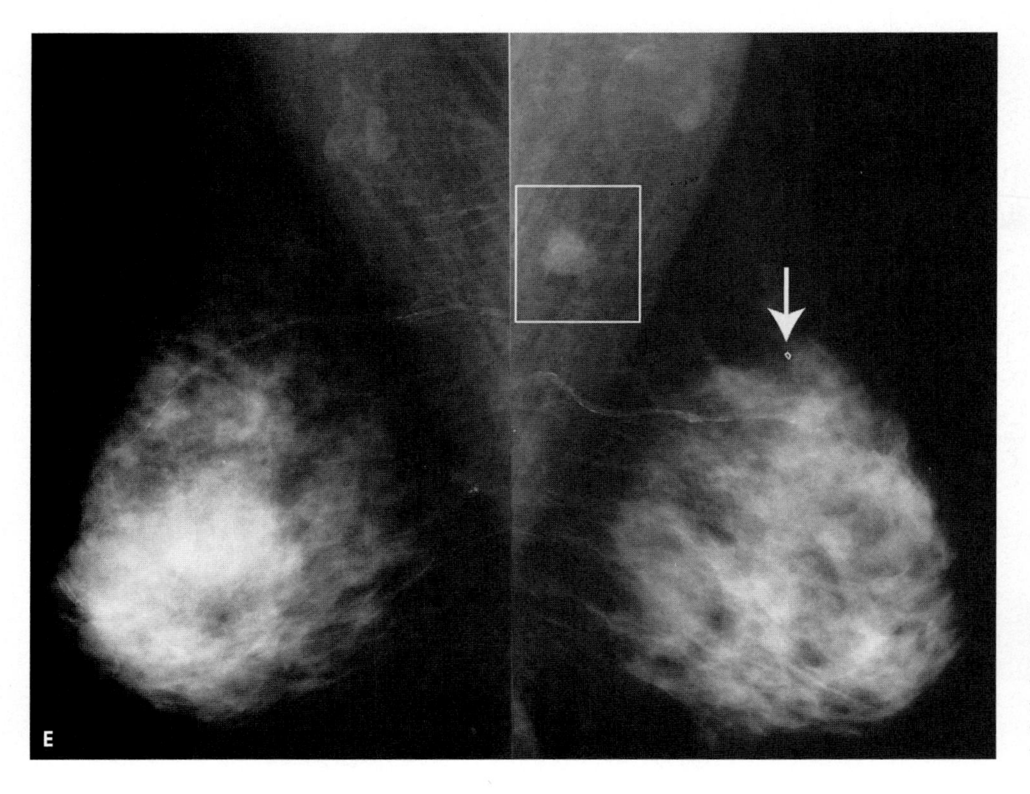

Figure 2.27. (*Continued*) Mediolateral oblique **(E)** views. Micromark clip (*arrow*) is seen in the left breast consistent with a prior stereotactically guided, vacuum-assisted biopsy for microcalcifications. The potential perceived lesion is within the box.

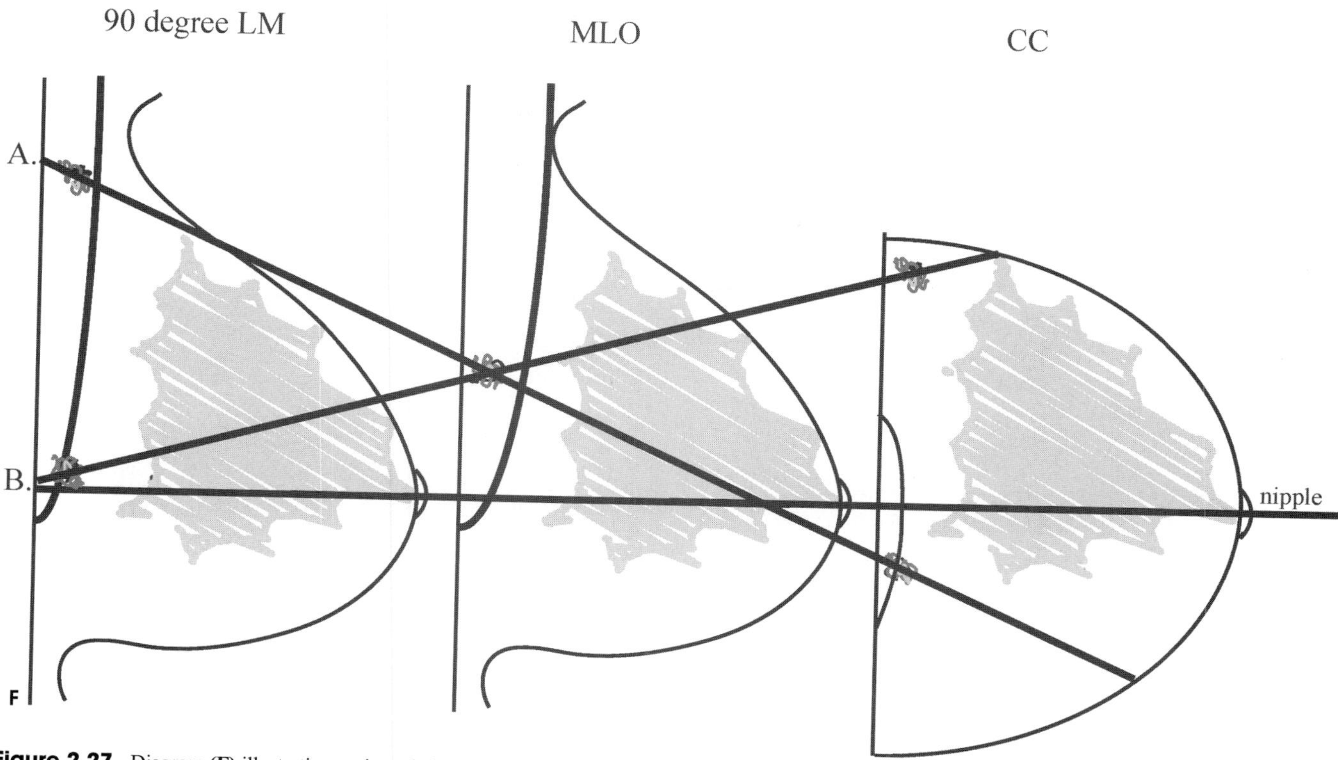

Figure 2.27. Diagram **(F)** illustrating a triangulation method described by Sickles to localize lesions on orthogonal views. Ninety-degree lateral, mediolateral oblique, and craniocaudal views are lined up using the nipple as the reference point. A line is then drawn connecting the lesion on the two views in which it is seen. The line is extended into the third image. The lesion can be expected along the course of this line. By measuring back from the nipple, you can approximate the location of the lesion along the course of the line.

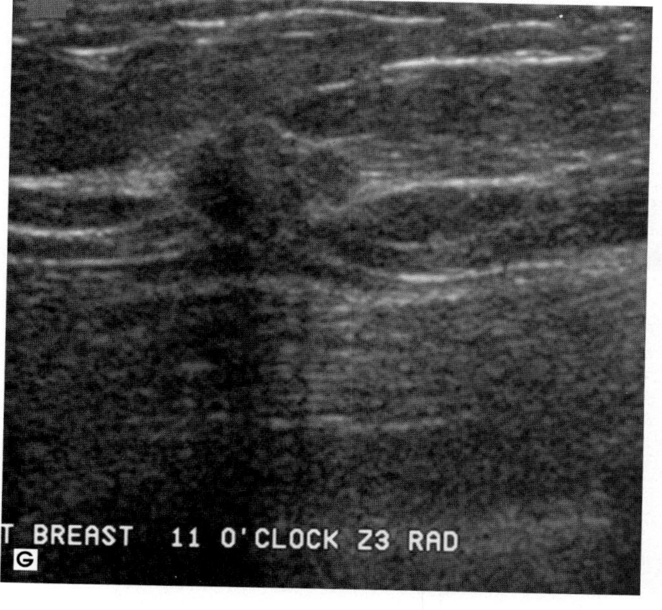

Oval, hypoechoic, indistinct margins shadowing

Figure 2.27. Ultrasound image **(G)** in the radial (RAD) projection of the lesion identified posteriorly (Z3) at the 11 o'clock position of the left breast.

PATIENT 25

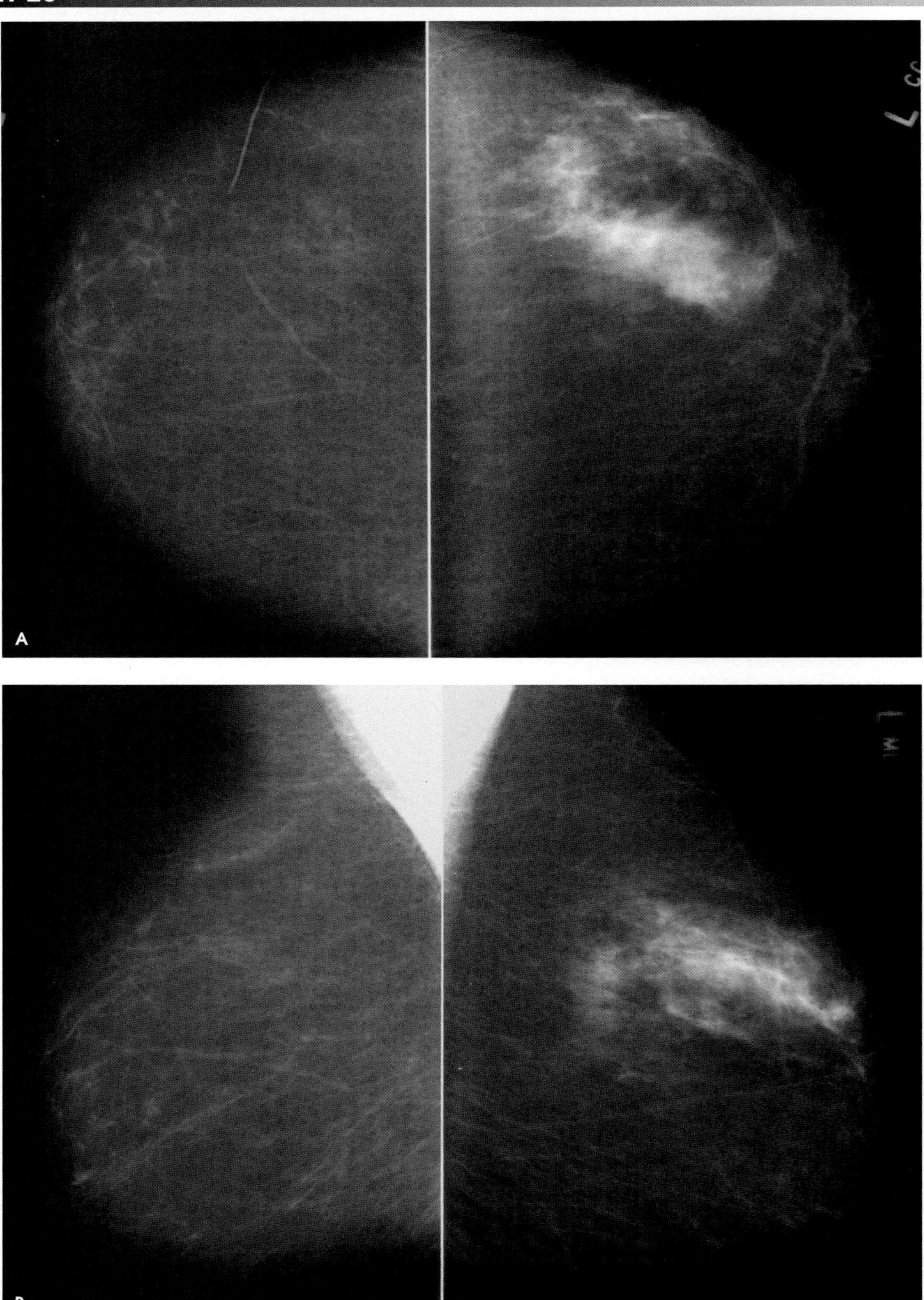

Figure 2.28. Screening study, 55-year-old woman. Craniocaudal **(A)** and mediolateral oblique **(B)** views.

What are the pertinent observations?

There is global parenchymal asymmetry in the left breast. Establishing the presence of global parenchymal asymmetry requires comparison with the contralateral side. A greater volume of tissue is present in the left breast compared to the same area in the right breast. As defined in the Fourth Edition of BI-RADS®, global asymmetry should involve at least one quadrant of the breast. Although breast tissue is more commonly symmetric, global asymmetry, as demonstrated here, can be seen in a small number of woman as a normal variant. No mass or distortion is noted in the area of increased tissue on the right. The tissue in this area is scalloped and contains associated areas of fatty lobulation. Abnormal, asymmetric changes may be the result of chest wall trauma (e.g., burns), congenital abnormalities (e.g., Poland syndrome), or surgery when the corresponding area of tissue in the contralateral breast has been excised. Invasive ductal carcinomas can present with global areas of parenchymal asymmetry, but these are usually clinically apparent and readily palpable. Invasive lobular carcinoma can also present with global areas of parenchymal asymmetry and progressive changes in breast size (either increases or decreases); palpable findings may be present, but they are often more subtle in patients with invasive lobular carcinomas. Rarely, lymphoma can present with diffuse, asymmetric involvement of one breast.

Based on your observations, what is your working hypothesis for this patient and what BI-RADS® category would you use?

In this woman, you can establish the iatrogenic cause of the asymmetry by making all pertinent observations. Did you notice the radio-opaque linear marker used on the right craniocaudal view at the site of a prior excisional biopsy? Did you notice that the right breast is slightly smaller than the left? The patient has had a prior biopsy in the upper outer quadrant of the right breast with resulting asymmetry of the remaining tissue on the left. Did you notice the suboptimal positioning on the mediolateral oblique views? An inadequate amount of pectoral muscle is included in the images.

How often do you see mammographic changes following an excisional biopsy? And what are the possible changes?

We do not routinely use scar markers on screening studies because no perceivable abnormality is apparent in more than 50% of women following a breast biopsy. Additionally, in those women in whom postoperative changes are noted, they can usually be characterized as such without the use of scar markers. Placing markers on the breast is time-consuming, can be distracting at the time of interpretation, and is relatively costly. Changes that can be seen following an excisional biopsy include a decrease in the size of the affected breast, localized skin thickening and retraction, architectural distortion, a spiculated or mixed-density mass, oil cyst(s), dystrophic calcifications, and areas of focal or global parenchymal asymmetry in the contralateral breast, as demonstrated with this patient's mammogram.

BI-RADS® category 1: negative, unless this is the first study following the biopsy, in which case BI-RADS® category 2: benign finding, can be used if the observation is described in the report. Annual screening mammography is recommended.

PATIENT 26

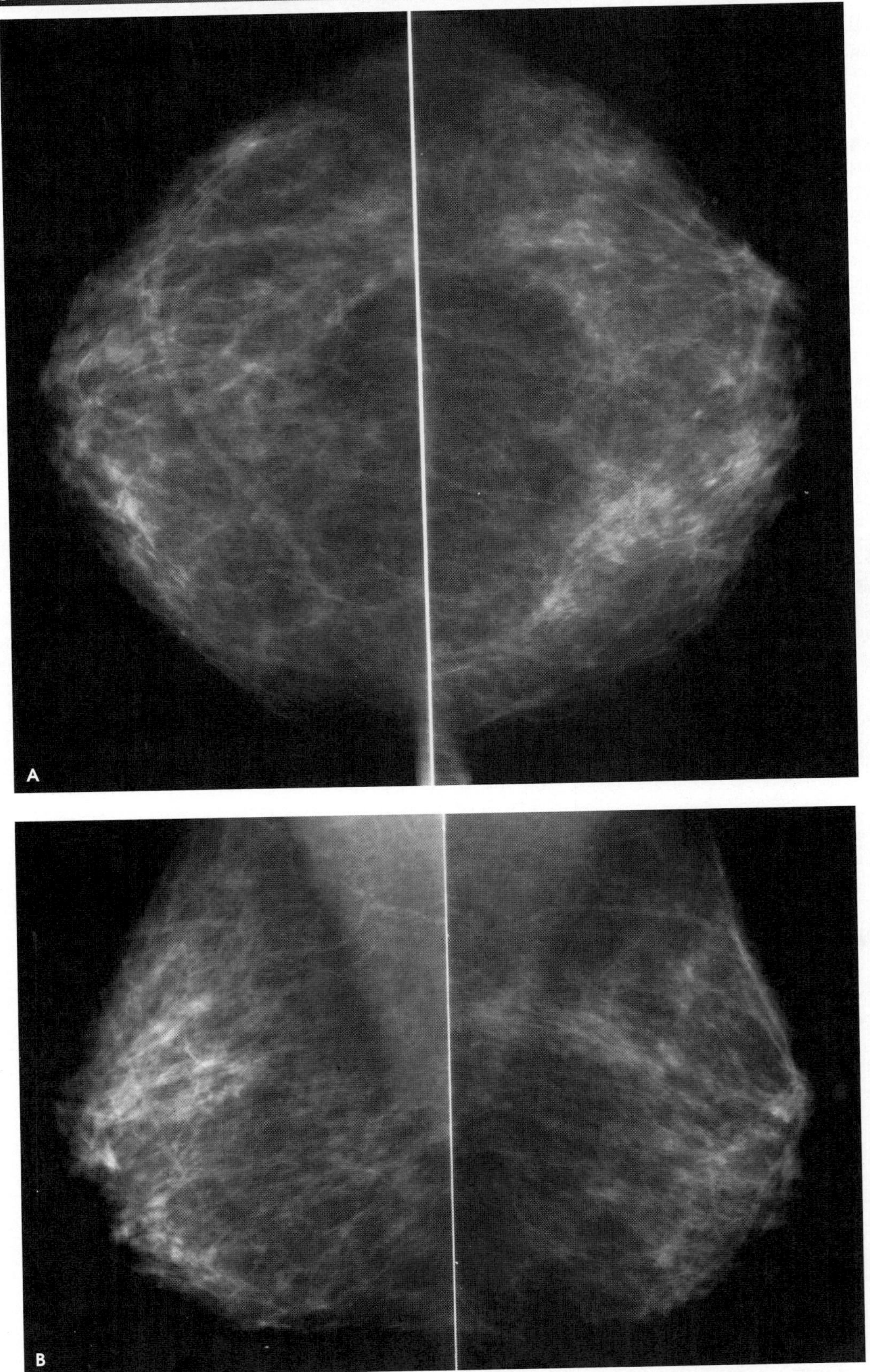

Figure 2.29. Screening study, 54-year-old woman. Craniocaudal **(A)** and mediolateral oblique **(B)** views.

What do you think? Do you see a potential lesion?

Review the images systematically. Do you see a potential mass? Split the craniocaudal and mediolateral oblique views into thirds to focus your attention as you go back and forth between the right and left breasts. Does something catch your eye in the left breast anterolaterally? With what degree of certainty can you say this is normal or abnormal? How would you dictate the report? Why not get additional information by comparing the current study with prior films, and depending on what the comparison shows, obtaining spot compression views, correlative physical examination, and sonography? Depending on what is found on the workup, a biopsy may be indicated.

BI-RADS® category 0: need additional imaging evaluation.

What is the goal when viewing and interpreting screening mammograms, and why place a high emphasis on additional imaging evaluations?

On screening studies our goal is to detect *potential* abnormalities. We make no effort to characterize potential or true lesions on screening studies. Additional evaluations increase our confidence in appropriate recommendations and often point to the proper diagnosis. They also provide us with the opportunity to establish a rapport with our patients and complete workups, including imaging guided biopsies, when indicated. Definitive and directive reports are generated. Consequently, the only BI-RADS® assessment categories we use on our screening studies are category 1: negative, category 2: benign finding(s), and category 0: need additional imaging evaluation or need prior mammograms for comparison.

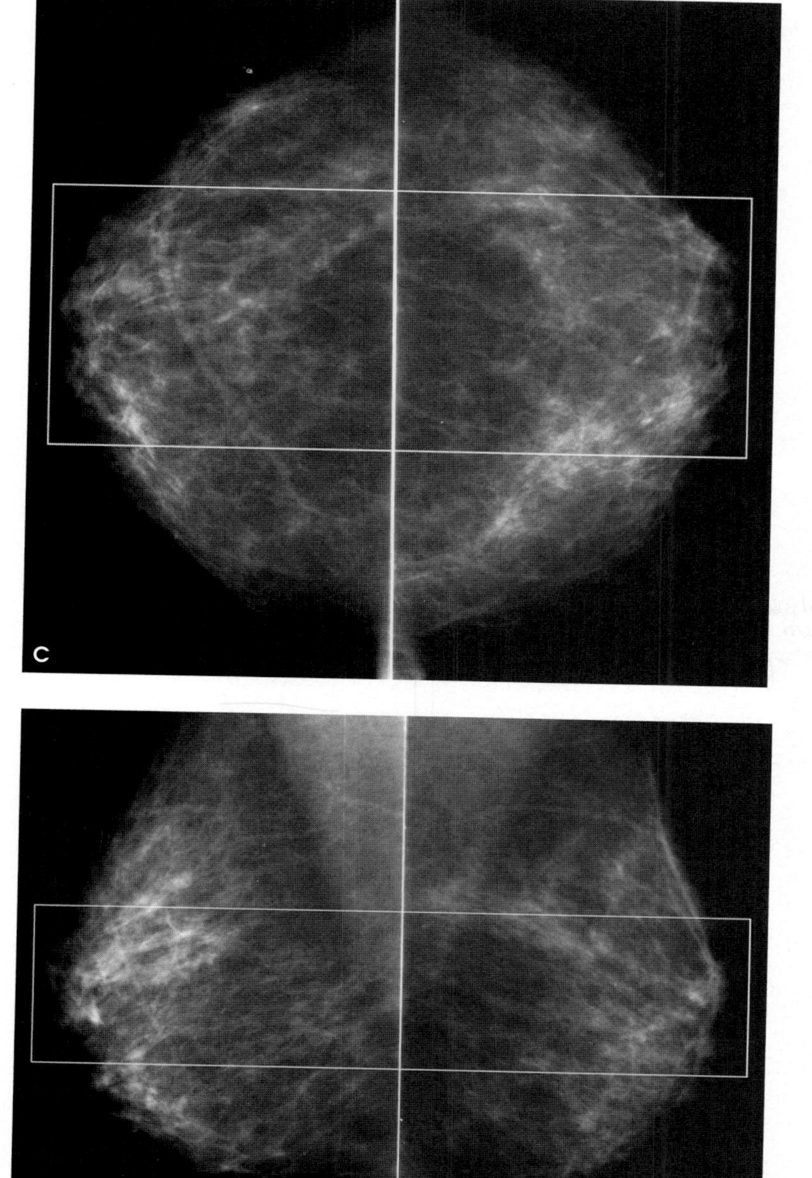

Figure 2.29. (*Continued*) Craniocaudal **(C)** and mediolateral oblique **(D)** focusing on the mid aspect of the breasts.

Do you see a possible mass in the left subareolar area?

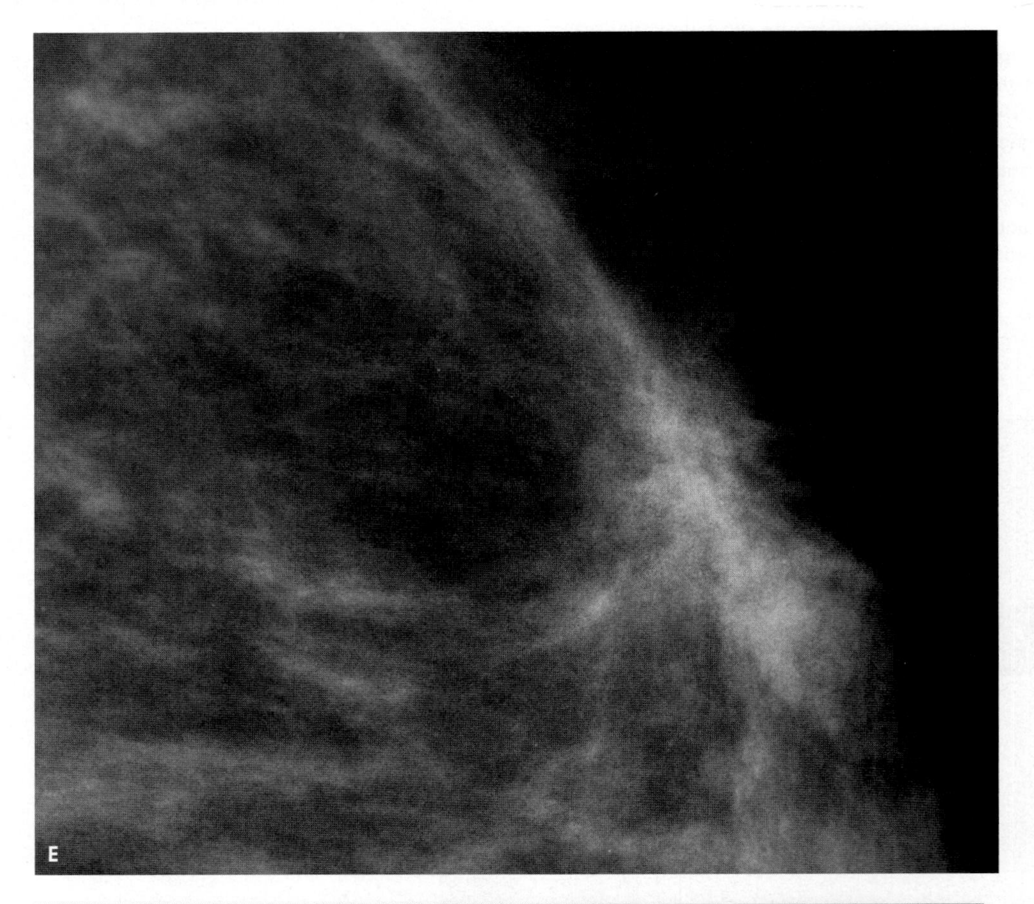

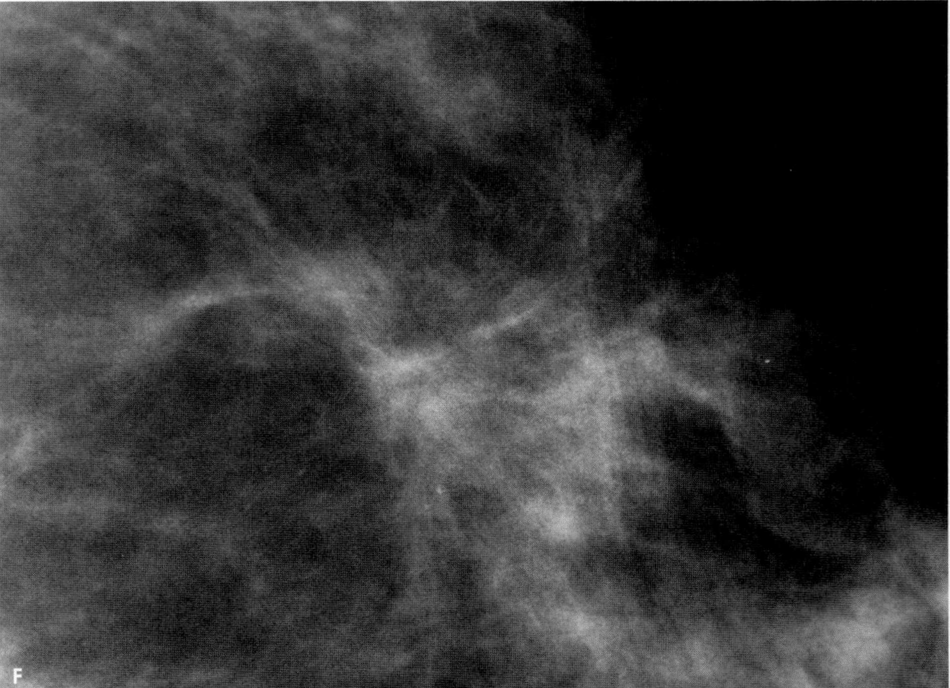

Figure 2.29. (*Continued*) Craniocaudal **(E)** and mediolateral oblique **(F)** spot compression views.

Do the spot compression views help you?
With what degree of certainty can you now say there is a significant abnormality in the left breast?

A 2-cm, irregular, spiculated mass is confirmed on the spot compression views. The ultrasound demonstrates a hypoechoic, intensely shadowing mass with vertical (i.e., not parallel or taller than wide) orientation and spiculation. If there is no history of surgery, significant trauma, or mastitis at this site, this finding requires a biopsy, which can be readily, easily, and safely undertaken at the time of the diagnostic evaluation using ultrasound guidance. The information provided by the additional views is critical in enabling us to make recommendations confidently and to dictate a succinct, definitive, and directive report (in essence, a 2-cm, spiculated, irregular mass is confirmed at the 2 o'clock position of the left breast 1 cm from the nipple. Biopsy is indicated. An imaging-guided biopsy is undertaken and reported separately).

BI-RADS® category 4: suspicious finding; biopsy is indicated. An ultrasound-guided core biopsy is done at the time of the diagnostic evaluation. An invasive mammary carcinoma, thought to be either an invasive ductal carcinoma with lobular features or an invasive lobular carcinoma, is reported on the core samples. A 2.3-cm invasive lobular carcinoma is reported histologically following the lumpectomy. The sentinel lymph node is normal [pT2, pN0(sn)(i−), pMX; Stage IIA].

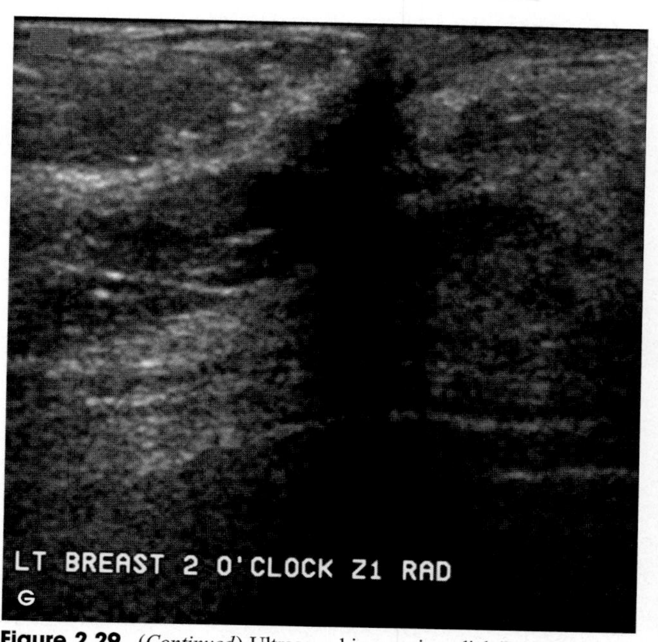

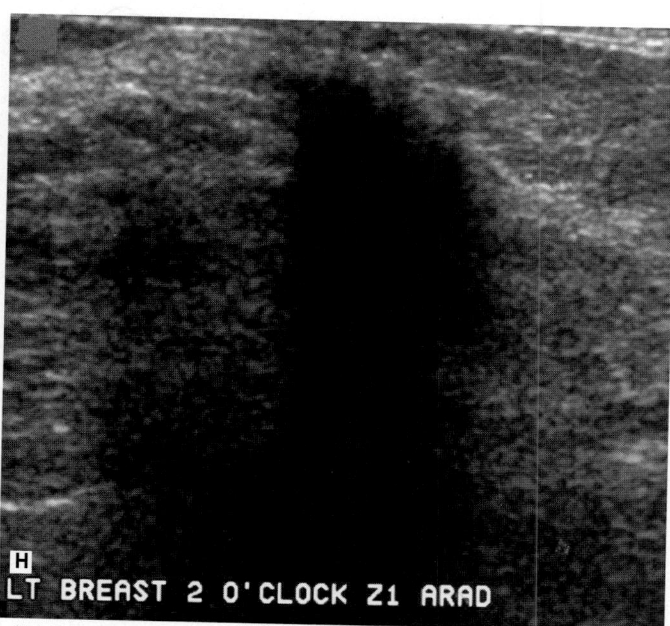

Figure 2.29. (*Continued*) Ultrasound images in radial (RAD) **(G)** and antiradial (ARAD) **(H)** projections, left breast at the 2 o'clock position, anteriorly (Z1).

PATIENT 27

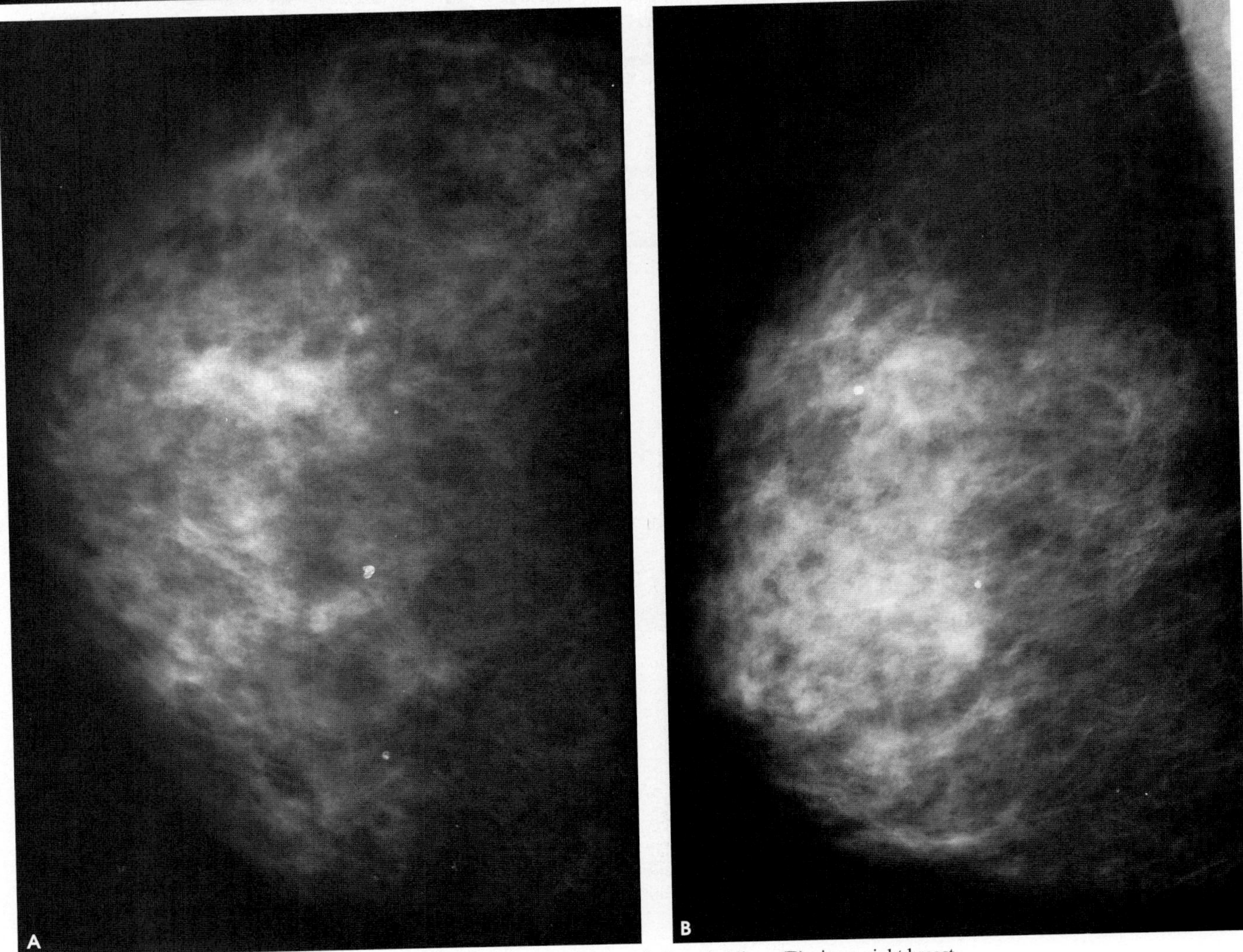

Figure 2.30. Screening study, 62-year-old woman. Craniocaudal **(A)** and mediolateral oblique **(B)** views, right breast.

Any observations?
Do you think additional views are indicated?

In reviewing this mammogram, consider the fat–glandular interfaces and medial tissue. Straight lines can be seen radiating out from an area of density in the upper inner quadrant of the right breast. If there is no history of surgery at this site, additional evaluation is indicated.

BI-RADS® category 0: need additional imaging evaluation.

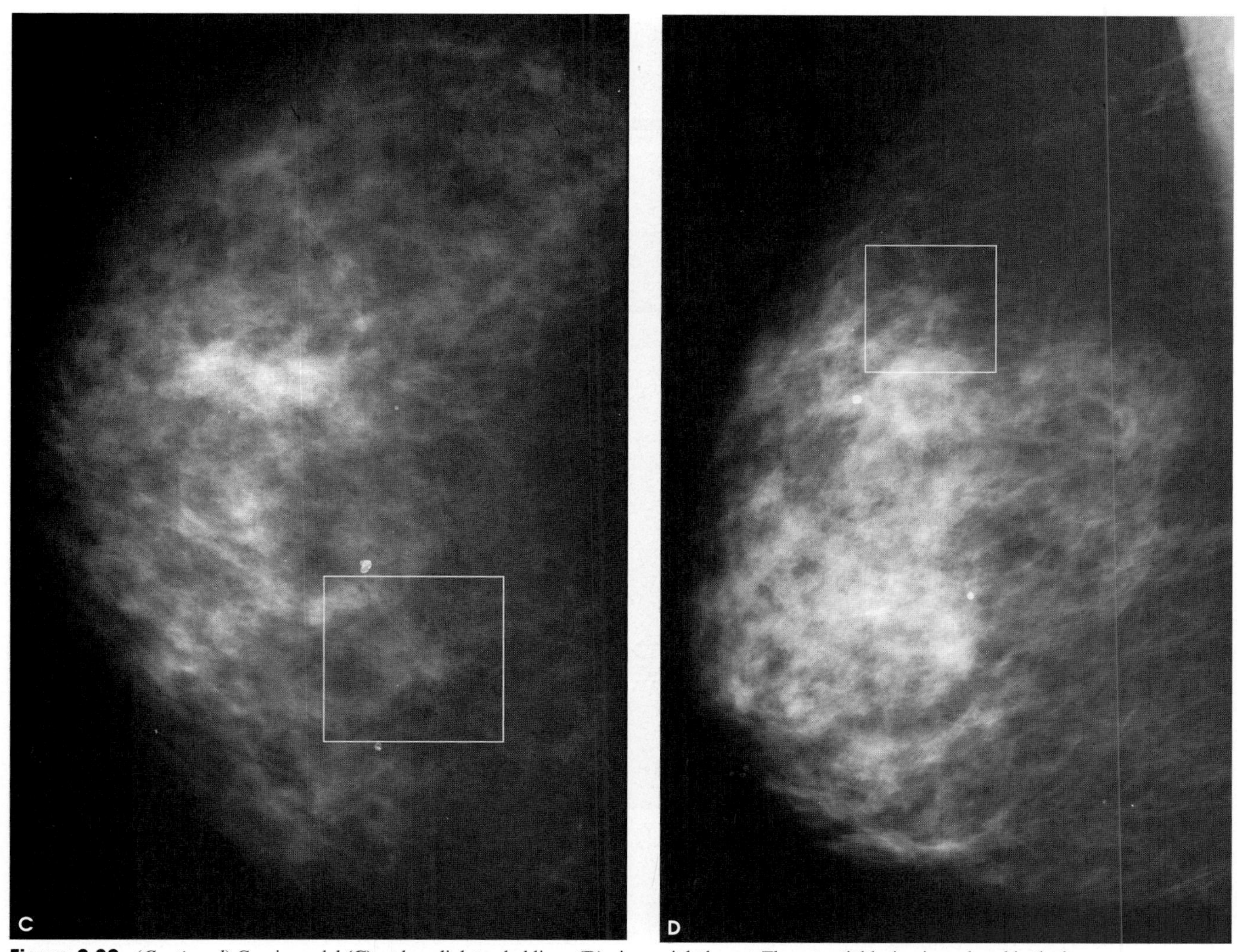

Figure 2.30. *(Continued)* Craniocaudal **(C)** and mediolateral oblique **(D)** views, right breast. The potential lesion is enclosed in the box.

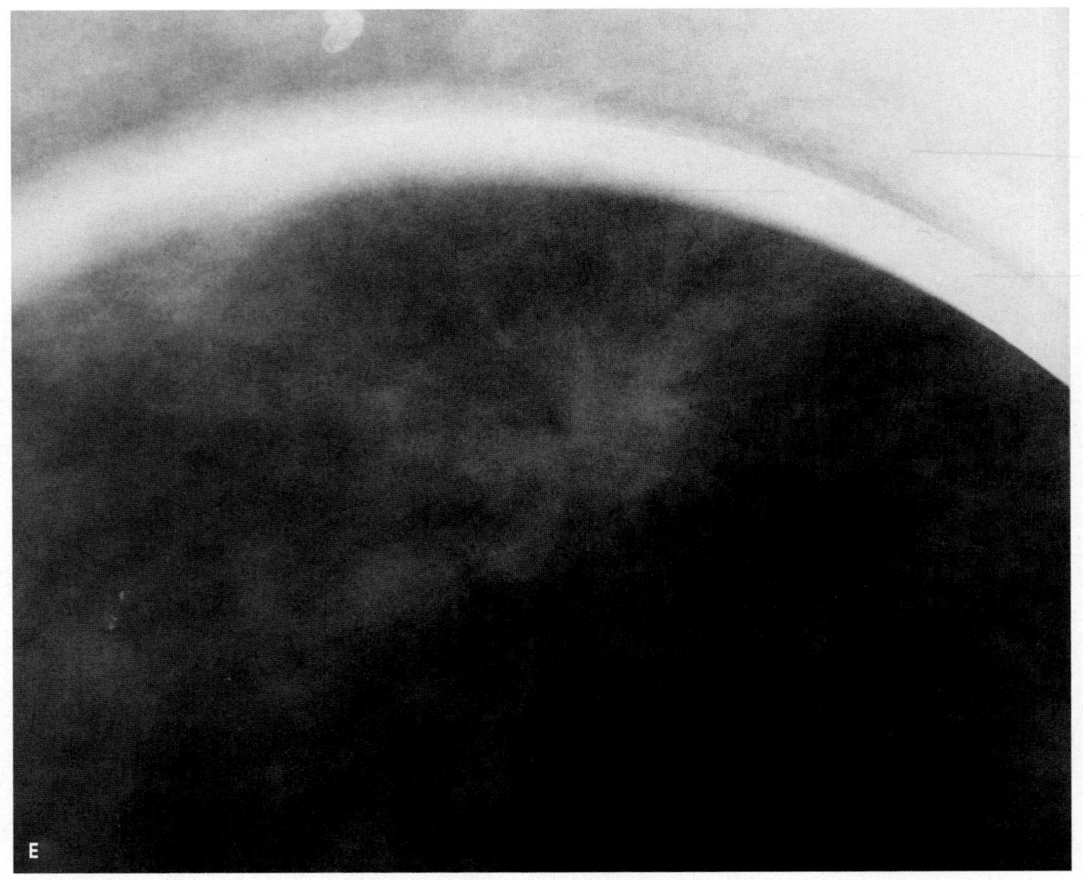

Figure 2.30. (*Continued*) Spot compression view **(E),** right craniocaudal projection.

What do you think now?

A spiculated mass is confirmed with the spot compression view. Based on the mammographic findings, a biopsy is indicated.

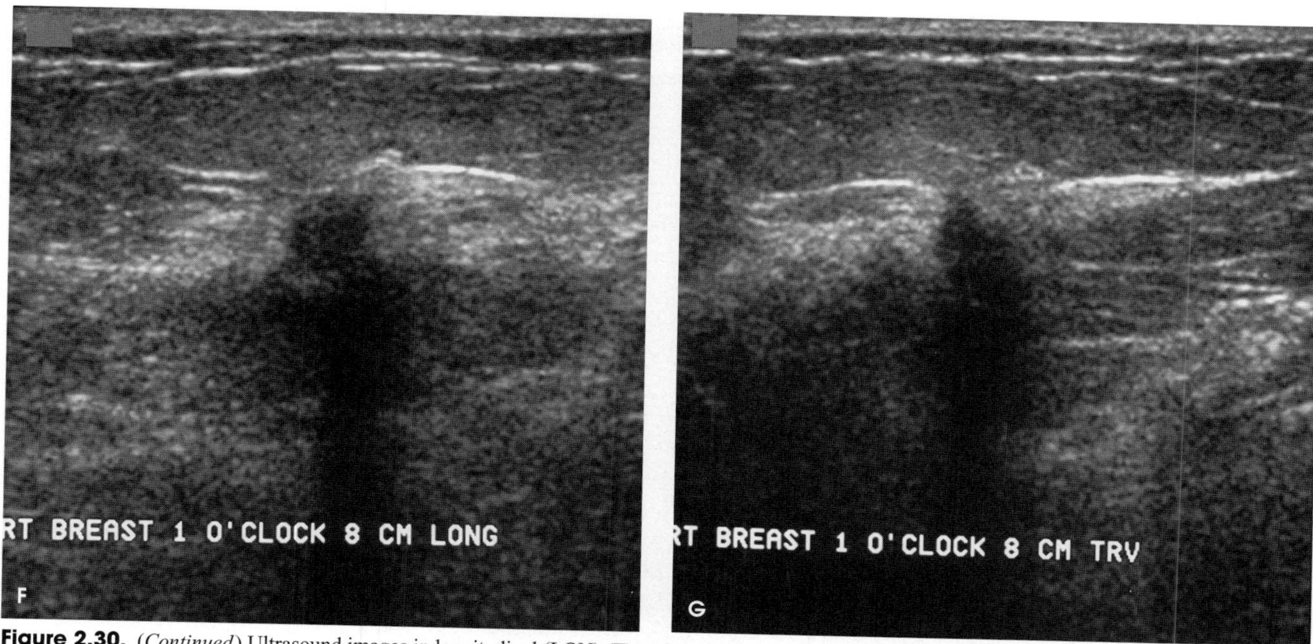

Figure 2.30. (*Continued*) Ultrasound images in longitudinal (LON) **(F)** and transverse (TRS) **(G)** orientations, right breast.

How would you describe the ultrasound findings?

A 1.5-cm irregular mass with indistinct and angular margins, shadowing, and associated disruption of the normal tissue planes (distortion) is imaged at 1 o'clock, 8 cm from the right nipple, corresponding to the area of mammographic concern.

BI-RADS® category 4: suspicious abnormality; biopsy should be considered. An invasive ductal carcinoma is reported histologically following an ultrasound-guided biopsy. A 2-cm grade I, invasive ductal carcinoma is reported on the lumpectomy specimen. Metastatic disease is diagnosed in one of five excised axillary lymph nodes (pT1c, pN1, pMX; Stage IIA).

What is the reported incidence of axillary nodal metastasis in patients with T1 tumors, and what factors have been suggested as predictors for nodal involvement?

The reported incidence of axillary nodal metastasis in patients with T1 tumors (2-cm-sized tumors or smaller) ranges from 6% to 36%. Predictors of axillary lymph node metastasis in patients with T1 tumors include tumor size, lymphovascular space involvement, and the histological grade of the lesion (e.g., in one report, 26.7% of patients with grade I, T1c tumors had metastatic disease to the axilla, compared with 35.7% of patients with grade III, T1c tumors).

PATIENT 28

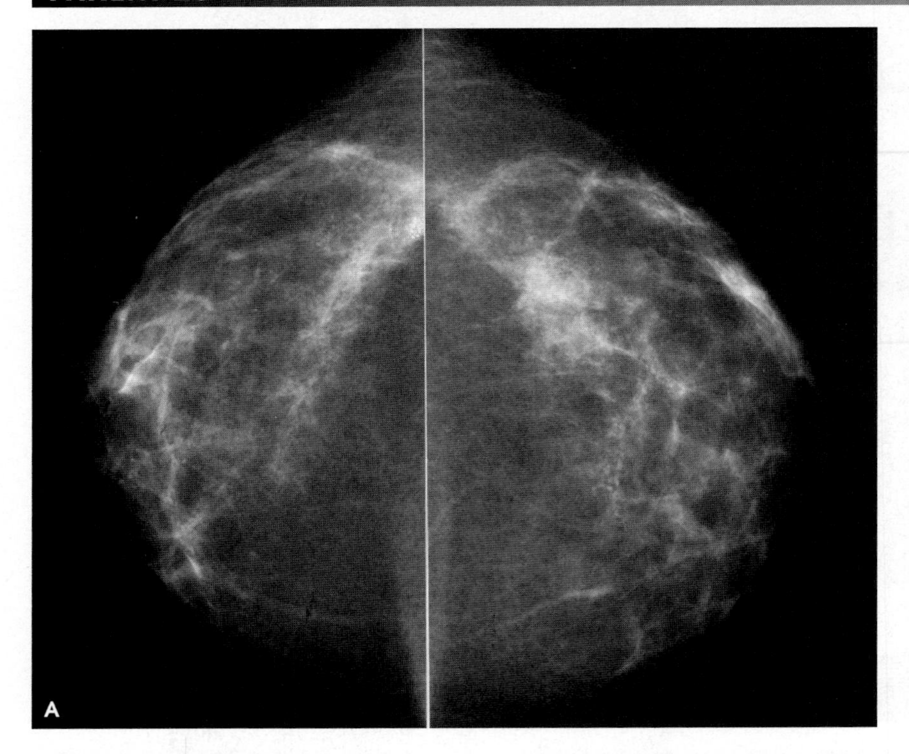

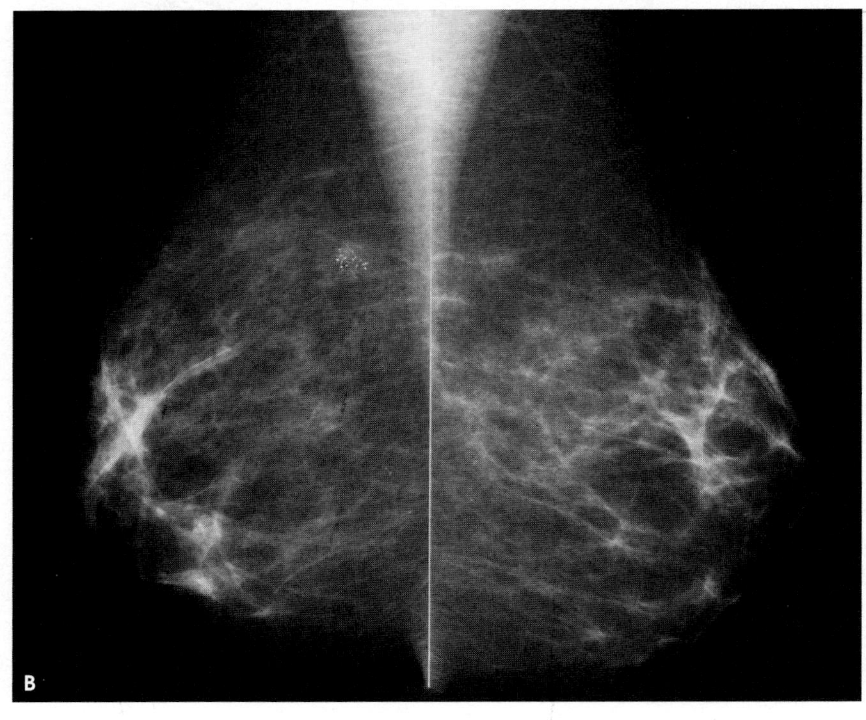

Figure 2.31. Screening study, 45-year-old woman. Craniocaudal **(A)** and mediolateral oblique **(B)** views.

Are there any findings in the right breast?
Are there any findings in the left breast?
What would you recommend next?

A cluster of calcifications is present in the right breast. The cluster is best imaged on the mediolateral oblique view; it is partially visualized laterally on the right craniocaudal view. No abnormality is appreciated in the left breast. Additional evaluation with magnification views is indicated on the right.

BI-RADS® category 0: need additional imaging evaluation.

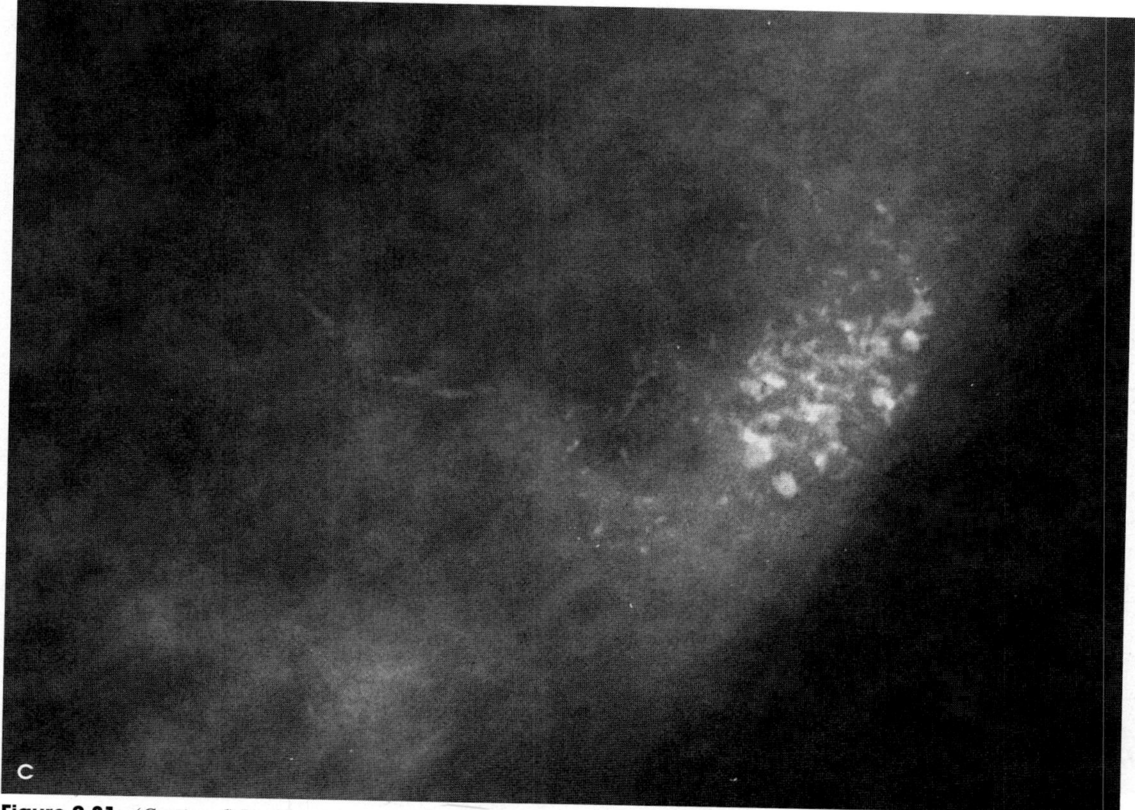

Figure 2.31. (*Continued*) Double spot compression magnification views, craniocaudal projection, exaggerated laterally (XCCL) **(C).**

A cluster of pleomorphic calcifications of variable density, imaged on the exaggerated craniocaudal views laterally (XCCL) magnification view, is shown here. Some of the calcifications are linear and some demonstrate linear orientation. This is likely to represent a ductal carcinoma in situ with central necrosis.

BI-RADS® category 5: Highly suspicious of malignancy; appropriate action should be taken.

Appropriate action, in the form of a stereotactially guided biopsy, is taken. A high-nuclear-grade ductal carcinoma with central necrosis is diagnosed following the core biopsy. As with all of our patients diagnosed with breast cancer, magnetic resonance imaging (MRI) is undertaken to evaluate for the presence of multifocal or multicentric disease in the ipsilateral breast and to assess the contralateral breast.

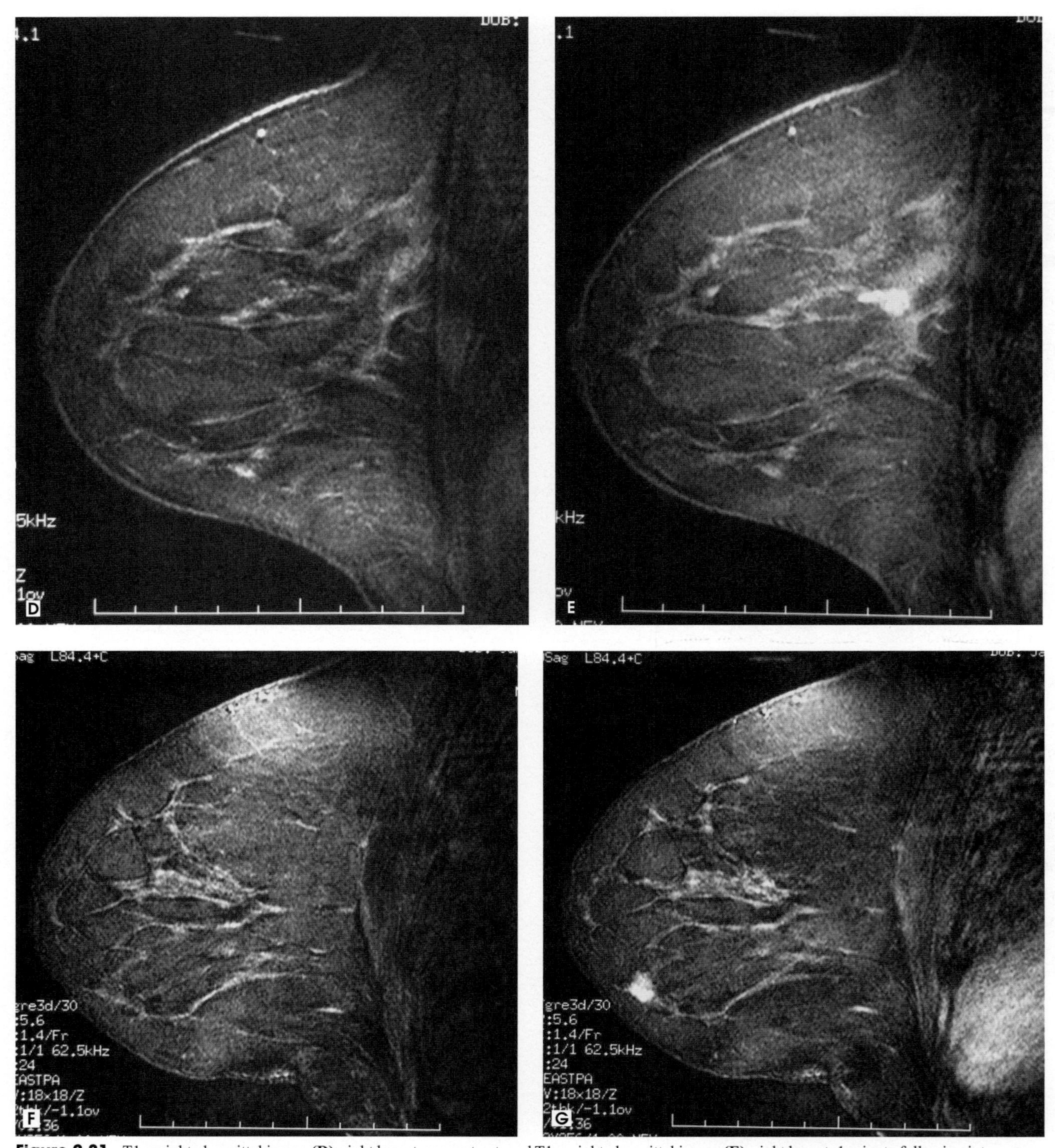

Figure 2.31. T1-weighted, sagittal image **(D),** right breast, precontrast, and T1-weighted, sagittal image **(E),** right breast, 1 minute following intravenous bolus of gadolinium, same tabletop position as shown in **(D).** T1-weighted, saggital image **(F)**, left breast precontrast, and T1-weighted image **(G)**, left breast, 1 minute following intravenous bolus of gadolinium, same table top position as shown in **(F).**

How would you describe the imaging findings?

A focus of enhancement is noted posteriorly in the right breast, corresponding to the area of ductal carcinoma in situ detected mammographically. Kinetically, there is rapid wash-in and wash-out of contrast, consistent with a malignant process. Unexpectedly, a mass, characterized by rapid wash-in and wash-out of contrast, is imaged in the left breast. The patient is called back following the MRI for ultrasound evaluation of the left breast. Based on the MR images (i.e., slice thickness and relationship of lesion to nipple), the expected location of the lesion can be approximated prior to the ultrasound.

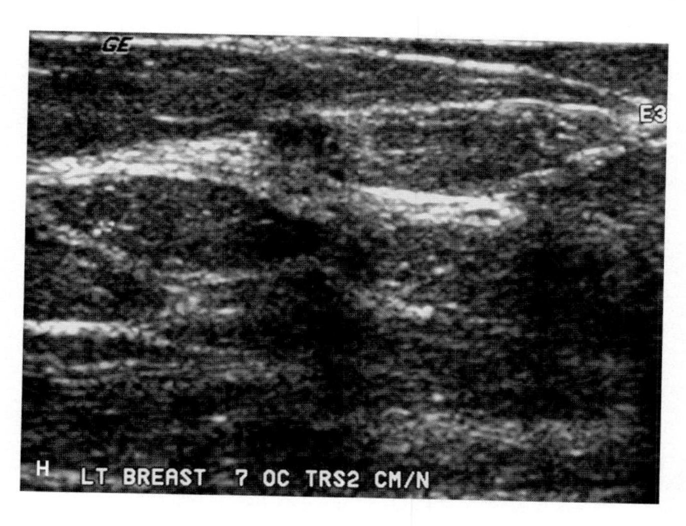

Figure 2.31. (*Continued*) Ultrasound image **(H),** lower inner quadrant, left breast.

What do you think, and what is your recommendation?

An irregular 1-cm mass with indistinct margins is identified at the 7 o'clock position, 2 cm from the left nipple.

BI-RADS® category 4: Suspicious abnormality; biopsy should be considered.

An invasive mammary carcinoma is diagnosed following ultrasound-guided core biopsy.

A high-nuclear-grade ductal carcinoma in situ, associated with necrosis and calcifications measuring 2 cm in size, is confirmed following a lumpectomy on the right. Three excised sentinel lymph nodes are normal [pTis(DCIS), pN0(sn)(i−), pMX; Stage 0]. A grade I invasive ductal carcinoma measuring 1 cm is confirmed following a lumpectomy on the left. Two excised sentinel lymph nodes are normal [pT1b, pN0(sn)(i−), pMX; Stage 1].

What is the potential role of magnetic resonance imaging in patients diagnosed with breast cancer?

The routine use of magnetic resonance imaging preoperatively in patients with a known breast cancer diagnosis is helpful in further characterizing the extent of the disease and directing appropriate surgical management in some patients. Women with multicentric lesions confirmed to be either intraductal or invasive disease may be more appropriately managed with a mastectomy, and those with more extensive or multifocal disease may require wider excisions than initially planned. In the 5% to 6% of women identified with synchronous contralateral cancers, bilateral procedures are indicated.

For patients with MRI-detected lesions, the location of the lesion is approximated based on the MRI and a targeted ultrasound is done. If the lesion is identified, an ultrasound-guided biopsy can be done; otherwise, MR-guided biopsy, clip placement, or wire localization may be indicated.

PATIENT 29

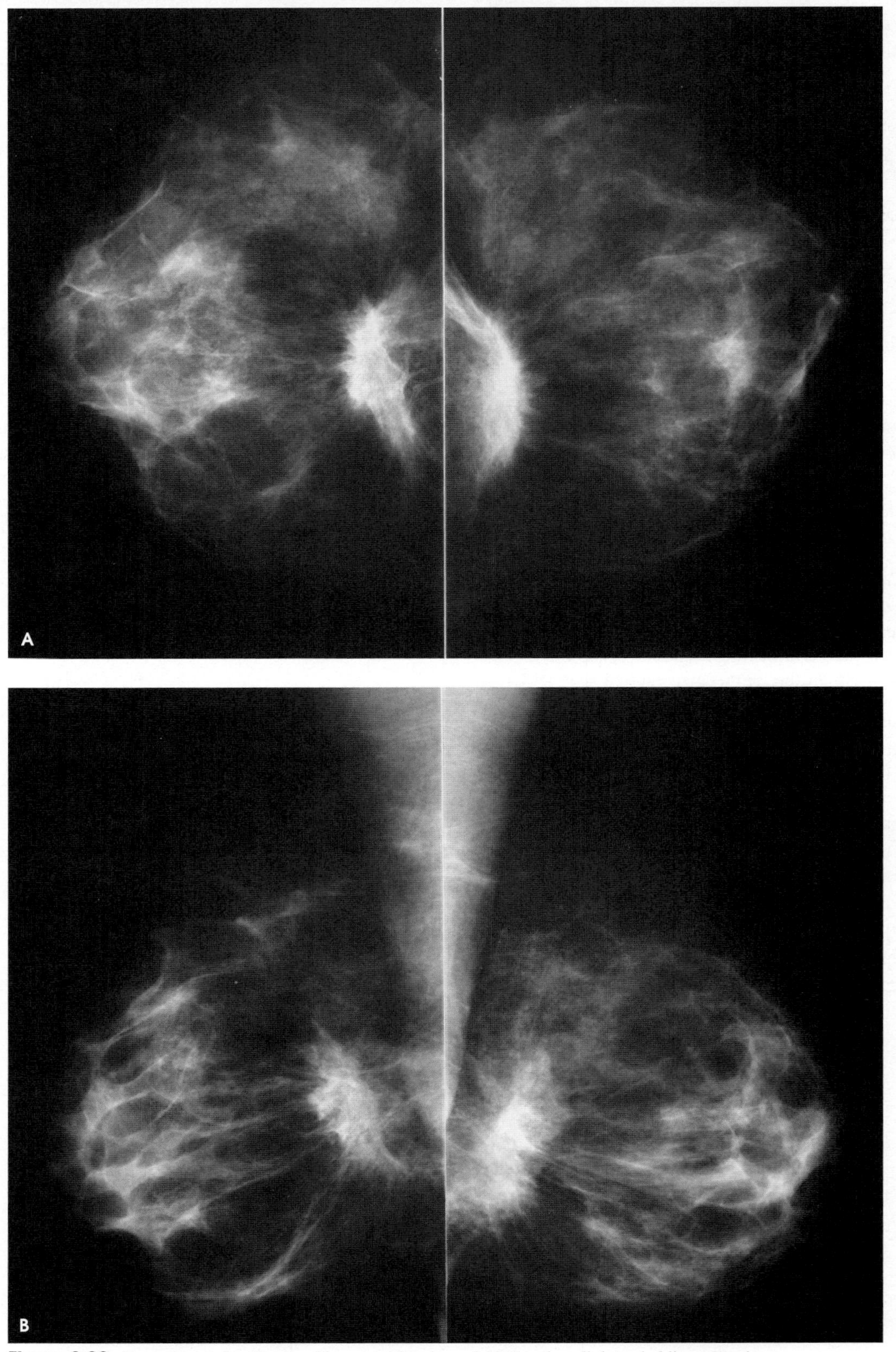

Figure 2.32. Screening study, 43-year-old woman. Craniocaudal **(A)** and mediolateral oblique **(B)** views.

What do you think?

Bilateral, symmetric spiculated masses are present with associated distortion. What could generate symmetric, almost identical findings in this location? What specific question would you ask the patient?

How about, did she have implants and were they removed?

Yes, she has had implants, and they have been removed. Mammographically, the findings following implant removal are variable. In some women, fluid collections may develop at the site of the implants; in others, portions of the capsule may be seen as curvilinear densities in the central aspect of the breasts posteriorly. Dense calcifications (dystrophic) may occur. Rarely, spiculated masses, presumably reflecting fat necrosis, may be present (as in this woman). Alternatively, the mammogram may be normal following implant removal.

BI-RADS® category 1: negative. BI-RADS® category 2: benign findings, is used if the observations are described in the report. Annual screening mammography is recommended.

PATIENT 30

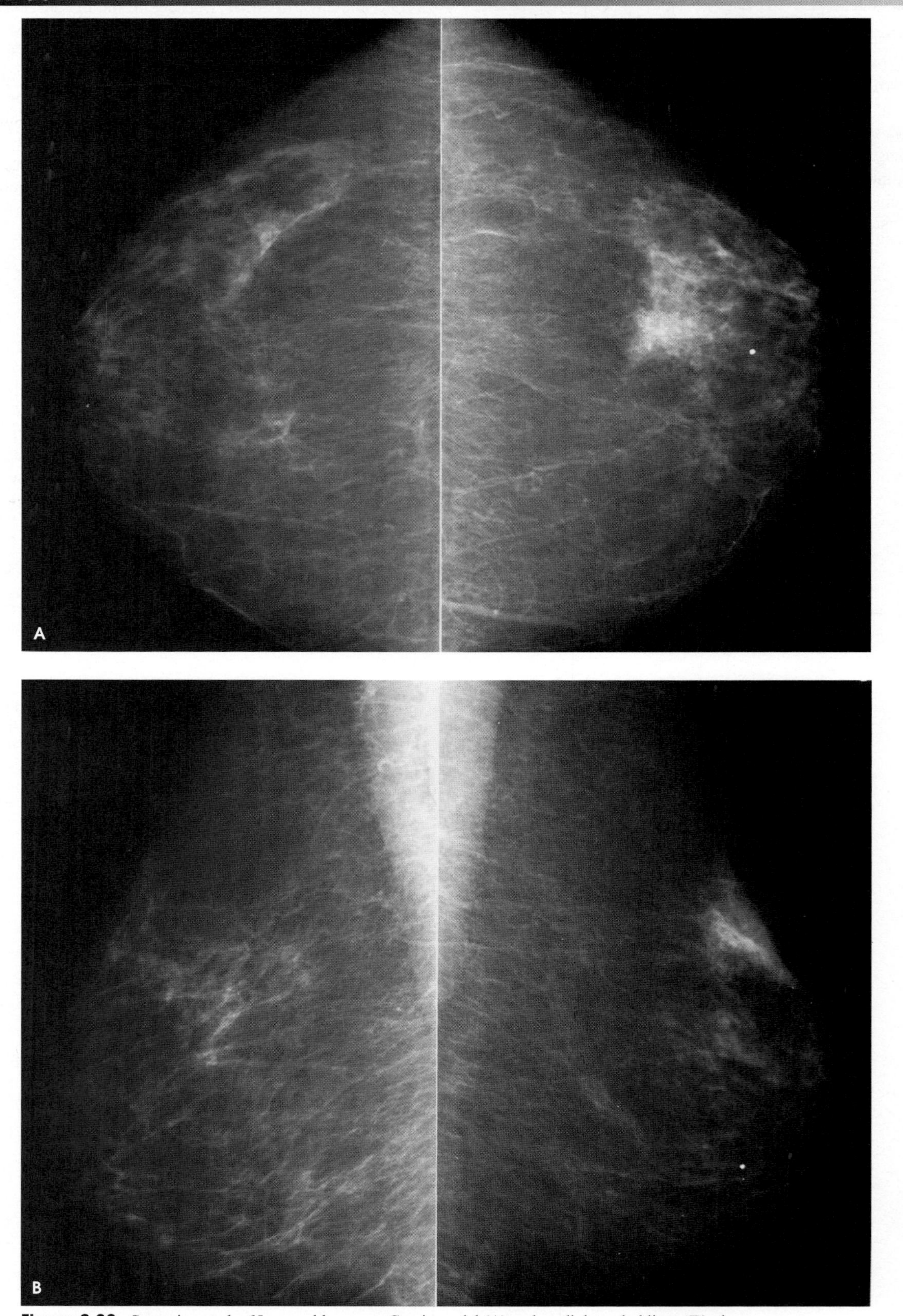

Figure 2.33. Screening study, 65-year-old woman. Craniocaudal **(A)** and mediolateral oblique **(B)** views.

What do you think, and what additional information would you like?

A focal area of parenchymal asymmetry is present in the upper central aspect of the left breast. It is in the same approximate distance from the nipple on both projections; however, it appears more spread out on the craniocaudal (CC) view. On the CC view, this area lacks the convex borders that are associated with most masses, and there is fat interspersed in the glandular tissue. In most patients, focal parenchymal asymmetry is a normal variant.

A good history is important. Has the patient had any breast surgery (e.g., a comparable area of tissue excised from the right breast), or does this finding reflect fat necrosis postsurgery at this site in the left breast? Is there any history of trauma to this site (e.g., hematoma)? Estrogen use? Presumably, if the patient had any focal tenderness, erythema, skin dimpling, or discoloration limited to this site, she would have been scheduled for a diagnostic evaluation or your technologist would have indicated this on the woman's history sheet.

What else would be helpful?

Comparison with prior studies is critical. If the area of focal parenchymal asymmetry represents a change, or if no prior studies are available for comparison, spot compression views and ultrasound with correlative physical examination are undertaken to exclude an underlying malignancy. If normal tissue is imaged on spot compression views and ultrasound, and there is no corresponding palpable abnormality on physical examination, no further intervention is recommended. Magnetic resonance imaging may also provide helpful information, particularly in high-risk patients in whom no definite mass is palpated but there is thickening or persistent concerns discerned during the physical examination at the site of the asymmetry. If concerns remain following the diagnostic evaluation, an imaging-guided biopsy can be undertaken.

Fibrosis or pseudoangiomatous stromal hyperplasia (PASH) is often the diagnosis on core biopsies done through these areas.

What is the differential diagnosis?

Differential considerations include normal variant, hormone replacement therapy effect, asymmetry secondary to prior surgical excision of the corresponding tissue in the right breast, focal fibrosis, pseudoangiomatous stromal hyperplasia (PASH), postsurgical or traumatic changes (evolving hematoma; fat necrosis), mastitis, fibroadenolipoma (hamartoma), invasive ductal carcinoma not otherwise specified, invasive lobular carcinoma, and lymphoma.

This area is unchanged from prior studies (not shown).

BI-RADS® category 1: negative. Annual screening mammography is recommended.

PATIENT 31

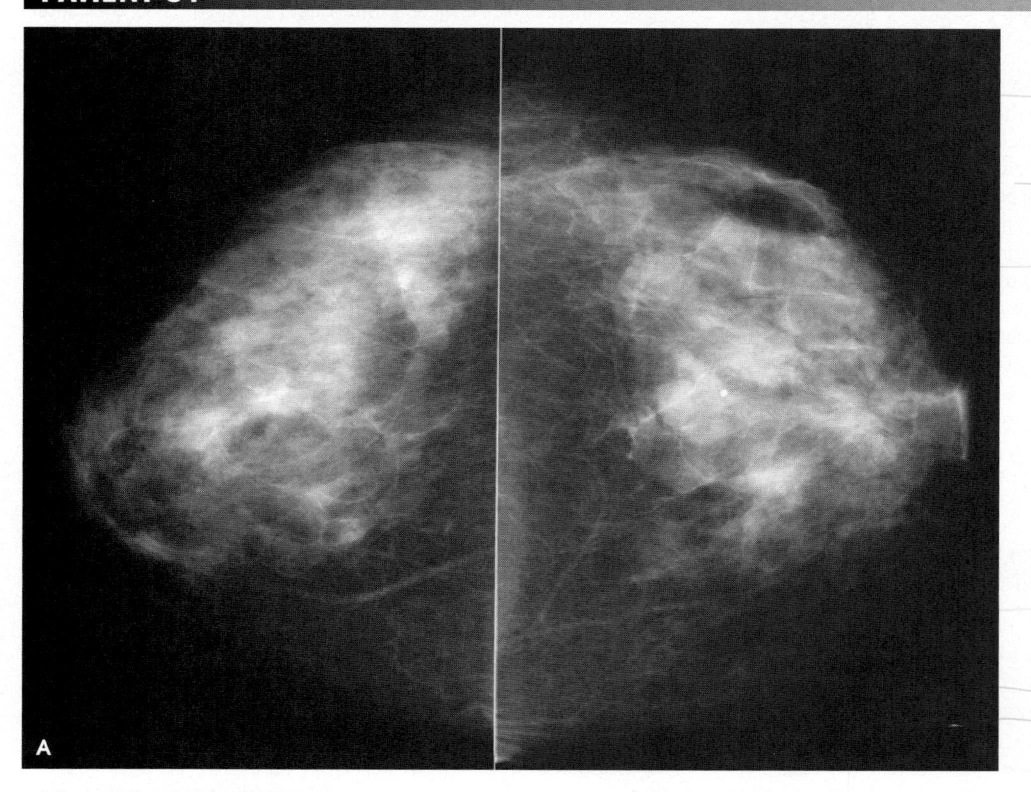

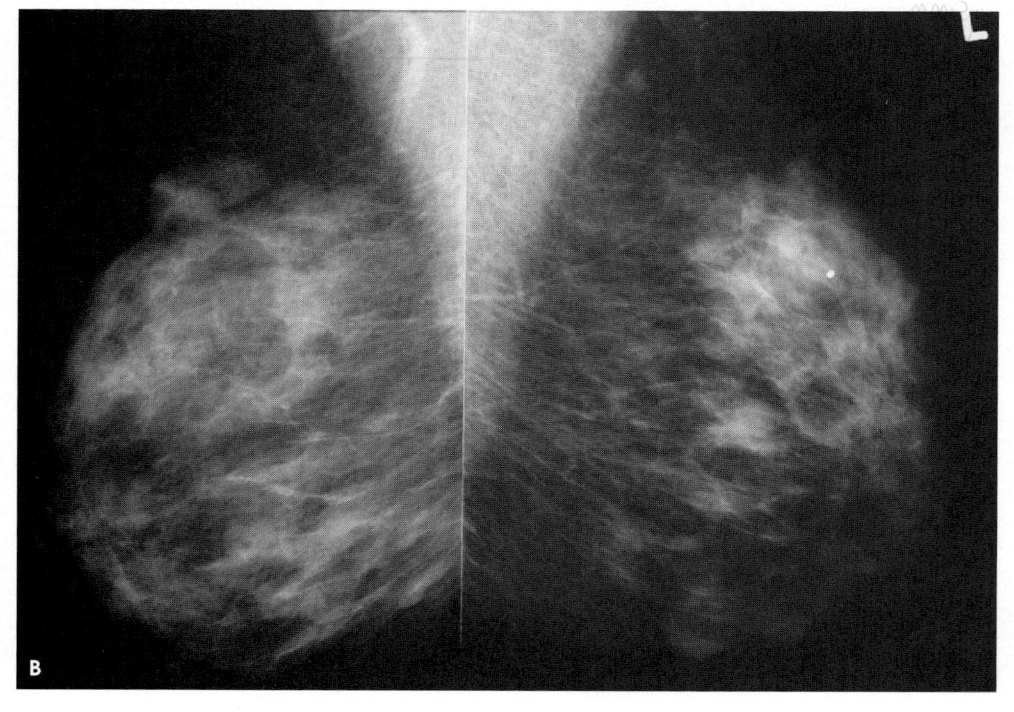

Figure 2.34. Screening study, 74-year-old woman. Craniocaudal **(A)** and mediolateral oblique **(B)** views. Metallic BB on skin lesion, left breast.

What do you think?

In this patient, the potential abnormality may not be readily apparent. In these situations, it is particularly important to review the films systematically, looking specifically for a mass, calcifications, distortion, or asymmetry. Evaluate specific locations including medial quadrants on the craniocaudal views, fat–glandular interfaces, the fatty stripe of tissue between the pectoral muscle and the glandular tissue on the mediolateral oblique (MLO) views, the upper cone of tissue on the MLO views and the subareolar areas. You need to focus carefully: Unlike most masses and calcifications, the perception of distortion is difficult and requires special attention.

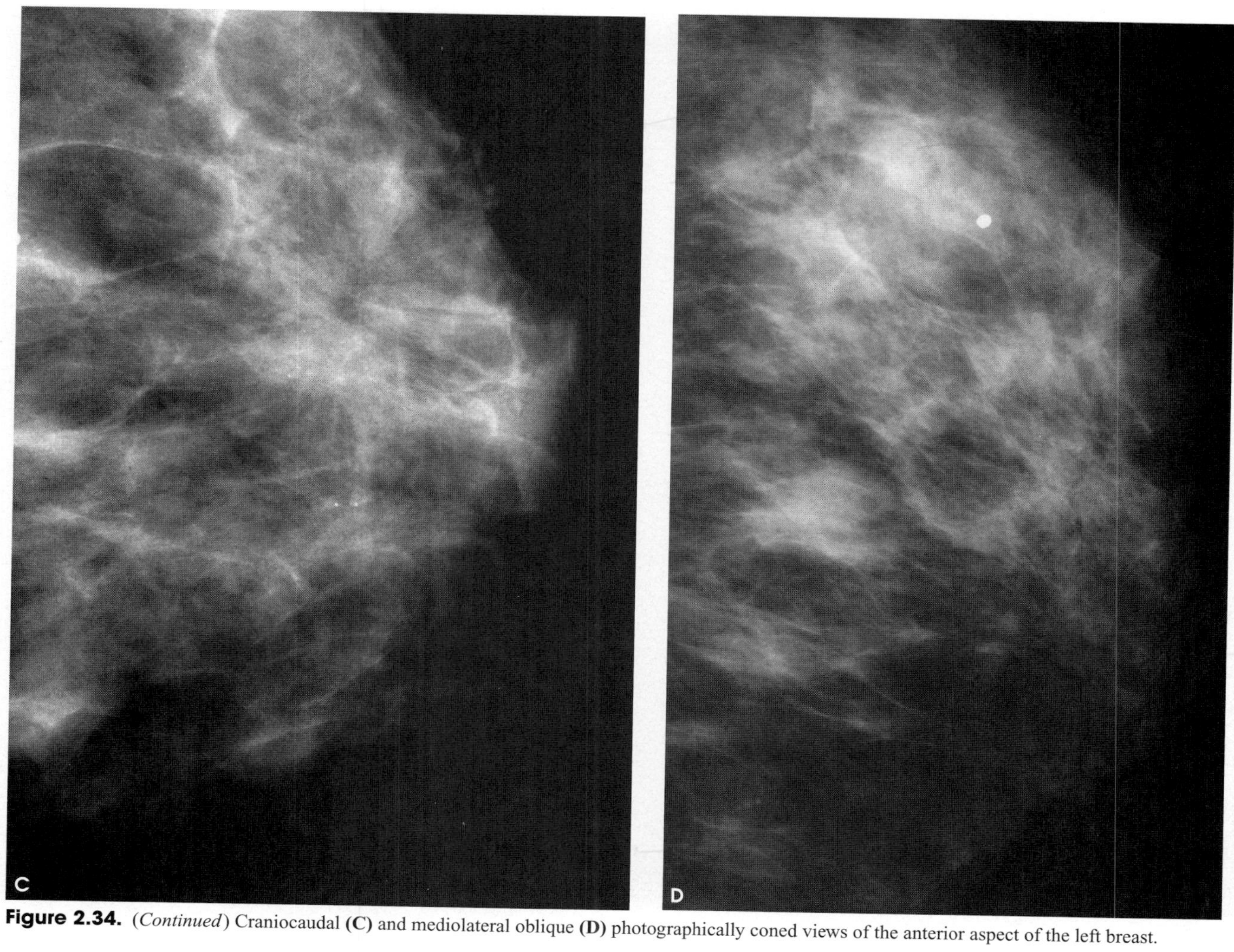

Figure 2.34. (*Continued*) Craniocaudal **(C)** and mediolateral oblique **(D)** photographically coned views of the anterior aspect of the left breast.

Focus your attention anteriorly. Look for straight lines and an overall disruption of tissue architecture. In some patients you may see what appear as small locules of fat clustered in the central aspect of the distortion as well as along the straightened trabecula. As you focus your search of the subareolar area, do you see the distortion?

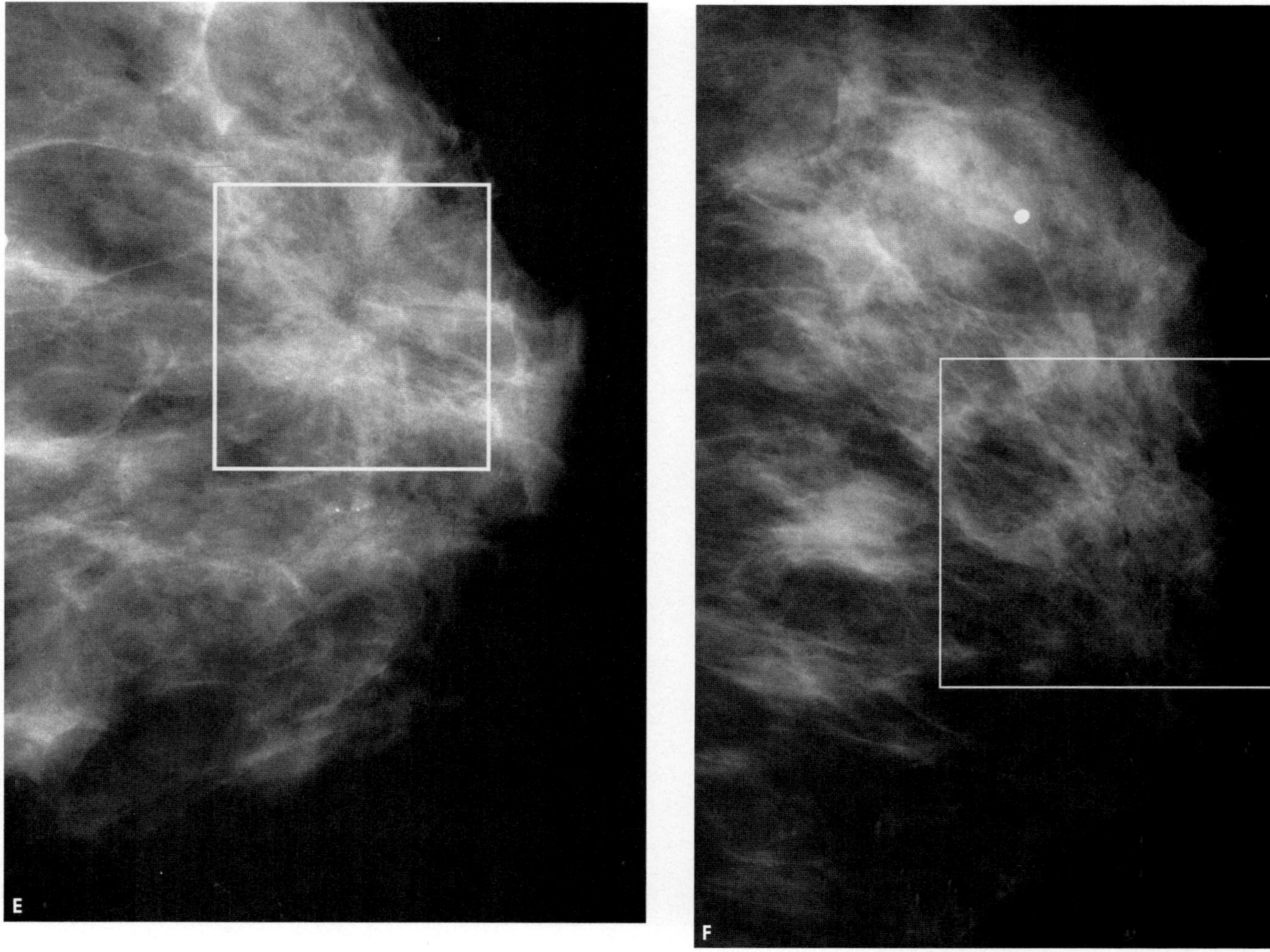

Figure 2.34. (*Continued*) Craniocaudal **(E)** and mediolateral oblique **(F)** photographically coned views of the anterior aspect of the left breast; area of distortion is delineated by box.

How can you increase your perception skills for distortion?

One way to enhance your perception of distortion is to evaluate the mammograms of women who have had a prior surgical biopsy. Although in many of these women no abnormality is apparent, in a small number, subtle distortion can be seen at the biopsy site; looking for it will help you enhance your perception skills for subtle distortion. Previous films and a history of prior breast biopsies or trauma should be obtained. If the patient has not had a prior breast biopsy or significant trauma to the left subareolar area and this finding represents an interval change, additional evaluation is indicated.

BI-RADS® category 0: need additional imaging evaluation.

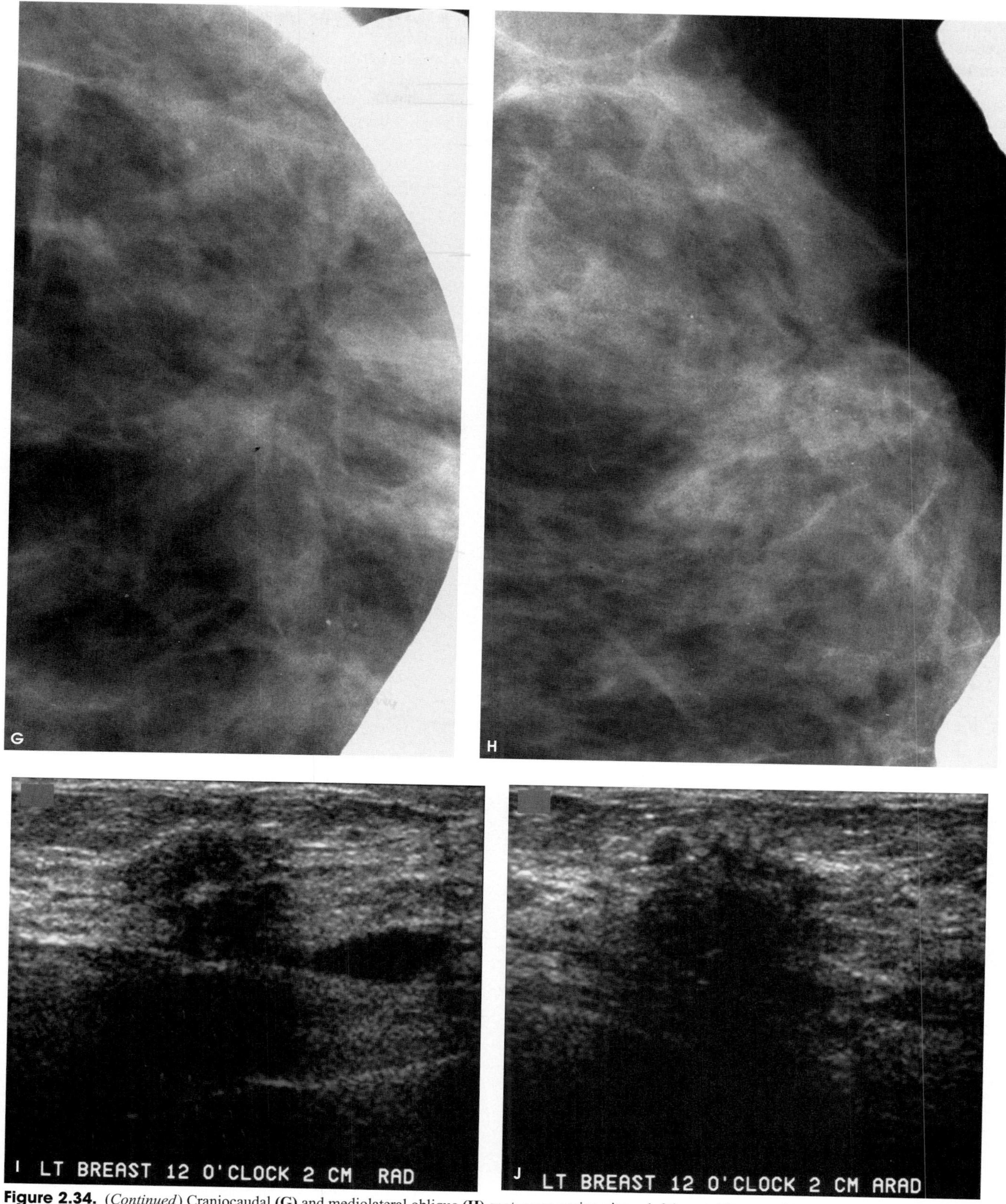

Figure 2.34. (*Continued*) Craniocaudal **(G)** and mediolateral oblique **(H)** spot compression views, left breast. Ultrasound images in radial (RAD) **(I)** and antiradial (ARAD) **(J)** projections, left breast, corresponding to the site of mammographic concern.

Do the compression views help? How would you describe the imaging findings?

Distortion is confirmed on the spot compression views. An irregular, vertically oriented, hypoechoic, 2-cm mass with indistinct, angular, and microlobulated margins and associated shadowing is imaged at the 12 o'clock position, 2 cm from the left nipple.

BI-RADS® category 4: suspicious abnormality; biopsy should be considered.

An invasive lobular carcinoma is reported on the core samples. A 2.2-cm, grade I invasive ductal carcinoma with prominent lobular features is reported on the lumpectomy specimen. Three excised sentinel lymph nodes are normal [pT2, pN0(sn)(i−), pMX; Stage IIA].

PATIENT 32

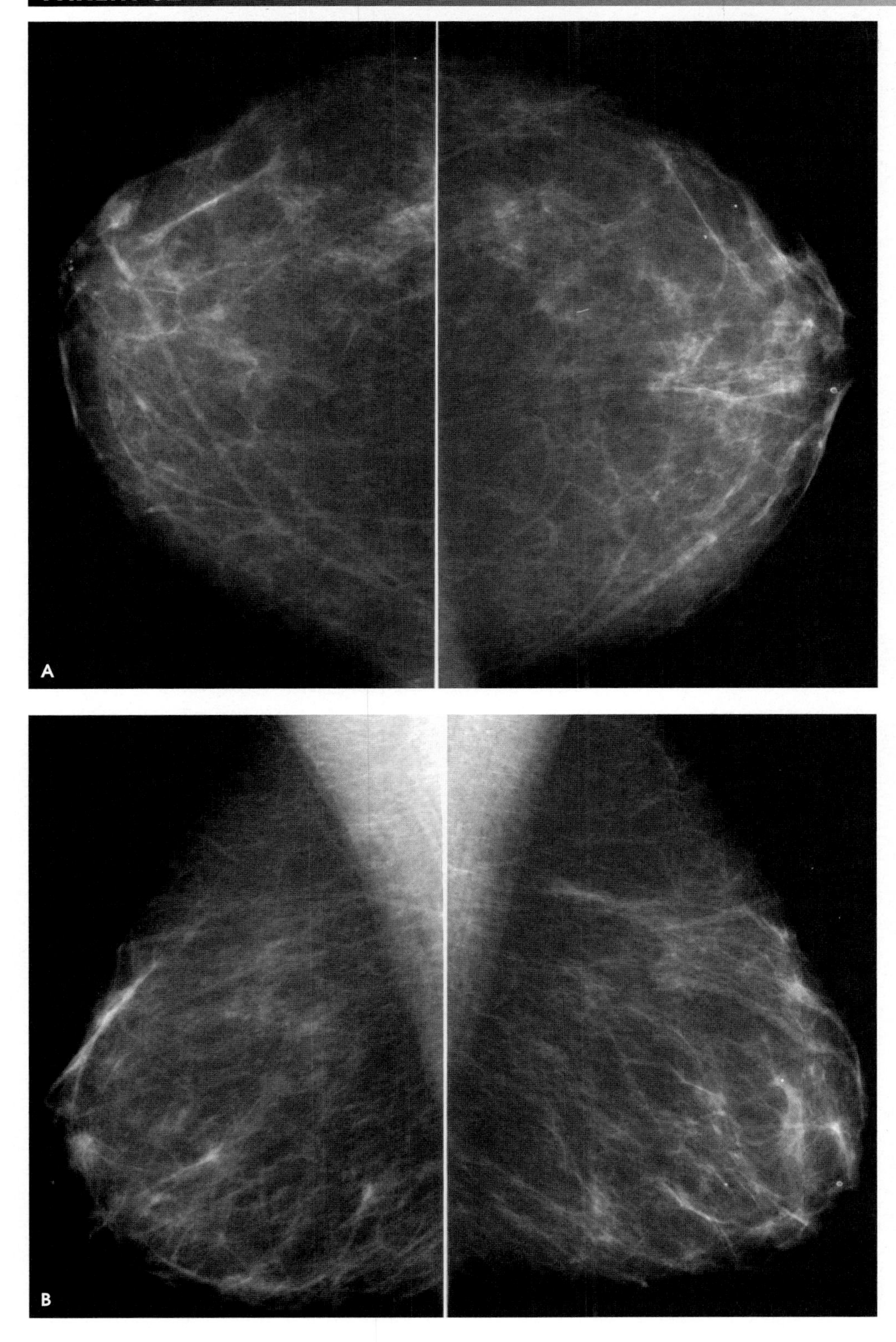

Figure 2.35. Screening study, 55-year-old woman. Craniocaudal **(A)** and mediolateral oblique **(B)** views.

Any observations?

A mass is present in the right subareolar area. If prior studies are available, comparison will be helpful. If this finding is new, additional evaluation is indicated. If this finding is stable, decreasing in size, or has previously been evaluated, additional evaluation may not be indicated.

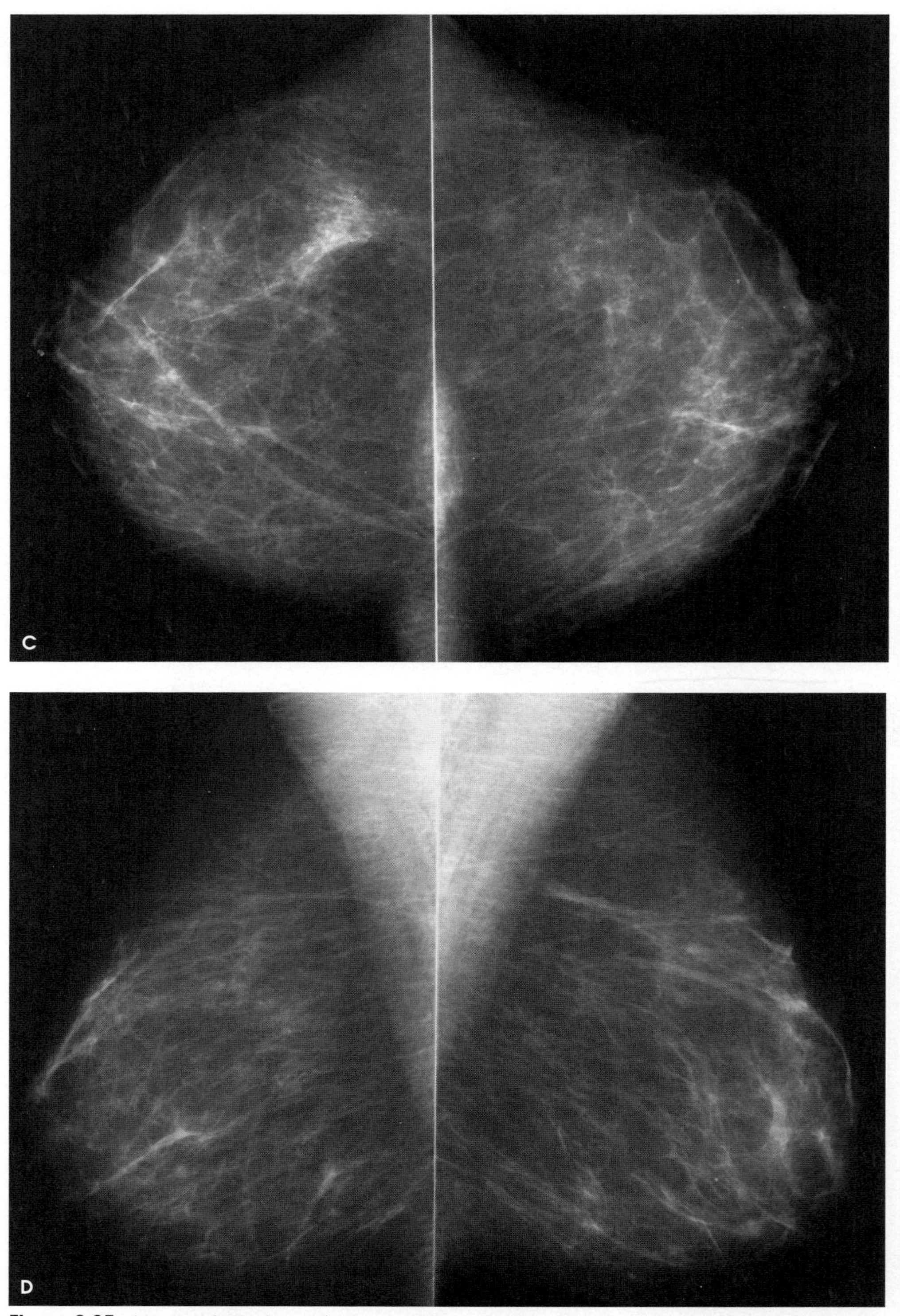

Figure 2.35. (*Continued*) Craniocaudal **(C)** and mediolateral oblique **(D)** views, 16 months prior to **(A)** and **(B)**.

What do you think, and what BI-RADS® assessment category would you assign?

The finding in the right breast represents a change. Additional evaluation with spot compression views and ultrasound is recommended.

BI-RADS® category 0: need additional imaging evaluation.

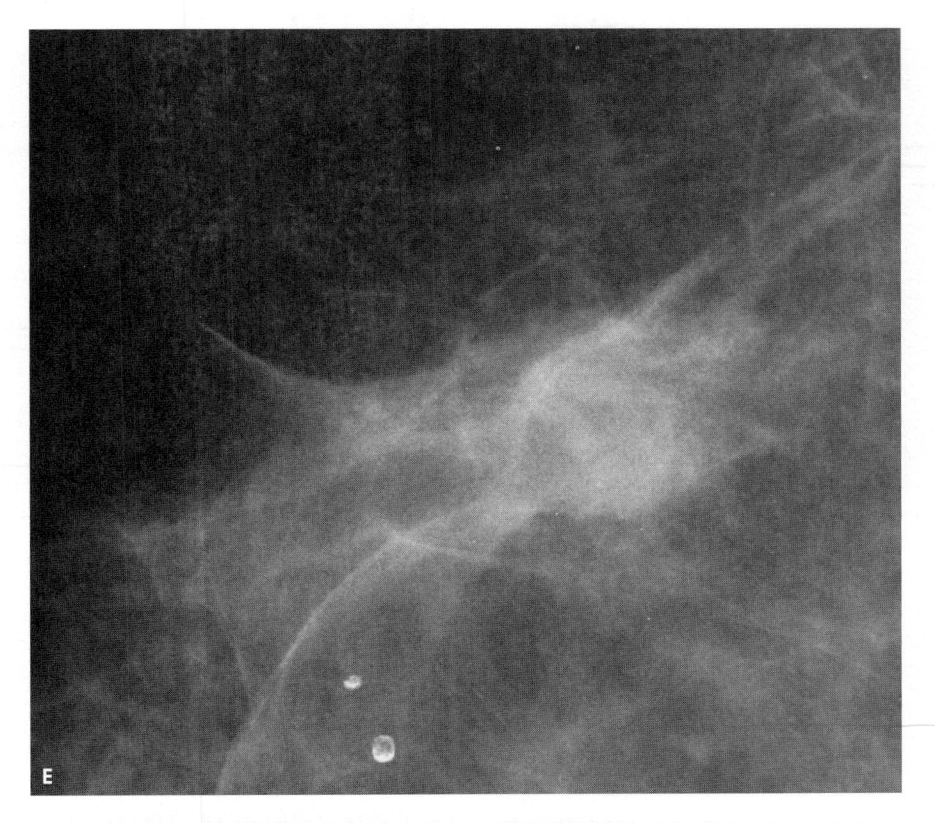

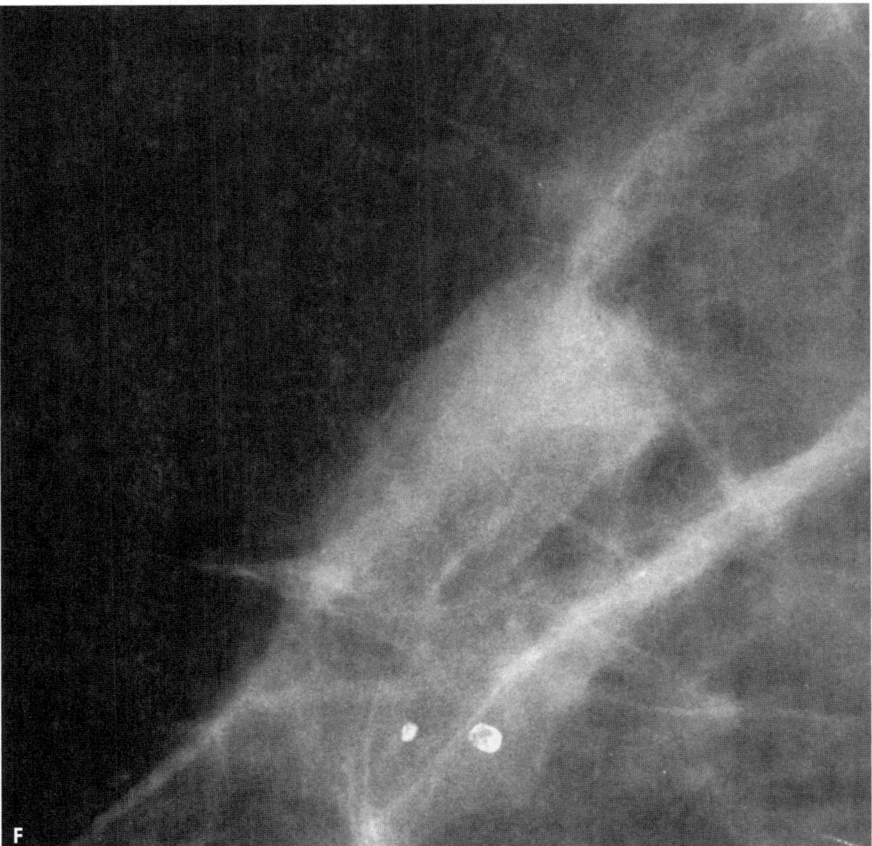

Figure 2.35. (*Continued*) Craniocaudal **(E)** and mediolateral oblique **(F)** spot compression views, right breast.

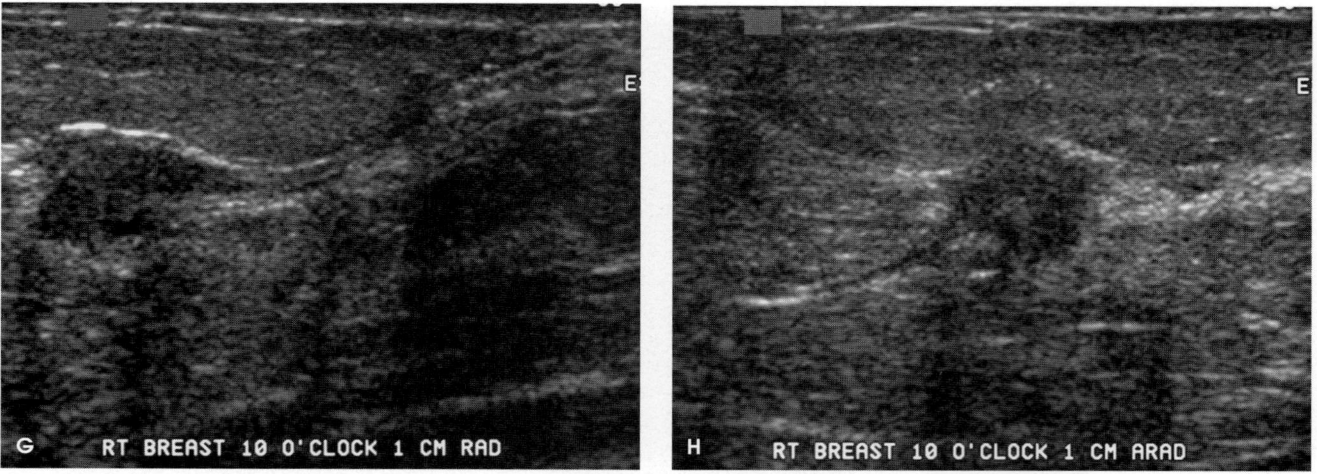

Figure 2.35. (*Continued*) Ultrasound images in radial (RAD) **(G)** and antiradial (ARAD) **(H)** projections, right subareolar area, corresponding to the site of mammographic concern.

How would you describe the imaging findings, and how would you sort through the differential?

A mass with indistinct and obscured margins is imaged on the spot compression views. A hypoechoic mass, with angular margins and associated prominent ducts extending toward the nipple and branching away from the nipple (Fig. 2.35I, J) is imaged at the 10 o'clock position, 1 cm from the right nipple. A fibroadenoma is unlikely to develop in a 55-year-old woman, particularly if she is not on hormones, and the imaging features are not typical of a fibroadenoma. Although the patient has no history of nipple discharge, and none is elicited during the ultrasound study, a papillary lesion is a significant consideration given the subareolar location and the associated ductal changes noted on the ultrasound study. Focal fibrosis, pseudoangiomatous stromal hyperplasia (PASH), invasive ductal carcinoma not otherwise specified, mucinous, medullary, or papillary carcinomas are additional considerations. The bottom line? A solid mass developing in a postmenopausal woman requires biopsy.

BI-RADS® category 4: suspicious abnormality; biopsy should be considered.

An ultrasound-guided biopsy is done at the completion of the diagnostic evaluation.

Invasive ductal and intraductal carcinomas are reported on the ultrasound-guided core biopsy. A 1.5-cm grade I invasive ductal carcinoma and associated solid and cribriform ductal carcinoma in situ without necrosis are reported on the lumpectomy specimen. Micrometastatic disease detected on the hematoxylin-eosin (H&E) slides ($>$0.2 mm but $<$2 mm in size) is reported in two of three excised sentinel lymph nodes (pT1c, pN1mi, pMX; Stage IIB).

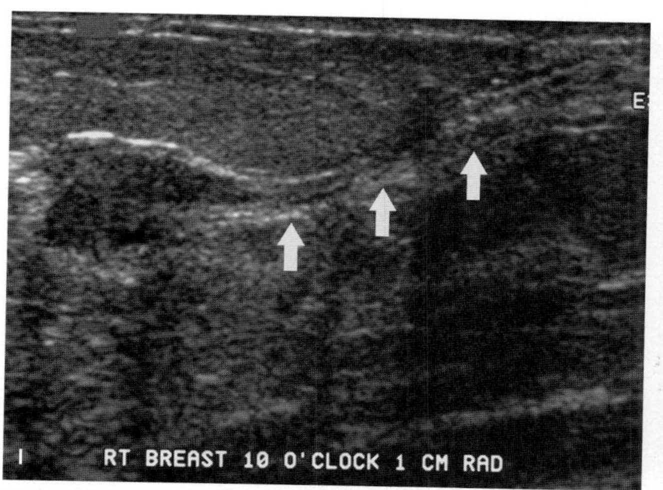

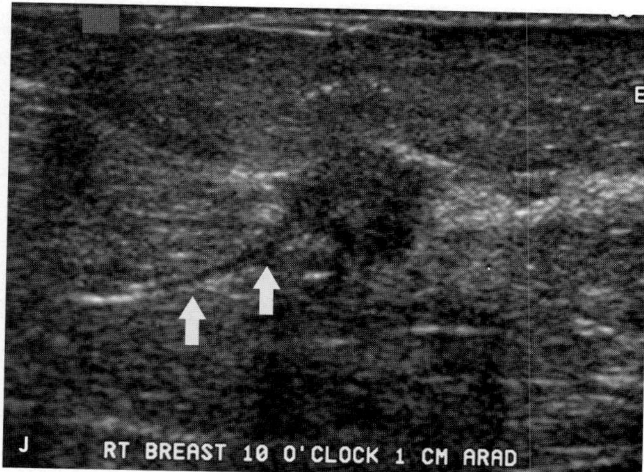

Figure 2.35. (*Continued*) Ultrasound image in (RAD) (**I**) projection demonstrating ducts (arrows) extending from the mass in the subareolar area towards the nipple ("duct extension"). Ultrasound image in antiradial (ARAD) (**H**) projection demonstrating ducts branching (arrows) away from the mass/nipple ("branch pattern").

What changes in the handling of lymph node specimens have been seen with the introduction of sentinel lymph nodes biopsies?

The advent and now widespread use of sentinel lymph node biopsy has resulted in a more meticulous evaluation of the excised lymph node(s). This includes serial sectioning of the entire lymph node (as opposed to sample sections from multiple lymph nodes) and a more focused histologic and immunohistochemical (IHC) evaluation of the excised lymph node. Some of the effects of this more thorough pathologic evaluation include the observation of isolated tumor cells and micromestatic disease. Consequently, the significance of these findings (isolated tumor cells and micrometastasis) involving excised sentinel lymph nodes is not yet clear, and there is no consensus on their prognostic significance. Currently, the use of IHC evaluation of sentinel lymph nodes is not encouraged; however, it is done at many institutions. The determination of micromestatic disease should be based on routine H&E histologic evaluation.

PATIENT 33

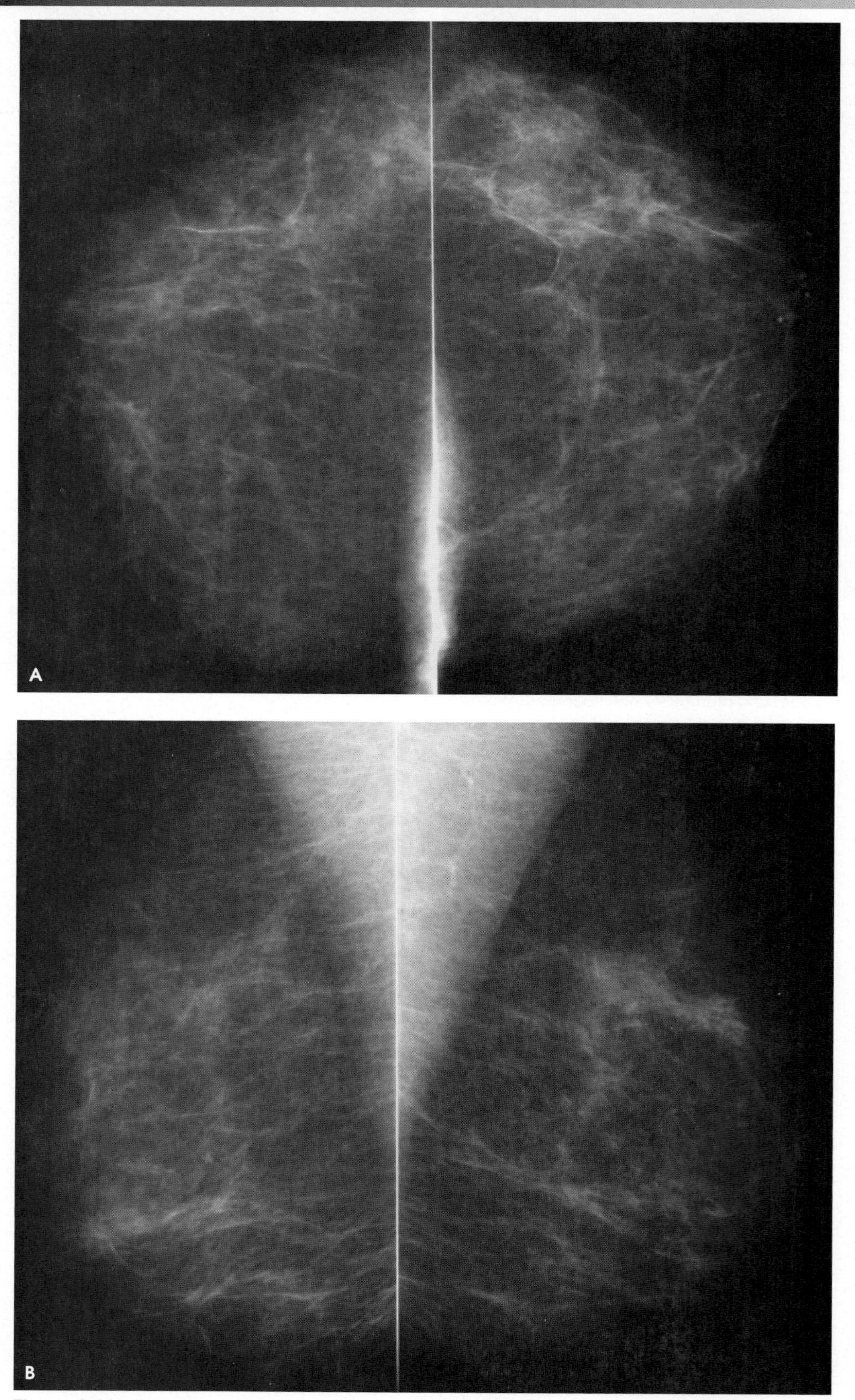

Figure 2.36. Screening study, 52-year-old woman. Craniocaudal **(A)** and mediolateral oblique **(B)** views.

What do you think?
Is this a normal mammogram, or do you think additional evaluation is indicated?

Review the images carefully, using a systematic approach. Divide the images in thirds so that you focus your attention on smaller portions of the mammograms and look specifically for masses, calcifications, asymmetric areas, distortion, and diffuse changes section by section. Do you notice anything? How about an area of asymmetry on the left, when you evaluate the upper third of the mediolateral oblique (MLO) views? Is there a comparable potential abnormality on the left craniocaudal (CC) view? How can you determine this? Although you can measure with a ruler, an easier way is to determine how many finger breadths behind the nipple the lesion is located on the MLO, making sure your fingers are positioned so that they are parallel to the edge of the pectoral muscle. For me, this lesion is three finger breadths posterior to the nipple ("X" cm, Fig. 2.36C). On the CC view, if I place my three fingers parallel to the edge of the film ("X" cm, Fig. 2.36D), the potential lesion will probably be somewhere along the course of my fingers (i.e., on a line drawn perpendicular to the arrow, Fig. 2.36D). This is obviously a rough measure, but it is helpful in determining if observations you make on one view have a corresponding potential finding on the other projection. In this patient, there is a potential abnormality noted on the CC view (box). This may be superimposed glandular tissue; however, with what degree of certainty can we establish this on the screening views? Do we mention it on the report, hedge and let it go, or do we call the patient back for additional views?

BI-RADS category 0: need additional imaging evaluation.

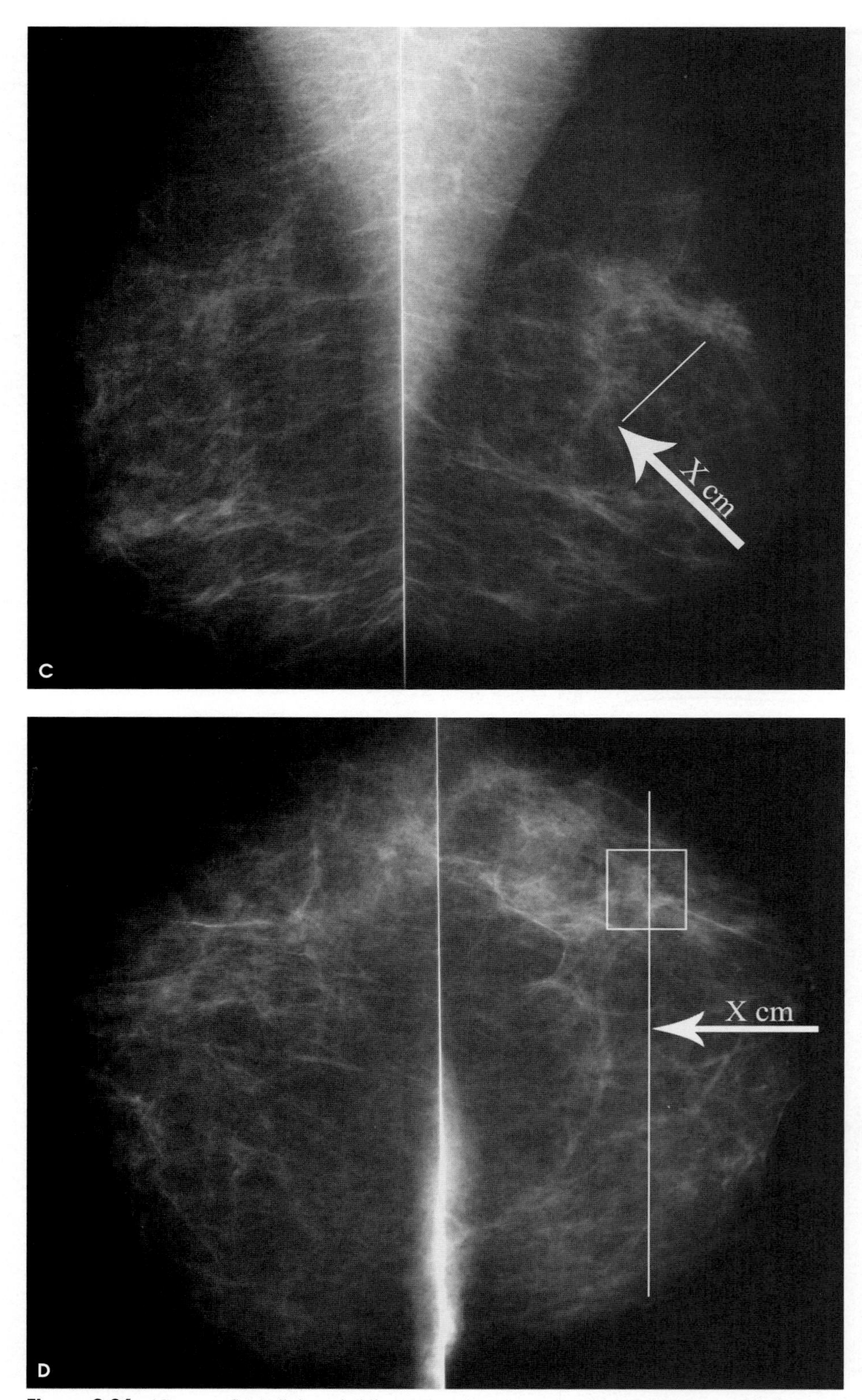

Figure 2.36. (*Continued*) Mediolateral oblique **(C)** and craniocaudal **(D)** views. The potential abnormality noted in the mediolateral oblique view is measured to be "X" cm posterior to the nipple. If there is a corresponding abnormality on the craniocaudal view, one can expect to find it along a line drawn to "X" cm from the nipple. A potential corresponding area of asymmetry is found in the craniocaudal view, within the box.

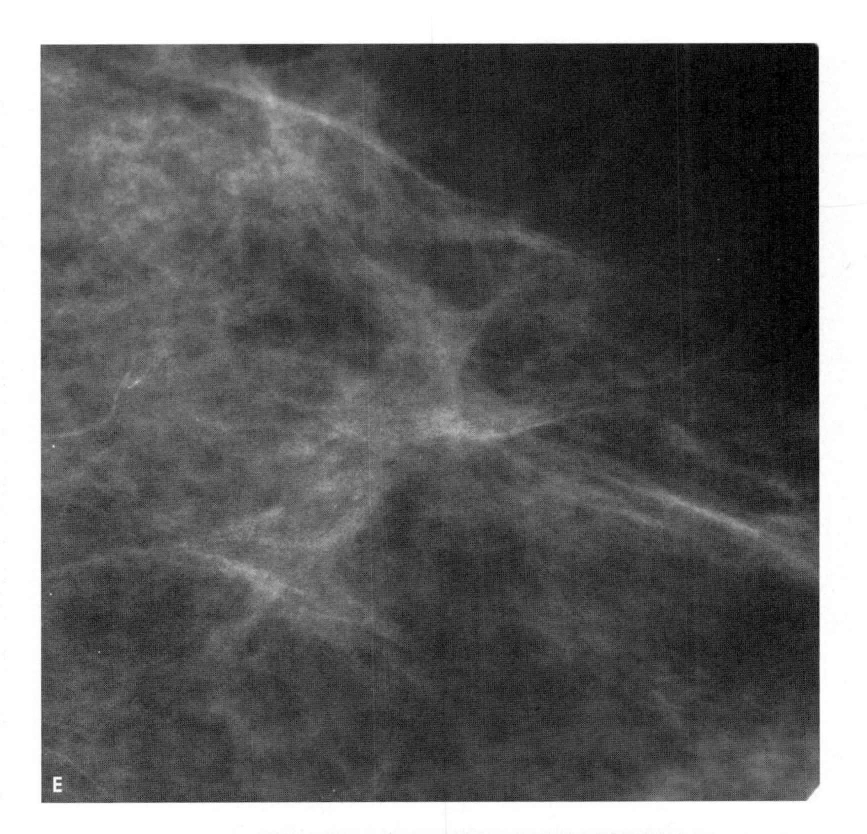

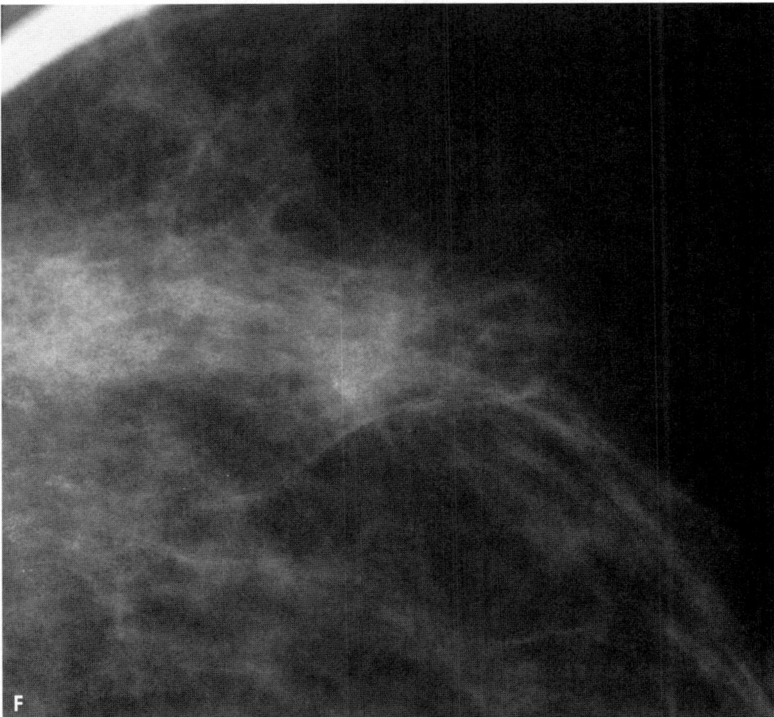

Figure 2.36. (*Continued*) Craniocaudal **(E)** and mediolateral oblique **(F)** spot compression views, left breast.

What do you think now?
Are you surprised?

The spot compression views demonstrate a 1-cm area of distortion corresponding to the area of concern on the screening study. In the absence of a history of a surgical biopsy or significant trauma at this site, correlative physical examination and ultrasound are undertaken.

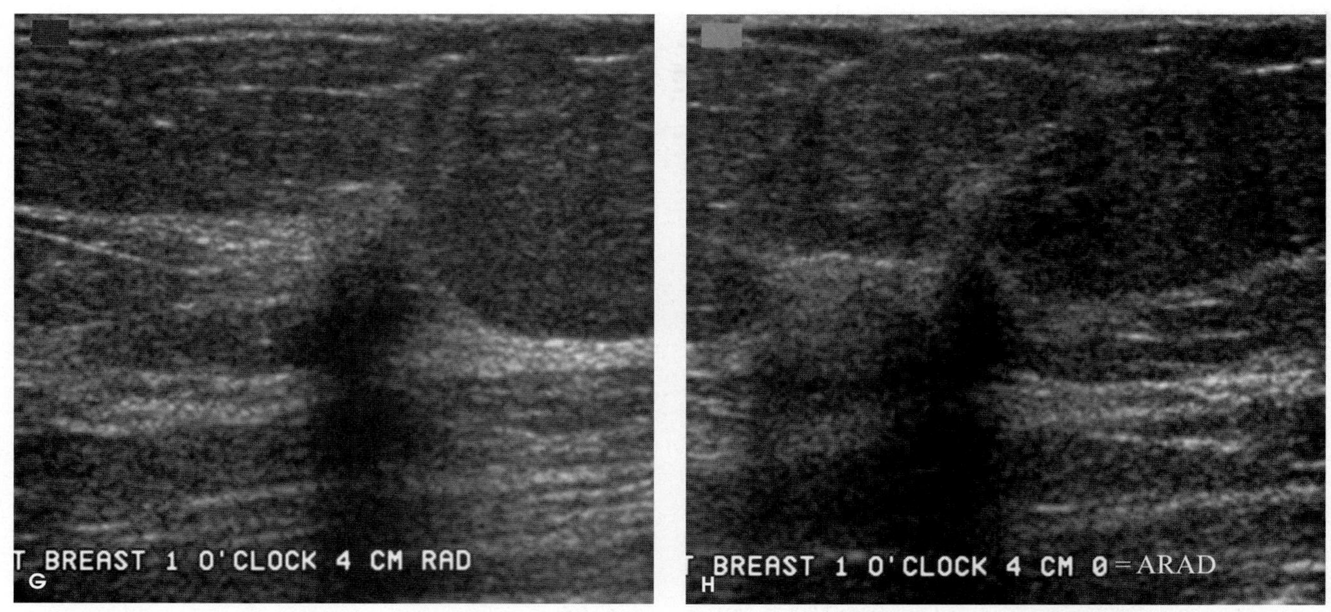

Figure 2.36. Ultrasound images, radial (RAD) **(G)** and antiradial (ARAD) **(H)** projections corresponding to the area of mammographic concern.

How would you describe the ultrasound findings, and what is your recommendation?

A vertically oriented, irregular, hypoechoic mass with indistinct margins and shadowing is consistently imaged at the 1 o'clock position, 4 cm from the left nipple. This corresponds to the area of mammographic concern. There is no corresponding palpable abnormality detected as this area is scanned.

BI-RADS® category 4: suspicious abnormality; biopsy should be considered.

An invasive lobular carcinoma is diagnosed following ultrasound-guided core biopsies. A 4.2-cm invasive lobular carcinoma is reported on the lumpectomy specimen; associated atypical lobular hyperplasia is present. No metastatic disease is diagnosed in two excised sentinel lymph nodes [pT2, pN0(sn)(i−), pMX; Stage IIA].

What do you think about the size described pathologically? Does this correlate with the imaging findings? Why not?

This is one of the reasons I call invasive lobular carcinoma the "sleaze disease." Small monomorphic cells that invade tissue in single files without forming nests of cells or disrupting surrounding structures characterize invasive lobular carcinoma histologically. Consequently, invasive lobular carcinomas can be clinically, mammographically, and pathologically (the invading cells can resemble lymphocytes) subtle. When we see something mammographically, the findings commonly underestimate the extent of disease found histologically (i.e., what we see mammographically is often the tip of the iceberg).

PATIENT 34

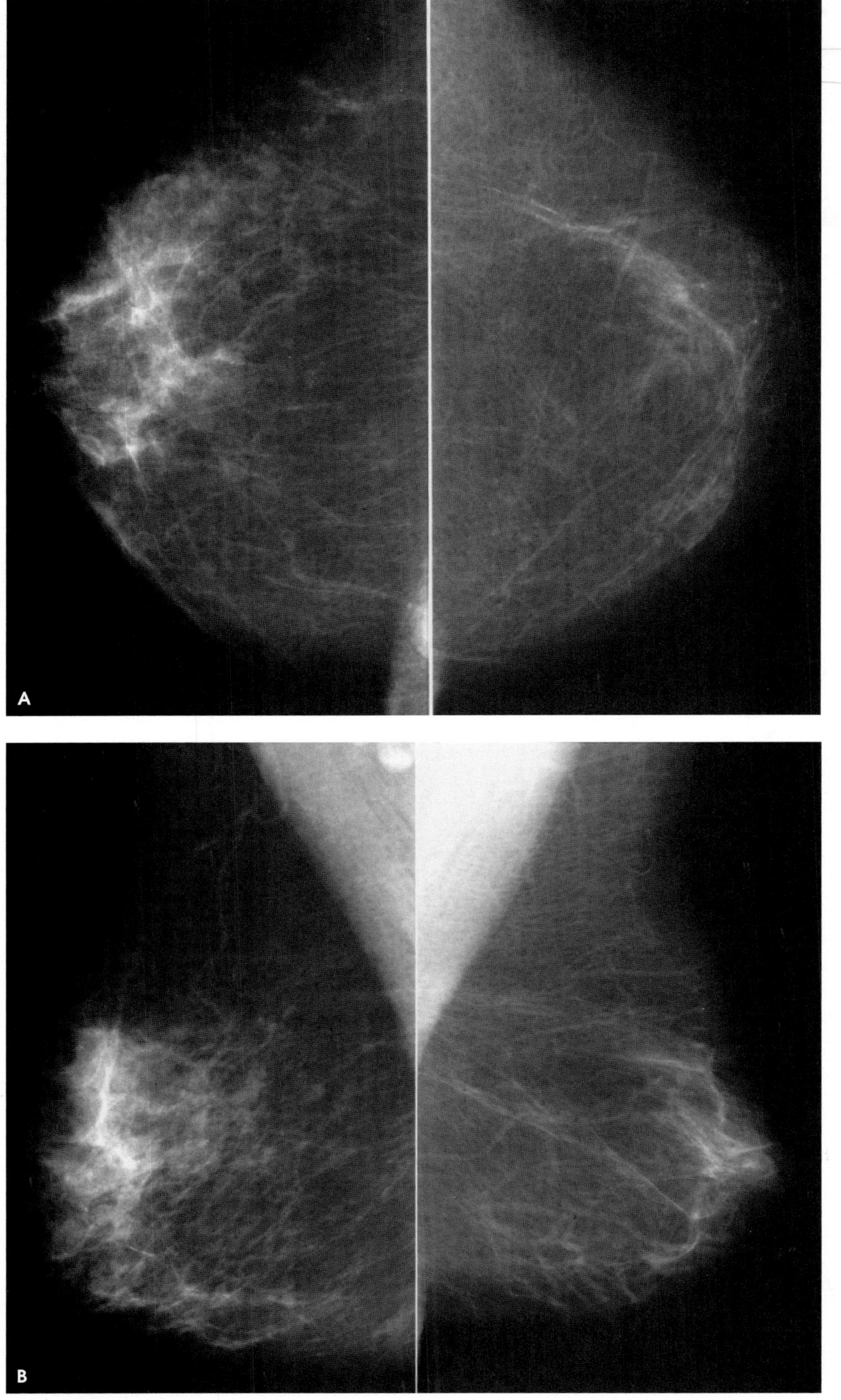

Figure 2.37. Screening study, 73-year-old woman. Craniocaudal **(A)** and mediolateral oblique **(B)** views.

What are the pertinent observations, and what is your working hypothesis?

Global parenchymal asymmetry is present in the right breast. The left breast is smaller and there is subtle distortion on the left, such that the prior breast surgical history should be reviewed. In this patient, the findings are iatrogenic. The patient has had a biopsy in the left breast, so the tissue on the right is now asymmetric. Following excisional biopsies, no mammographic abnormality is apparent in >50% of the patients. Changes that can be seen following an excisional biopsy include a decrease in size of the affected breast, localized skin thickening and retraction, architectural distortion, a spiculated or mixed-density (fat containing) mass, oil cysts, dystrophic calcifications, and areas of focal or global parenchymal asymmetry in the contralateral breast.

BI-RADS® category 1: negative. In general, for benign findings, if the observations represent a change from the prior mammogram, I describe them in the report and use BI-RADS® category 2: benign finding. If the findings are stable compared with prior mammograms, I do not describe them and use category 1 for the assessment. Annual screening mammography is recommended.

PATIENT 35

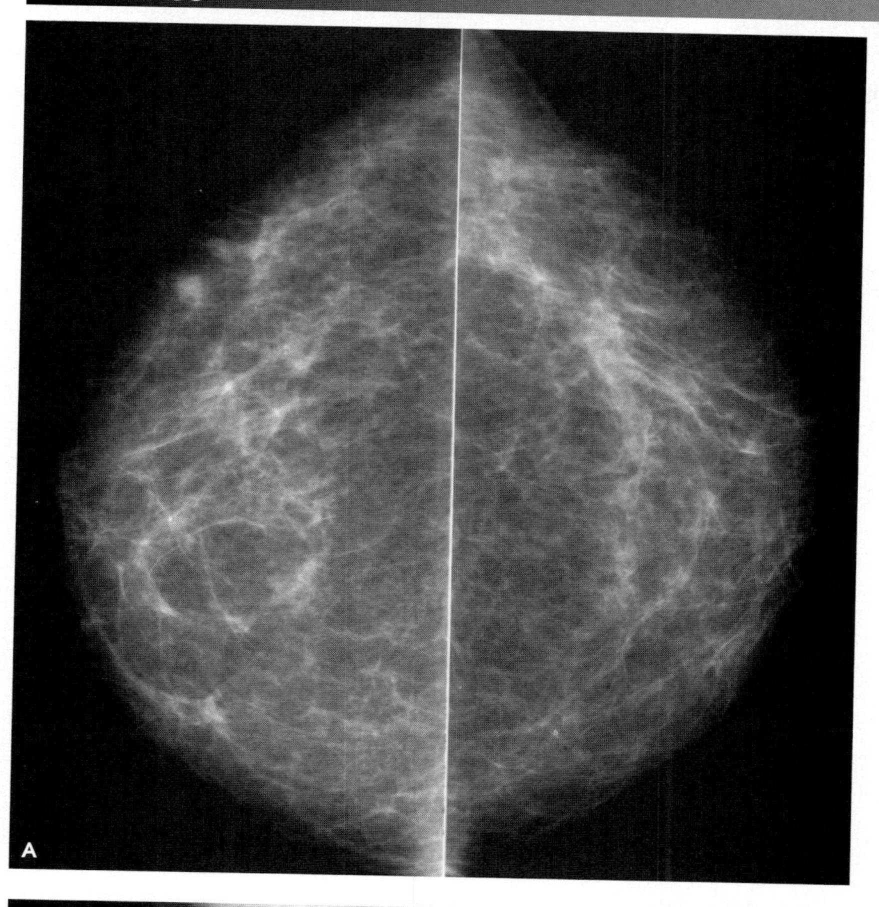

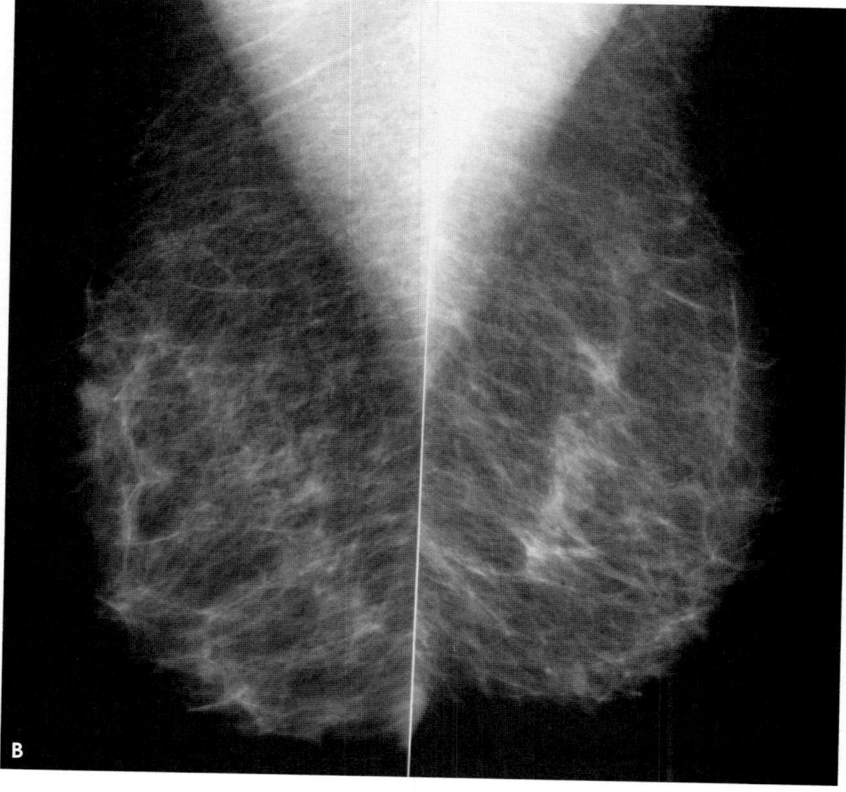

Figure 2.38. Screening study, 73-year-old woman. Craniocaudal **(A)** and mediolateral oblique **(B)** views.

Is this a normal mammogram, or is it potentially abnormal? How many lesions do you think may be present, and with what degree of certainty can you determine the significance of any finding?

A mass is present in the upper outer quadrant of the right breast (or, given the craniocaudal view, are there two?). Although you might be tempted to think that this is an intramammary lymph node, remember—make no assumptions! Is this mass well circumscribed? Can you unequivocally identify a fatty hilum? Can you establish the stability of this finding? Without prior films, which are not available, the stability of this finding cannot be determined. On the current study, it is not possible to confidently describe the margins as well circumscribed, nor can the presence of a fatty hilum be established; consequently, additional evaluation is indicated.

BI-RADS® category 0: need additional imaging evaluation.

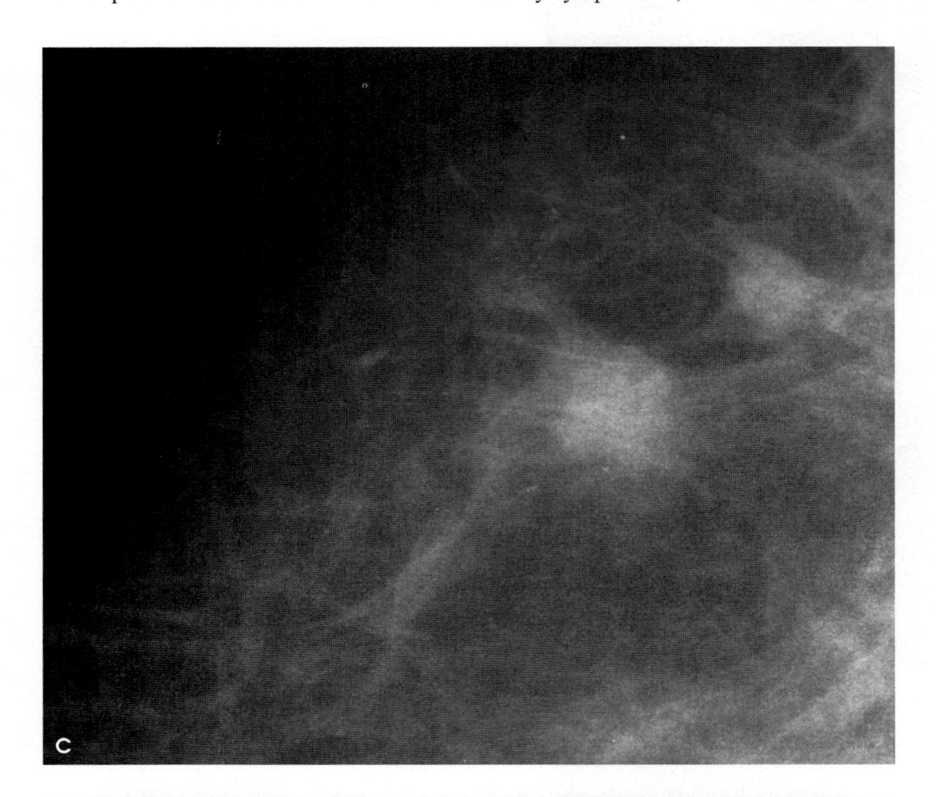

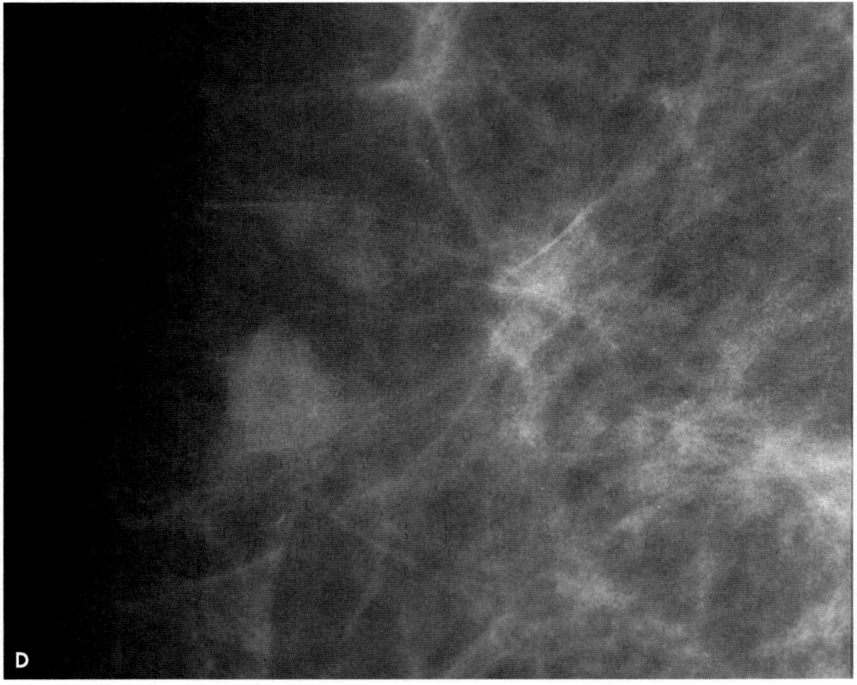

Figure 2.38. (*Continued*) Craniocaudal **(C)** and mediolateral oblique **(D)** spot compression views, right breast.

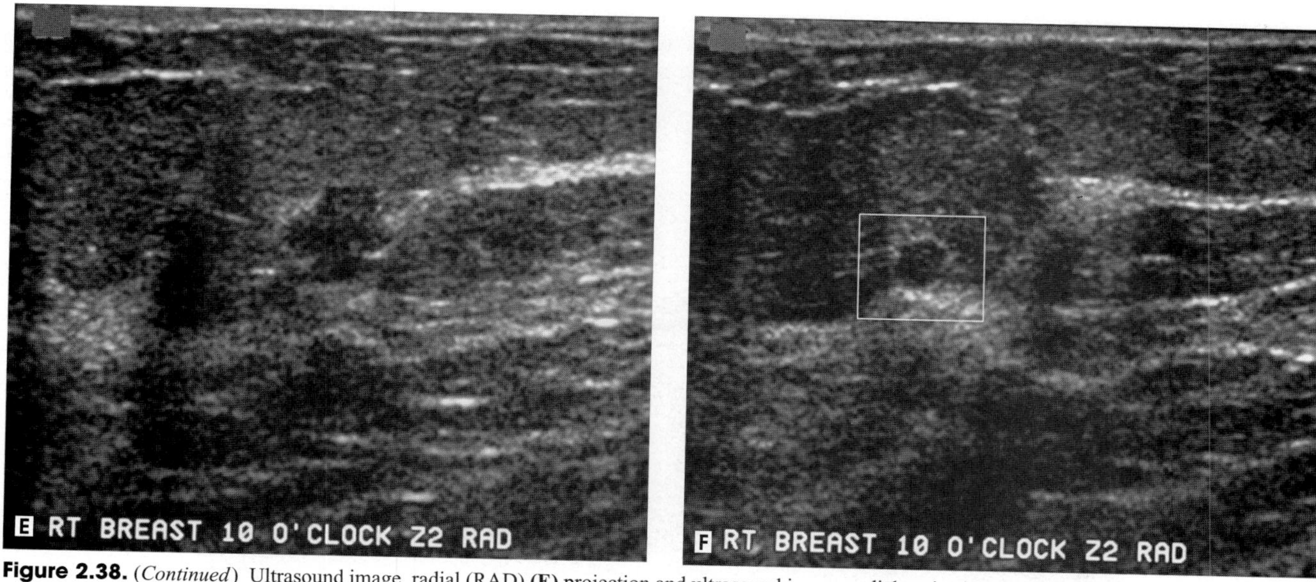

Figure 2.38. *(Continued)* Ultrasound image, radial (RAD) **(E)** projection and ultrasound image, radial projection **(F)**.

How would you describe the findings, and what is your recommendation?

The spot compression views confirm the presence of two masses with indistinct margins. On ultrasound, the larger of the two masses (Fig. 2.38E) is irregular in shape, vertically oriented, and characterized by angular margins. The smaller of the two masses (within box, Fig. 2.38F) is round with small spiculations. Both masses are at the 10 o'clock position, zone 2 in the right breast.

BI-RADS® category 4: suspicious abnormality; biopsy should be considered.

An invasive mammary carcinoma is reported on the core biopsy samples. A 1.2-cm grade III invasive mammary carcinoma, micropapillary type, is reported on the lumpectomy specimen. No metastatic disease is diagnosed in one excised sentinel lymph node [pT1c, pN0(sn)(i−), pMX; Stage I].

Invasive micropapillary carcinoma is a recently described entity. Unlike this patient, most of the patients described in the literature with this type of tumor have associated involvement of the axillary lymph nodes. As a result, this type of carcinoma has been associated with a poor prognosis.

PATIENT 36

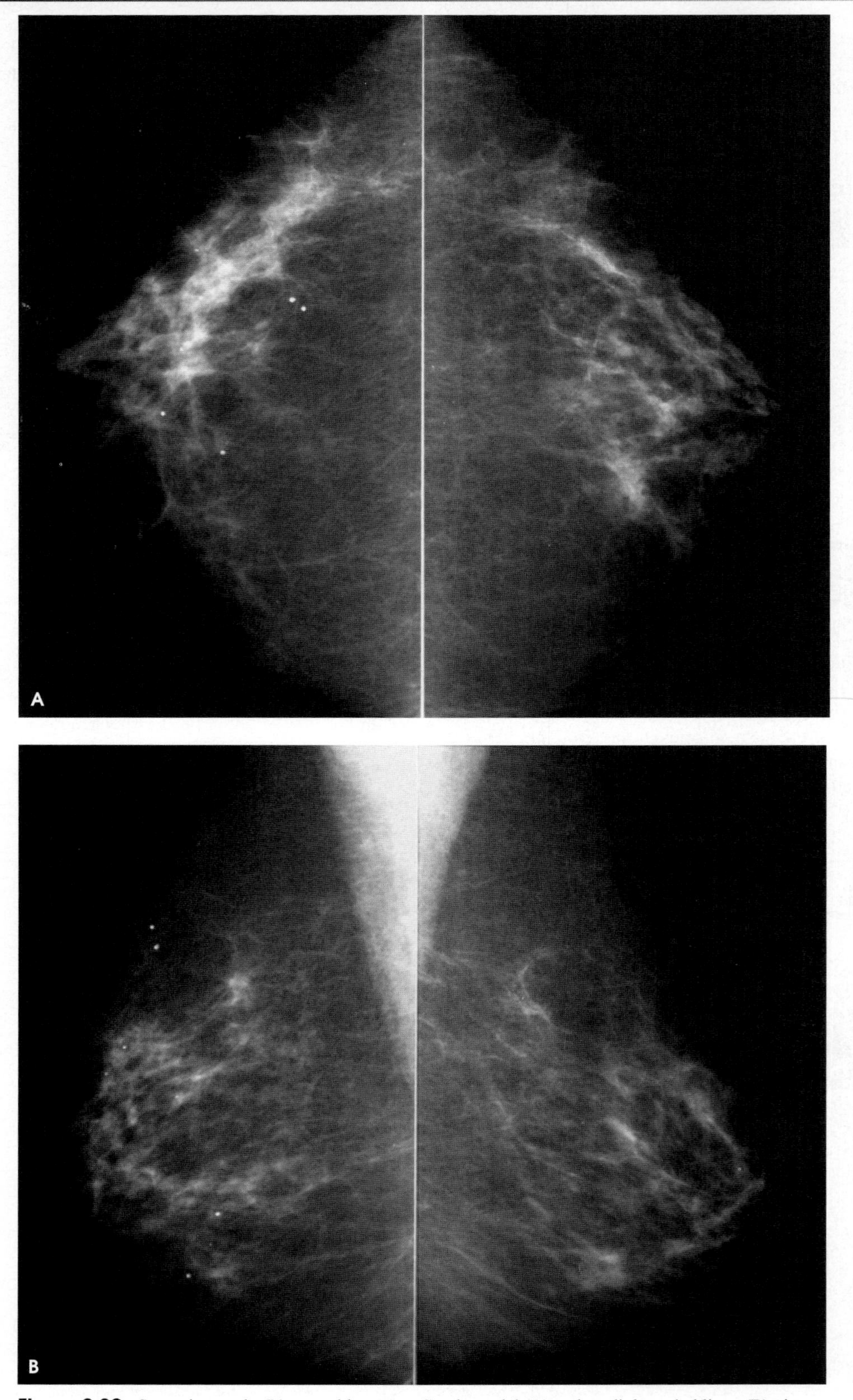

Figure 2.39. Screening study, 74-year-old woman. Craniocaudal **(A)** and mediolateral oblique **(B)** views.

What is the main observation?

Divide the images in thirds (Fig. 2.39C, D) so that you focus your attention on smaller portions of the mammograms and look specifically for masses, calcifications, asymmetric areas, distortion, and diffuse changes in a systematic progression. Asymmetric tissue is imaged medially in the left breast on the craniocaudal view.

Is there a corresponding area on the left mediolateral oblique view?

Use your fingers to approximate the distance from the nipple back to the asymmetric area on the craniocaudal (CC) view (Fig. 2.39E).

Now, go to the mediolateral oblique (MLO) view and, angling your fingers (Fig. 2.39F) so that they are parallel to the obliquity of the pectoral muscle, look for a corresponding abnormality at the edge of your finger—do you see it? Before calling the patient back, prior films (not shown) are reviewed and indicate that this is an interval change.

BI-RADS® category 0: need additional imaging evaluation.

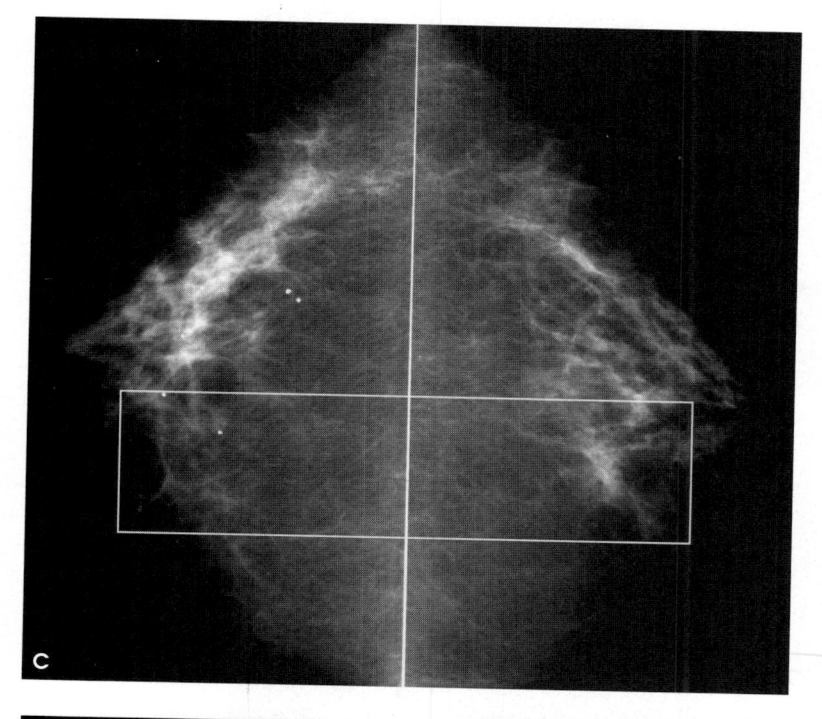

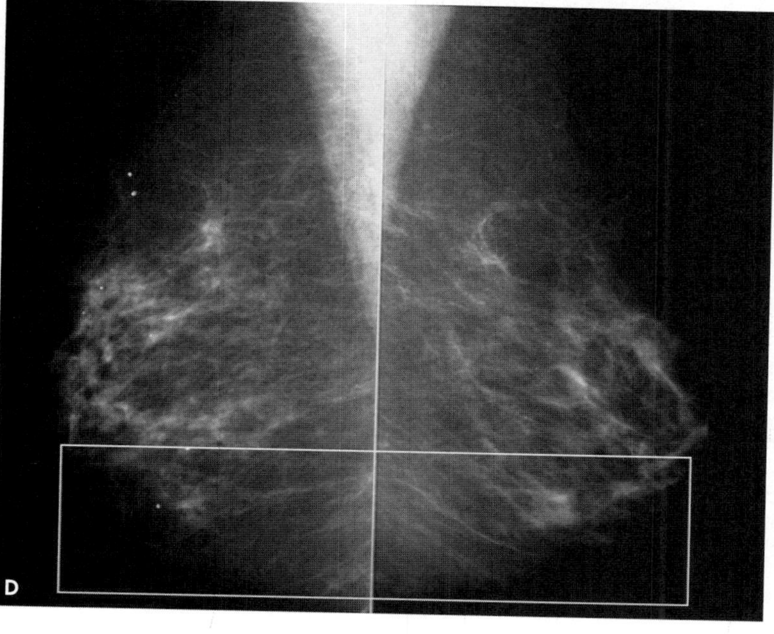

Figure 2.39. (*Continued*) Craniocaudal **(C)** and mediolateral oblique **(D)** views, limiting the evaluation to the medial and inferior thirds of the breasts. This helps focus attention on smaller amounts of tissue and enables you to go back and forth between the right and left breasts looking for masses, areas of parenchymal asymmetry, distortion, and calcifications.

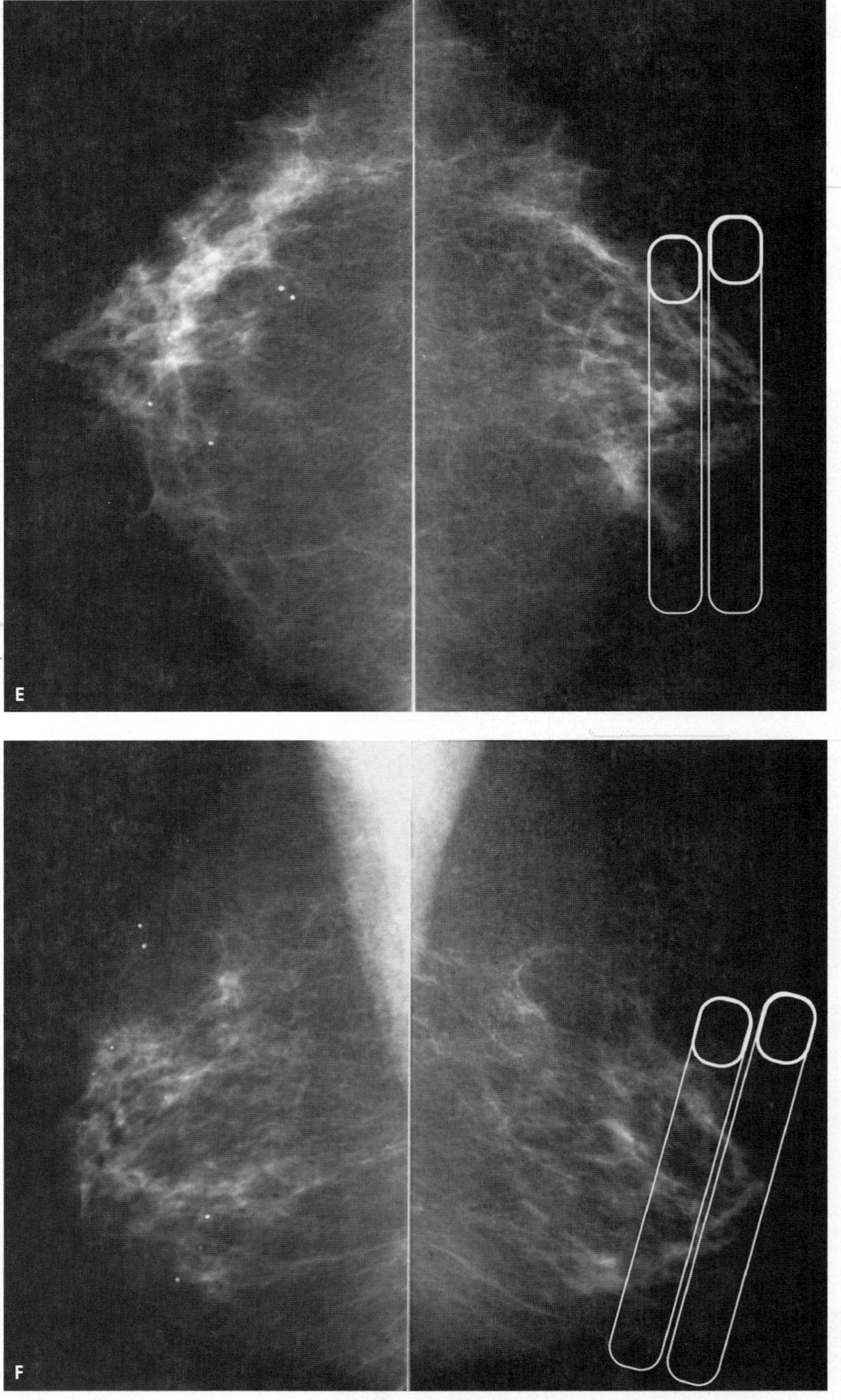

Figure 2.39. Craniocaudal **(E)** and mediolateral oblique **(F)** views. With the identification of an area of parenchymal asymmetry, medially in the left craniocaudal view, you can use your fingers to estimate the distance of this area from the nipple. Now, go to the mediolateral oblique view and, angling your fingers so that they are parallel to the obliquity of the pectoral muscle, you can identify a corresponding abnormality at the edge of your finger inferiorly on the mediolateral oblique view.

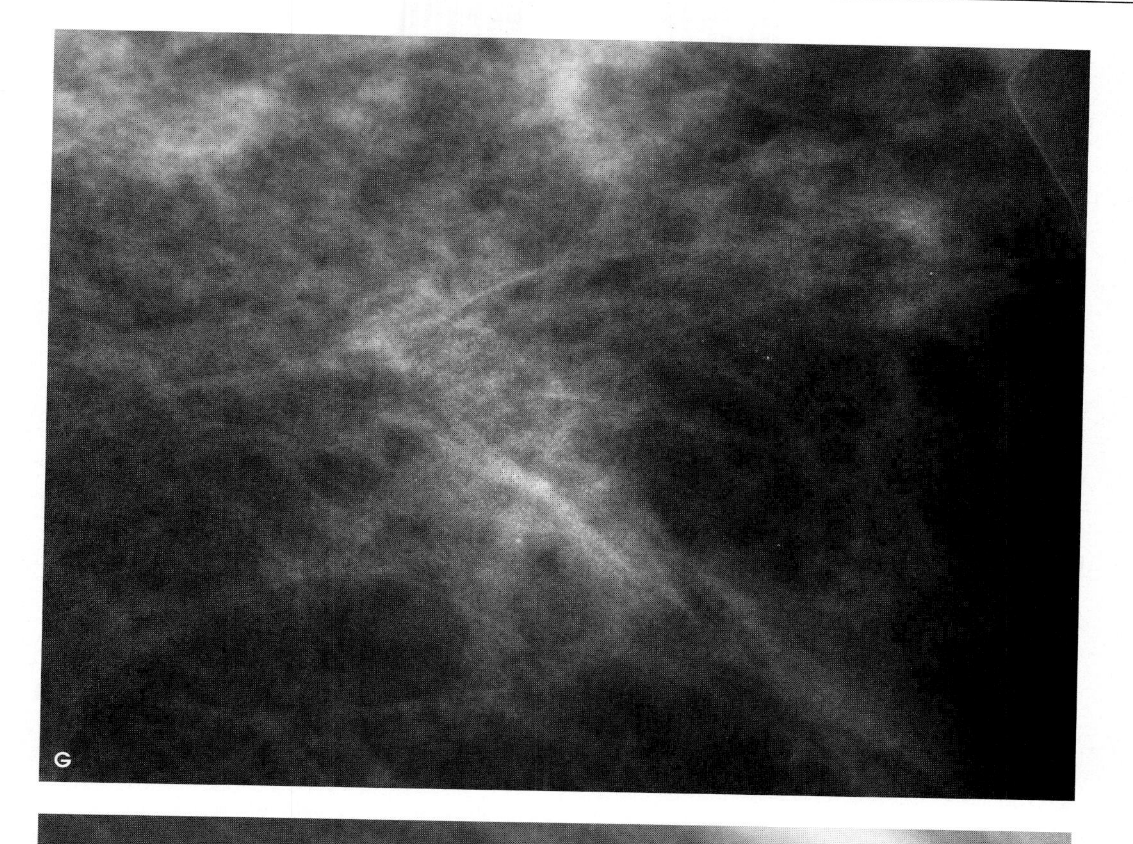

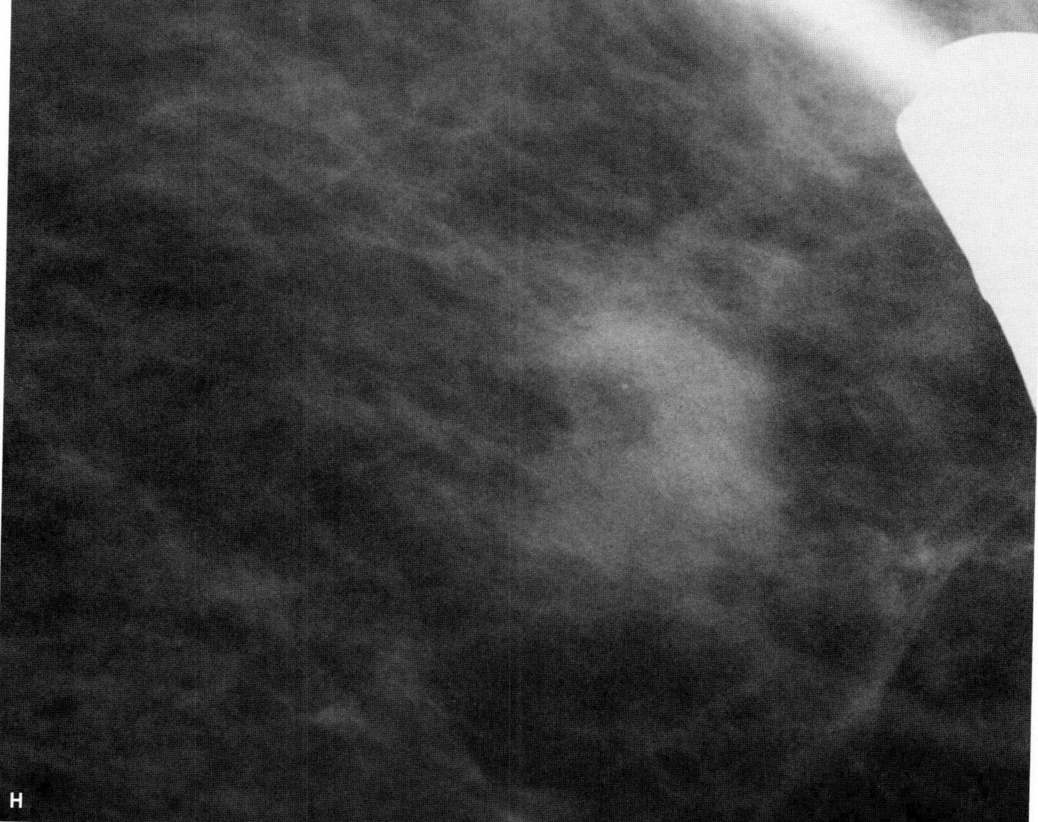

Figure 2.39. (*Continued*) Craniocaudal **(G)** and mediolateral oblique **(H)**, spot compression views.

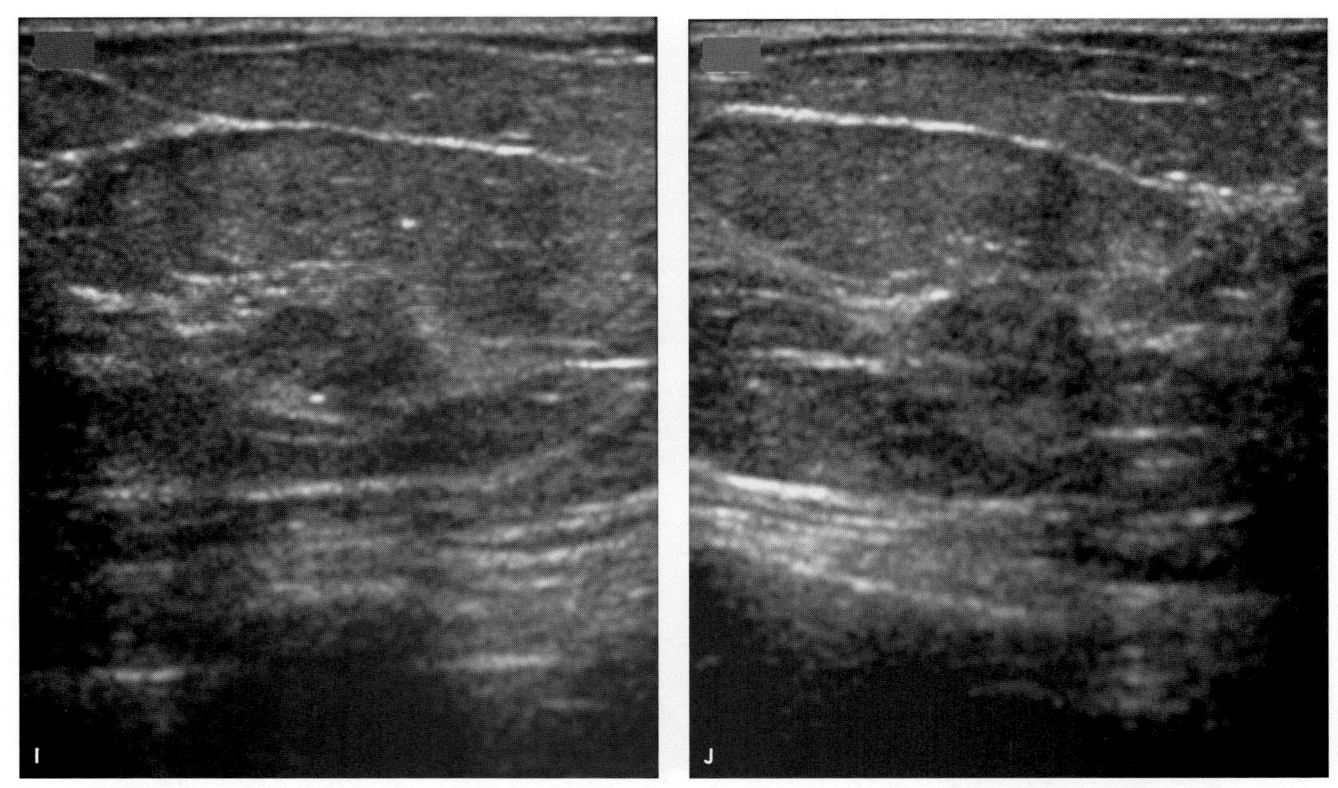

Figure 2.39. (*Continued*) Ultrasound images in radial **(I)** and antiradial **(J)** projections at the 7 o'clock position, 4 cm from the left nipple.

How would you describe the imaging findings, and what is your recommendation?

The spot compression views confirm the presence of a 1.5-cm mass with indistinct margins. On ultrasound, the mass is nearly isoechoic; however, it is detected and characterized by an irregular shape and angular margins.

BI-RADS® category 4: suspicious abnormality; biopsy should be considered.

An invasive mammary carcinoma with focal mucinous features is reported on the core biopsies. A 1.2-cm, grade II invasive ductal with mucinous features is reported on the lumpectomy specimen. Associated solid and cribriform ductal carcinoma in situ with no necrosis is also reported. The sentinel lymph node is normal [pT1c, pN0(sn)(i−), pMX; Stage I].

PATIENT 37

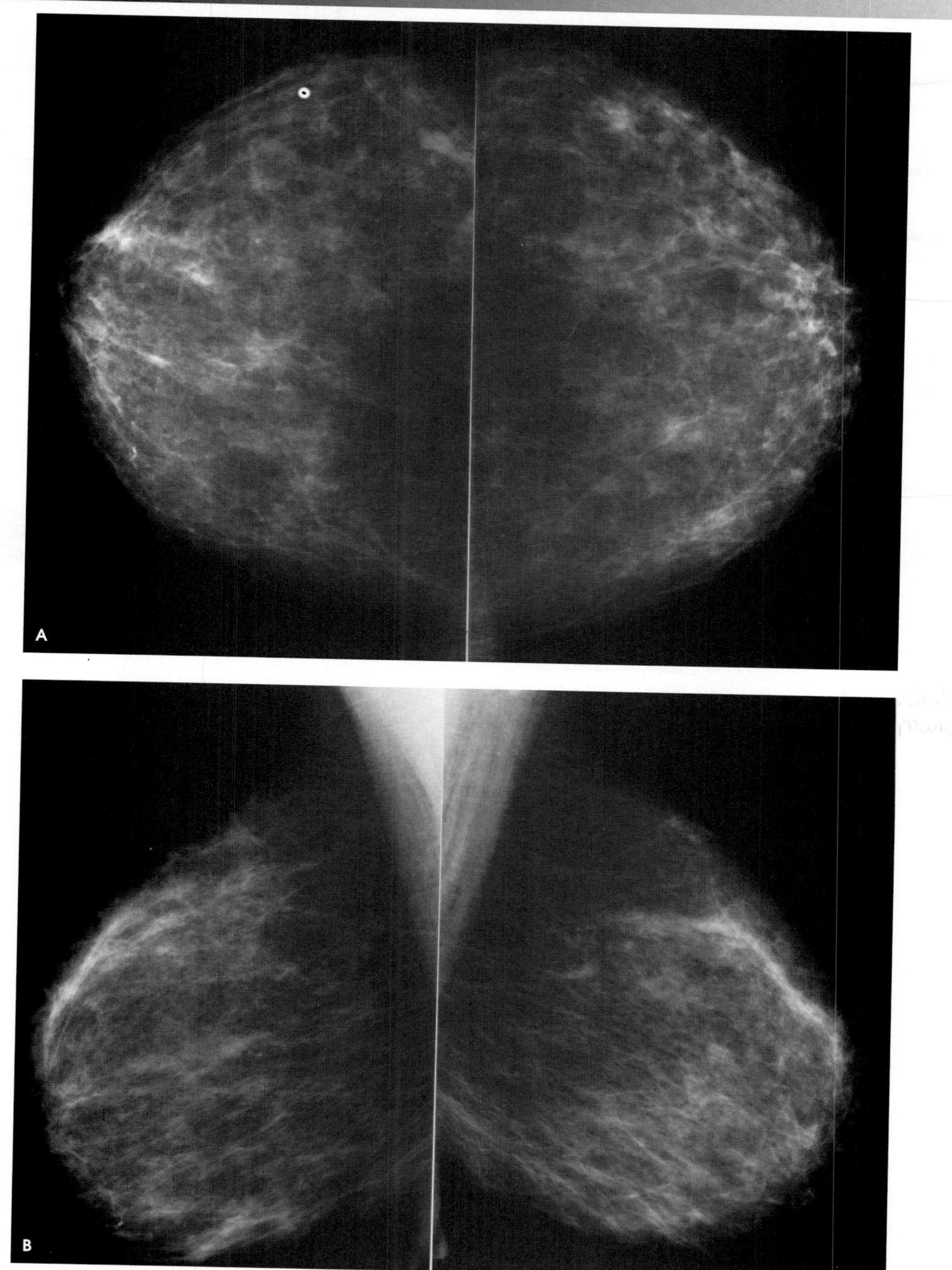

Figure 2.40. Screening study, 59-year-old woman. Craniocaudal **(A)** and mediolateral oblique **(B)** views.

Is this mammogram normal?

Review the images systematically:

1. Technically, is this an adequate study? Positioning is not optimal, particularly on the mediolateral oblique (MLO) views; however, the images are adequate.
2. Are there diffuse changes?
3. Evaluate specific locations: (a) medial quadrants on the craniocaudal views; (b) fat–glandular interfaces; (c) fatty stripe of tissue between anterior edge of pectoral muscle and glandular tissue on the MLO views; (d) subareolar areas; and (e) superior cone of tissue on the MLO views.
4. Splitting the images in thirds, look for specific lesions: (a) masses; (b) calcifications; (c) distortion; and (d) islands of asymmetry.

Is this a normal study? What is indicated next (be specific)?

BI-RADS® category 0: need additional imaging evaluation. Magnification views in two projections are indicated for further evaluation.

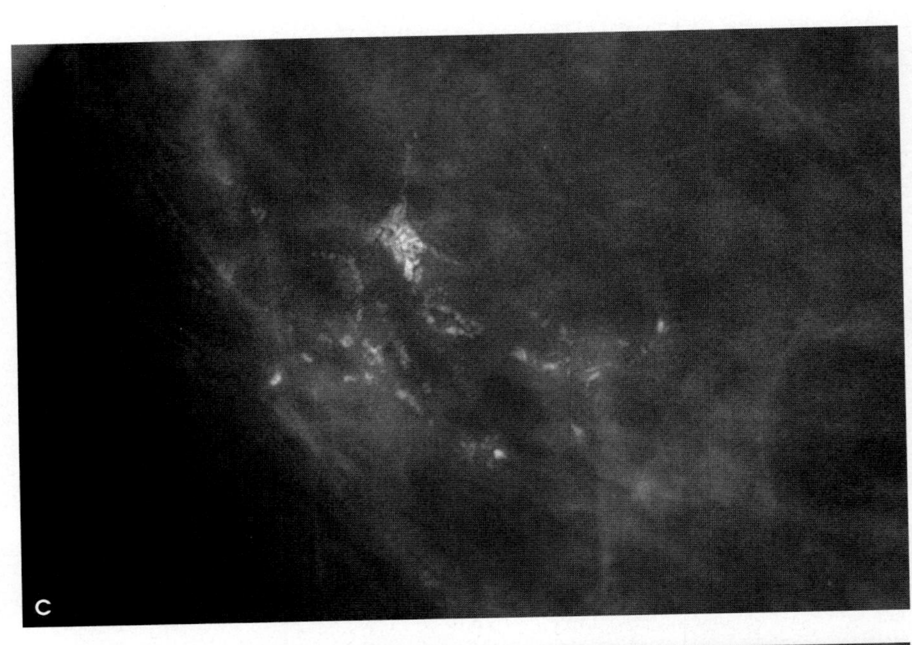

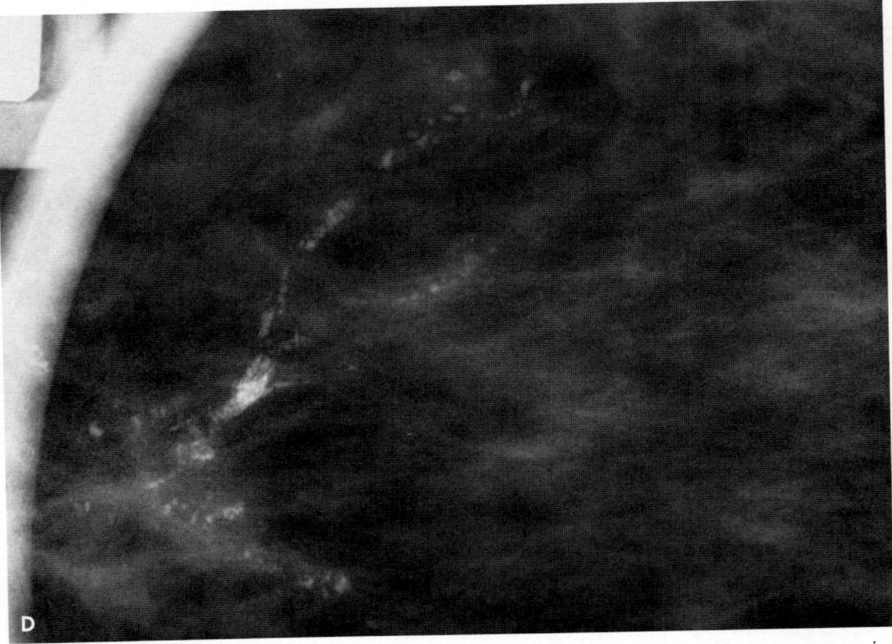

Figure 2.40. (*Continued*) Craniocaudal **(C)** and mediolateral oblique **(D)** double spot compression magnification views, right breast.

A cluster of pleomorphic calcifications is confirmed on the double spot compression magnification views. There are linear calcifications characterized by irregular margins and clefts. Additionally, linear and round calcifications demonstrate linear orientation. This represents at least ductal carcinoma in situ until proven otherwise.

BI-RADS® category 5: Highly suggestive of malignancy; appropriate action should be taken.

Appropriate action is taken in the form of a stereotactically guided biopsy. A high-nuclear-grade ductal carcinoma in situ with associated central necrosis is reported. This diagnosis is confirmed on the lumpectomy specimen [pTis(DCIS), pNX, pMX; Stage 0]. No invasive disease is diagnosed. No sentinel lymph node biopsy is done.

PATIENT 38

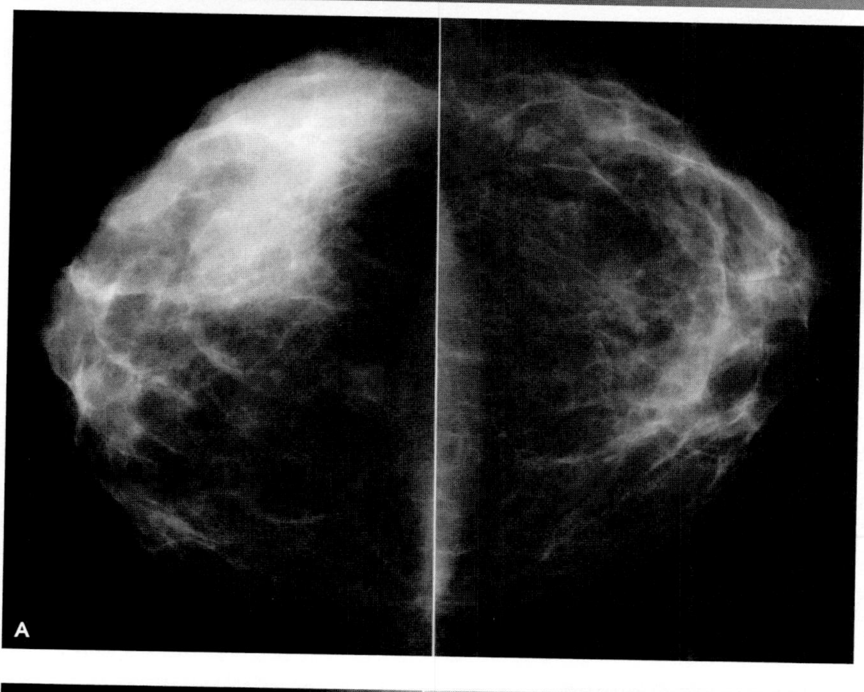

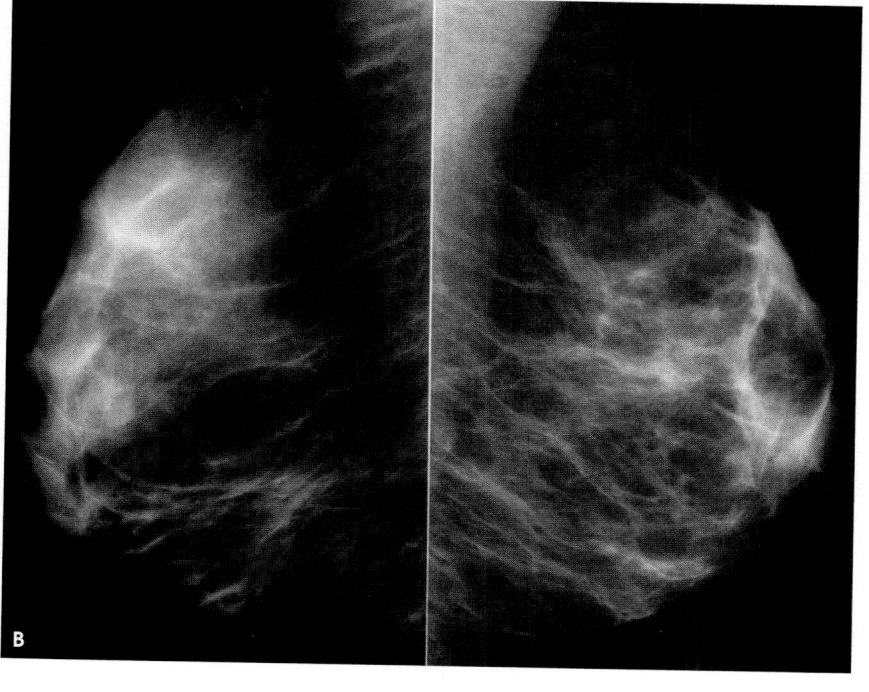

Figure 2.41. Screening study, 41-year-old woman. Craniocaudal **(A)** and mediolateral oblique **(B)** views.

How would you describe the findings on this mammogram?

Global parenchymal asymmetry can be described in the right breast. Establishing the presence of global parenchymal asymmetry requires comparison with the contralateral side. A greater volume of tissue is present in the right breast compared to the same area in the left breast. As defined in the Fourth Edition of BI-RADS®, global asymmetry should involve at least a quadrant of the breast. Although breast tissue is more commonly symmetric, global asymmetry, as demonstrated here, can be seen in a small number of woman as a normal variant. No mass or distortion is noted in the area of increased tissue on the right. The tissue in this area is scalloped and contains associated areas of fatty lobulation. Comparison with prior studies is helpful in assessing the stability of this finding.

What piece of information is critical in this patient? What BI-RADS® category would you use for this mammogram?

In women with global or focal parenchymal asymmetry, it is critical to establish that there is no palpable abnormality corresponding to the area of parenchymal asymmetry. If there is any question about a corresponding palpable abnormality, the patient can be asked to return for correlative physical examination and, if needed, additional mammographic images, ultrasound, or, occasionally, magnetic resonance imaging.

BI-RADS® category 1: negative. In general, for benign findings, if the observations represent a change from the prior mammogram, I describe them in the report and use BI-RADS® category 2: benign finding. If the findings are stable compared with prior mammograms, I do not describe them and use category 1 for the assessment. Annual screening mammography is recommended for this patient.

PATIENT 39

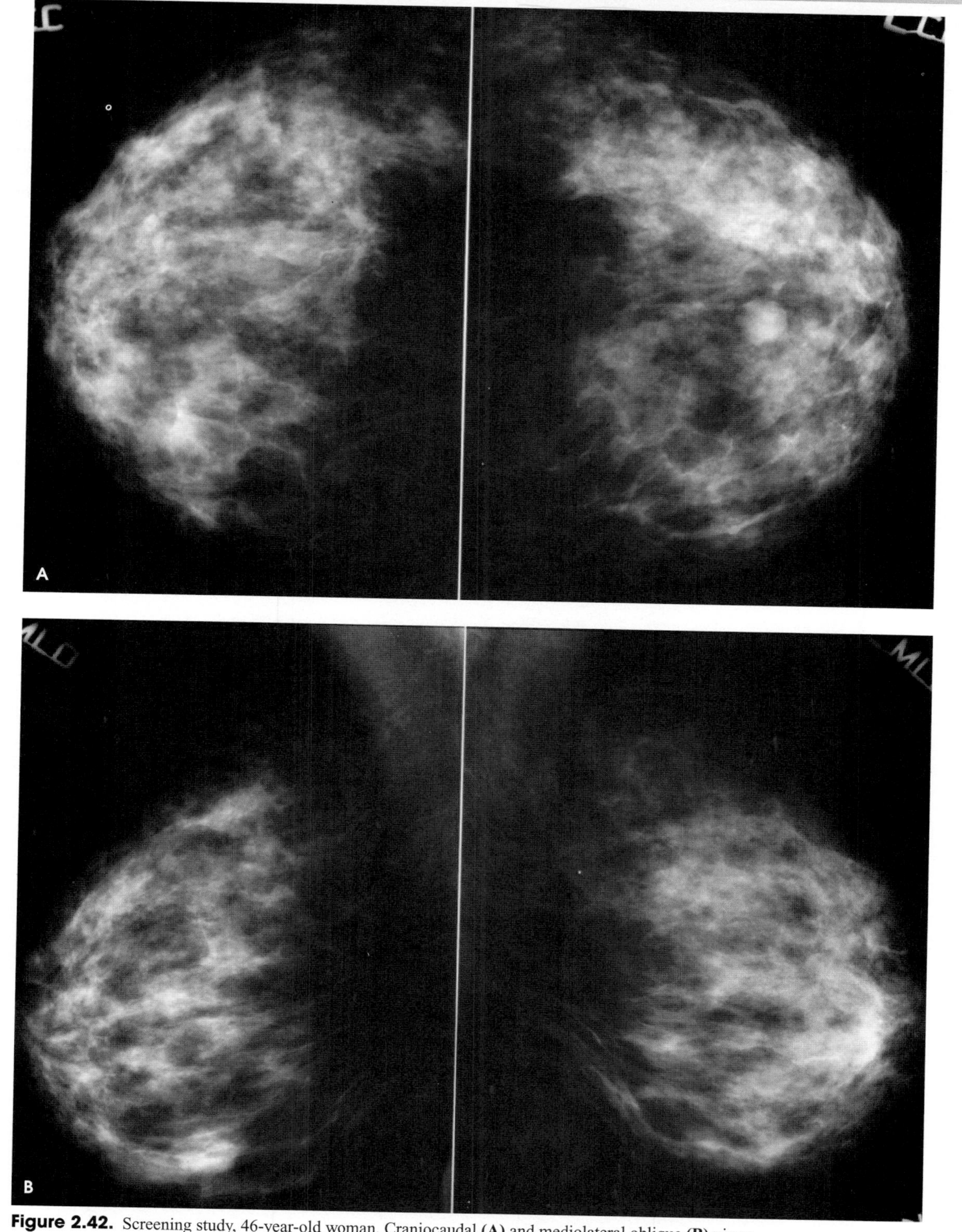

Figure 2.42. Screening study, 46-year-old woman. Craniocaudal **(A)** and mediolateral oblique **(B)** views.

What observations can you make, and what would you like to do next?

A mass is present in the left breast, best seen on the craniocaudal (CC) view, directly posterior to the nipple. Are there any other observations? Review the images systematically. Focus your attention on smaller amounts of tissue by splitting the CC and mediolateral oblique (MLO) views into thirds. Look for specific findings, including diffuse changes, masses, distortion, asymmetry, and calcifications. Review areas on the mammograms where breast cancers are likely to develop, specifically, fat–glandular interfaces, the fatty stripe of tissue between pectoral muscle and glandular tissue on MLO views, the superior cone of tissue on MLO views, medial tissue on CC views, and subareolar areas. Focus down with a magnification lens, particularly when looking for small masses, distortion, and clusters of calcifications. Is there a potential mass with distortion in this patient? Where? On the CC views, review the fat–glandular interfaces particularly abutting the retroglandular area on the right (Fig. 2.42C). On the MLOs, look at the upper thirds of the MLOs and more specifically at the upper cone of tissue on the right MLO (Fig. 2.42D). Do you see the mass? Do you see the distortion? Additional evaluation is indicated bilaterally.

BI-RADS® category 0: need additional imaging evaluation.

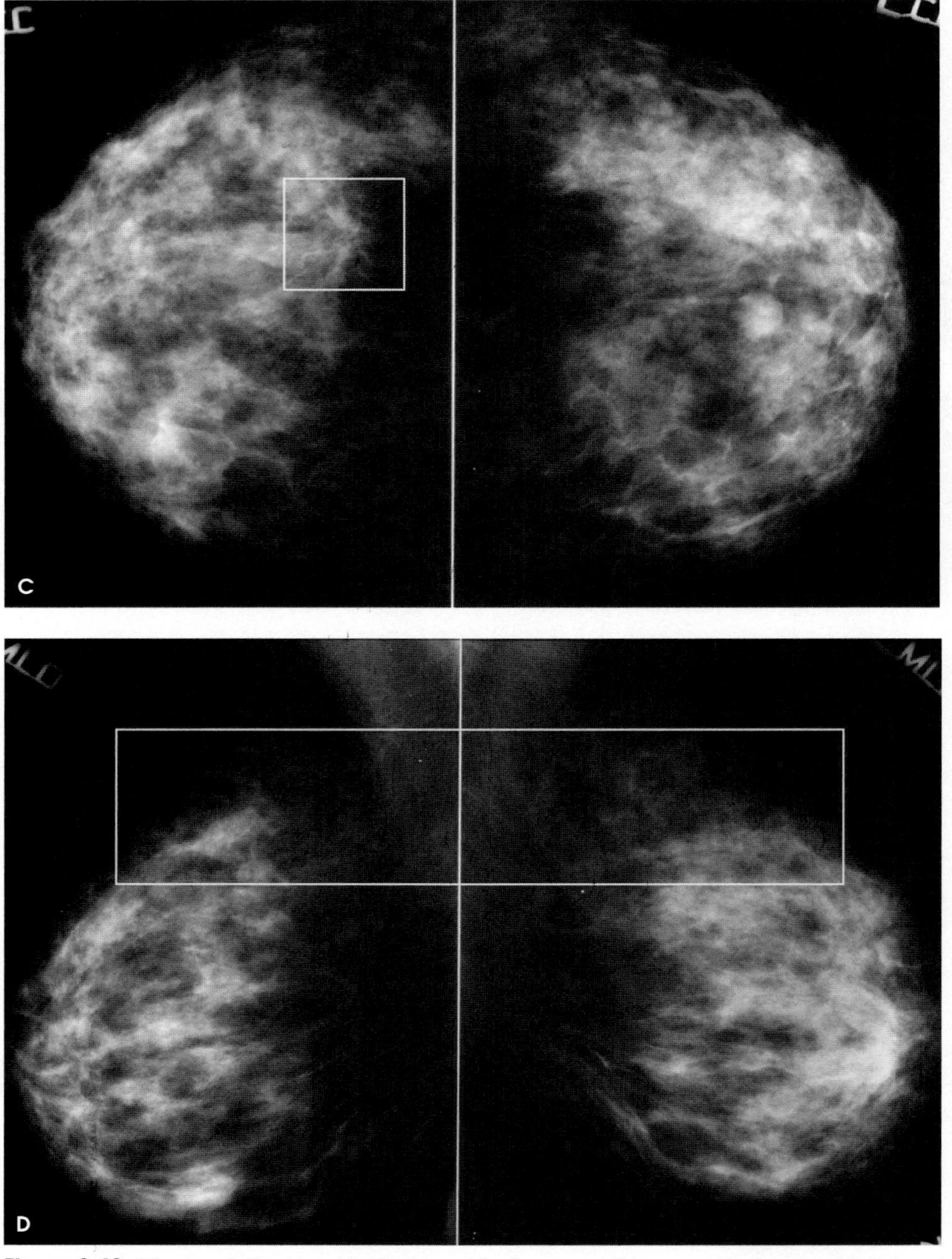

Figure 2.42. (*Continued*) Craniocaudal **(C)** views with a box on possible mass with distortion. Mediolateral oblique views **(D),** with box delineating asymmetry involving the upper cone of tissue on the right breast.

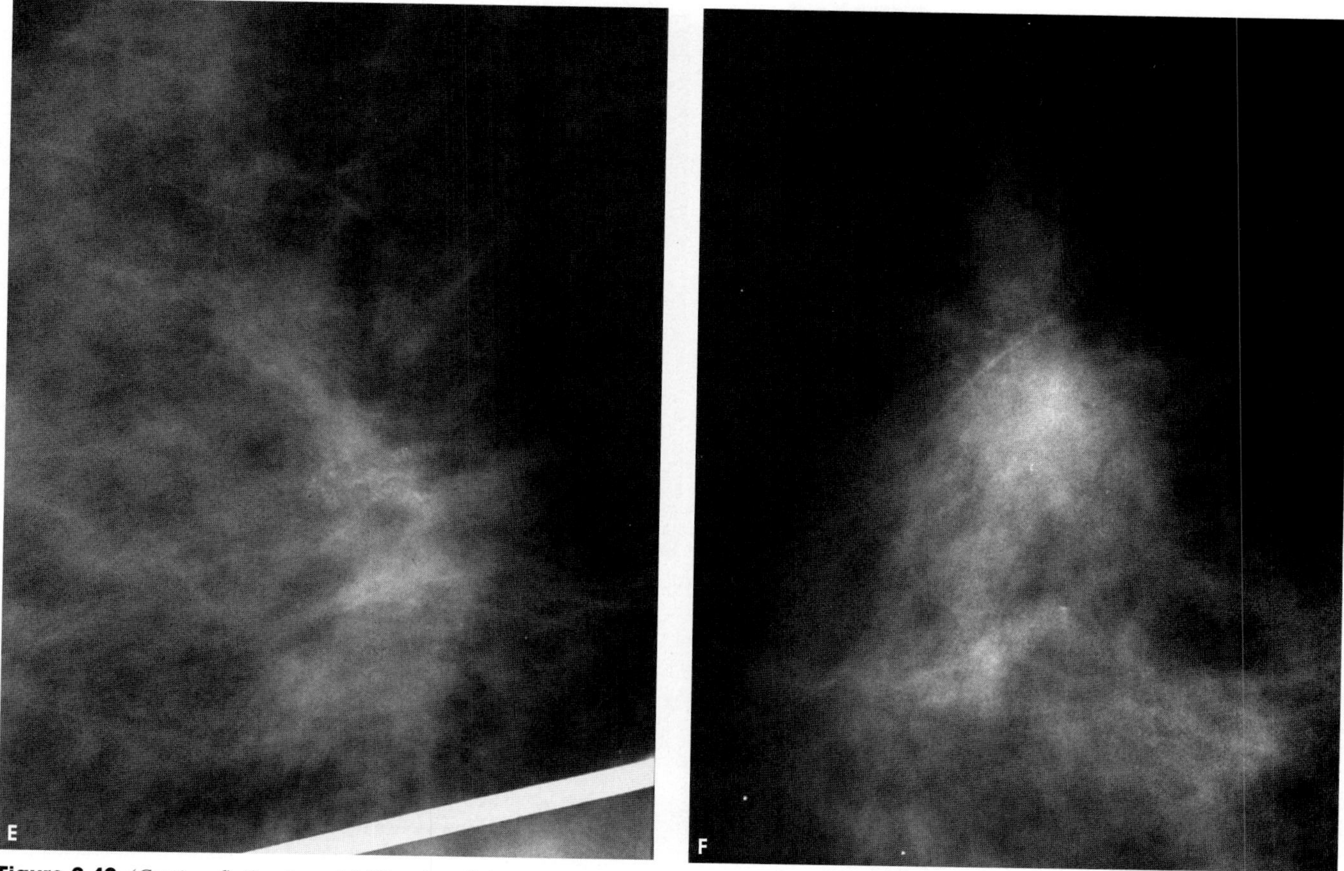

Figure 2.42. (*Continued*) Craniocaudal **(E)** and mediolateral oblique **(F)** spot compression views, right breast.

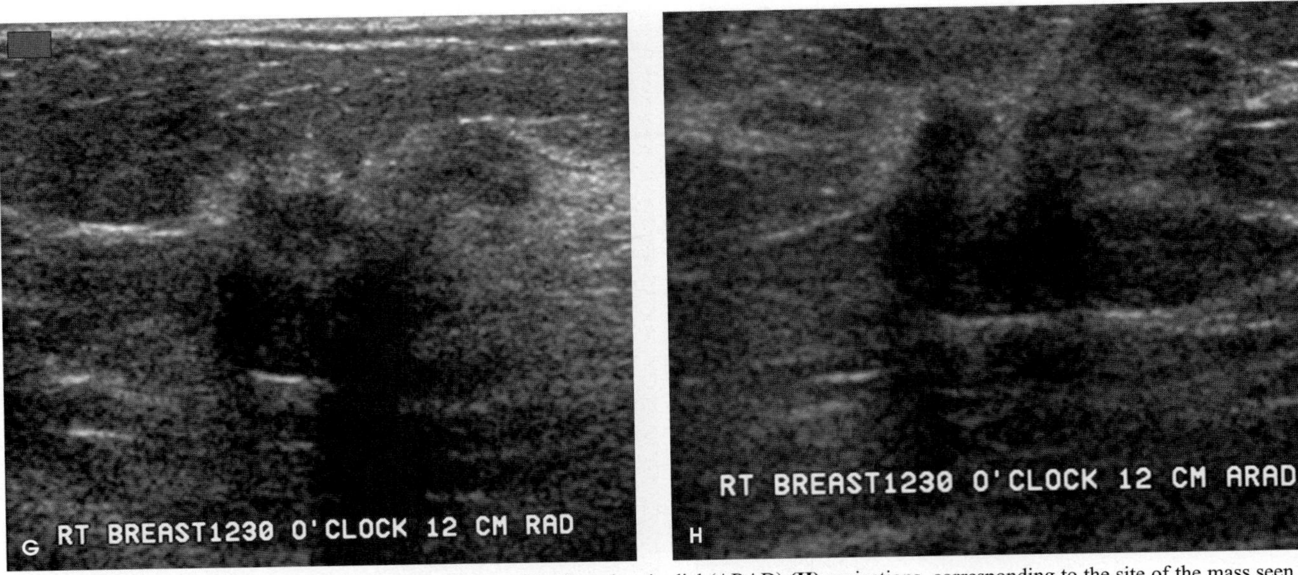

Figure 2.42. (*Continued*) Ultrasound images, radial (RAD) **(G)** and antiradial (ARAD) **(H)** projections, corresponding to the site of the mass seen mammographically in the right breast.

How would you describe the findings, and what is your recommendation?

The 1.2-cm mass in the left breast is a cyst (images not shown) and requires no further intervention. The spot compression views on the right confirm the presence of an irregular 2.5-cm mass with associated distortion and low-density amorphous calcifications (Fig. 2.42E, F). On ultrasound, an irregular, hypoechoic mass with areas of shadowing is imaged at the 12:30 o'clock position, 12 cm from the right nipple (Fig. 2.42G, H).

BI-RADS® category 5: Highly suggestive of malignancy; appropriate action should be taken.

Appropriate action is taken in the form of an ultrasound-guided core biopsy. Histologically, an invasive mammary carcinoma is reported on the cores. A grade II, invasive ductal carcinoma measuring 2.7 cm is reported on the lumpectomy specimen. Associated intermediate-grade, solid-type ductal carcinoma in situ is also present. Two excised sentinel lymph nodes are negative for metastatic carcinoma [pT2, pN0(sn)(i−), pMX; Stage IIA].

PATIENT 40

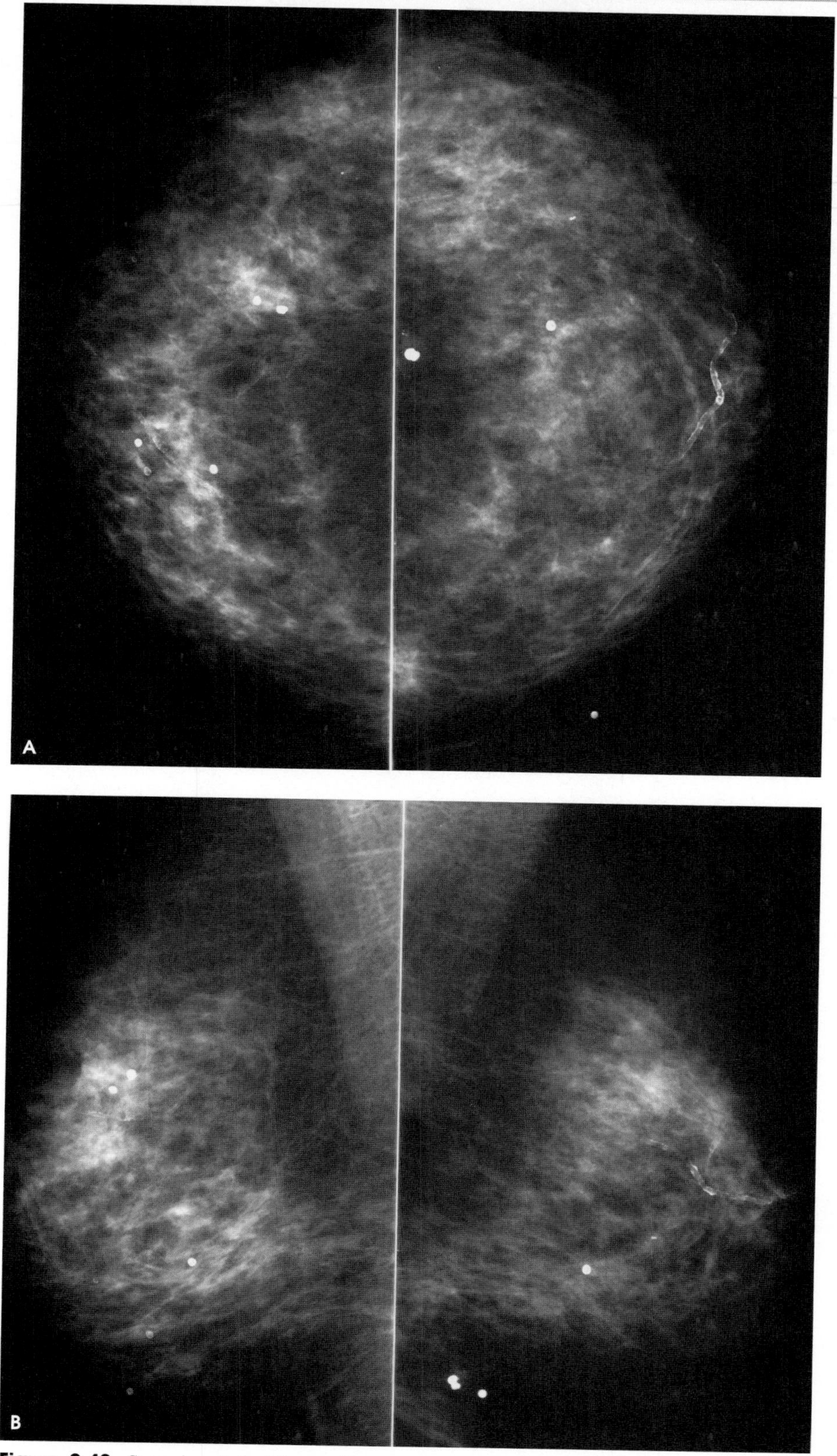

Figure 2.43. Screening study, 76-year-old woman. Craniocaudal **(A)** and mediolateral oblique **(B)** views. A metallic BB on the left marks a skin lesion.

What do you think?
What, if anything, would you like to do next?

Review the films systematically. There are scattered dystrophic calcifications and arterial calcifications bilaterally. Focus your attention on smaller amounts of tissue by splitting the craniocaudal (CC) and mediolateral oblique (MLO) views into thirds. Look for specific findings, including diffuse changes, masses, distortion, asymmetry, and calcifications. Review areas on the mammograms where breast cancers are likely to develop, specifically, fat–glandular interfaces, the fatty stripe of tissue between pectoral muscle and glandular tissue on MLO views, the superior cone of tissue on MLO views, medial tissue on CC views, and subareolar areas. Focus down with a magnification lens, particularly when looking for small masses, distortion, and clusters of calcifications. Do you notice anything when you evaluate medial tissue on the CC views (Fig. 2.43C)? How about at the edge of the film on the left? Because there is nothing readily apparent on the MLO view, are you comfortable describing this as a normal mammogram? With what degree of certainty can you dictate a report on this screening study? Could a lesion have been excluded on the MLO view?

BI-RADS® category 0: need additional imaging evaluation.

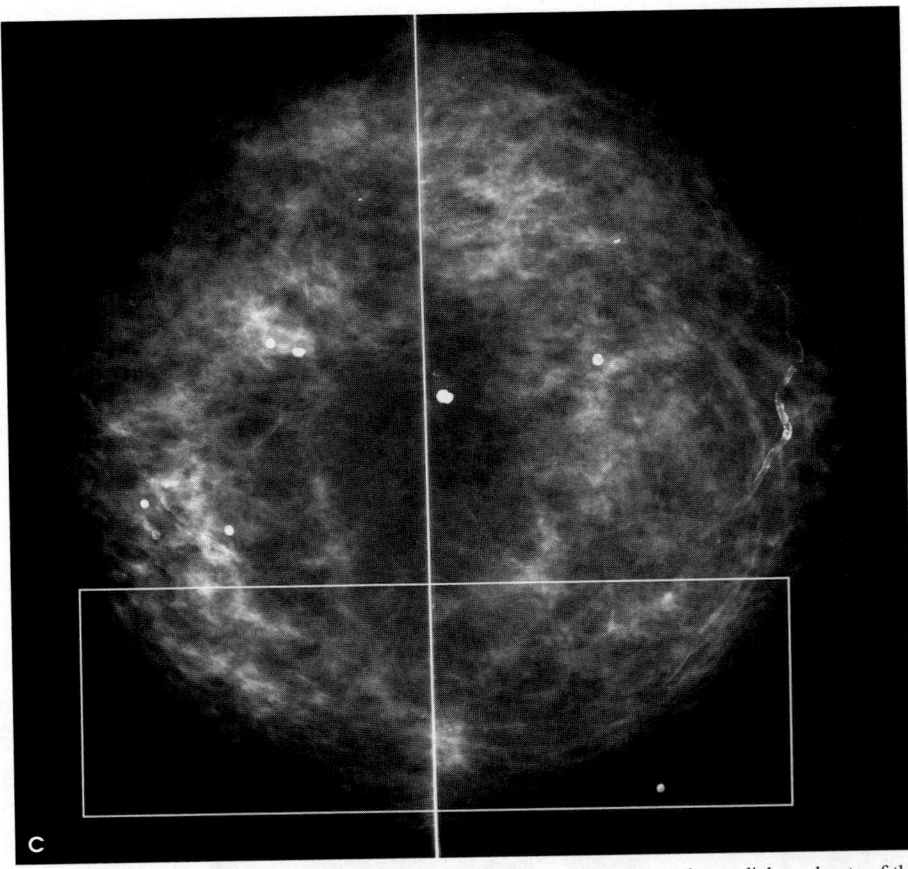

Figure 2.43. *(Continued)* Craniocaudal **(C)** views. Limiting evaluation to the medial quadrants of the breasts focuses your evaluation on smaller amounts of tissue. Now look specifically for a possible mass.

Do you see it?

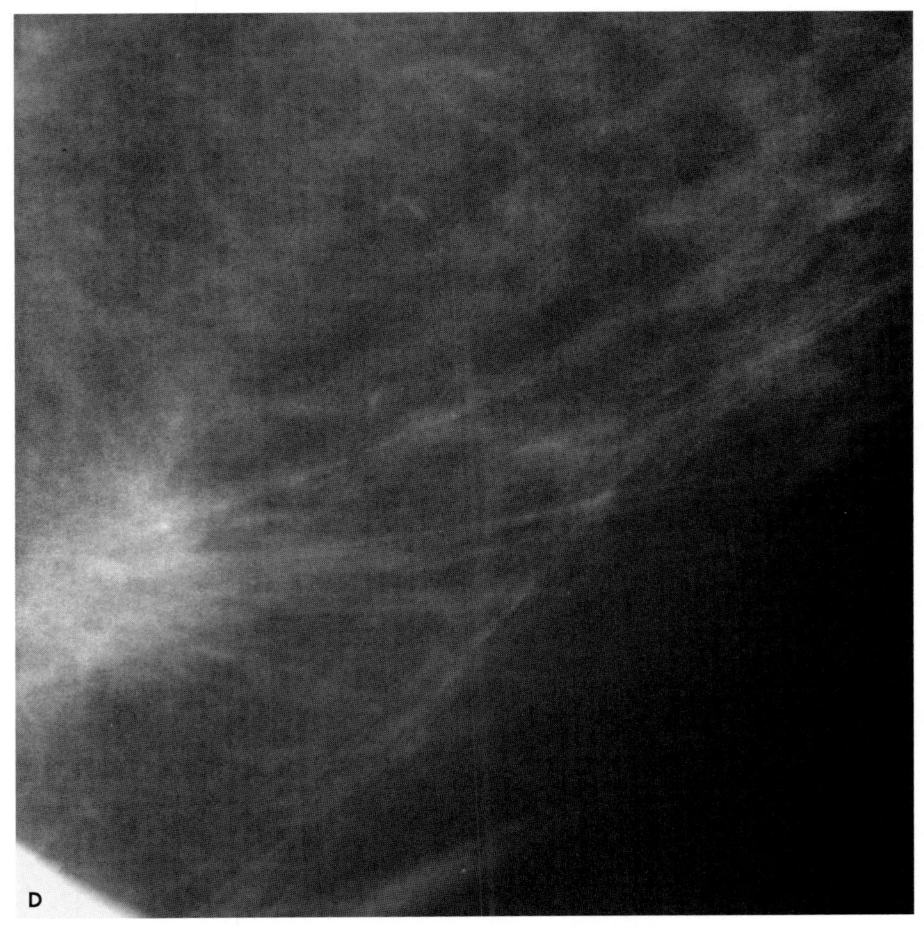

Figure 2.43. (*Continued*) Craniocaudal **(D)** spot compression view, left breast.

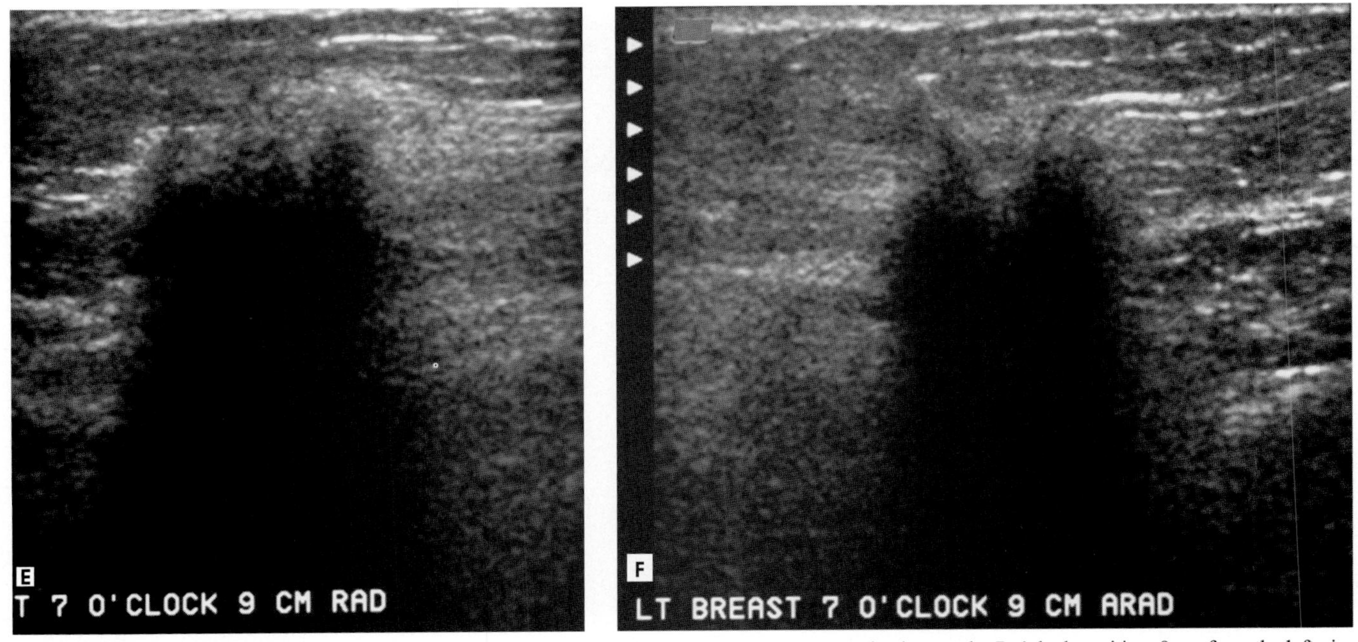

Figure 2.43. (*Continued*) Ultrasound images, in radial (RAD) **(E)** and antiradial (ARAD) **(F)** projections at the 7 o'clock position, 9 cm from the left nipple.

How would you describe the findings?

The spot compression view confirms the presence of a spiculated mass posteromedially in the left breast. Based on this information, what is your degree of certainty that there is a significant abnormality and that a biopsy is indicated? Is it now possible to dictate a succinct, definitive, and directive report? On ultrasound, a hypoechoic spiculated mass, with intense shadowing and vertical orientation, is identified at the 7 o'clock position, 9 cm from the left nipple.

Time and time again, you will find that by following a simple, logical process, and completing the image workup, you will deliver optimal patient care that minimizes the likelihood of delaying the diagnosis of breast cancer.

This patient illustrates the need to focus keenly on tissue extending to the edge of the films. The fact that this lesion is not imaged on the MLO view should not dissuade you from calling the patient back. With far posteromedial lesions, it is common to partially (barely) image them on only one of the two routine views. Usage of the spot compression paddle often allows more tissue to be included on the image.

With respect to imaging this lesion on the orthogonal view, what view might be helpful and why? Be specific.

When considering 90-degree lateral views, there are two possibilities: a 90-degree lateromedial (LM) or a 90-degree mediolateral (ML) view. For the 90-degree LM view, the bucky is placed up against the sternum so that a maximal amount of medial tissue is included on the image and, because medial tissue is closest to the film, resolution of medial lesions is improved. For the 90-degree ML view, the bucky is placed laterally and compression is applied medially. In this patient, a 90-degree LM view provides the best chance to image the lesion on the orthogonal view.

BI-RADS® category 4: suspicious abnormality; biopsy should be considered.

Rather than just consider biopsy, one is undertaken using ultrasound guidance. An invasive ductal carcinoma is diagnosed on the core samples. A 1.2-cm, grade I invasive ductal carcinoma is reported on the lumpectomy specimen. No metastatic disease is reported in three excised sentinel lymph nodes [pT1c, pN0(sn)(i−), pMX; Stage I].

90° LM - see MEDIAL
90° ML - LATERAL

PATIENT 41

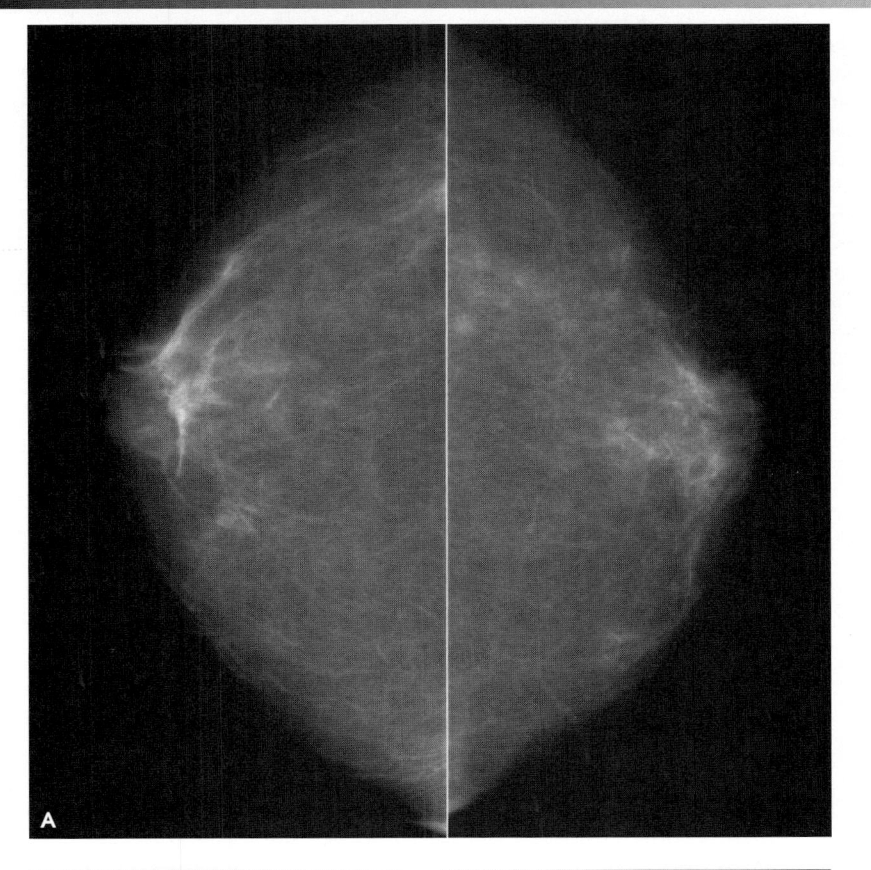

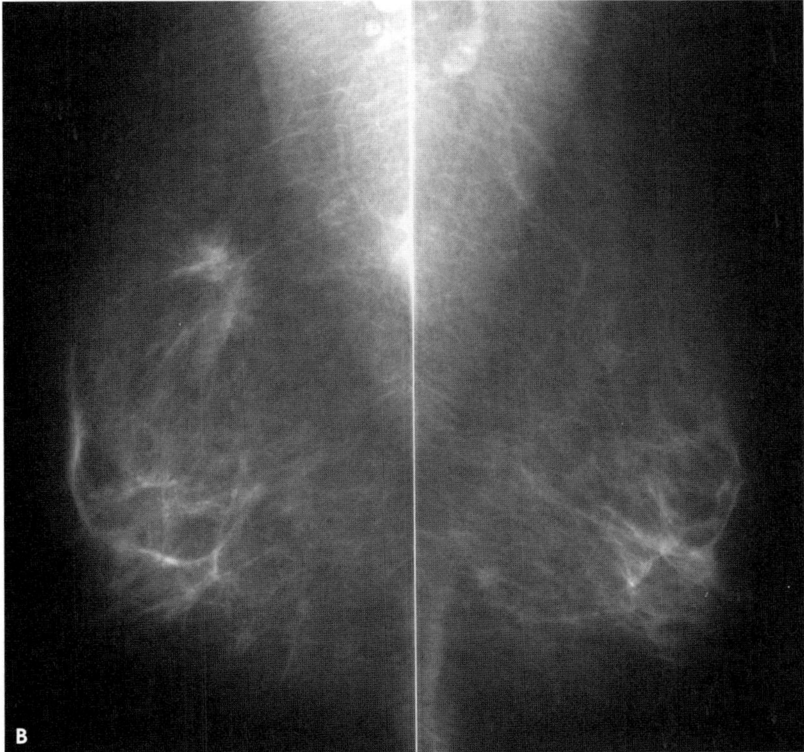

Figure 2.44. Screening study, 57-year-old woman. Craniocaudal **(A)** and mediolateral oblique **(B)** views.

What are your observations?

An asymmetry with irregular margins is imaged in the right mediolateral (MLO) view anterior to the pectoral muscle; however, there is no corresponding abnormality on the craniocaudal (CC) view. Are there any other observations? Is breast positioning optimal on the CC views? How can you tell? Do you see pectoral muscle in either CC view? Do you see cleavage in either CC view? *When you cannot see pectoral muscle or cleavage on CC views, you must consider the possibility that posterior tissue has been excluded from the image.* Under these circumstances, you should measure the posterior nipple line (PNL). The PNL measurement on the CC view should be within 1 cm of that measured on the MLO view (Fig. 2.4E, F). If the measurements are not within a centimeter of each other, posterior tissue has been excluded and the CC image needs to be repeated. In this patient, posterior tissue has been excluded from both CC views and, with it, possibly a lesion. The CC views need to be repeated.

Do you have any other observations? What else would you like at this point?

How about prior studies? Ideally, when you observe a potential abnormality on a screening study, you should review prior films and determine if the patient has had any surgery or trauma localized to the site of concern. Although it would be appropriate to call this patient back for further evaluation if there are no prior studies or they are unavailable, you do not want to recall patients in whom the potential abnormality has decreased in size, been previously evaluated, or if it reflects postoperative changes.

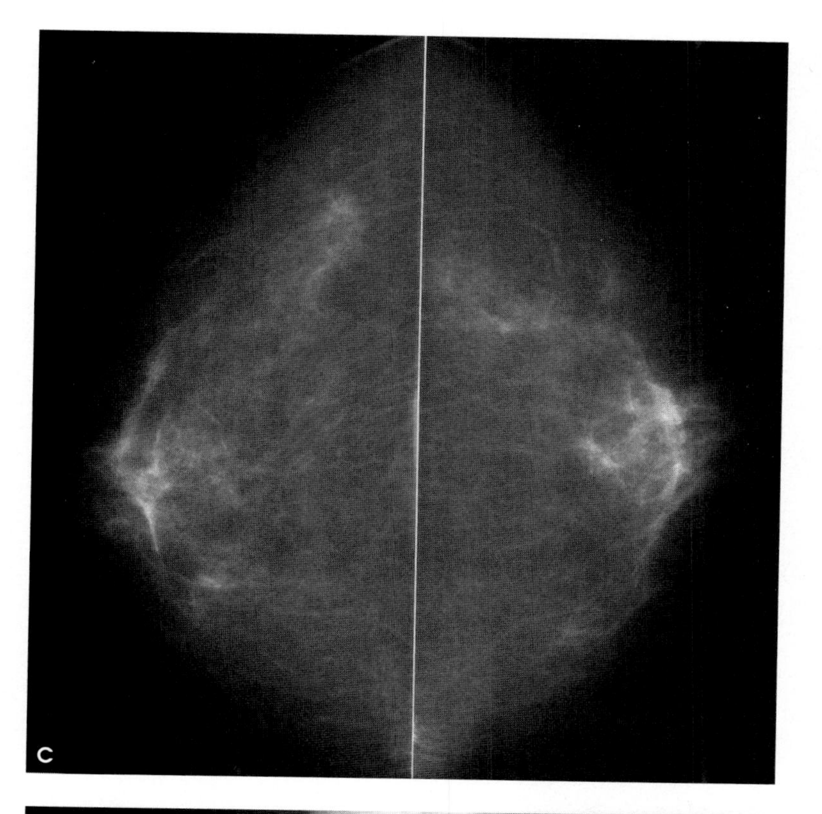

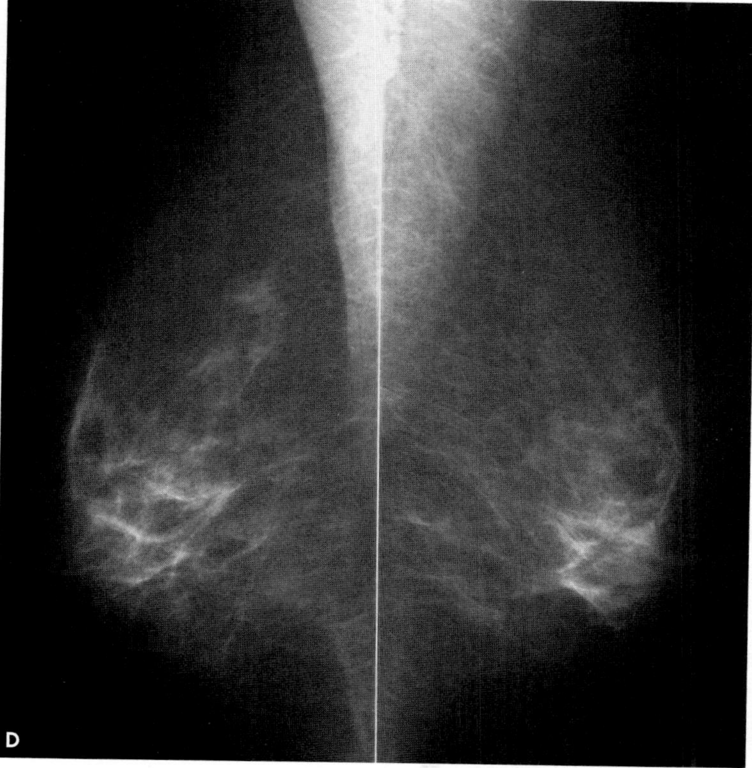

Figure 2.44. (*Continued*) Craniocaudal **(C)** and mediolateral oblique **(D)** views, screening study 2 years prior to **(A)** and **(B)**. No history of breast surgery or trauma.

What do you think? Does the patient need additional evaluation?

The area of asymmetry has increased in size compared to the prior study and, with better positioning on the CC views, it can be seen on the prior CC view. In comparing the two studies, do you have any other observations? What is the next step?

BI-RADS® category 0: need additional imaging evaluation.

The patient is called back for further evaluation. Did you notice the new nodule in the left breast (Fig. 2.44E, F, arrows)? What will you ask the technologist to do on the right? How about on the left?

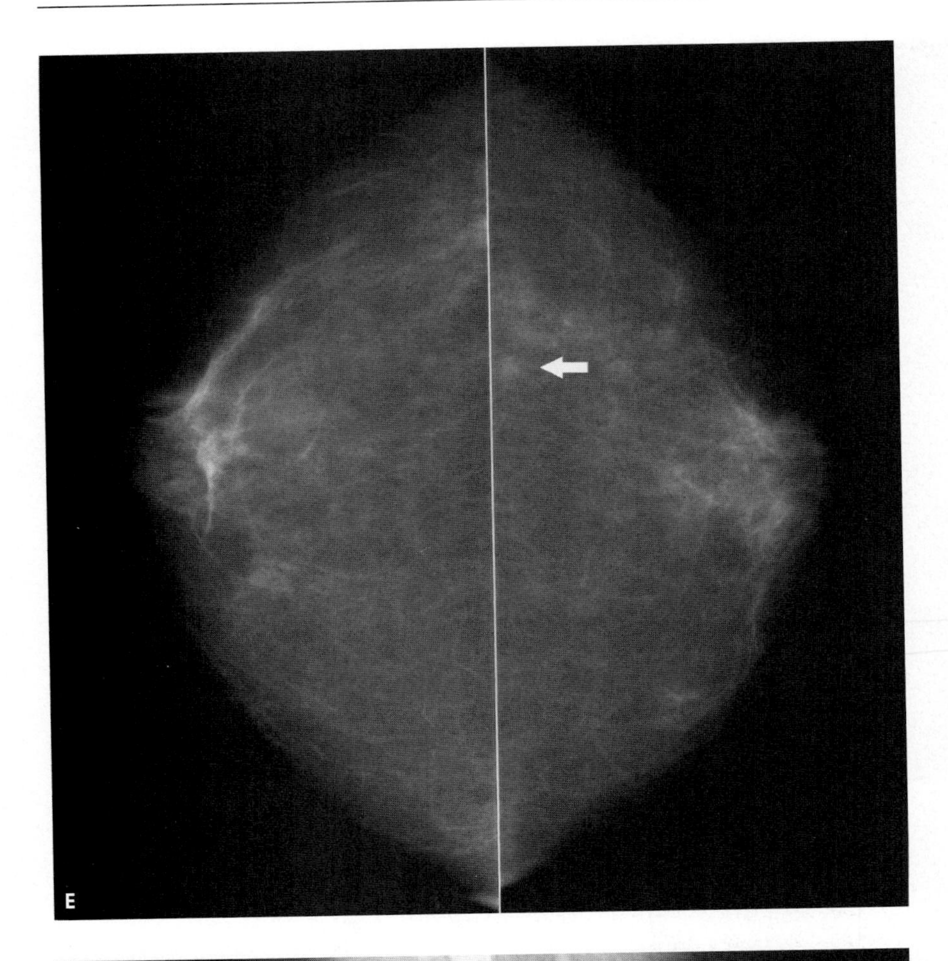

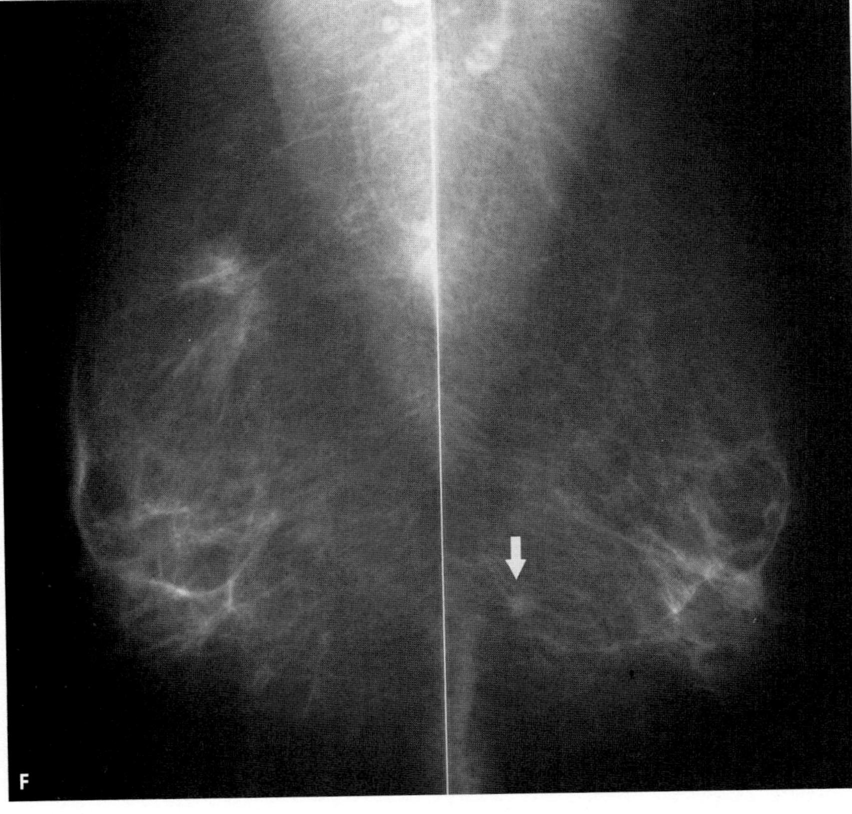

Figure 2.44. (*Continued*) Craniocaudal **(E)** and mediolateral oblique **(F)** views. There is a mass in the left breast *(arrows)*. This represents a change from the prior study and therefore also requires evaluation.

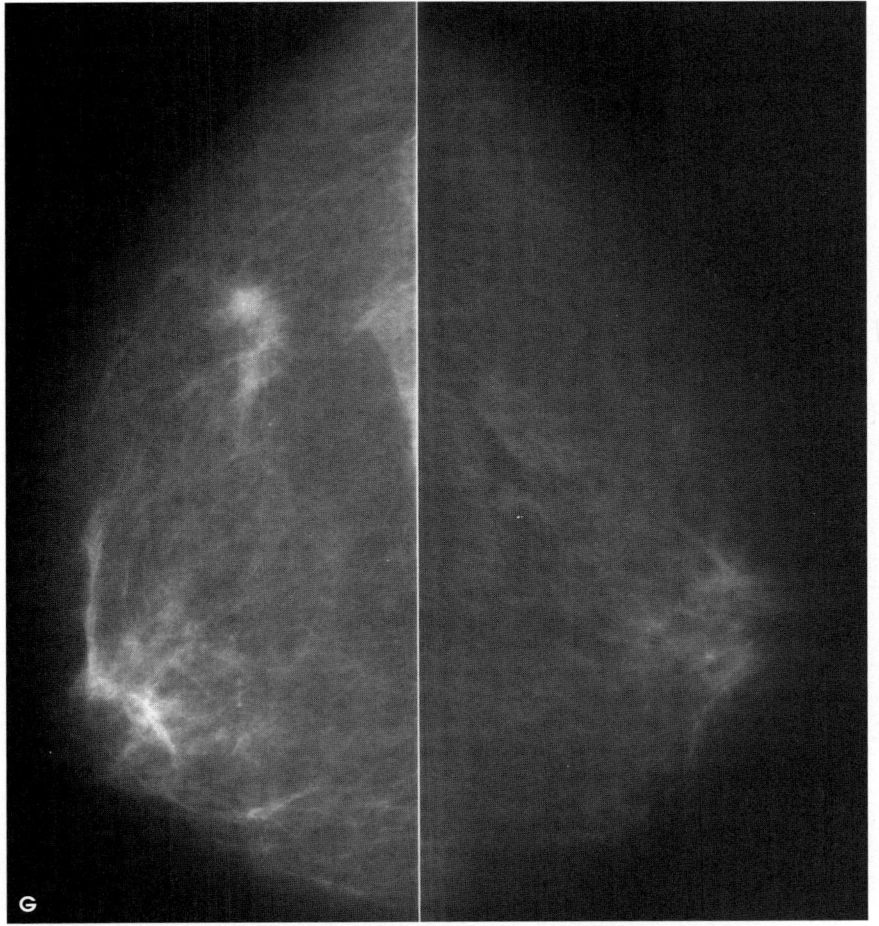

Figure 2.44. (*Continued*) Repeat craniocaudal **(G)** views. With better positioning, the lesion is now seen in this projection laterally.

What can be done to maximize visualization of lateral tissue on craniocaudal views?

The lesion in the right breast was excluded from the field of view on the initial craniocaudal (CC) view. Repeat CC views, with a tug on the lateral aspect of the breast, will maximize the amount of lateral tissue included on the images. Alternatively, an exaggerated craniocaudal view, laterally (XCCL), can be done. The XCCL view can be done using the large compression paddle or a spot compression paddle. When positioning patients for CC views, it is important for the mammographic technologist to identify the inframammary fold (IMF) and lift the breast as much as the natural mobility of the IMF permits. Additionally, the technologist needs to pull the tissue out away from the body and routinely tug on the lateral aspect of the breast to maximize the amount of posterolateral tissue included on the images. If, after the lateral tug is done, tissue is still seen extending to the edge of the film laterally, and there is tissue posteriorly superimposed on the pectoral muscle on the MLO view, an XCCL view may be indicated.

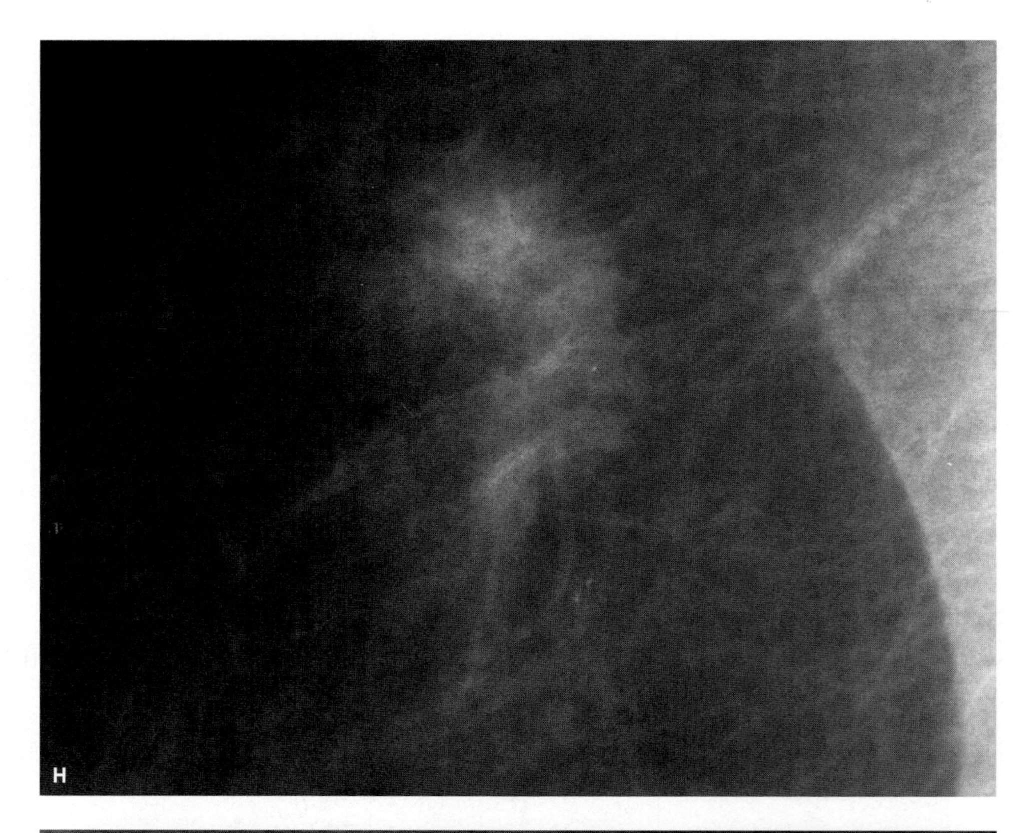

Figure 2.44. (*Continued*) Mediolateral oblique **(H)** spot compression view, right breast. Craniocaudal **(I)** and mediolateral oblique **(J)** spot compression views, left breast.

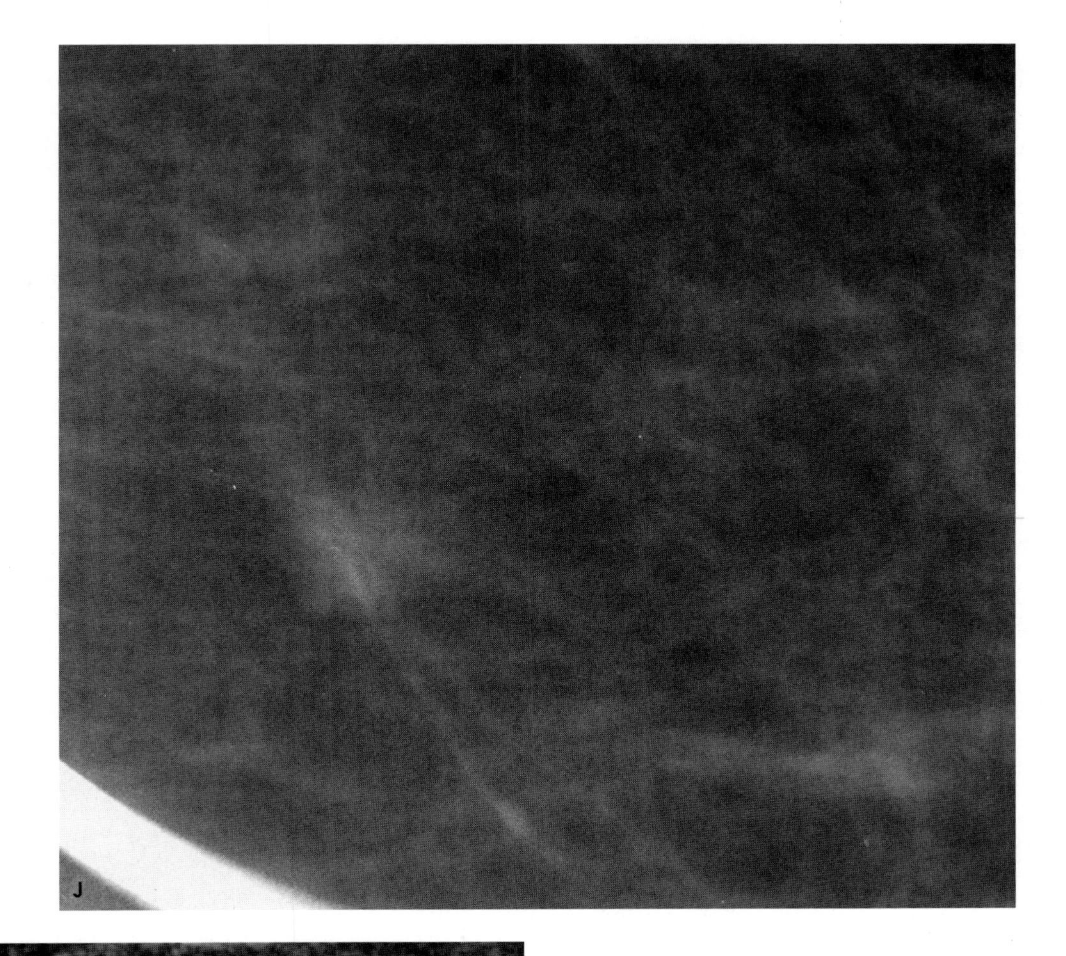

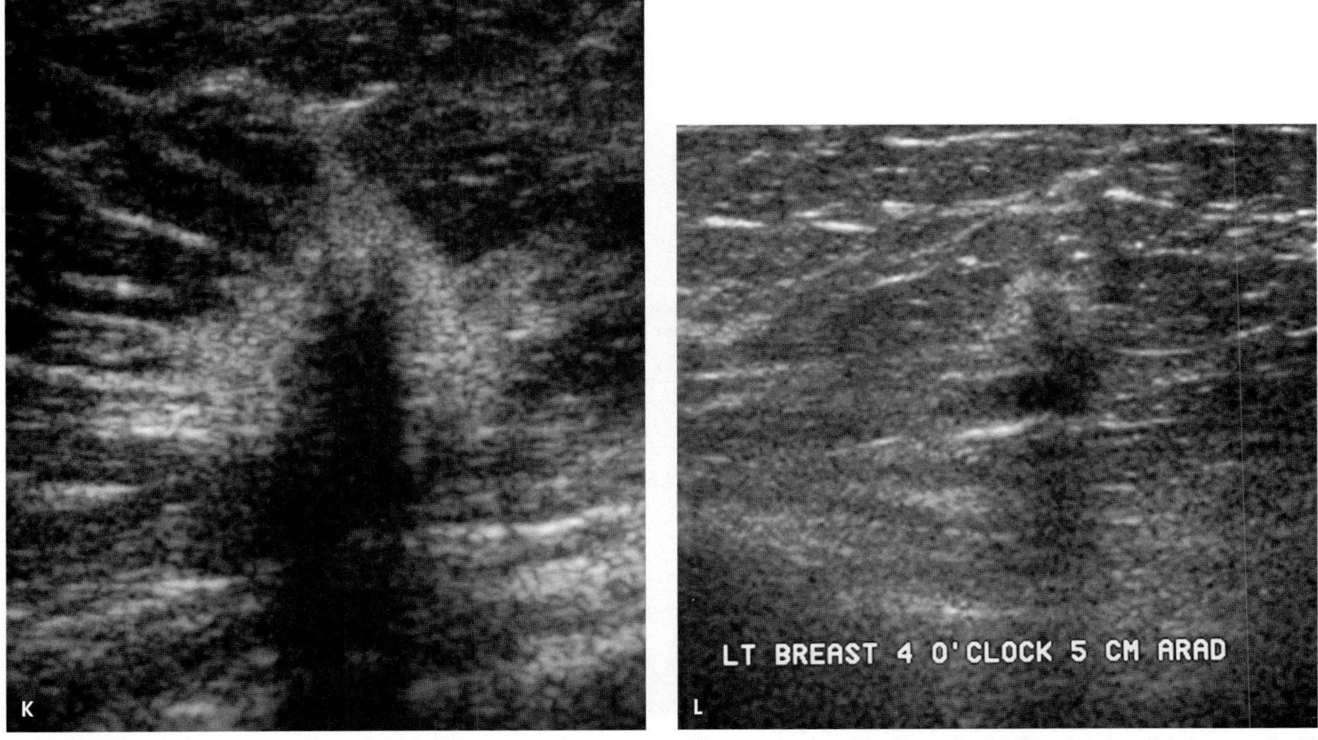

Figure 2.44. (*Continued*) Mediolateral oblique **(J)** spot compression views left breast. Ultrasound image, antiradial **(K)** projection, right breast at the 10 o'clock position approximately 8 cm from the right nipple. Ultrasound image, antiradial (ARAD) **(L)** projection, left breast.

How would you describe the findings?

Spot compression views, bilaterally, confirm the presence of bilateral lesions. The mass on the right is irregular with spiculated margins and some associated calcifications and measures approximately 2 cm. A hypoechoic mass with intense shadowing, an echogenic halo, vertical orientation, and spiculation is identified on ultrasound at the 10 o'clock position, 8 to 10 cm from the right nipple. The mass on the left is round with indistinct and possibly microlobulated margins and measures approximately 0.7 cm. An irregular, hypoechoic mass, with angular margins and an echogenic halo, is found in the left breast at the 4 o'clock position, 5 cm from the nipple. This corresponds to the expected location of the lesion seen mammographically in the left breast. Biopsies are indicated bilaterally. *Be mindful of any developing solid mass in postmenopausal women, particularly if they are not on hormone replacement therapy.*

BI-RADS® category 4: suspicious finding; biopsy should be considered.

Imaging-guided biopsies are done bilaterally. Invasive and intraductal carcinomas are reported bilaterally on the ultrasound-guided core samples.

How are multifocality and multicentricity defined? How about synchronous and metachronous lesions? What is emerging as the modality of choice in evaluating patients diagnosed with breast cancer?

If you identify one suspicious (and obvious) finding, be sure to continue looking at the mammogram for other lesions bilaterally. Multifocal lesions occur in the same quadrant and multicentric lesions are found in different quadrants in the same breast. Bilateral breast cancers are synchronous if they are diagnosed at the same time and metachronous if they are diagnosed after an arbitrary interval (e.g., 6 or 12 months from the initial cancer diagnosis). The published literature relative to the incidence of multifocality and multicentricity is limited and difficult to review because there are significant differences in how the terms are defined and how tissue is evaluated histologically. There are now good data supporting the use of magnetic resonance imaging (MRI) in evaluating patients for multifocal, multicentric, and synchronous contralateral lesions, all of which could change the surgical management of the patient. We recommend bilateral breast MRI in all of our patients with a new diagnosis of breast cancer.

PATIENT 42

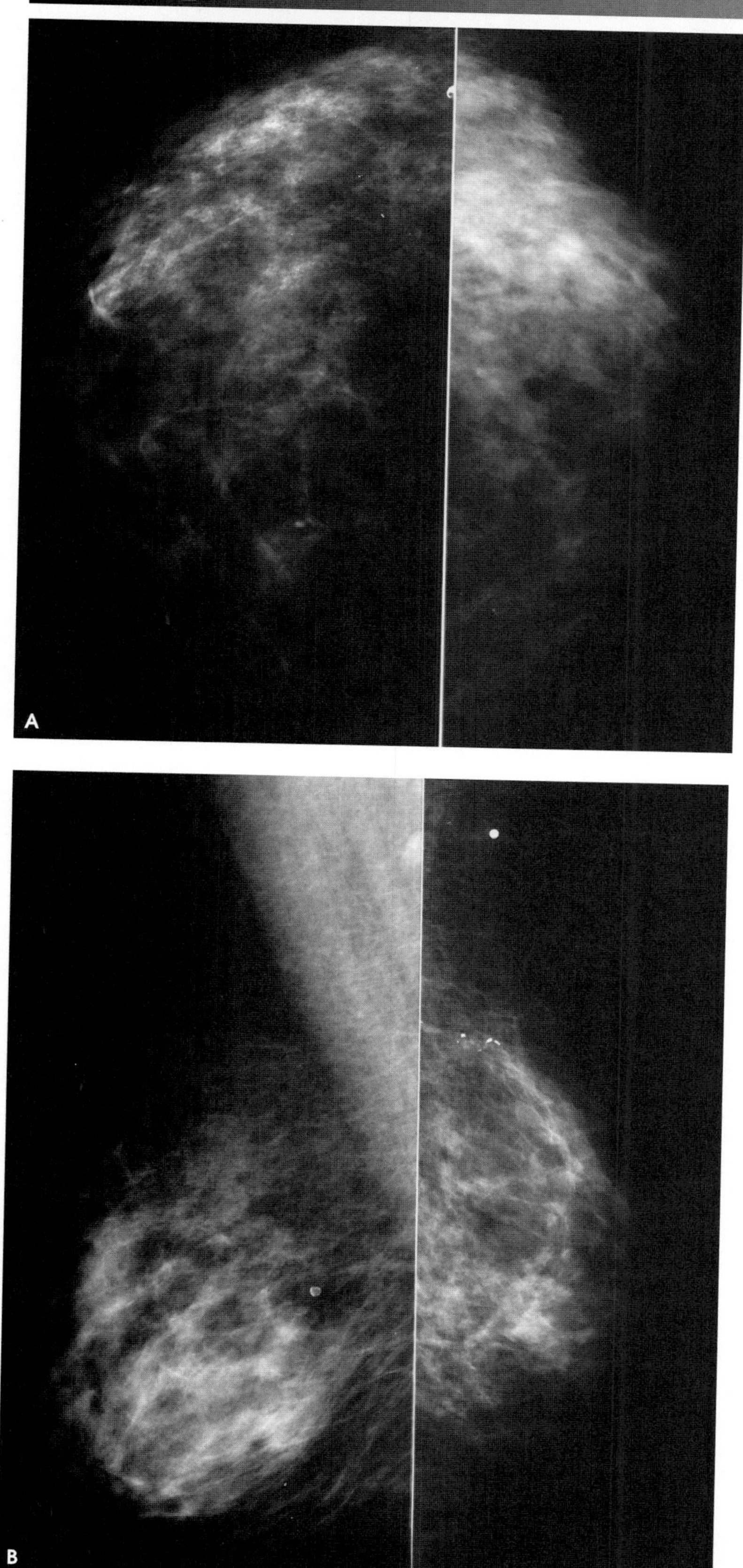

Figure 2.45. Screening study, 40-year-old woman. Craniocaudal **(A)** and mediolateral oblique **(B)** views.

What observations can you make, and what underlying condition do you think the patient has?

The left breast is smaller than the right, and there is no pectoral muscle imaged on the left. In some patients, the pectoral muscle may not be imaged secondary to a history of prior trauma (e.g., a burn) to the chest wall or shoulder, or a stroke, such that the patient is unable to cooperate with positioning. Alternatively, Poland's syndrome should be considered. This patient has no history of trauma or stroke. She has Poland's syndrome.

Poland's syndrome is a rare, sporadic congenital malformation with unilateral hypoplasia of the chest wall, ipsilateral hand abnormalities, absence of the costosternal portion of the pectoralis major muscle, absence of the pectoralis minor muscle, and absence of the second, third, and fourth or third, fourth, and fifth costal cartilages or ribs. The clinical manifestations of Poland's syndrome are variable. It is postulated that hypoplasia or damage to the subclavian artery, or its branches, in utero leads to the range of developmental abnormalities reported in these patients. Mammographic manifestations in this syndrome include hypoplasia of the ipsilateral breast, inability to visualize the pectoralis muscle, and absence of a nipple. Association with malignancies including leukemia, lymphoma, and leiomyosarcoma has been reported in these patients. There have also been several case reports of breast cancer identified in women with Poland syndrome.

BI-RADS® category 1: negative. In general, for benign findings, if the observations represent a change from the prior mammogram, I describe them in the report and use BI-RADS® category 2: benign finding. If the findings are stable compared with prior mammograms, I do not describe them and use category 1 for the assessment. Annual screening mammography is recommended in this patient.

PATIENT 43

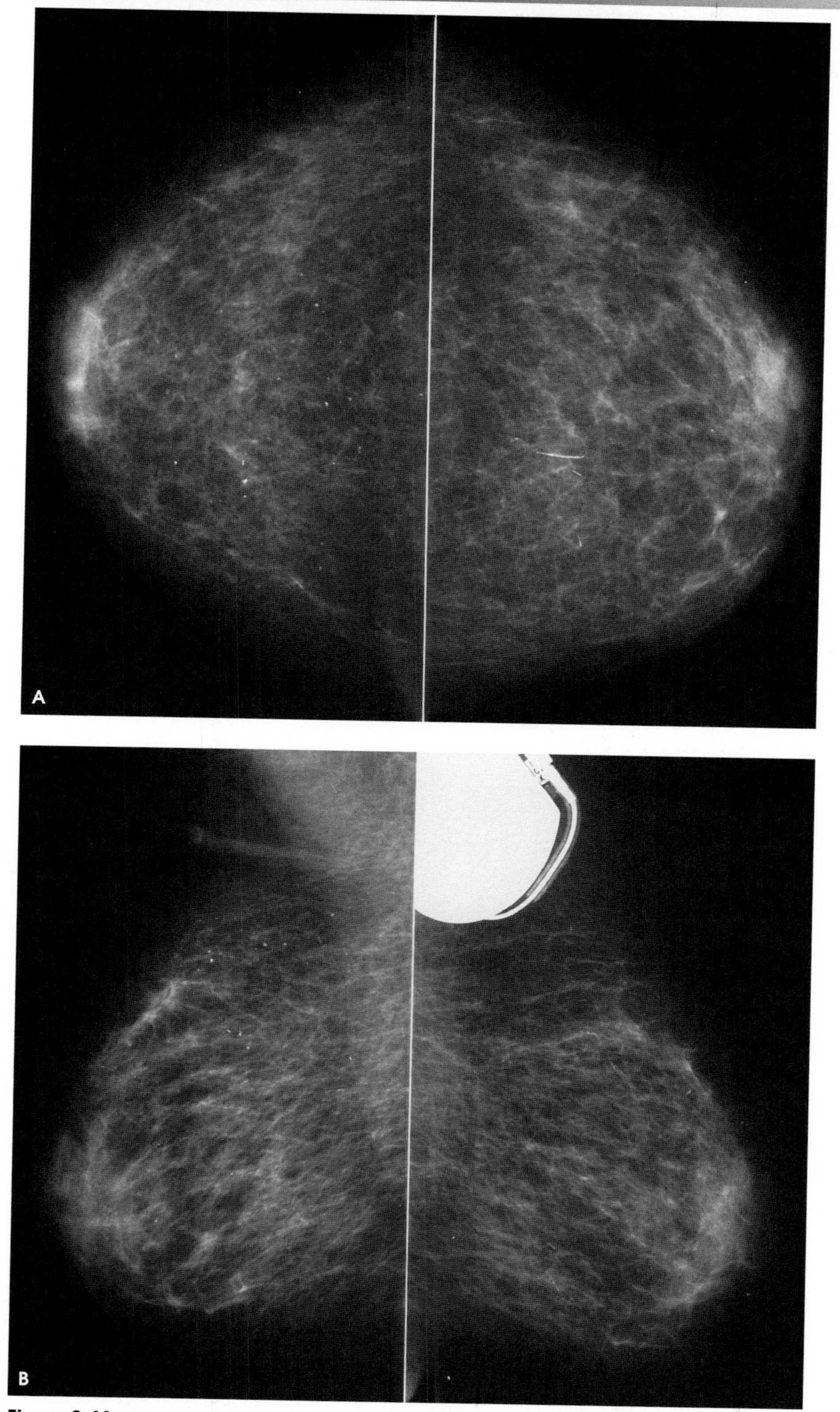

Figure 2.46. Screening study, 78-year-old woman. Craniocaudal **(A)** and mediolateral oblique **(B)** views.

Is this a normal mammogram?

A pacemaker is present in the left subpectoral region and there are scattered dystrophic and vascular calcifications. Before focusing your attention on the search for subtle signs of breast cancer, consider evaluating the study for technical adequacy and the presence of diffuse changes. When they are bilateral, diffuse changes can be hard to perceive. Did you notice the prominence of the trabecular markings? This becomes particularly striking when you compare with a study from 2 years previously.

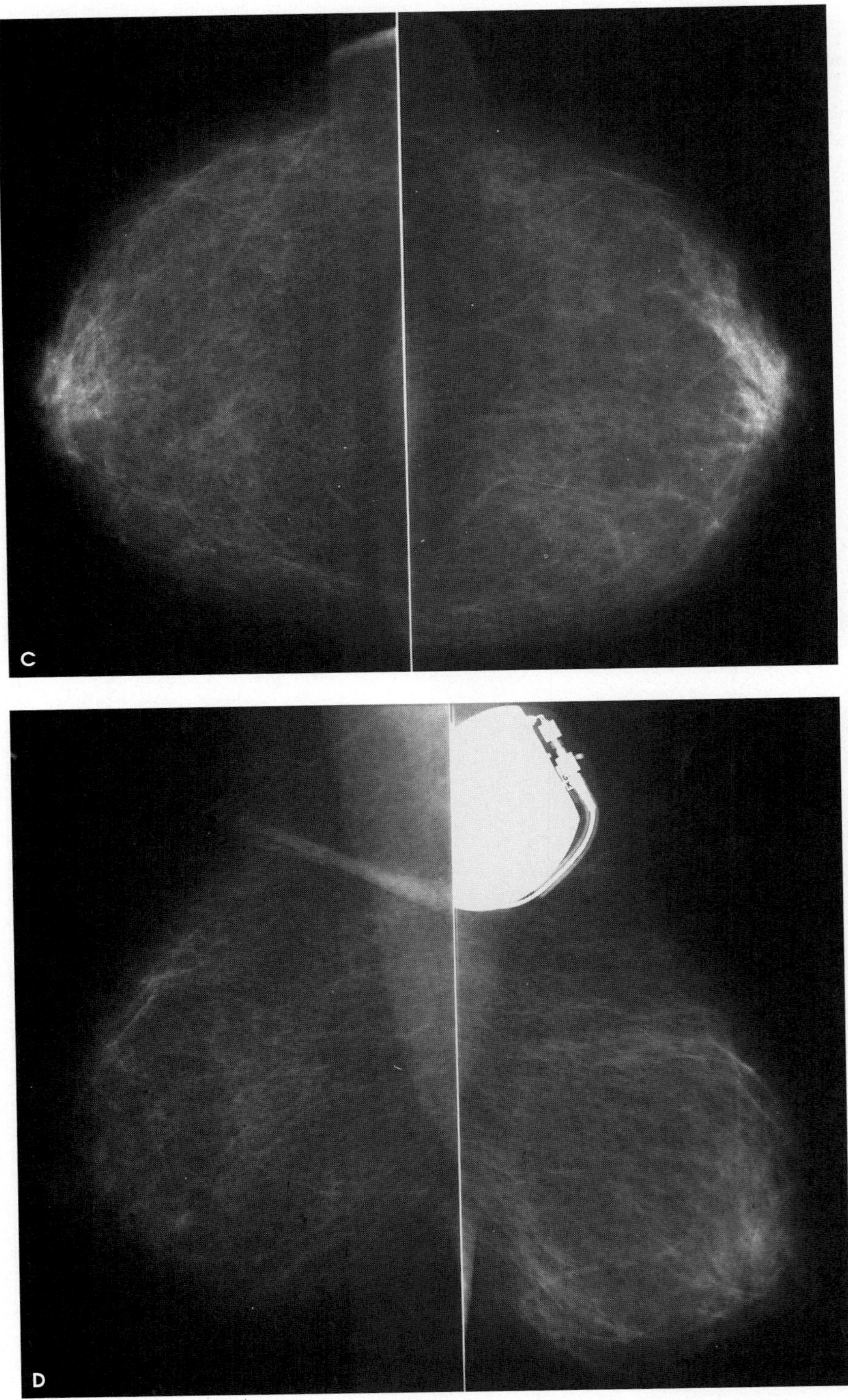

Figure 2.46. (*Continued*) Comparison screening study, 2 years previously. Craniocaudal **(C)** and mediolateral oblique **(D)** views.

What is your differential?

Differential considerations for diffuse changes that are usually unilateral, although rarely can be bilateral, include radiation therapy effect, inflammatory changes (e.g., mastitis), trauma, ipsilateral axillary adenopathy with lymphatic obstruction, dialysis shunt in the ipsilateral arm with fluid overload, invasive ductal carcinoma not otherwise specified, inflammatory carcinoma, invasive lobular carcinoma, or lymphoma. Invasive lobular carcinoma can lead to increases in breast density and size or a decrease in breast size (the shrinking breast). Differential considerations for diffuse changes that are usually bilateral, although they can be unilateral, include hormone replacement therapy (e.g., estrogen), weight change, congestive heart failure, renal failure with fluid overload, and superior vena cava syndrome. Additional rare benign causes include granulomatous mastitis, coumadin necrosis, arteritis, and autoimmune disorders (e.g., scleroderma). Obtaining a thorough history, examining the patient, and an ultrasound are often helpful in sorting through the differential considerations.

In this patient, the findings reflect congestive heart failure with fluid overload. Signs and symptoms improve significantly with diuretics; this applies to the mammographic changes as well.

BI-RADS® category 2: benign finding. Next screening mammogram is recommended in 1 year.

PATIENT 44

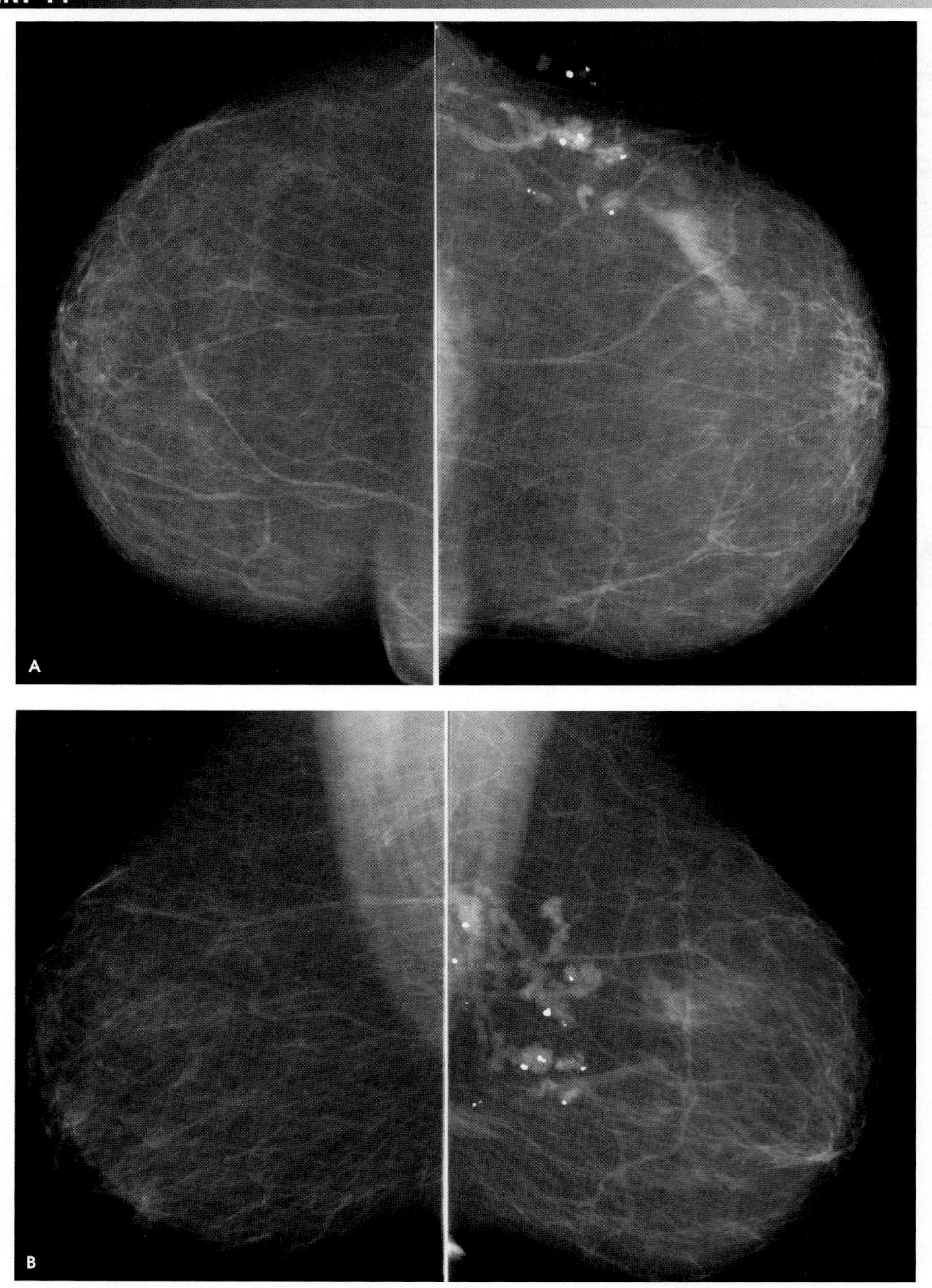

Figure 2.47. Screening study, 66-year-old woman. Craniocaudal **(A)** and mediolateral oblique **(B)** views.

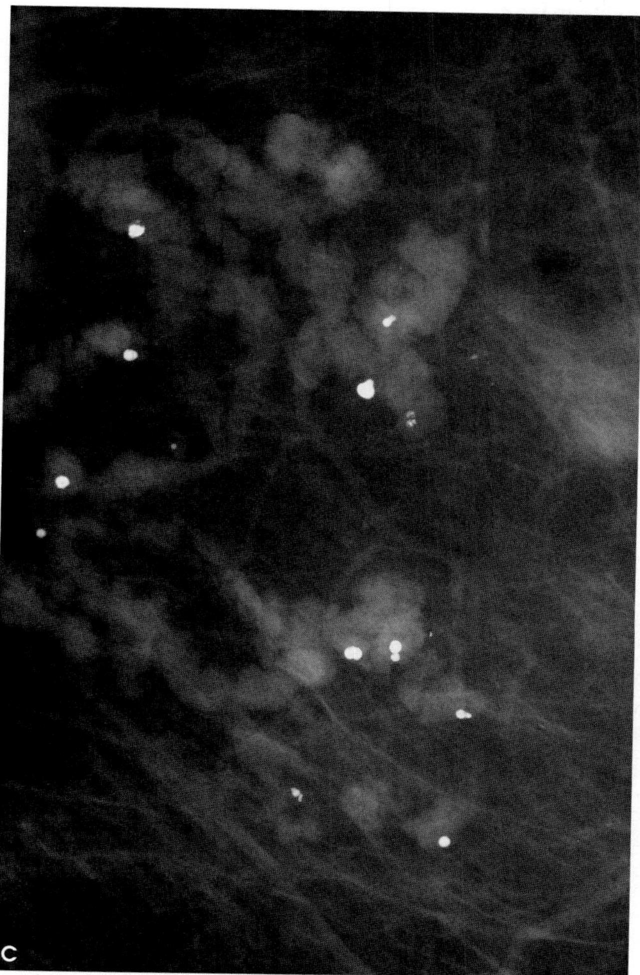

Figure 2.47. (*Continued*) Mediolateral oblique, photographically coned view **(C)**, left breast.

What is the diagnosis?

A serpiginous tubular structure is imaged in the upper outer quadrant of the left breast associated with scattered coarse calcifications. This is most likely a thrombosed vein (varix) reflecting healed Mondor's disease. In most patients, Mondor's disease resolves completely, with no residual imaging finding. Rarely, calcification may be seen outlining the thrombosed vein.

What is Mondor's disease?

Mondor's disease is a self-limiting, uncommon trombophlebitis involving one of the superficial veins in the breast. The thoracoepigastric and lateral thoracic veins are the most commonly involved. In most patients, the cause is idiopathic. However, reported causes of Mondor's disease include breast trauma, breast surgery, imaging-guided biopsies, sentinel lymph node biopsy, dehydration, excessive physical activity, an inflammatory process, and, rarely, breast cancer.

What is the clinical presentation of Mondor's disease, and what imaging findings can be seen? What is the treatment of choice?

Acutely, patients with Mondor's disease describe a tender cord that is often associated with linear dimpling, accentuated when the ipsilateral arm is raised, or superficial serpiginous nodularity (simulating the appearance of a varicose vein) corresponding to the course of the involved vein. Mammographically, the affected vein may have a rope- or beadlike appearance. On ultrasound, a superficial beaded tubular structure may be imaged, corresponding to the linear dimpling. Mondor's disease typically resolves spontaneously. Patients are reassured of the likely benign nature of this condition and supported with nonsteroidal, anti-inflammatory agents for symptomatic relief of associated tenderness.

BI-RADS® category 1: negative. Next screening mammogram is recommended in 1 year.

PATIENT 45

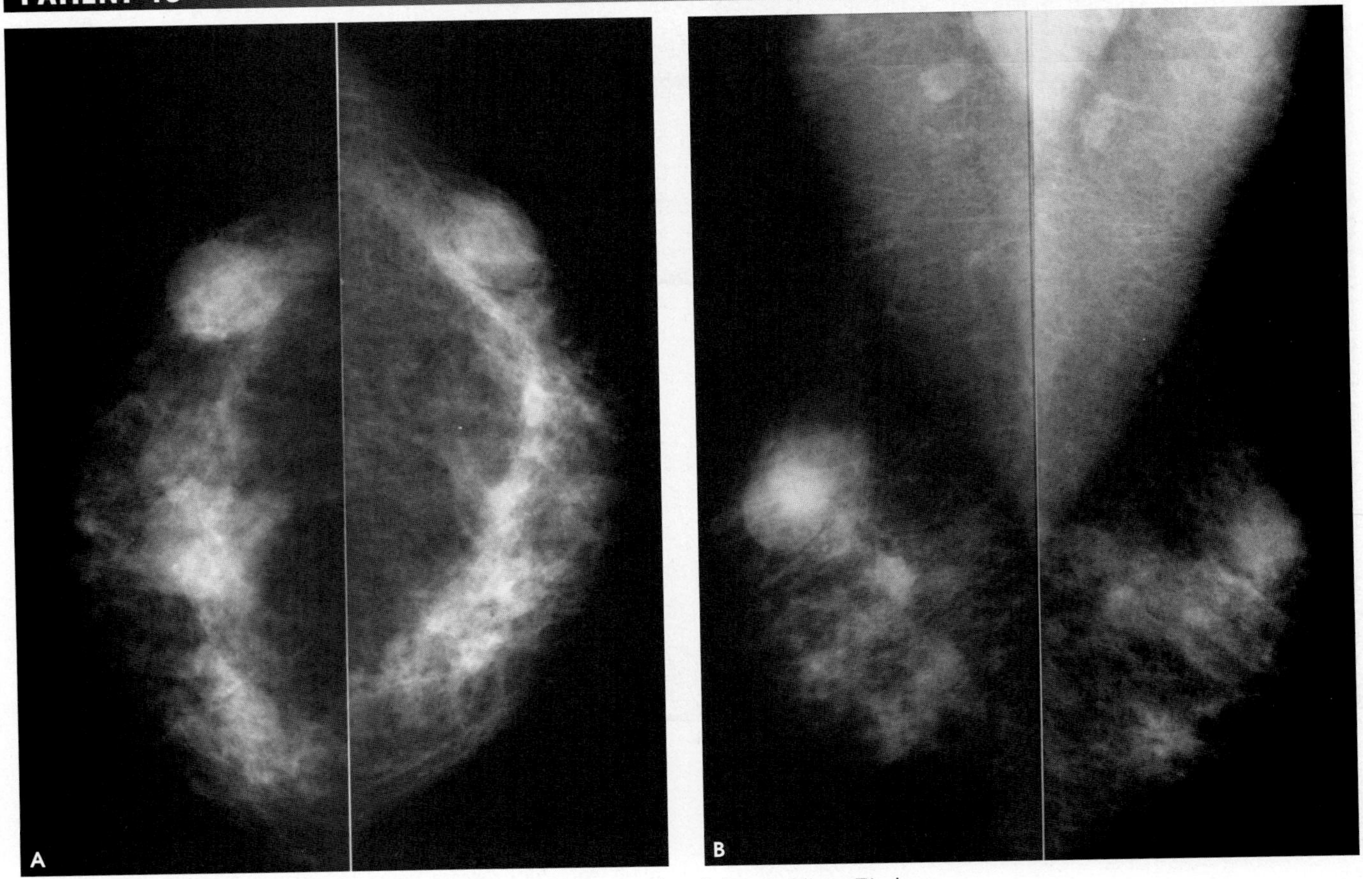

Figure 2.48. Screening study, 54-year-old woman. Craniocaudal **(A)** and mediolateral oblique **(B)** views.

What observations can you make, and what would you like to do next?

Lymph nodes and the pectoralis minor muscles (triangular densities at the edge of the mediolateral oblique views) are imaged bilaterally, superimposed on the pectoralis major muscles. More important, masses are present bilaterally. Comparison with prior studies is important to determine if these represent an interval change, in which case additional evaluation is indicated. If the masses are stable or decreasing in size, or if they have been previously evaluated, no further evaluation may be needed.

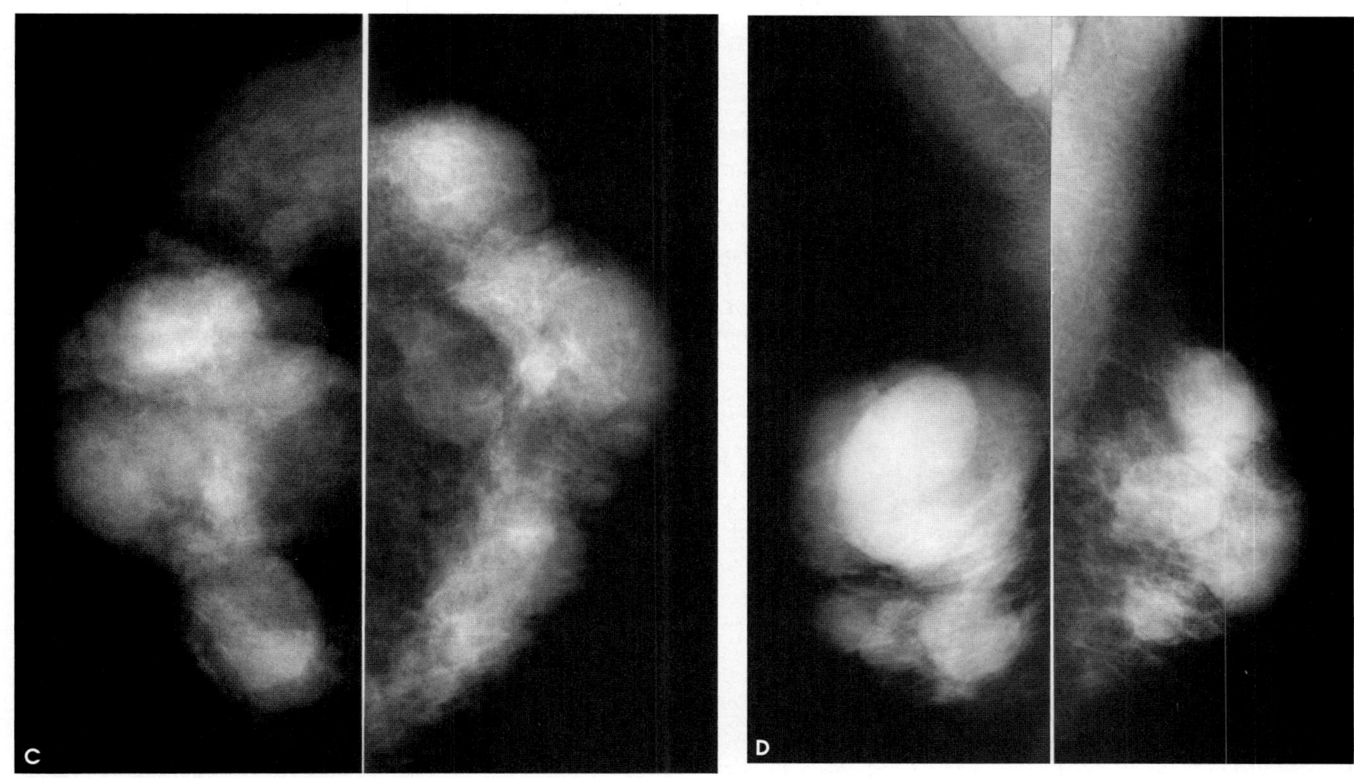

Figure 2.48. *(Continued)* Craniocaudal **(C)** and mediolateral oblique **(D)** views, 2 years previously.

Based on the prior studies, what would you recommend next?

When compared with sequential prior studies (only one prior study is shown), multiple masses are seen bilaterally with notable size fluctuations. These have been evaluated with ultrasound previously and therefore no further evaluation is indicated at this time, particularly because they have almost completely regressed. Cysts are common and can occur at any age, including during adolescence. In many women, however, cysts develop, or become more prominent, during the perimenopausal period. If no hormone replacement is used, most cysts regress spontaneously following menopause. A second, smaller peak of cyst development is seen in women in their mid to late 70s and early 80s.

How should women with multiple similar masses on a screening mammogram be managed?

The management of women with multiple masses on screening mammograms is controversial. Given a low yield of malignancy, some suggest that no evaluation is indicated, provided the masses are similar in appearance mammographically. My approach to women with multiple masses is to evaluate them at the first presentation with spot compression views and ultrasound. If the masses are cysts, annual screening mammography is recommended. Thereafter, only new masses are evaluated with spot compression views and ultrasound. If one or more likely benign solid masses are imaged on ultrasound, a follow-up ultrasound is recommended in 6 months. A biopsy is done when a mass is solid and does not fit the criteria for a probably benign lesion following a complete workup.

BI-RADS® category 1: negative. Next screening mammogram is recommended in 1 year. (If for some reason the masses are described in the report, a BI-RADS® category 2: benign findings assessment is used and annual mammography is recommended).

BIBLIOGRAPHY

American College of Radiology (ACR). ACR BI-RADS®—Mammography. 4th ed. In: *ACR Breast Imaging Reporting and Data System, Breast Imaging Atlas.* Reston, VA: American College of Radiology; 2003.

American College of Radiology. *Mammography Quality Control Manual.* Reston, VA: American College of Radiology; 1999.

American Joint Commission on Cancer. *Cancer Staging Manual.* 6th ed. New York: Springer-Verlag; 2002.

Bassett LW, Hirbawi IA, DeBruhl N, et al. Mammographic positioning: evaluation from the view box. *Radiology.* 1993;188:803–806.

Bassett LW, Jackson VP, Fu KL, Fu YS. *Diagnosis of Diseases of the Breast*. 2nd ed. Philadelphia: Elsevier Saunders; 2005.

Cardenosa G, Eklund GW. Rate of compliance with recommendations for additional mammographic views and biopsies. *Radiology*. 1991;181(2):359–361.

Catania S, Zurrida S, Veronesi P, et al. Mondor's disease and breast cancer. *Cancer*. 1992;69:2267–2270.

Conant EF, Wilkes AN, Mendelson EB, Feig SA. Superficial thrombophlebitis of the breast (Mondor's disease): mammographic findings. *AJR Am J Roentgenol*. 1993;160:1201–1203.

Cooper RA, Johnson MS. Mammographic depiction of Poland's syndrome. *Br J Radiol*. 1990;63:302–303.

Doyle AJ. Unilateral breast edema in congestive heart failure—a mimic of diffuse carcinoma. *Australas Radiol*. 1991;35: 274–275.

Eklund GW, Cardenosa G. The art of mammographic positioning. *Radiol Clin North Am*. 1992;30:21–53.

Eklund GW, Cardenosa G, Parsons W. Assessing adequacy of mammographic image quality. *Radiology*. 1994;190:297–307.

Fokin AA, Robicsek F. Poland's syndrome revisited. *Ann Thorac Surg*. 2002;74:2218–2225.

Fukushima T, Otake T, Yashima R, et al. Breast cancer in two patients with Poland's syndrome. *Breast Cancer*. 1999;6:127–130.

Giuliano AE, Barth AM, Spivack B, et al. Incidence and predictors of axillary metastasis in T1 carcinoma of the breast. *J Am Coll Surg*. 1996;183:185–189.

Harris AT. Mondor's disease of the breast can also occur after sonography-guided core biopsy. *AJR Am J Roentgenol*. 2003;180:284–285.

Jaberi M, Willey SC, Brem RF. Stereotactic vacuum-assisted breast biopsy: an unusual cause of Mondor's disease. *AJR Am J Roentgenol*. 2002;179:185–186.

Jemal A, Murray T, Ward E, et al. Cancer statistics, 2005. *CA Cancer J Clin*. 2005;55:10–30.

Kriege M, Brekelmans CT, Boetes C, et al. Efficacy of MRI and mammography for breast cancer screening in women with a familial or genetic predisposition. *N Engl J Med*. 2004;51:427–437.

Leung JW, Sickles EA. Multiple bilateral masses detected on screening mammography: assessment of need for recall imaging. *AJR Am J Roentgenol*. 2000;175:23–29.

Liberman L, Morris EA, Kim CM, et al. MR imaging findings in the contralateral breast of women with recently diagnosed breast cancer. *AJR Am J Roentgenol*. 2003;180:333–341.

Markopoulos C, Kouskos E, Mantas D, et al. Mondor's disease of the breast: is there any relation to breast cancer. *Eur J Gynaecol Oncol*. 2005;26:213–214.

Mendelson EB. Evaluation of the postoperative breast. *Radiol Clin North Am*. 1992;30:107–138.

Miller CL, Feig SA, Fox JW. Mammographic changes after reduction mammoplasty. *AJR Am J Roentgenol*. 1987;149:35–38.

Morris EA, Liberman L, Ballon DJ, et al. MRI of occult breast carcinoma in a high-risk population. *AJR Am J Roentgenol*. 2003; 181:619–626.

Oraedu CO, Pinnapureddy P, Alrawi S, et al. Congestive heart failure mimicking inflammatory breast carcinoma: a case report and review of the literature. *Breast J*. 2001;7:117–119.

Piccoli CW, Feig SA, Palazzo JP. Developing asymmetric breast tissue. *Radiology*. 1999;211:111–117.

Robertson CL, Kopans DB. Communication problems after mammographic screening. *Radiology*. 1989;172(2):443–444.

Samuels TH, Haider MA, Kirkbride P. Poland's syndrome: a mammographic presentation. *AJR Am J Roentgenol*. 1996;166:347–348.

Schneidereit NP, Davis N, Mackinnon M, et al. T1a breast carcinoma and the role of axillary dissection. *Arch Surg*. 2003;138: 832–837.

Shetty MK, Watson AB. Mondor's disease of the breast: sonographic and mammographic findings. *AJR Am J Roentgenol*. 2001;177:893–896.

Shoup M, Malinzak L, Weisenberger J, Aranha GV. Predictors of axillary node metastasis in T1 breast carcinoma. *Am Surg*. 1999; 65:748–752.

Sickles EA. Findings at mammographic screening on only one standard projection: outcome analysis. *Radiology*. 1998;208:471–475.

Sickles EA. The subtle and atypical mammographic features of invasive lobular carcinoma. *Radiology*. 1991;178:25–26.

Sickles EA. Practical solutions to common mammographic problems: tailoring the examination. *AJR Am J Roentgenol*. 1988; 151:31–39.

Smith RA, Cokkinides V, Eyre HJ. American Cancer Society guidelines for the early dectection of cancer, 2005. *CA Cancer J Clin*. 2005;55:31–44.

Smith RA, Saslow D, Sawyer KA, et al. American Cancer Society guidelines for breast cancer screening. *CA Cancer J Clin*. 2003; 53:141–169.

Stacey-Clear A, McCarthy KA, Hall DA, et al. Mammographically detected breast cancer: location in women under 50 years old. *Radiology*. 1993;186:677–680.

Stahl-Kent V, Sandbank J, Halevy A. Mondor's disease of the axilla: a rare complication of sentinel lymph node biopsy. *Breast J*. 2004;10:253–255.

Swann CA, Kopans DB, McCarthy KA. Localization of occult breast lesions: practical solutions to problems of triangulation. *Radiology* 1987; 163:557.

Tabar L, Dean PB. *Teaching Atlas of Mammography*. 3rd ed. New York: Thieme; 2001.

Tabar L, Tot T, Dean PB. *Breast Cancer: The Art and Science of Early Detection with Mammography*. New York: Thieme; 2005.

Tabar L, Vitak B, Chen HH, et al. The Swedish two-county trial twenty years later. *Radiol Clin North Am*. 2000; 38:625-651.

Urschel HC. Poland's syndrome. *Chest Surg Clin North Am*. 2000; 10:393–403.

Vitucci C, Tirelli C, Graziano F, Santoro E. Results of conservative surgery for limited-sized infiltrating breast cancer: analysis of 962 tested patients: 24 years experience. *J Surg Oncol*. 2000;74: 108–115.

Warner E, Plewes DB, Hill KA, et al. Surveillance of BRCA1 and BRCA2 mutation carriers with magnetic resonance imaging, ultrasound, mammography and clinical breast examination. *JAMA*. 2004;292:1317–1325.

Woo CS, Silberman H, Nakamura SK, et al. Lymph node status combined with lymphovascular invasion creates a more powerful tool for predicted outcome in patients with invasive breast cancer. *Am J Surg*. 2002;184:337–340.

Yiangou C, Shousha S, Snnett HD. Primary tumor characteristics and axillary node status in breast cancer. *Br J Cancer*. 1999;80: 1974–1978.

Diagnostic Breast Imaging

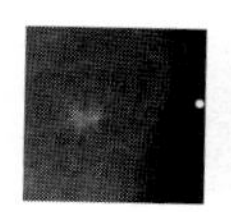
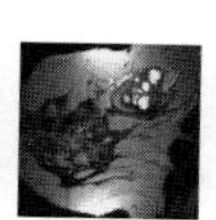
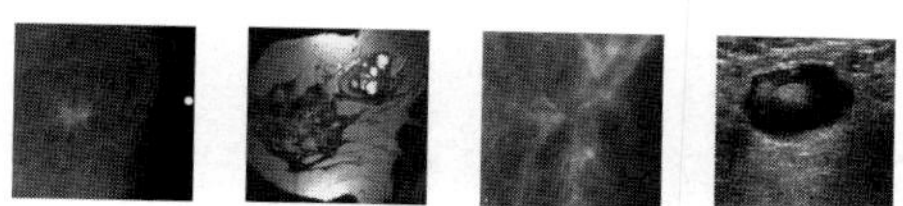
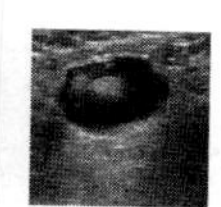

TERMS

Adenosis tumor
Air gap
Axillary lymph node dissection (ALND)
Cat scratch disease
Columnar alteration with prominent apical snouts and secretions (CAPSS)
Complex fibroadenoma
Complex sclerosing lesion (CSL)
Cyst
Diabetic fibrous mastopathy
Double spot compression magnification views
Ductal carcinoma in situ (DCIS)
Epidermal inclusion cyst
Extensive intraductal component (EIC)
Extra-abdominal desmoid
Extracapsular tumor extension
Fat necrosis
Fibroadenoma
Fibromatosis
Focal fibrosis
Focal spot
Galactocele
Granular cell tumor
Gynecomastia
Hematoma
Invasive ductal carcinoma not otherwise specified (NOS)
Invasive lobular carcinoma
Lactational adenoma
Lipoma
Lobular neoplasia
Lymphovascular space involvement
Male breast cancer
Mastitis
Medullary carcinoma
Metachronous carcinoma
Metaplastic carcinoma
Metastatic disease
Milk of calcium
Mucinous carcinoma
Multiple peripheral papillomas
Neoadjuvant therapy
Oil cyst
Papillary carcinoma
Papilloma
Perineural invasion
Peripheral abscess
Phyllodes tumor
Port-a-catheters
Posttraumatic change
Pneumocystography
Probably benign lesion
Psammoma bodies
Pseudoangiomatous stromal hyperplasia (PASH)
Radial scar
Sclerosing adenosis
Sebaceous cyst
Secretory calcification
Sentinel lymph node biopsy (SLNB)
Shrinking breast
Spot compression views
Spot tangential views
Subareolar abscess
Synchronous carcinoma
Touch imprints
Triangulation of lesion location
Tubular adenoma
Tubular carcinoma
Tubulolobular carcinoma
Tumor necrosis
Vascular calcification

INTRODUCTION

The diagnostic patient population is made up of women called back for potential abnormalities detected on a screening mammogram, patients who present with signs and symptoms of disease localized to the breast(s), patients with a history of breast cancer treated with lumpectomy and radiation therapy, and those undergoing follow-up during neoadjuvant chemotherapy for breast cancer. At some facilities, and according to the American College of Radiology (ACR) Practice Guideline for the Performance of Diagnostic Mammography, women with implants may also be included in the diagnostic patient population.

This chapter describes *one* approach to the diagnostic evaluation of patients with breast related findings, which I have developed and fine-tuned through years of experience and thousands of patient encounters. I provide the rationale for a *common-sense,* streamlined approach and illustrate principles that I think you will find practical, efficient, and helpful in minimizing a delay in a breast cancer diagnosis. Simplicity, creativity, and resourcefulness in problem solving are all components of the approach. Obviously, there are many different ways of approaching this patient population, and again my recommendation is that you select a method that works in your hands, and *use it consistently.* Do not short-circuit evaluations for the sake of expediency, be flexible and creative (but keep it simple) in sorting through dilemmas, make no assumptions, and demand the highest quality possible from yourself and those around you.

Although I provide the imaging algorithms I use, a dedicated breast imaging radiologist directs all diagnostic evaluations and can tailor the exam to the patient and the problem being evaluated. Results, impressions, and recommendations are discussed with the patient directly at the time of the evaluation. Tools available to evaluate patients include mammographic images, correlative physical examination, ultrasound, cyst aspiration, pneumocystography, ductography, imaging-guided fine-needle aspiration, and imaging-guided needle biopsy. If indicated, magnetic resonance imaging of the breast is scheduled at the time of the patient's diagnostic evaluation, including all patients diagnosed with breast cancer following an imaging-guided procedure.

ADDITIONAL MAMMOGRAPHIC VIEWS

For patients called back after screening, additional mammographic images are almost always taken. Virtually all of the additional views imaged during diagnostic evaluations involve the use of the spot compression paddle and include spot compression, rolled spot compression, spot tangential, and double spot compression magnification views. Spot compression and rolled compression views are taken when trying to determine if a lesion is present (or is it merely an "imaginoma"), when establishing the marginal characteristics of a mass, or, with rolled views, for triangulating the location of a lesion seen initially on only one of the routine views. Spot tangential views are taken routinely in evaluating focal signs and symptoms. They are also used when a lesion is thought to be localized to the skin or to position postoperative skin changes following lumpectomy and radiation, in tangent to the x-ray beam so that they are not superimposed and potentially obscuring significant changes at the lumpectomy bed. Double spot compression magnification views are indicated when evaluating calcifications. The only diagnostic images that are sometimes done with the large compression paddle are lateral views (90-degree lateromedial or 90-degree mediolateral views) used to triangulate the location of a lesion on the orthogonal view. As with screening views, high-quality, well-exposed, high-contrast diagnostic images, with no blur or artifacts, are essential to minimize the likelihood of delaying or missing a breast cancer diagnosis.

DIAGNOSTIC EVALUATION OF PATIENTS OVER THE AGE OF 30 YEARS WHO PRESENT WITH FOCAL FINDINGS

When women over the age of 30 years present with a "lump" or other focal symptom (focal pain, skin change, nipple retraction, etc.), a metallic BB is placed at the site of focal concern. Then craniocaudal (CC) and mediolateral oblique (MLO) views are imaged bilaterally, as well as a spot tangential view of the focal abnormality. A unilateral study (CC and MLO views) of the symptomatic breast with the spot tangential view at the site of focal concern is done if the patient has had a mammogram within the preceding 6 months. Based on what is seen on these initial images, additional spot compression, or double spot compression magnification views, may be oftained. Depending on the location of the focal finding, and the appearance of this area on the spot tangential view, correlative physical examination and an ultrasound are usually indicated. The ultrasound may be deferred in patients in whom there is no chance that the lesion has been excluded from the field of view and completely fatty tissue, or a benign lesion (e.g., an oil cyst or a dystrophic calcification), is imaged corresponding to the area of concern.

DIAGNOSTIC EVALUATION OF PATIENTS UNDER AGE 30 YEARS, PREGNANT, OR LACTATING, WITH FOCAL FINDINGS

For women under the age of 30 years, or who are pregnant or lactating, who present with a "lump" or other focal symptom, we start by doing a physical examination and an ultrasound. In most of these patients, this is all that is required for an appropriate disposition. Rarely, if a breast cancer is suspected based on the physical exam and ultrasound findings, a biopsy may be indicated in this patient population. If cancer is suspected, a full bilateral mammogram is also done.

OUR GOAL AND APPROACH RELATIVE TO DIAGNOSTIC EVALUATIONS

When patients present for diagnostic evaluations, our goal is to establish the correct diagnosis, accurately and efficiently, so we do as much as is indicated and the patient desires, in one visit. For some women this may include mammographic images only, or additional views and an ultrasound; for other patients, additional mammographic views, an ultrasound, and a core biopsy are performed. In my experience, if a biopsy is indicated, the patient's immediate question is "How soon can I have it done?" and they are appreciative (and in many ways relieved) when I respond, "If you would like, we can do the biopsy now and have results by tomorrow." Rarely, a patient requests time to discuss the recommendation with her family; in that case, we schedule the biopsy for a date that is convenient for the patient.

Histologic findings are discussed by the radiologist and the pathologist who review the cores within 24 hours of the core biopsy, so patients are asked to return the following business day to receive their results. The biopsy site is examined, biopsy results are discussed, and, based on the results, our recommendations regarding the need to return to screening guidelines, short-interval follow-up, excisional biopsy, or surgical consultation are discussed with the patient. If a surgical consultation is indicated, this is scheduled for the patient before she leaves our center. With a commitment from the breast surgeon, patients are seen within 48 hours of a breast cancer diagnosis.

BI-RADS® ASSESSMENT CATEGORIES USED FOLLOWING DIAGNOSTIC EVALUATIONS

Under the Mammography Quality Standards Act (MQSA), all reports involving mammographic images require an assessment category. Our approach, however, is to provide an assessment that reflects our recommendation following the completed diagnostic evaluation. This usually incorporates the findings and impression formulated following the physical examination, mammogram, and ultrasound (or other studies that may be done). So, in addition to using BI-RADS® categories 1 and 2, and category 3 (probably benign, short-interval follow-up), we also use category 4 (suspicious abnormality, biopsy should be considered) and category 5 (highly suggestive of malignancy—appropriate action should be taken), based on what is determined following the completed diagnostic evaluation. Based on the likelihood of malignancy, category 4 lesions can be subclassified into 4A (low suspicion for malignancy), 4B (intermediate suspicion for malignancy), or 4C (moderate concern, but not classic as in category 5). Category 0 is used for patients for whom we schedule magnetic resonance imaging for further evaluation, and BI-RADS® category 6 (known malignancy) is used primarily for patients with a breast cancer diagnosis who are receiving chemotherapy (e.g., neoadjuvant therapy) and are undergoing monitoring of chemotherapy response. Although in this text I use the ACR lexicon terminology, in our practice we have chosen to vary the verbiage provided with categories 4 and 5 to indicate that a "biopsy is indicated" rather than "should be considered" or "appropriate action should be taken" (more on this below).

SOME PHILOSOPHICAL CONSIDERATIONS REGARDING PATIENT CARE AND DIAGNOSTIC EVALUATIONS: ARE WE FILM READERS OR CONSULTANTS?

Before going further, please indulge me in a short philosophical discussion about how we, as radiologists, choose to practice breast imaging. Although some are likely to disagree with several (and maybe all) of the concepts presented here, in generating a reaction, one way or the other, I accomplish my goal of getting you to think about issues that are not usually thought about—but perhaps should be.

As radiologists, we can effectively choose to delegate many of our responsibilities as physicians to others, thereby minimizing our direct role in the care of patients. We work hard during screening to identify small breast cancers, yet we routinely relegate the role of discussing our findings with patients to others. With this comes an obfuscation of our critical role in the detection of clinically occult early-stage breast cancer and possible misrepresentations to patients relative to the limitations of mammography and the generation of unrealistic expectations regarding the appropriateness of ultrasound and magnetic resonance imaging. We struggle during diagnostic evaluations to arrive at an answer, yet we dismiss patients with lines such as "You will get the results from your doctor," as though we are incapable (or unwilling) to do it, or we avoid *all* direct contact with the patient and have one of our surrogates tell the patient that she should contact her physician for the results. We identify potential cancers, yet we won't do the biopsy while the patient is in our facility because it is not practical or expedient. Patients are asked to wait for days and sometimes weeks for a biopsy to be done and then for results. If we do the biopsy, we often relegate patient follow-up and the discussion of results to the referring physician or surgeon. How can this be acceptable? Imagine the anguish. Is it any wonder that radiologists are the physicians most commonly named in malpractice lawsuits for delays in the diagnosis of breast cancer? I would argue that, in breast imaging, we are in a position to revolutionize and substantially improve patient care. *Carpe diem.*

What, then, should our role be? Should our role be to interpret films in isolation, or should it be that of clinicians and consultants who interpret breast images? I consider my role to be that of a clinical consultant in breast imaging (rather than a radiology report, I dictate "breast imaging consultations"), and as such, the patients who come to see me are *my* patients. In the diagnostic setting, rather than accept the history and physical examination described by others, I talk to the patients directly and, when indicated, undertake a physical examination. As opposed to delegating the breast ultrasound study to a technologist, I view this as an opportunity to establish effective rapport with the patient, review the history provided, and undertake correlative physical examination (in effect, placing eyeballs at the tips of my fingers). Why not take this opportunity? We place a significant amount of importance on what our images show, but shun the information provided by the physical examination and by talking directly with the patient. This information can be just as critical and important in arriving at the right answer as any finding on our imaging studies. There are times when the imaging studies are negative or equivocal and a biopsy is indicated based on clinical findings.

As I scan during the ultrasound study, I examine and talk with the patient. In addition to the visual information from the ultrasound, I find that use of the ultrasound coupling gel to examine a patient enhances my ability to find, feel, and characterize palpable findings. During the real-time portion of the study, as I scan and examine the patient, I determine if a lesion is present. After making this determination, I take the images needed to adequately and appropriately document the features of the lesion and that support the impression I formulate during the real-time portion of the study (i.e., directed image taking). I do not take pictures of normal tissue. Time and time again, I am impressed with how often the history obtained during these interchanges yields critical information used to establish the "true" nature and significance of what is going on. The other critical aspect of these interchanges is that it allows me to gauge the reaction of the patient to my recommendations. I want patients to understand and feel comfortable with what is happening. There are some who say we cannot afford to do this (i.e., it is not cost-effective). My response is to ask how can we afford *not* to do this? I would argue that it is more efficient and cost-effective, and I am convinced that this approach actually expedites high-quality patient care.

For a moment, consider patients referred to any specialist for a consultation. If a gastroenterologist detects a polyp during a colonoscopy, does he pull the scope out and dictate: "suspicious abnormality, biopsy should be considered?" or "finding highly suggestive of malignancy—appropriate action should be taken"? Likewise, if a cardiologist detects a significant coronary lesion that can be managed effectively with an angioplasty, does she call the referring physician for "permission" to proceed with an indicated procedure? No, they go ahead and do what needs to be done to take care of the patient. Why do we not consider a patient being sent to a breast imaging radiologist for evaluation in a similar light as a patient being sent to a breast surgeon for evaluation? Surgeons routinely do fine-needle aspirations and excisional biopsies on patients referred to them for clinical findings, even when fatty tissue is imaged mammographically and sonographically. This is acceptable, yet, on a mammogram with pleomorphic, linear casting-type calcifications, or a clinically occult 6-mm spiculated mass, we are expected to say "biopsy should be considered" or "appropriate action should be taken"? Considered by whom and when? Appropriate action to be taken by whom and when?

As a consultant, therefore, I exercise the right to discuss all aspects of a patient's breast-related findings, options for diagnosis (and treatment when appropriate), and, most important, I make specific recommendations and manage patients accordingly. In conjunction with the patient's physician, I make referrals when indicated. Following biopsies, I provide all patients with my business card and cell phone number so they can contact me if they have questions or concerns, and I ask them to return the following business day for the results of the biopsy. During the post biopsy visit, I examine the biopsy site and, most important, discuss the results of the biopsy directly with the patient. I discuss all options with the patient, but I follow this with a specific recommendation for what I think is the next appropriate step. When indicated, and following a discussion with the patient's physician, I make referrals so that the patient is helped and expedited through the system. Our patients are hungry for time, a warm touch, information, guidance, and yes, what we think is indicated.

CONSIDERING YOUR APPROACH TO PATIENTS

Consider how you approach patients. I suggest that proper attire, including a white coat with your name badge clearly visible, is critical in sending a powerful message to patients. Scrubs belong in the operating room or the interventional suite, not when approaching a patient relative to a possible breast cancer diagnosis. Also, although things like jeans and chewing gum may be acceptable in recreational venues, they are not when you are doing an ultrasound or an imaging-guided biopsy on a patient who is watching you like a hawk, waiting for some feedback. Address patients by their title and last name; unless specifically requested by the woman, patients should not be addressed by their first name, and terms of endearment should not be used (this applies to the technologists as well). Introduce yourself to the patient and shake her hand. Before starting the examination, ask her one or two questions relative to her concerns. If the patient has been called back for a potential abnormality on the screening study, and you have done additional mammographic images, tell her what you have seen so far and explain what you would like to do next. If you are doing an ultrasound, let the patient watch the screen, and keep an eye on her. If she is watching the screen as you scan, involve her in the study by educating her on what you are looking at. The ribs can be used to show her what a "tumor" would look like. Try to make sure the patient understands and is comfortable with what you recommend, and never let an angry patient leave your facility. Talk to her and find out what you can do to make things better.

I think it is also important to consider some of the language that permeates our work. Although this sounds trivial, I think it negatively colors our perspective and helps impersonalize and distance us from our patients. Consider terms such as "cases," "complaints," "denies," and "refuses." Does it not subtly affect us if we view "cases as complainers who deny and refuse"? I see *patients*, not cases. Why do we choose to view what a patient presents with as a complaint? If you have a legitimate concern about something, does it not bother you even slightly if someone says you are complaining about it? If you have legitimate fears about something and want time to think and consider your options, or if you are afraid, is this refusing? Does it not turn us off when someone says, "She is refusing"? First, it is a patient's right not to want something done, and this should always be respected and never judged negatively. Second, maybe if we worked harder to understand the patient's concerns, we might be able to help her more effectively. Rather than close the door, leave it open so she feels she can walk back through it and you will be there to help her. Try never to judge patients and what they have chosen to do. Comments such as "How could she have let this go?" or "Can you believe that she is saying this just came up?" are not acceptable. Who are we to know what a patient is going through and what her reasons may be for making a decision? Little is accomplished, and I think we stand to lose much, by having a patient feel guilty about what she has chosen to do. Our job is not to judge her, but to help her today and put her in as positive a frame of mind as possible to deal with what she is facing. I urge you to consider and analyze everything that you say and do in approaching patients. Work hard and creatively to spin things in a positive light; rather than viewing what we do as a chore, we should view the trust patients place in us as an incredible privilege unlike few others afforded us in life. We should feel honored that patients have enough confidence in us to share some of their most personal information, fears, and concerns.

You set the tone for your facility, and insisting that everyone in your facility think of patients as presenting with legitimate concerns and having the right to forgo a procedure has a positive effect on how everyone approaches his or her job and our patients.

COMMUNICATION AND DOCUMENTATION

Lastly, I want to emphasize the need for communication and appropriate documentation. Communicate directly with patients, referring physicians, pathologists, surgeons, and medical oncologists. Demand to speak directly with the physician ("I do not take no for an answer."). It is critical that referring physicians be kept in the loop, particularly in relation to a breast cancer diagnosis in one of their patients. Relative to pathology results, talk directly with the pathologist signing out a fine-needle aspiration or core biopsy. If possible, visit the pathology lab and review the histology of some of the more interesting cases you may diagnose. These interchanges can be incredibly valuable learning tools, and by working together, decisions can be made as to the adequacy of sampling or any lingering concerns the pathologist may have that might alter your management of the patient. Discuss specimen radiography results directly with the surgeon while the patient is still in the operating room (e.g., are you concerned that a lesion may extend to the margins, or are you concerned that the lesion, or your localization wire, has not been excised?).

I document the date, time, and nature of all communication (if possible with direct quotes) on the patient's history form (not in the breast imaging consultation report). Invest time in teaching your clerical and technical staff how to document encounters with patients properly. Months or years down the road, appropriate documentation can be critical in dealing with unresolved patient issues. Documentation needs to be appropriate, factual, and nonjudgmental. Documentation should not be a reflection of how your employee felt or saw a situation but rather a narrative of what happened. Provide the information accurately and let the reader formulate the impression. These simple steps cost little and yet the rewards in good patient care, goodwill, and public relations can be significant (as intangible as they may seem).

PATIENT 1

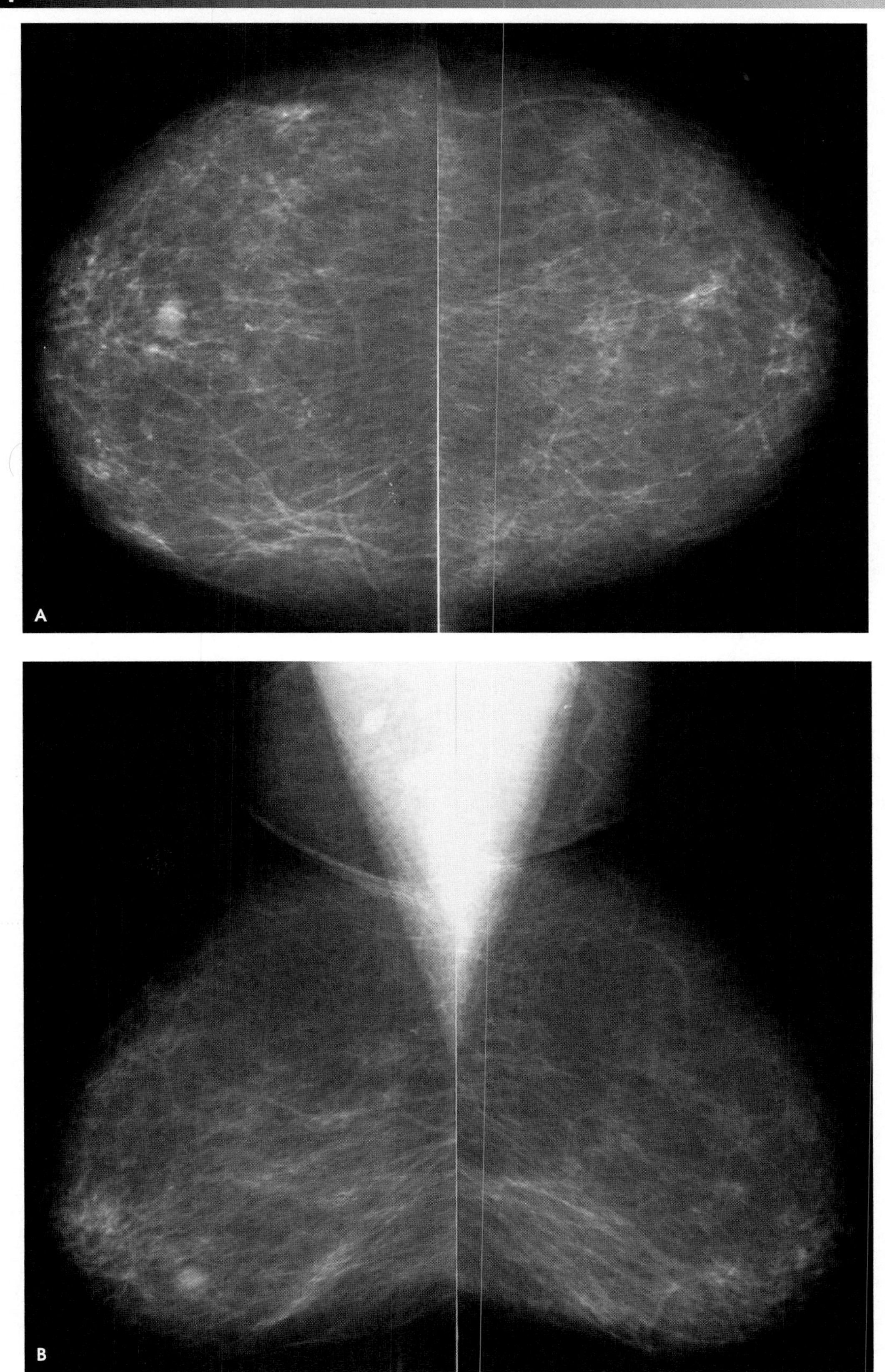

Figure 3.1. Screening study, 52-year-old woman. Craniocaudal **(A)** and mediolateral oblique **(B)** views.

What do you think, and what would you do next?

A mass is present in the right breast. Before recommending any additional evaluation, you should inquire about prior films. If prior films are available, and this mass is stable, decreasing in size, or has been previously evaluated, no additional intervention may be warranted at this time. Because this patient has no prior films, she is called back for additional evaluation, including spot compression views, correlative physical examination, and sonography.

BI-RADS® category 0: need additional imaging evaluation.

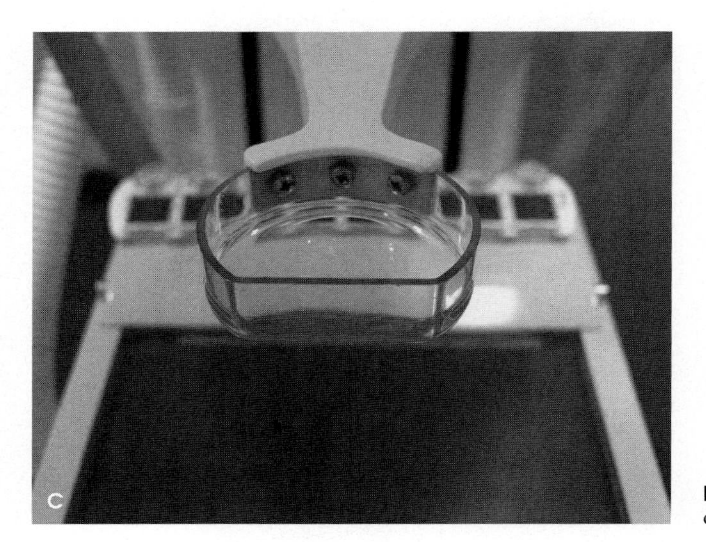

Figure 3.1. (*Continued*) Spot compression paddle **(C)** used in my practice for diagnostic evaluations.

Why use a spot compression paddle, and what are the indications for spot compression views? What is critical to consider when evaluating the adequacy of spot compression views? Why?

The spot compression paddle enables the application of maximal compression to a small area of the breast so that tissue is spread out and the area of radiographic concern is brought closer to the film, thereby improving resolution and image quality; it can help reach areas that are otherwise difficult to include when the large compression paddle is used. Spot compression views are helpful in several different situations in the diagnostic evaluation of patients. In some patients, spot compression views are used to distinguish a mass or distortion from normal superimposed glandular tissue. If a mass is detected on routine views, spot compression views can help characterize the marginal characteristics of the mass by displacing obscuring superimposed tissue.

In screening and diagnostic situations, spot compression views can be helpful in evaluating the subareolar area, particularly if compression of the anterior aspect of the breast is limited by the thickness of the base of the breast. If there is an area of relatively dense tissue that is underexposed, using the spot compression paddle may be helpful in improving the exposure by effectively decreasing the thickness of the tissue requiring penetration. In evaluating spot compression views, it is important to ensure that the area in question is included on the view; masses can sometimes be "squeezed" (or pulled) out from under the paddle and not imaged. As with routine views, spot compression views need to be well exposed, high in contrast, and free of motion blur.

When are rolled spot compression views used?

Rolled spot compression (i.e., change-of-angle) views are an additional tool available for establishing the existence of a lesion. Most tumors are three-dimensional and maintain their tumorlike shape as tissue is rolled. In contrast, breast tissue and focal areas of parenchymal asymmetry change in size, shape, and overall density as tissue is moved. Rolled spot compression views can also be used to move (roll) lesions away from surrounding tissue so that the marginal characteristics can be demonstrated to better advantage (Fig. 3.1D–F). Lastly, rolled spot compression views can be used to establish the approximate location of a lesion in the breast. If a lesion is located in the medial aspect of the breast, it will move with medial tissue. Similarly, if a lesion is in the lower outer quadrant of the breast, it will move with the tissue in the lower outer quadrant of the breast.

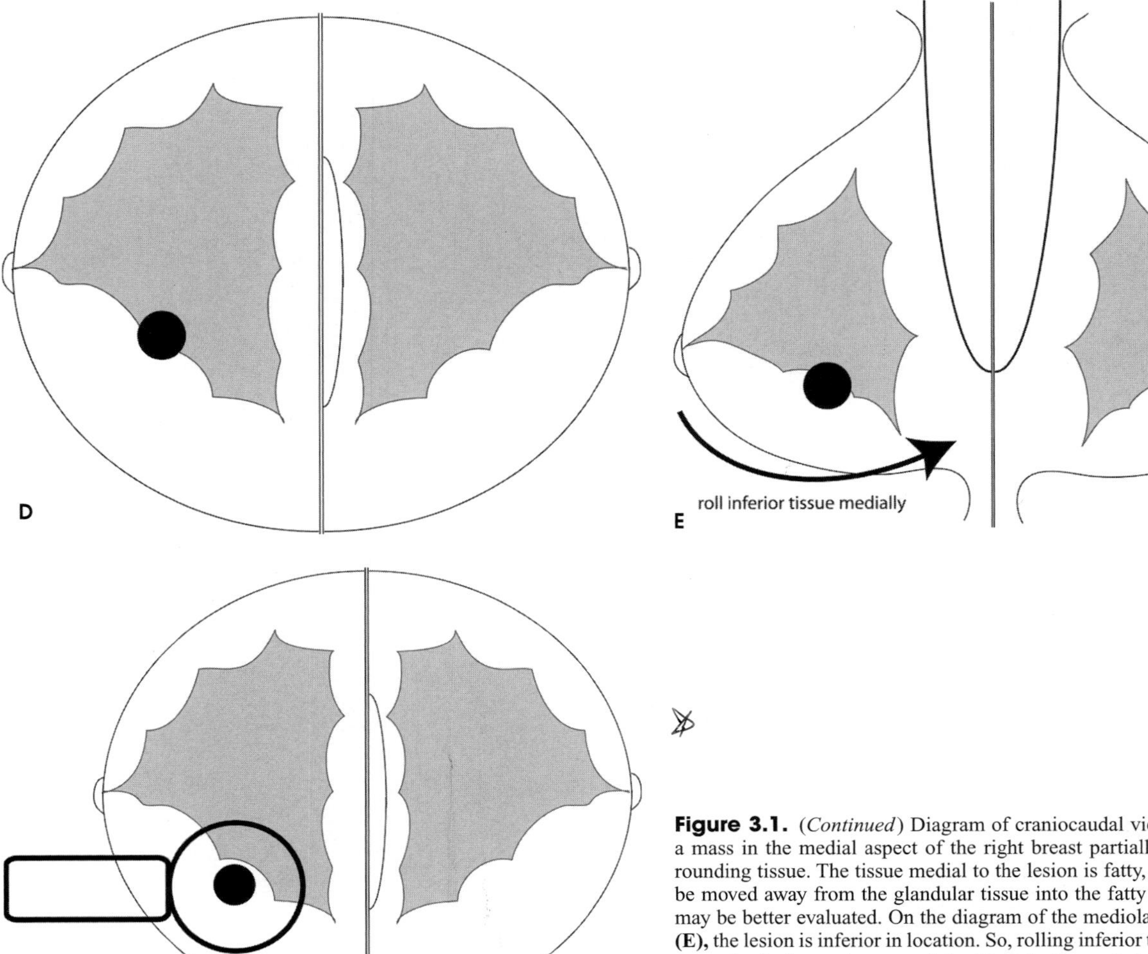

Figure 3.1. (*Continued*) Diagram of craniocaudal views **(D)** illustrating a mass in the medial aspect of the right breast partially obscured by surrounding tissue. The tissue medial to the lesion is fatty, so if the lesion can be moved away from the glandular tissue into the fatty tissue, the margins may be better evaluated. On the diagram of the mediolateral oblique views **(E),** the lesion is inferior in location. So, rolling inferior tissue medially may move the lesion and surround it with fatty tissue. Inferior tissue is rolled medially, and a spot compression view is done **(F).** The lesion is now surrounded by fat so that more of the margins can be evaluated.

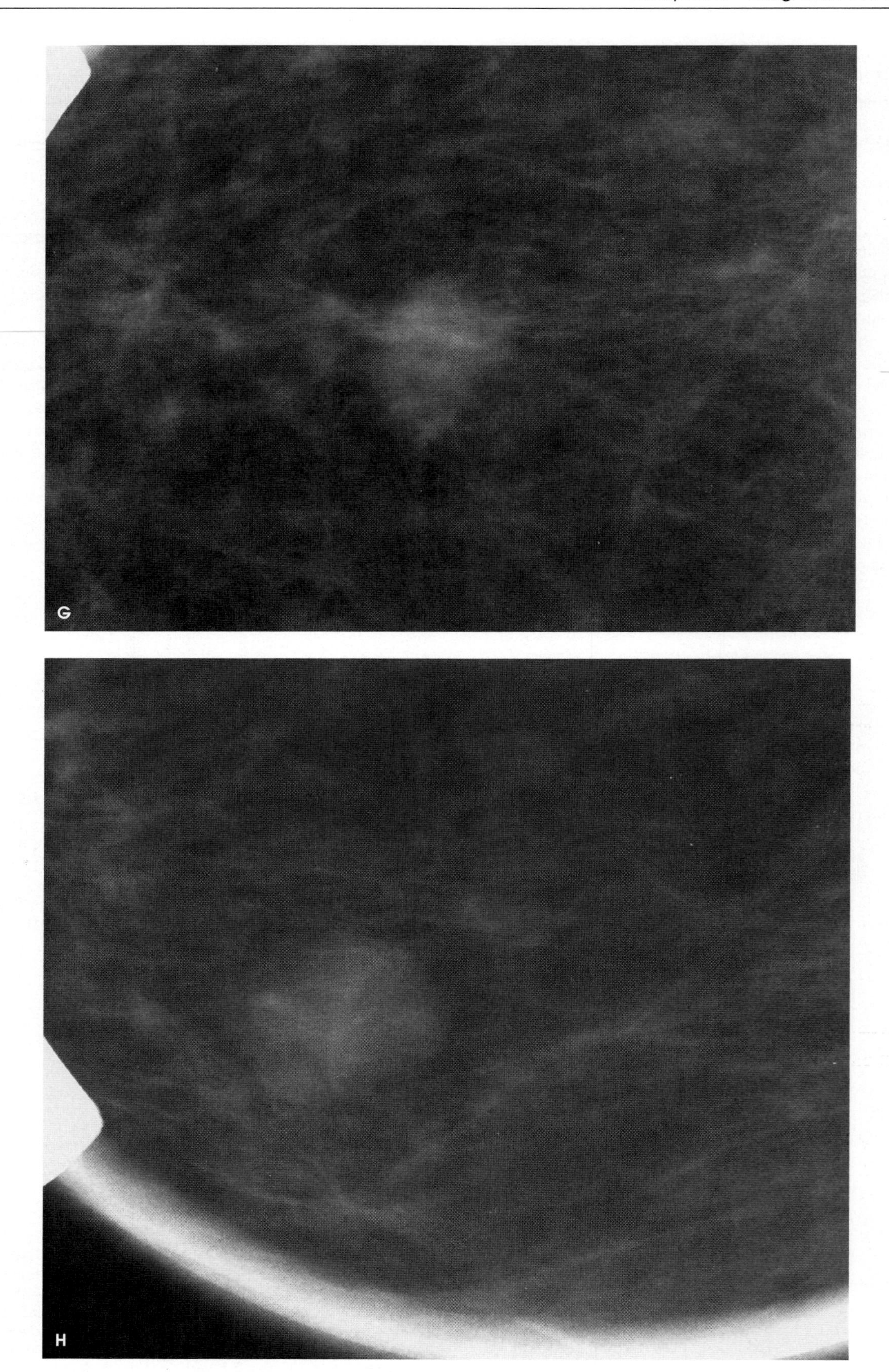

Figure 3.1. (*Continued*) Craniocaudal **(G)** and mediolateral oblique **(H)** spot compression views.

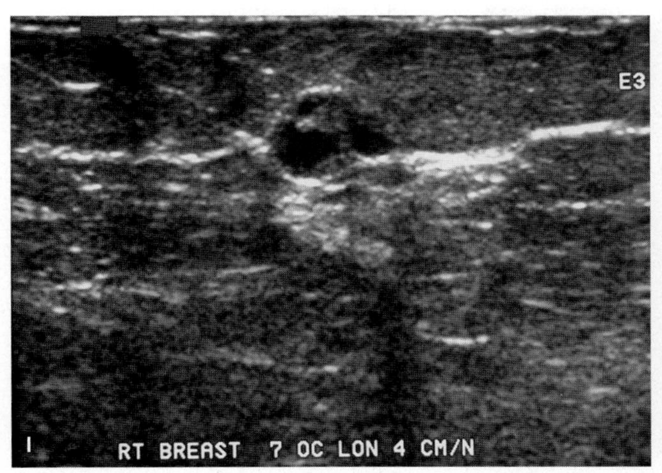

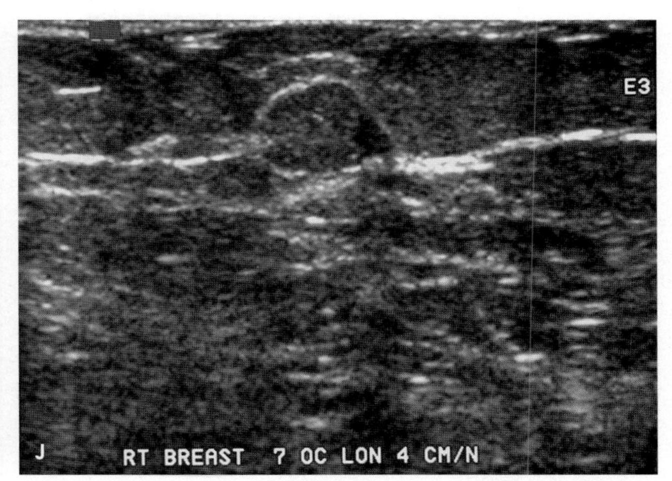

Figure 3.1. (*Continued*) Ultrasound images **(I, J)** through separate portions of the lesion at the 7 o'clock position, 4 cm from the nipple in the longitudinal (LON) projection.

How would you describe the imaging findings, and what differential would you consider?

The margins of this 1-cm mass are indistinct on the craniocaudal spot compression view and more circumscribed on the mediolateral oblique spot compression view. On ultrasound, this nearly isoechoic oval mass is well circumscribed with posterior acoustic enhancement and associated cystic changes.

Benign diagnostic considerations include fibroadenoma (tubular adenoma, complex fibroadenoma), phyllodes tumor, pseudoangiomatous stromal hyperplasia (PASH), focal fibrosis, papilloma, an inflammatory lesion, or, in certain clinical contexts (recent trauma or surgery), a hematoma. A granular cell tumor is a rare possibility. Malignant considerations include invasive ductal carcinoma not otherwise specified, mucinous carcinoma, papillary carcinoma, or a metastatic lesion. A biopsy is indicated.

BI-RADS® category 4: suspicious abnormality, biopsy should be considered.

Rather than just consider a biopsy, one is performed, and a complex fibroadenoma is diagnosed. The patient is asked to return in 1 year for her next screening mammogram.

Complex fibroadenomas are defined as fibroadenomas with superimposed fibrocystic changes including cysts >3 mm in size, sclerosing adenosis, epithelial calcifications, and papillary apocrine changes. They can be anticipated when cystic changes are noted in an otherwise well-circumscribed oval mass such as the one demonstrated here, or when round, punctuate, or amorphous calcifications are identified in an otherwise well-circumscribed mass mammographically (i.e., the punctate and amorphous calcifications reflect the presence of sclerosing adenosis). In some patients, no distinctive imaging features are identified to suggest a complex fibroadenoma. These lesions are benign and do not warrant any additional intervention following core biopsy. Approximately 33% of all fibroadenomas have been reported as complex. When proliferative changes are present in the stroma surrounding a complex fibroadenoma, the risk of breast cancer has been reported to be increased 3.88 times.

PATIENT 2

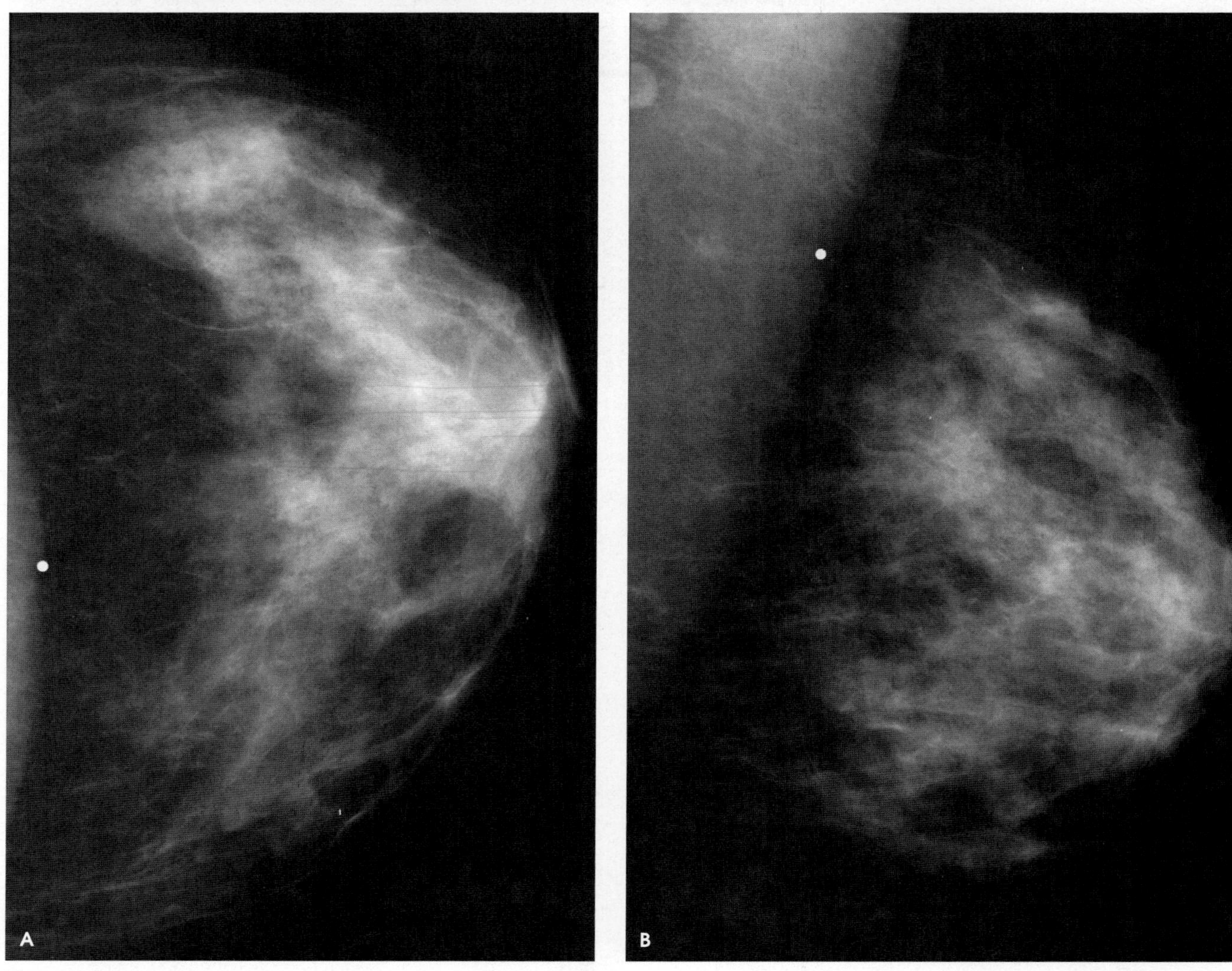

Figure 3.2. Diagnostic evaluation, 50-year-old patient who presents describing a "lump" in her left breast. She was told at another imaging facility that her mammogram and ultrasound are normal; she is adamant in wanting an explanation for what she feels. Craniocaudal **(A)** and mediolateral oblique **(B)** views, left breast.

What is an appropriate approach to patients who describe a localized concern (a "lump," focal skin changes, pinpoint tenderness, etc.)?

For patients who are 30 years of age or older and who present with a palpable abnormality (or other localized finding), a metallic BB is placed at the site of the focal finding and a bilateral mammogram is done; a unilateral study of the symptomatic breast is done if the patient has had a mammogram within the last 6 months. A spot tangential view at the site of the focal abnormality is obtained in conjunction with the routine views. In many patients, the tangential view is helpful in either partially or completely outlining the lesion with subcutaneous fat, enabling better visualization and characterization of the lesion. If needed, additional spot compression or spot compression magnification views can be done. Depending on the location of the focal finding, and the appearance of this area on the spot tangential view, correlative physical examination and an ultrasound are usually indicated. The ultrasound may be deferred in patients in whom there is no chance the lesion has been excluded from the field of view and completely fatty tissue, or a benign lesion (oil cyst, dystrophic calcification, etc.), is imaged corresponding to the area of concern. Aspiration or core biopsy may be indicated, depending on the clinical and imaging features of the lesion.

How would you describe the findings on the routine views of this patient, and with what degree of certainty can you make any recommendations?

Although there is a small island of tissue superimposed on the left pectoral muscle in close proximity to the metallic BB, no definite abnormality is apparent on the routine views of the left breast. At this point, we have an inadequate amount of information to make any justifiable recommendations. We need to review the spot tangential view of the "lump," talk to the patient, undertake correlative physical examination, and do an ultrasound.

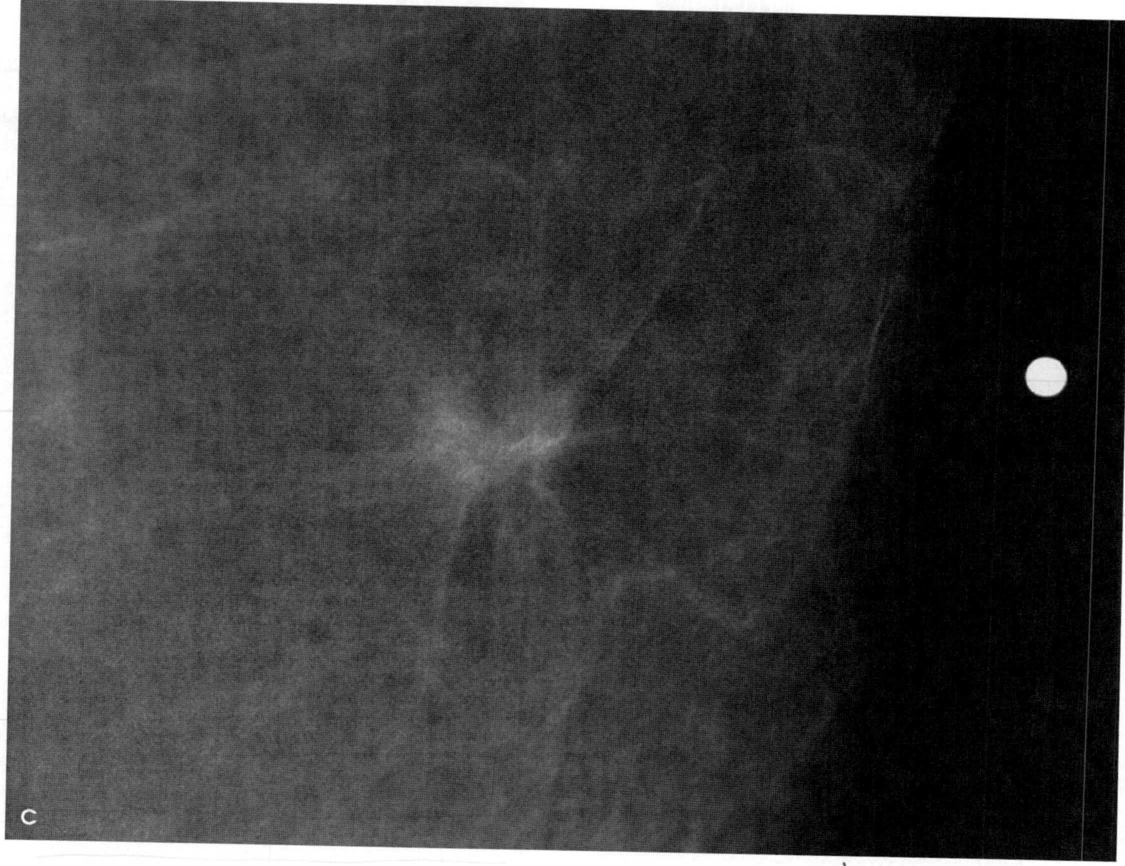

Spot tangential view

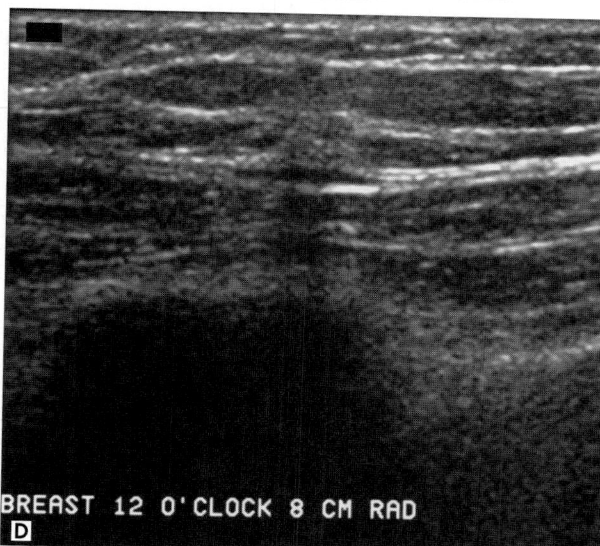

Figure 3.2. (*Continued*) Spot tangential **(C)** view, palpable finding left breast. Ultrasound image in the radial (RAD) **(D)** projection at the site of the palpable finding in the left breast.

What do you think now?

A 7-mm spiculated mass associated with punctate, low-density calcifications is imaged on the spot tangential view corresponding to the palpable finding. A discrete, hard mass is palpated at the site indicated by the patient in the left breast. She has not had a prior biopsy or trauma to this site, and no tenderness is elicited on palpation. On ultrasound, a small hypoechoic mass with disruption of the Cooper ligament is identified at the 12 o'clock position, 8 cm from the left nipple, corresponding to the palpable abnormality. Although the finding is subtle on ultrasound, with careful and meticulous technique it is discernable and reproducibly imaged as the palpable area is scanned. In positioning patients for the ultrasound study, I try to thin the area of the breast being evaluated as much as possible. In evaluating lateral lesions, the patient is placed in an oblique position with a wedge under the ipsilateral arm, and for medial lesions she is supine. If the patient says she feels the "lump" more when she is upright, I will palpate and scan the area with her sitting as well as lying down. During the ultrasound study, I hold the transducer with my right hand and I place the pads of my left index, ring, and middle fingers at the leading edge of the transducer so that I am palpating the tissue as I rotate and move the transducer with my right hand. I apply varying amounts of compression as I manipulate the transducer directly over the area of clinical or mammographic concern.

What is your differential diagnosis, and what recommendation should you make to the patient?

Differential considerations for the findings include invasive ductal carcinoma not otherwise specified (NOS), tubular carcinoma, and invasive lobular carcinoma. Benign considerations include fat necrosis (posttrauma or postsurgery), sclerosing adenosis, papilloma, focal fibrosis, a complex sclerosing lesion, and inflammatory changes (mastitis). Other rare benign causes include granular cell tumor or an extra-abdominal desmoid.

A biopsy is indicated.

BI-RADS® category 4: suspicious abnormality, biopsy should be considered.

An ultrasound-guided biopsy is done, and an invasive mammary carcinoma with features suggestive of tubular carcinoma is described on the core samples. A tubular carcinoma is confirmed following the lumpectomy. Sampled lymph nodes are normal (pT1b, pN0, pMX; Stage I).

In considering tubular carcinoma, what associated lesions may be seen and what should you look for mammographically?

The reported incidence of tubular carcinomas varies depending on detection method, tumor size, and the definition used to classify these tumors. Pure tubular carcinomas probably represent 1% to 2% of all breast cancers. Tubular carcinomas are usually detected mammographically as a small spiculated mass; less commonly, patients present with a palpable mass. Associated round, punctate, and amorphous calcifications may be seen, reflecting the presence of low-nuclear-grade ductal carcinoma in situ (solid, cribriform, and micropapillary), in an average of 65% of patients. Satellite lesions may also be seen, because these lesions may be multifocal or multicentric in 10% to 20% (reportedly as high as 56% in one small series) of patients. Lobular neoplasia (lobular carcinoma in situ), contralateral invasive ductal carcinomas NOS, and a history of breast cancer in a first-degree relative have been reported in as many as 15% (range 0.7% to 40%), 38%, and 40% of patients diagnosed with tubular carcinoma, respectively.

What distinguishes the glands seen in tubular carcinomas from normal glands? Histologically, what are the differential considerations for this lesion?

Histologically, these lesions are characterized by the presence of oval and round, open tubules some with angulation. The glands in tubular carcinomas are lined by a single epithelial cell layer and, in contrast to normal glands, lack myoepithelial cells. Desmoplastic changes are noted in the surrounding stroma and probably explain the imaging features of these lesions (i.e., spiculation). Tubular carcinomas may be difficult to distinguish from radial scars/complex sclerosing lesions (in some patients, tubular carcinomas arise in radial scars/complex sclerosing lesions), sclerosing adenosis, and microglandular adenosis. Special immunohistochemical stains are sometimes needed to assess the presence of myoepithelial cells. These tumors are often diploid, estrogen- and progesterone-receptor-positive, and only rarely over-express HER-2 neu.

Why is listening, correlating physical and imaging findings, and establishing rapport with your patients so important?

Complete, thoughtful evaluations are indicated for all patients, but particularly those presenting with focal signs and symptoms. Radiologists as a group are the most commonly sued physicians, and delays in the diagnosis of breast cancer are the most common causes of malpractice claims filed. Interestingly, the suits are not usually (at least not yet) for missing subtle mammographic findings, but rather for clinically apparent findings the patient feels were ignored. I urge you to establish a good rapport with your patients, listen to their concerns, and make every effort possible to help them. Not only is this good medicine, it makes for a rewarding and fulfilling practice opportunity. You do not want patients leaving your facility angry and feeling that their concerns were ignored or not adequately evaluated. Do not short-circuit appropriate and logical mammographic workups. Make sure that what is seen mammographically correlates with the clinical findings. In making sure that what is seen on ultrasound correlates with the mammographic findings you are evaluating, determine the expected clock position of the lesion and its approximate distance from the nipple *before* going into the ultrasound room; this location should be the starting point for the ultrasound study.

While examining the patient and correlating clinical, mammographic, and ultrasound findings, I obtain a more detailed history from the patient. This is also a good time to convey to the patient what I am doing on her behalf, to discuss recommendations, determine if the patient is comfortable with my recommendations, and answer her questions. Although some consider it inefficient for a radiologist to do the ultrasound studies personally, I argue that it is more efficient and it makes for good patient care.

During the real-time scan, and before taking any images, I determine if there is an identifiable abnormality by examining the patient as I rotate the transducer and apply varying amounts of compression over the area of concern. The 360-degree rotation of the transducer is critical in excluding pseudolesions created by areas of fatty lobulation, which in one plane may look round or oval but elongate and fuse with surrounding tissue as you rotate the transducer. A real mass maintains a round or oval shape as you rotate the transducer directly over it. Applying variable amounts of compression over an area can help eliminate critical angle shadowing that may limit the evaluation of deeper tissue. If I determine that a lesion is present, I take orthogonal images (with and without measurements) that demonstrate representative features of the lesion. In some women, this may require radial and antiradial projections, whereas in others, transverse and longitudinal (i.e., sagittal) orientations show the lesion and its characteristics to better advantage. I use the images taken to support my impression and justify my recommendations. I take no images of normal tissue. In annotating the images, the breast being scanned is indicated, as is the clock position of the lesion and its distance in centimeters from the nipple.

PATIENT 3

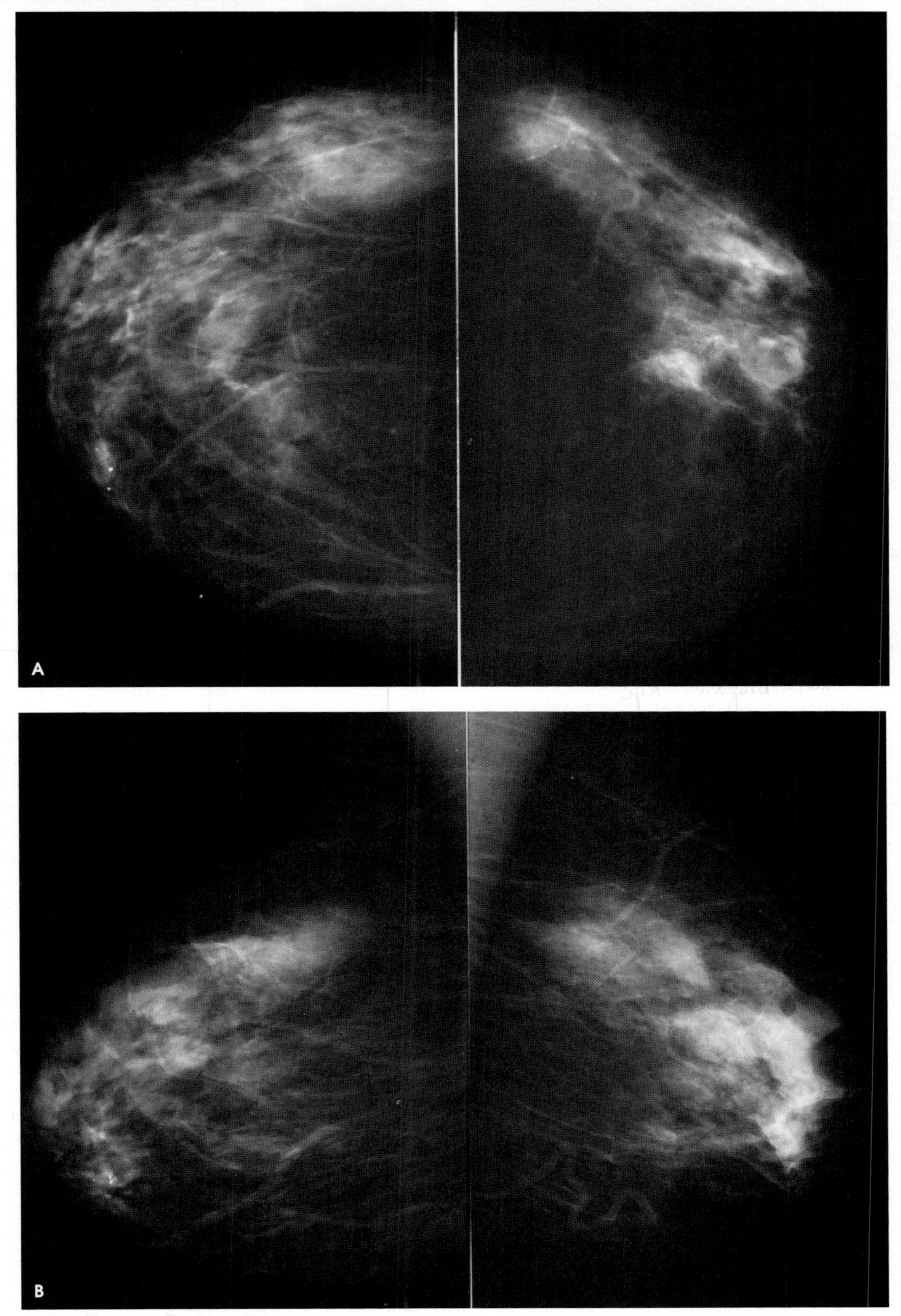

Figure 3.3. Diagnostic evaluation, 80-year-old patient presenting with a "lump" in the right breast. Craniocaudal **(A)** and mediolateral oblique **(B)** views.

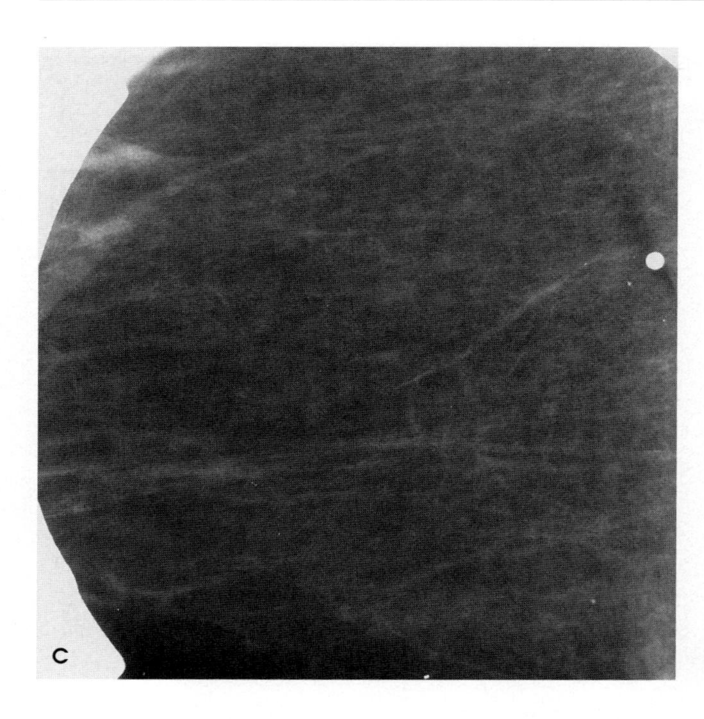

Figure 3.3. (*Continued*) Spot tangential **(C)** view taken of the palpable finding (metallic BB on palpable finding).

What is an acceptable approach to patients who present with focal findings?
In evaluating the adequacy of spot tangential views, what should you consider?

In patients who are 30 years of age or older and who present with a palpable abnormality (or other localized finding), a metallic BB is placed at the site of concern, and routine views are done bilaterally unless the patient has had a mammogram in the preceding 6 months, in which case a unilateral mammogram of the symptomatic breast is done. In addition, a spot tangential view of the focal finding is done. In many patients, the tangential view is helpful in either partially or completely outlining the lesion, with subcutaneous fat facilitating characterization. Depending on the location of the focal finding, and the appearance of this area on the spot tangential view, correlative physical examination and an ultrasound are usually indicated. Ultrasound may be deferred in patients in whom there is no chance the lesion has been excluded from the tangential view and completely fatty tissue, or a benign lesion, is imaged corresponding to the palpable abnormality.

In this patient, do you see the metallic BB on the routine views of the right breast? Why not? In this patient, the palpable finding is deep in the breast, just above the inframammary fold. The metallic BB was placed on the "lump" but has been excluded from the field of view. The metallic BB is seen on the spot tangential view, and predominantly fatty tissue is imaged on the spot tangential view. In this patient, the possibility that the lesion has been excluded from the images is a real concern. As with all spot compression views, you need to consider the possibility that the lesion has been squeezed out of the field of view or, because of its location, is not included on the images. Correlative physical examination in this patient confirms the presence of a palpable mass fixed at the inframammary fold. Also noted are arterial calcifications in the left breast and coarse, dense, benign-type calcifications anteriorly in the right breast.

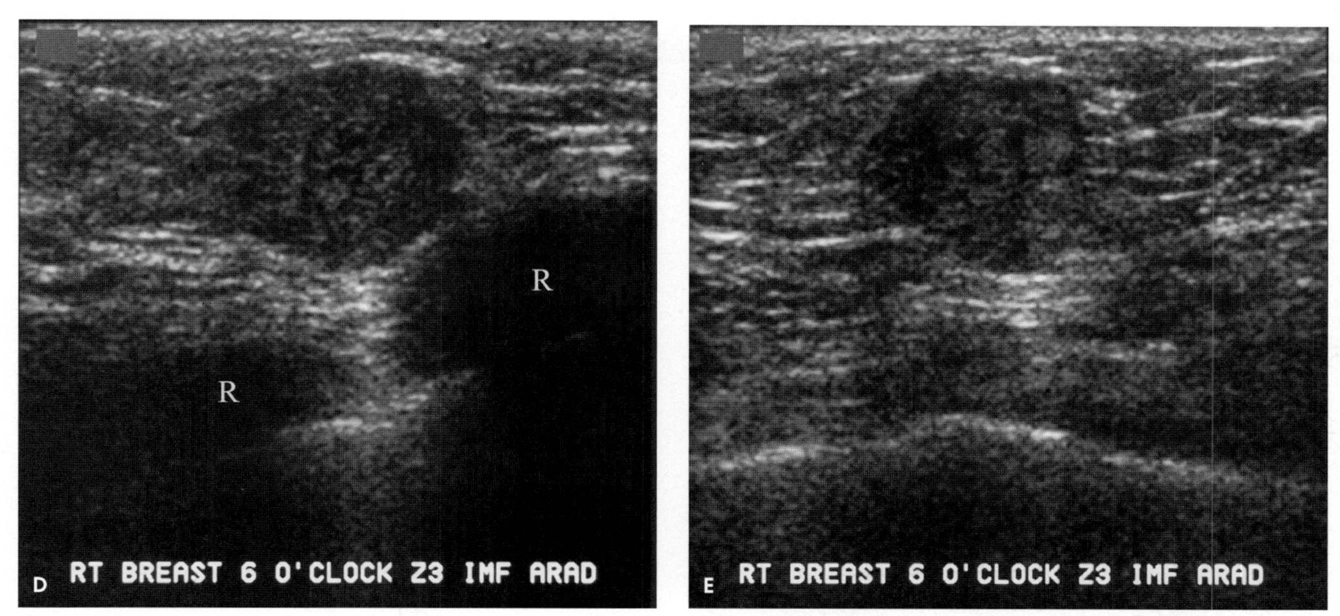

Figure 3.3. Ultrasound images **(D, E)** of the palpable mass at the inframammary fold of the right breast in an antiradial (ARAD) projection.

How would you describe the ultrasound findings, and what is indicated in this patient?

A round, 1.2-cm hypoechoic mass with partially indistinct margins and associated posterior acoustic enhancement is imaged corresponding to the palpable finding at the 6 o'clock position, posteriorly (Z3) in the right breast. The lesion is just below the skin and snuggled in close proximity to the ribs (R). An invasive ductal carcinoma not otherwise specified, mucinous carcinoma, papillary carcinoma, or a metastatic lesion are the primary considerations in an 80-year-old patient presenting with these findings.

BI-RADS® category 4: suspicious abnormality, biopsy should be considered.

A mucinous carcinoma is diagnosed on the ultrasound core biopsy. A 1.3-cm mucinous carcinoma with associated intermediate-grade ductal carcinoma in situ is confirmed on the lumpectomy specimen. The sentinel lymph node is negative for metastatic disease (pT1c, pN0(sn) (i−), pMX; Stage I).

What are some of the tools available in evaluating lesions possibly excluded from the routine views?

Lesions close to the chest wall (far superior, inferior, lateral, or medial) and lesions high in the axilla may not be included on routine or spot compression views of the breast. Anytime you suspect that a lesion is potentially excluded from the mammographic images, or there are potential factors limiting compression, correlative physical examination and ultrasound are wonderful adjunctive tools. Also, capitalize on basic concepts such as the use of various projections to position tissue as close to the film as possible. If you think a lesion is medial in location, consider a 90-degree lateromedial (LM) spot compression so that medial tissue is placed up against the film; this minimizes the possibility of exclusion because medial tissue is up against the film, and it improves resolution by placing the area of concern closest to the film. Likewise, if you think a lesion is high up in the breast, have the technologist do a from-below (FB) view such that superior tissue is now closest to the film. If you suspect a lesion is at, or just below, the inframammary fold (IMF), tell the technologist not to lift the breast as she positions for the craniocaudal (CC) view. She should place the film holder at the neutral position for the IMF, because as the breast is lifted at the IMF for the routine CC view, the mass may be able to slip out and not be included on the image. Remember, the use of the spot compression paddle usually makes it easier to include more posterior, superior, or axillary tissue in the field of view. In evaluating potential lesions in the axillary tail, an axillary view can be useful.

PATIENT 4

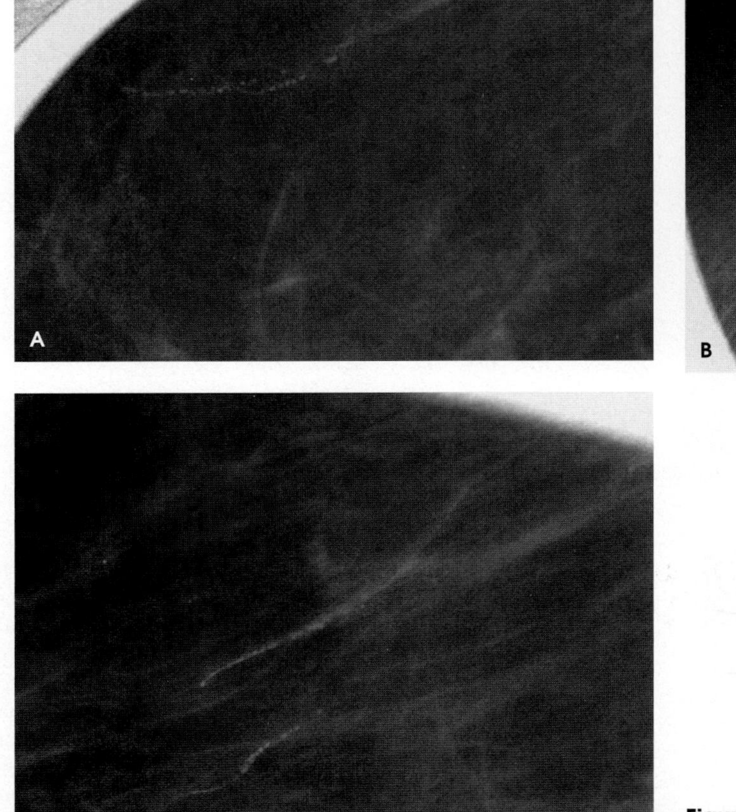

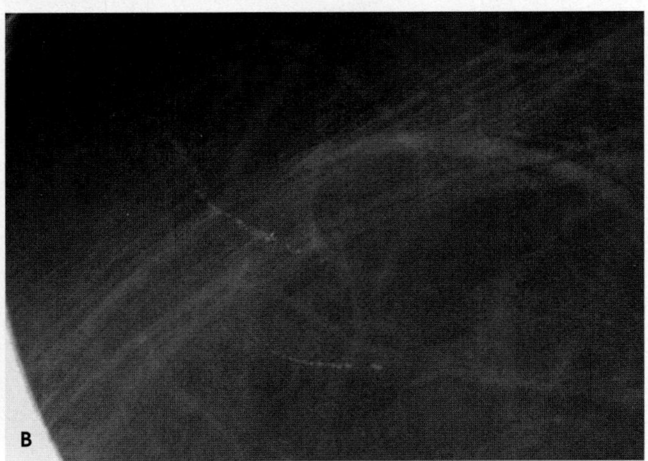

Figure 3.4. Diagnostic evaluation, 62-year-old woman called back for calcifications detected in the right breast on her screening study. Double spot compression magnification views **(A–C)** of calcifications, right breast.

What is an appropriate evaluation of patients with screening-detected calcifications that cannot be classified as benign on the routine views?

The next step should be magnification views. Specifically, our protocol uses double spot compression magnification views in orthogonal projections to evaluate women with indeterminate calcifications detected on routine mammographic views.

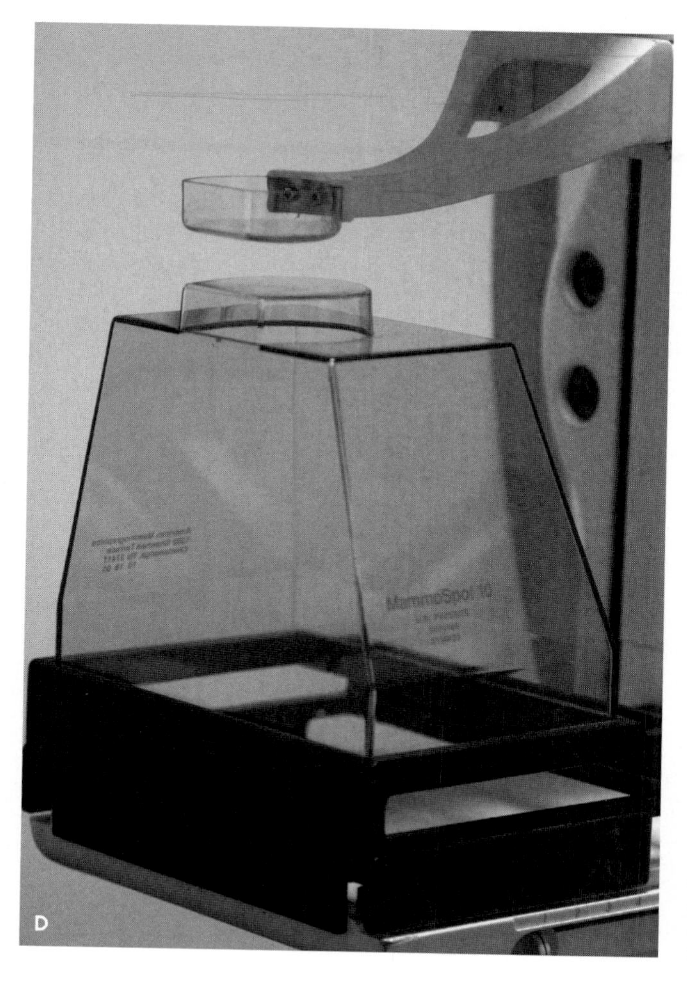

Figure 3.4. Setup for double spot compression magnification views **(D).** A Lexan® top magnification stand is used to minimize the amount of radiation absorbed by the stand itself. The built-in spot compression is combined with a spot compression paddle to obtain double spot compression of the tissue being evaluated. By reducing the amount of radiation absorbed by the magnification stand, maximizing compression by applying from above and below the lesion, and making adjustments in kilovoltage, well-exposed, high-contrast magnification views with no motion artifact can be obtained routinely.

How is magnification obtained, and what are the resulting effects?

Magnification technique is accomplished by increasing the distance between the breast (i.e., object) and film. The resulting air gap helps to eliminate scatter radiation, so a grid is not needed for magnification views. Compared with the 0.3-mm focal spot used for routine (nonmagnified) mammographic views, a 0.1-mm focal spot is used for magnification views. The small focal spot is needed to minimize the penumbra effect that results as you increase the breast (object)-to-film distance. The use of the small focal spot, however, results in increased exposure times, so motion becomes a significant issue that may limit the usefulness of magnification views.

What can be done to minimize the likelihood of motion blur on magnification views?

Optimizing the system to obtain an adequate exposure in a short period of time is critical for routinely obtaining high-quality magnification views. An appropriate selection of voltage, a magnification stand that minimizes the amount of radiation absorbed, optimal focal compression, and working with the patient on controlling her breathing are simple steps that can improve overall image quality significantly.

As a general rule, the voltage used for exposure on magnification views is increased by 2 kV over that used for the routine, nonmagnified views. We do all of our magnification views using a Lexan®-top magnification stand (MammoSpot®, American Mammographics, Chattanooga, TN). Compared to standard carbon-top magnification stands, those made of Lexan® absorb less radiation, so exposure times can be decreased by as much as 40%.

Optimal compression is also critical for obtaining high-quality magnification views. This is why we advocate the use of double spot compression. The magnification stand has a built-in spot compression, which, when combined with the spot compression paddle, enables maximal compression of the tissue being evaluated (i.e., double spot compression). The technologist is also encouraged to work with the patient on breath holding (i.e., the patient should stop breathing when requested rather than taking a deep breath in) to minimize the likelihood of motion.

If you have determined that there is a need for magnification views, don't settle for suboptimal quality and hide behind disclaimers. If the magnification views are not optimal, step back and review what the technologist is doing. Does the voltage need to be increased further (accepting that as you increase voltage, contrast is decreased)? Is the correct focal spot being used? Can compression be increased? Can you work with the patient to improve breath holding? High-contrast, well-exposed, artifact-free magnification views are critical for assessing the morphology and extent of calcifications that may reflect the presence of ductal carcinoma in situ. Recognize that the ability to detect and characterize calcifications and small masses is significantly compromised (and may be eliminated) on images with blurring.

How would you describe these calcifications in this patient, and what is your differential diagnosis? What is indicated?

Round, punctate, and linear calcifications demonstrating linear orientation are confirmed on the double spot compression magnification views. The differential is limited but includes fibrocystic changes including columnar alteration with prominent apical snouts (CAPPS), ductal hyperplasia and atypical ductal hyperplasia, fibrosis, and ductal carcinoma in situ. In the absence of any other change related to trauma (e.g., mixed-density mass, oil cyst), or a specific history of trauma or surgery to the site of the calcifications, these calcifications are unlikely to represent an early stage of fat necrosis. Given the linear orientation of the calcifications, biopsy is indicated.

BI-RADS® category 4: suspicious abnormality, biopsy should be considered.

Ductal carcinoma in situ is reported on the stereotactically guided biopsy and confirmed on the lumpectomy [Tis(DCIS), pNX, pMX; Stage 0].

PATIENT 5

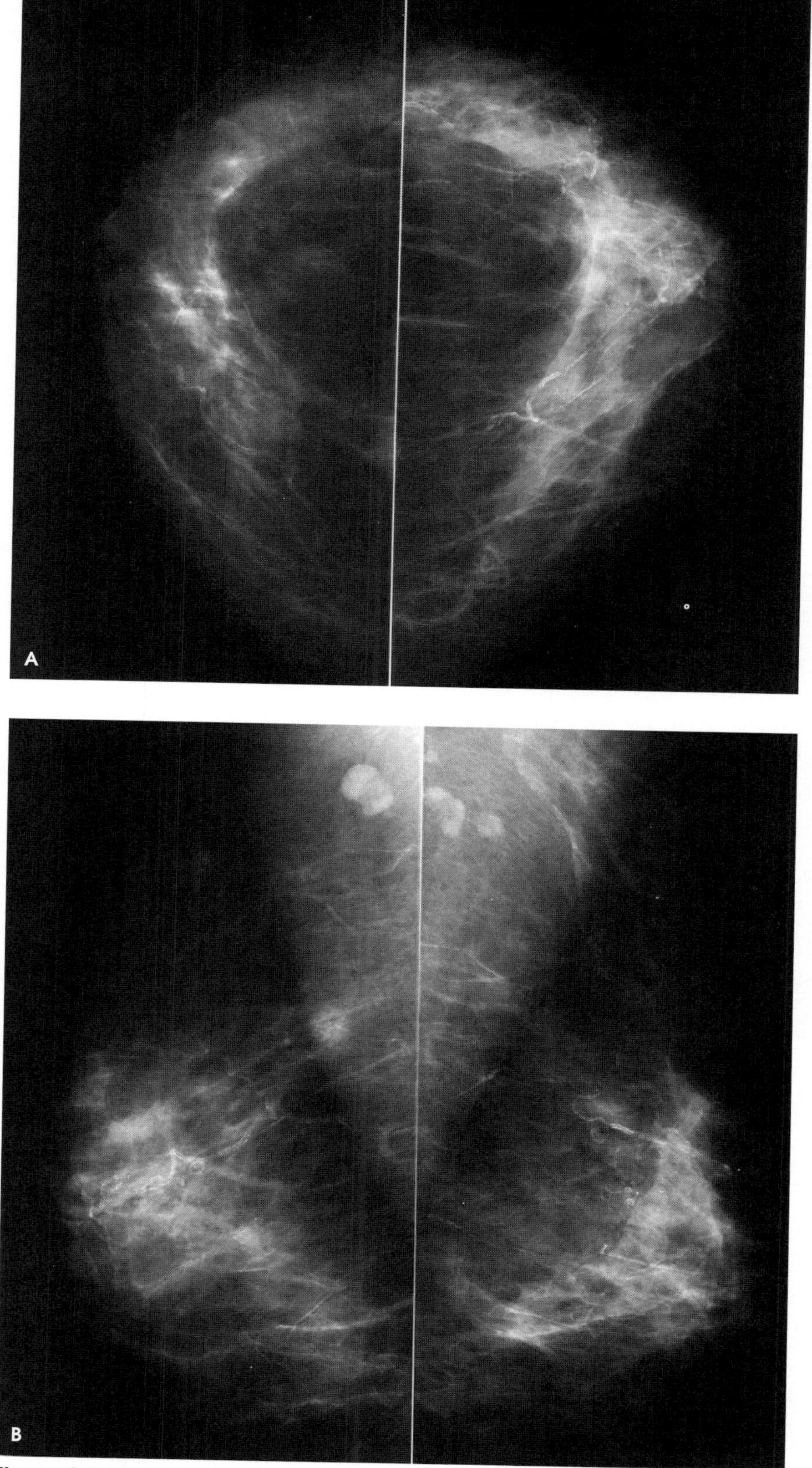

Figure 3.5. Screening study, 65-year-old woman. Craniocaudal **(A)** and mediolateral oblique **(B)** views.

What do you think, and what is your recommendation at this point?

Arterial calcifications are present bilaterally. A possible mass is present on the right mediolateral oblique (MLO) view superimposed on the pectoral muscle inferiorly. This should be distinguished from several well-circumscribed, mixed-density masses (i.e., lymph nodes) superimposed on the pectoral muscles, bilaterally. No definite corresponding abnormality is apparent on the right craniocaudal (CC) view. Comparison with prior studies is the starting point. If no prior films are available, or if this potential mass represents a change, additional evaluation is indicated.

BI-RADS® category 0: need additional imaging evaluation.

How would you approach the diagnostic evaluation of this patient? Be specific in describing the steps you would follow.

When a potential abnormality is seen in only one of the two standard views, we start by determining if the finding is real in the view in which it is initially perceived. In this patient, a spot compression view in the MLO projection is obtained. If no abnormality persists on the spot compression view, no additional views are done; if a question remains, rolled spot compression views can be done. In this patient, a 1.2-cm mass with indistinct margins is confirmed on the MLO spot compression view (Fig. 3.5C). We must now establish the location of this abnormality in the CC projection using a logical approach. We make no assumptions as to the lateral, central, or medial location of the lesion on the CC view. Rather, a 90-degree lateral view (usually a lateromedial view) is done to determine how this lesion moves with respect to its location on the MLO view. If the lesion moves up, it is located medially and a spot cleavage view is done; if the lesion moves down, it is located laterally such that a spot craniocaudal view exaggerated laterally is done; and if it does not move significantly, the lesion is central in location and a spot compression view directly behind the nipple is obtained. In this patient the lesion moves up (image not shown), consistent with a medial location. Upon further review of the CC view, a density is partially noted on the craniocaudal view at the edge of the film medially (box, Fig. 3.5D). A follow-up image with the spot compression paddle enables visualization of more tissue so that the lesion is imaged in its entirety (Fig. 3.5E) in the CC projection.

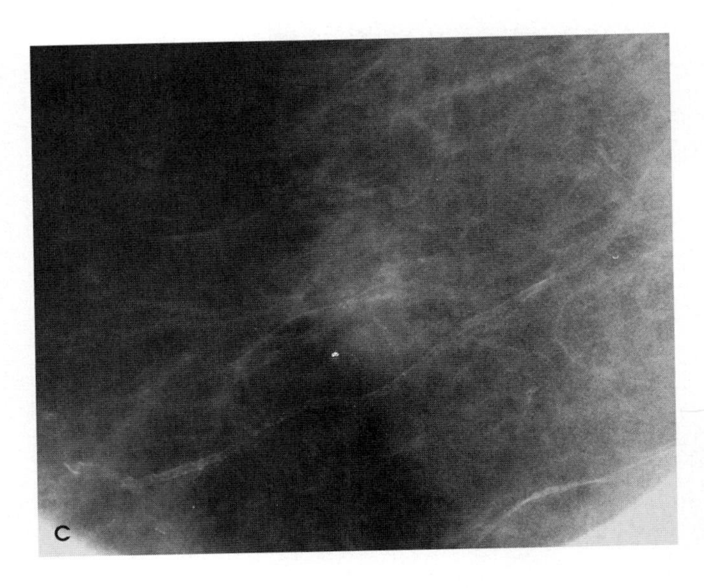

Figure 3.5. (*Continued*) Mediolateral oblique **(C)** spot compression view confirms the presence of a mass with indistinct and spiculated margins in the right breast. On a 90-degree lateromedial (LM) view (not shown), the lesion moves up with respect to its position on the mediolateral oblique view, consistent with a medial location for the lesion.

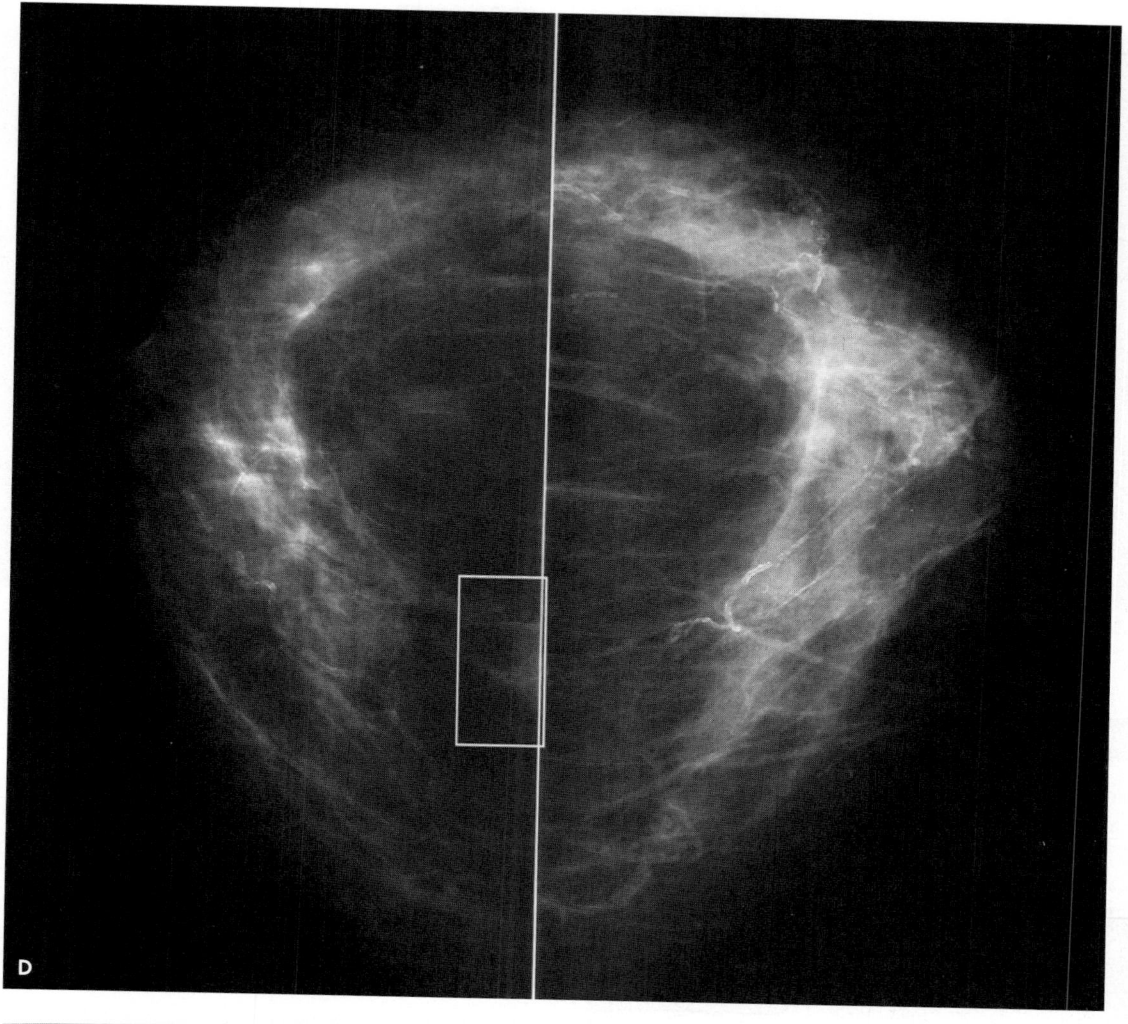

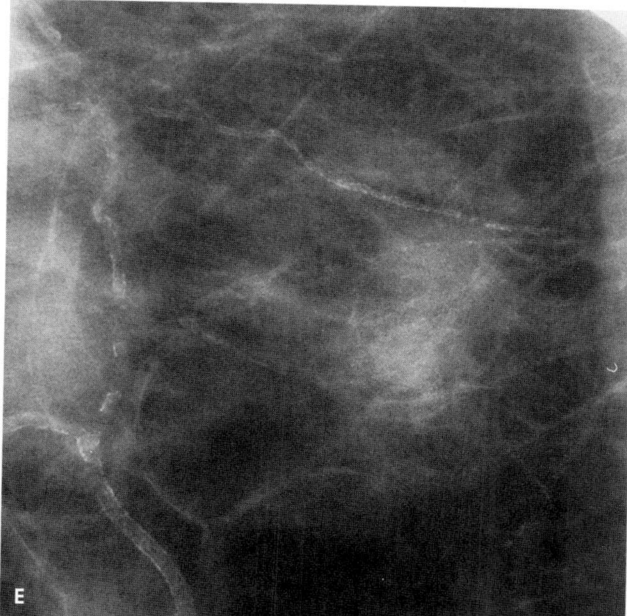

Figure 3.5. (*Continued*) Further review of the craniocaudal **(D)** views demonstrates a possible mass at the edge of the right craniocaudal view medially (*box*). Spot compression **(E)** view of the medial aspect of the right breast in the craniocaudal projection demonstrates a mass with indistinct and spiculated margins. Some punctate calcifications may be present. Pectoral muscle is now also seen at the edge of the spot compression view posteriorly. The spot compression paddle often enables visualization of otherwise hard-to-reach areas such as the upper inner quadrants posteriorly

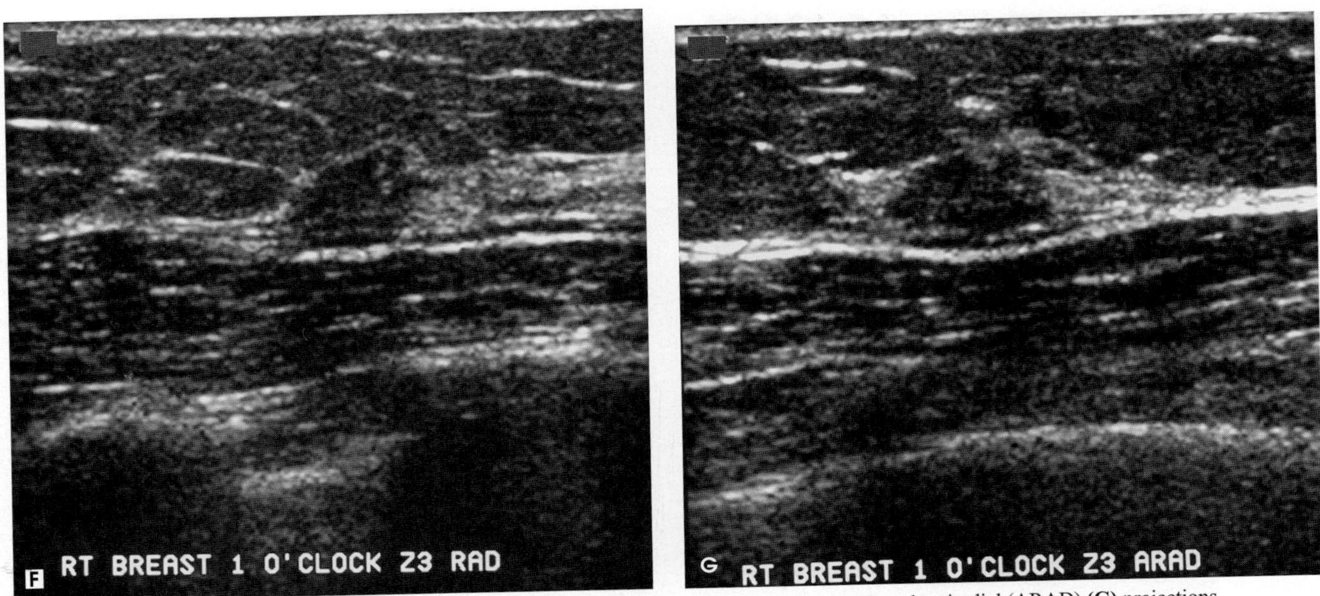

Figure 3.5. (*Continued*) Ultrasound images, upper inner quadrant, right breast, in radial (RAD) **(F)** and antiradial (ARAD) **(G)** projections.

How would you describe the ultrasound findings?

An irregular, 1.2-cm mass with indistinct, angular, and spiculated margins is imaged at the 1 o'clock position posteriorly (Z3), abutting the deep pectoral fascia (arrowheads, Fig. 3.5H). Straightening, thickening, and disruption of Cooper ligaments are noted. This mass corresponds to the mass seen mammographically.

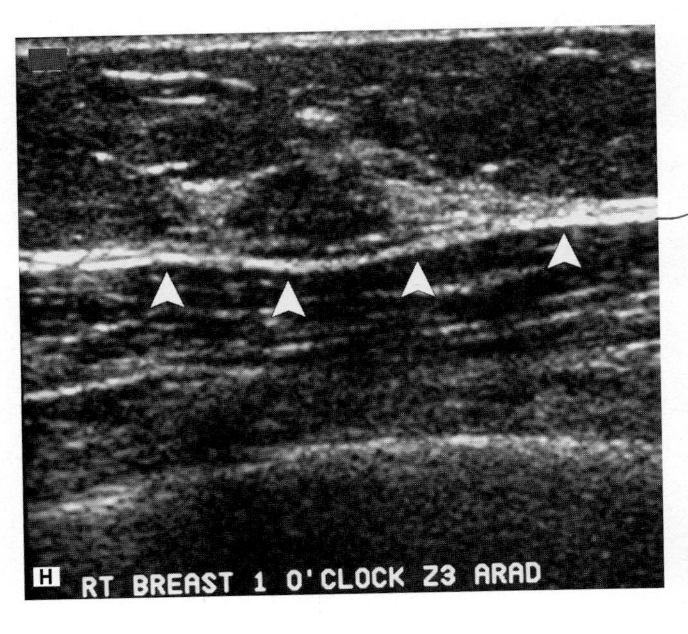

Figure 3.5. Ultrasound image **(H)** in the antiradial (ARAD) projection at the 1 o'clock position of the right breast, posteriorly, demonstrating gentle mass effect on the deep pectoral fascia (*arrowheads*).

What is your differential diagnosis, and what recommendation do you make to the patient?

Differential considerations include invasive ductal carcinoma not otherwise specified, invasive lobular carcinoma, or lymphoma. Rarely, ductal carcinoma in situ can present as a mass, asymmetric density, or distortion in the absence of microcalcifications. Benign considerations include an inflammatory process or posttraumatic changes, focal fibrosis, a papilloma, sclerosing adenosis, pseudoangiomatous stromal hyperplasia, granular cell tumor, or an extra-abdominal desmoid. Given the imaging features of this lesion, a biopsy is indicated.

BI-RADS® category 4: suspicious abnormality, biopsy should be considered.

An ultrasound-guided biopsy is done. An invasive ductal carcinoma with associated ductal carcinoma in situ is diagnosed on the core biopsy.

A 1.5-cm, grade I invasive mammary carcinoma, with apocrine differentiation and an associated extensive, intermediate-grade (solid, cribriform patterns) ductal carcinoma in situ is reported on the lumpectomy specimen. Malignant cells are reported on a touch imprint of the sentinel lymph node done intraoperatively. Twenty additional nodes removed at the time of the lumpectomy are negative for metastatic disease (pT1c, pN1a, pMX; Stage IIA).

What are touch imprints, and how are they used at the time of the lumpectomy and sentinel lymph node biopsy?

Touch imprints of the excised sentinel lymph node(s) are commonly done intraoperatively at the time of the lumpectomy and sentinel lymph node biopsy. The lymph node is sectioned and the cut edge is blotted on slides. The cytologic material on the slides is fixed, stained, and reviewed by the pathologist. If malignant cells are identified on the touch imprints, a complete axillary lymph node dissection is done at the time of the lumpectomy. However, metastatic disease is not excluded if the imprints are reported as benign; false-negative touch imprints are commonly associated with invasive lobular carcinoma. In patients in whom the imprint is negative but metastatic disease is identified in the permanent, hematoxylin and eosin–stained sections of the sentinel lymph node, a full axillary dissection is usually undertaken as a second operative procedure.

How is an extensive intraductal component defined, and what is its significance?

An extensive intraductal component (EIC) is described when an invasive ductal carcinoma has a prominent intraductal component within it or intraductal carcinoma is present in sections of otherwise normal adjacent tissue. This term also applies to lesions that are predominantly intraductal but have foci of invasion. An EIC may indicate the presence of residual disease 2 cm beyond the primary lesion in as many as 30% of patients and is associated with an increased incidence of local recurrence following breast-conserving surgery and radiation therapy. Patients with tumors characterized by an extensive intraductal component may benefit from a wider resection. Tumors with EIC are reportedly more common in younger women.

PATIENT 6

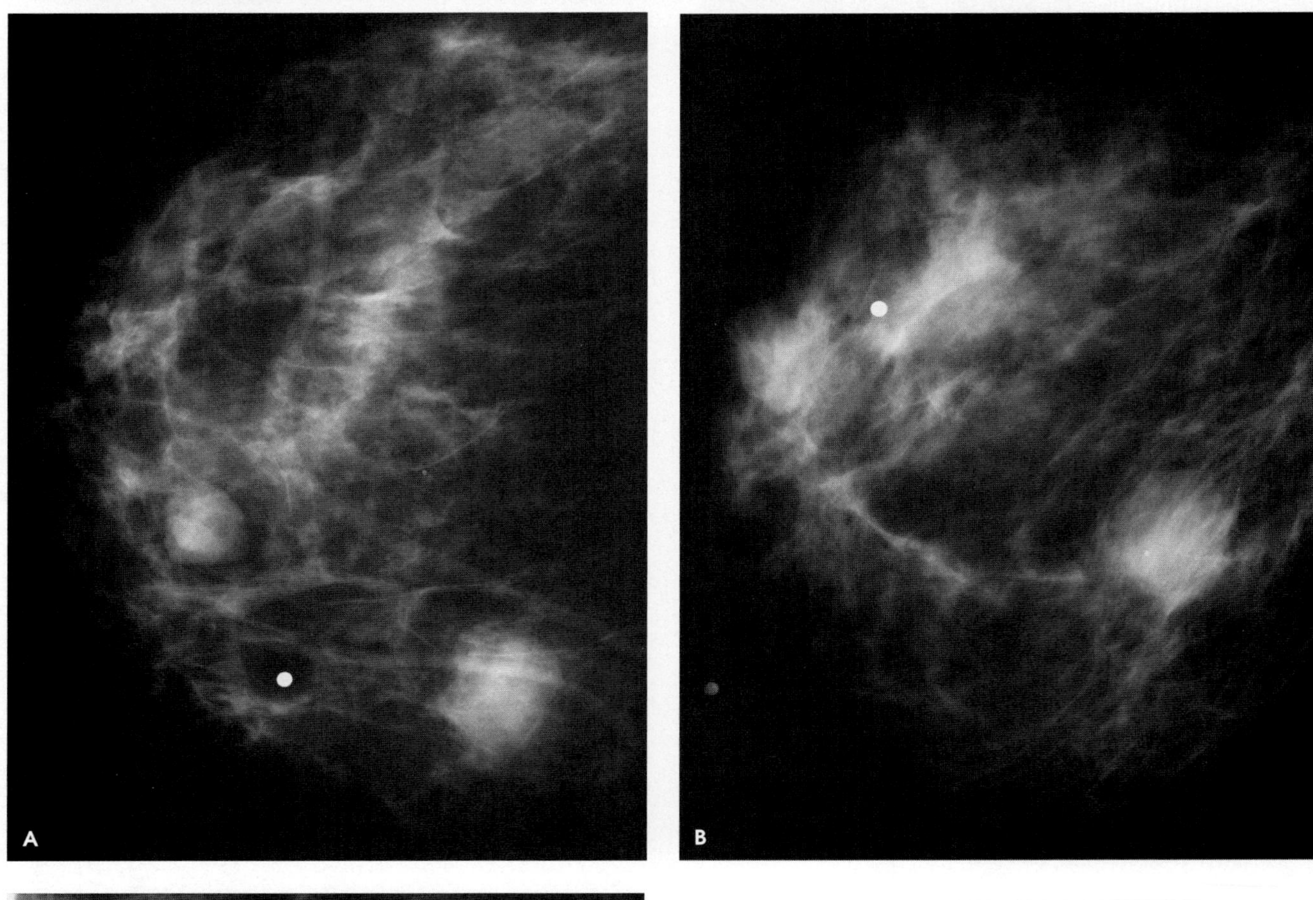

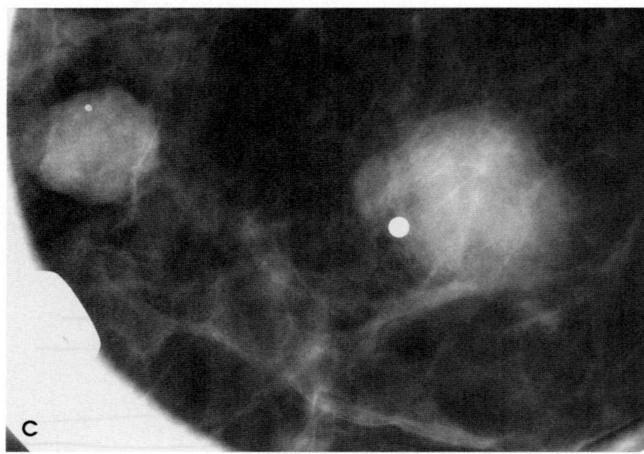

Figure 3.6. Diagnostic evaluation, 49-year-old patient presenting with two "lumps" in the right breast. Craniocaudal **(A)** and mediolateral oblique **(B)** views, right breast; metallic BBs used to mark "lumps." Spot compression **(C)** view (orthogonal view not shown), right breast.

How would you describe the two masses? What would you do next?

Two masses are present in the right breast, corresponding to the "lumps" described by the patient. The margins of the anterior mass are well circumscribed on the spot compression views (only one shown). In comparison, the margins of the larger, posterior mass are not as sharp and, for a portion of the mass, are indistinct. In entertaining a differential, you need to consider that these may reflect the same or, possibly, different processes. Cyst(s), fibroadenoma(s), tubular adenoma(s), phyllodes tumor(s) papilloma(s), pseudoangiomatous stromal hyperplasia (PASH), focal fibrosis, abscess(es), posttraumatic or postsurgical fluid collections, invasive ductal carcinoma(s), medullary carcinoma(s), mucinous carcinoma(s), papillary carcinoma(s), and metastatic lesion(s) are included in the differential. Correlative physical examination and an ultrasound are indicated for further characterization of these lesions.

Although these masses are palpable, based on their location on the mammogram, at what clock position do you expect to find these lesions? Be specific.

The anterior mass is located at the 12:30 o'clock position, 4 cm from the right nipple. It is a 1.2-cm oval, well-circumscribed mass characterized by areas of enhancement and shadowing. Although projecting below the level of the nipple on the mediolateral oblique view, the posterior mass is located in the upper inner quadrant of the right breast at the 2 o'clock position, 8 cm from the nipple, and measures 3 cm. It is vertically oriented, markedly hypoechoic, with indistinct margins and some spiculation. Some posterior acoustic enhancement is present. The imaging features of the anterior mass suggest a benign process and those of the posterior mass suggest a malignancy. Biopsies are recommended for both lesions.

BI-RADS® category 4: suspicious abnormality, biopsy should be considered.

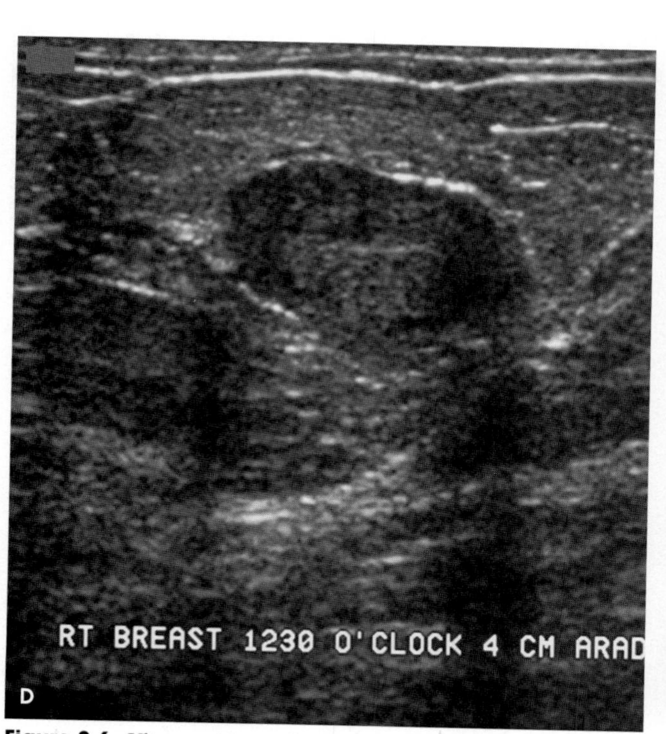

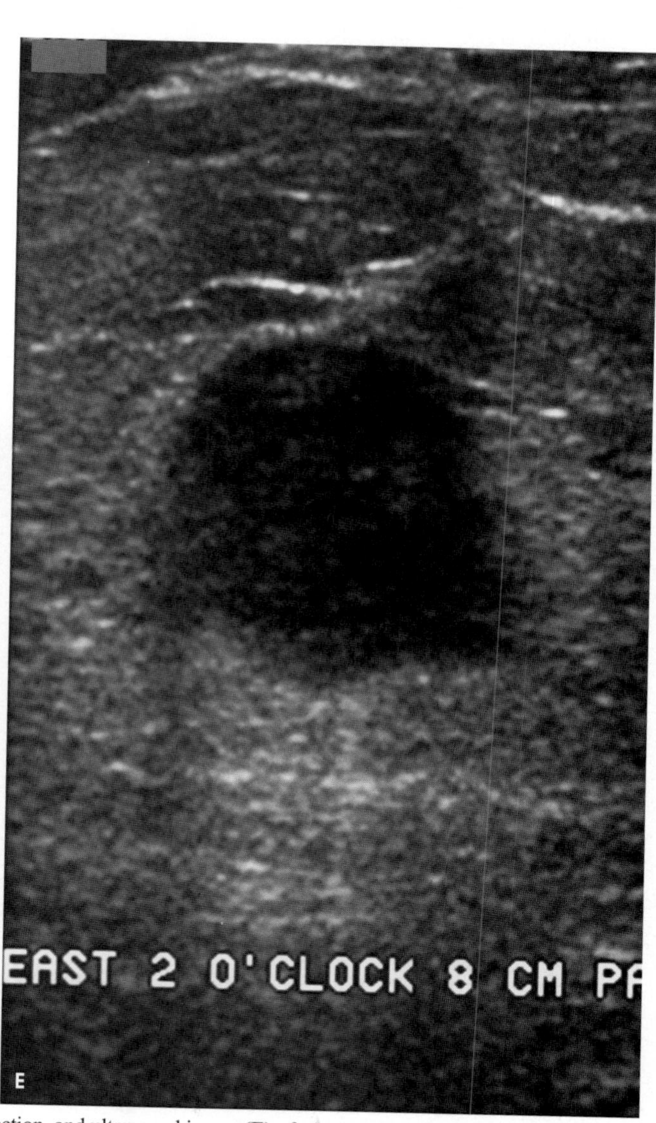

Figure 3.6. Ultrasound image **(D)** of anterior mass, antiradial (ARAD) projection, and ultrasound image **(E)** of posterior mass, ARAD projection.

A complex fibroadenoma is reported histologically for the anterior mass. An invasive mammary carcinoma is diagnosed for the posterior lesion. A 4-cm, metaplastic carcinoma with no heterologous elements and a normal sentinel lymph node biopsy are reported following surgery [pT2, pN0(sn) (i−), pMX, Stage IIB].

As you progress from the mammogram to doing the ultrasound, consider carefully and focus your attention on the anatomic location of the lesion being evaluated. Obviously, it is critically important to assure that the lesion seen on the mammogram correlates with what you find on the ultrasound study. To this end, review the mammographic images before scanning the patient, so that when you walk in to evaluate the patient you have the expected clock position and approximate distance from the nipple for the lesion being evaluated as your starting point.

On craniocaudal and 90-degree lateral views (LM and ML), the location of a lesion is anatomic with respect to the nipple. Medial, lateral, and central findings on craniocaudal views are located medially, laterally, and centrally (i.e., behind the nipple) in the breast. Superior and inferior findings with respect to the nipple are located in the upper and lower quadrants, respectively, on the 90-degree lateral view (Fig. 3.6F). On mediolateral oblique views, however, it is important to recognize that some lesions projecting below the level of the nipple are in an upper quadrant of the breast and some that project above the level of the nipple are in a lower quadrant (Fig. 3.6G–I).

Based on the CC and MLO views, the anatomic location of the lesion needs to be determined, to assure accurate correlation between what is seen on the mammogram and anything that may be found on the ultrasound study. The information on the CC and MLO views (taken with the patient upright and tissue pulled out away from the body) needs to be transposed to a patient who is now supine, or in a slight oblique position, for the ultrasound study. Approximating the clock position of a lesion in the breast can be facilitated (and learned) by using frontal diagrams of the breast, in conjunction with the location of the lesion on the CC and MLO views.

On a frontal diagram of the breast, the posterior nipple line (PNL) is drawn as extending from the upper inner quadrant to the lower outer quadrant of the breast, transecting the nipple (this defines the course of the x-ray beam when an MLO view is done). Next, reference the location of the lesion on the MLO view (Fig. 3.6J) with respect to the PNL. The lesions are how far above or below the posterior nipple line on the MLO view? The lines describing the location of the lesion, with respect to the PNL on the MLO view, are drawn on the frontal diagram (Fig. 3.6K). Using the location of the lesions on the CC view (Fig. 3.6L), you can now narrow down the clock location of the lesion along the course of the lines drawn on the frontal view (Fig. 3.6J). You can now walk into the ultrasound room and place the transducer at the expected clock position for each lesion and find them easily with the assurance that what you are imaging on ultrasound correlates with what is being seen mammographically.

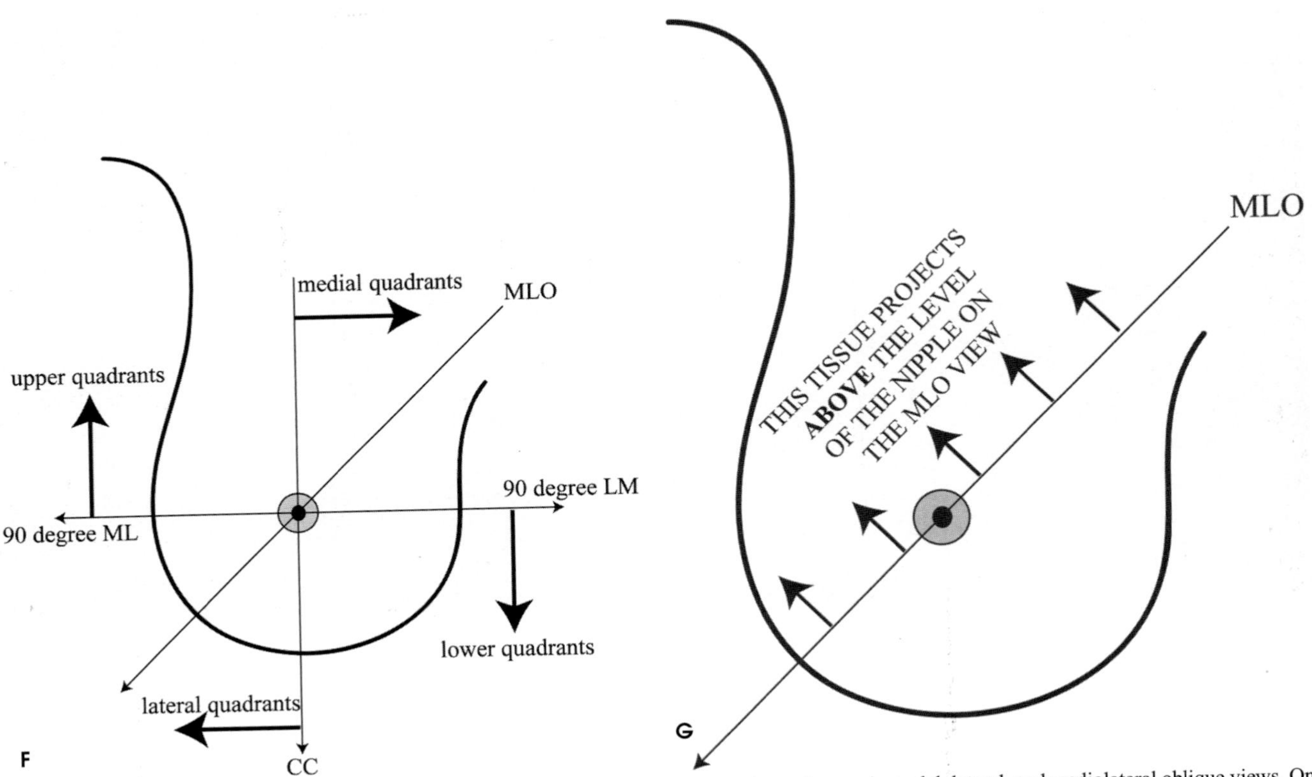

Figure 3.6. Frontal diagram **(F)** of the right breast, illustrating the course of the x-ray beam for craniocaudal, lateral, and mediolateral oblique views. On craniocaudal views, the location of lesions is anatomic: those projecting laterally or medially are in the lateral and medial aspects of the breast, respectively. Similarly, on true lateral views, lesions projecting superiorly or inferiorly are located in the upper or lower quadrants, respectively. On mediolateral oblique views, however, some of the tissue that projects above the level of the nipple is inferior to the nipple **(G)**, and some tissue projecting below the level of the nipple is superior to the nipple **(H)**.

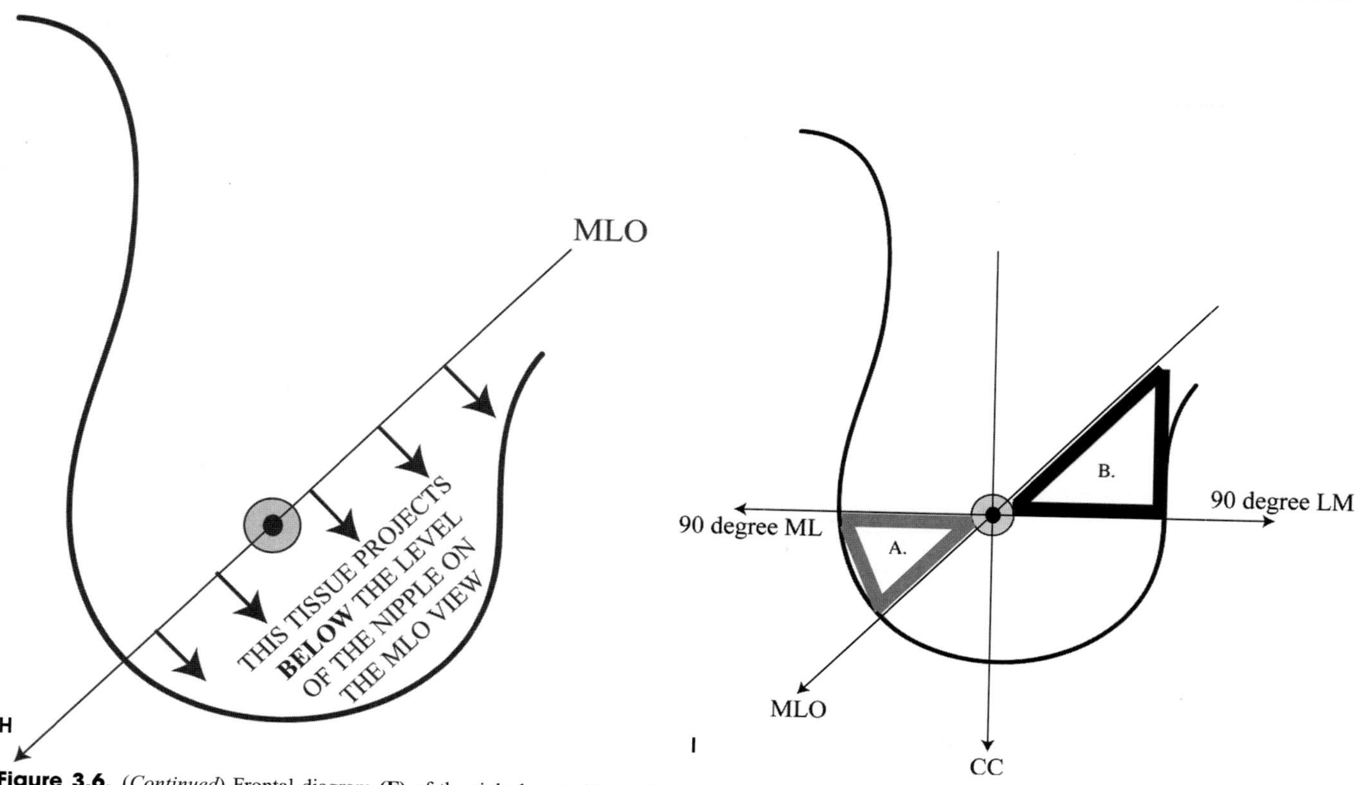

Figure 3.6. (*Continued*) Frontal diagram **(F)** of the right breast, illustrating the course of the x-ray beam for craniocaudal, lateral, and mediolateral oblique views. On craniocaudal views, the location of lesions is anatomic: those projecting laterally or medially are in the lateral and medial aspects of the breast, respectively. Similarly, on true lateral views, lesions projecting superiorly or inferiorly are located in the upper or lower quadrants, respectively. On mediolateral oblique views, however, some of the tissue that projects above the level of the nipple is inferior to the nipple **(G)**, and some tissue projecting below the level of the nipple is superior to the nipple **(H)**. Consequently, on a mediolateral oblique **(I)** view, some lesions projecting above the level of the nipple (gray triangle, "A") are anatomically in the lower outer quadrant, and some lesions projecting below the level of the nipple (black triangle, "B") are anatomically in the upper inner quadrant of the right breast.

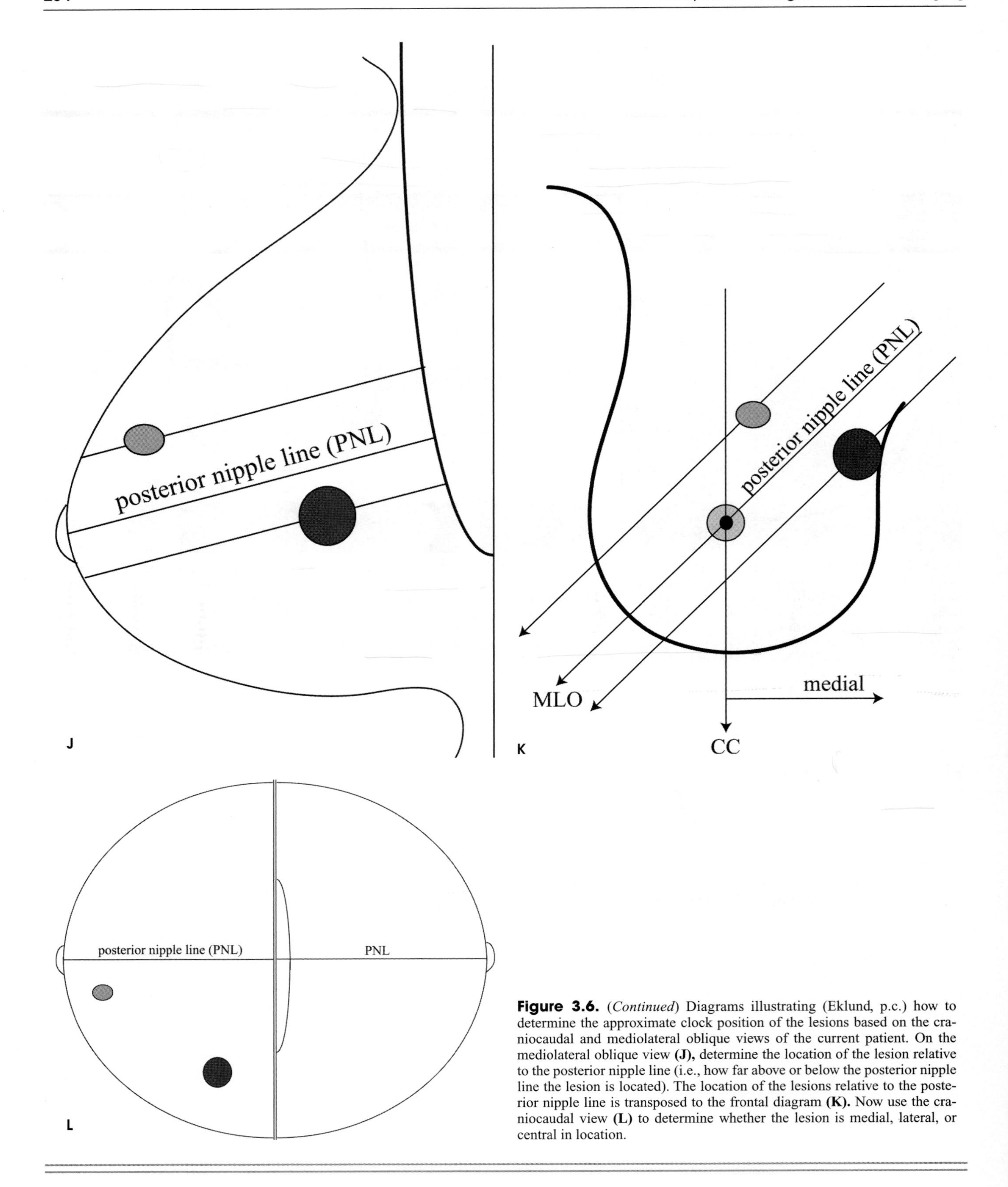

Figure 3.6. (*Continued*) Diagrams illustrating (Eklund, p.c.) how to determine the approximate clock position of the lesions based on the craniocaudal and mediolateral oblique views of the current patient. On the mediolateral oblique view **(J),** determine the location of the lesion relative to the posterior nipple line (i.e., how far above or below the posterior nipple line the lesion is located). The location of the lesions relative to the posterior nipple line is transposed to the frontal diagram **(K).** Now use the craniocaudal view **(L)** to determine whether the lesion is medial, lateral, or central in location.

PATIENT 7

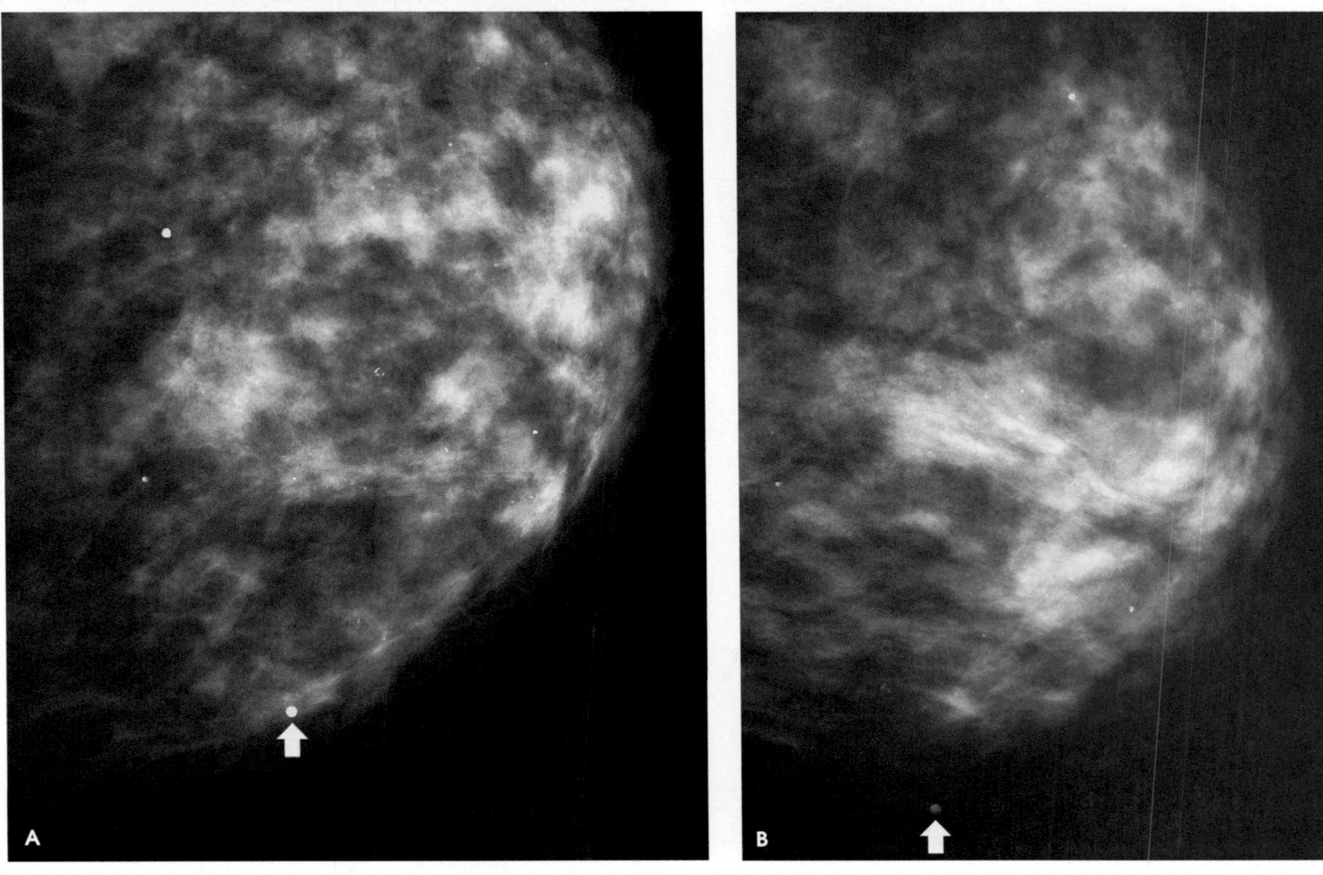

Figure 3.7. Diagnostic evaluation, 82-year-old patient presenting with a "lump" in the left breast. Craniocaudal **(A)** and mediolateral oblique **(B)** views photographically coned to the area of concern in the left breast. Metallic BB (*arrows*) indicate the location of the palpable mass.

At this point, what can you say and with what degree of certainty?
What else would you tell the technologist to do?

Scattered and some clustered round and punctate calcifications, as well as more dense, coarse, and some lucent-centered calcifications, are present. However, no definite abnormality is apparent on the craniocaudal and mediolateral oblique views that corresponds to the site of concern to the patient. At this point, we have insufficient information to say anything definitive. A spot tangential view of the palpable finding may be helpful; if it is not, correlative physical examination and an ultrasound are indicated.

When women who are over the age of 30 years present with a "lump" or other focal symptom (focal pain, skin change etc.), a metallic BB is placed at the site of focal concern. This is followed by craniocaudal and mediolateral oblique views, bilaterally, as well as a spot tangential view of the focal abnormality (a unilateral study of the symptomatic breast is done if the patient has had a mammogram within the last 6 months). Based on these initial images, additional spot compression or double spot compression magnification views may be done. Depending on the location of the focal finding, and the appearance of this area on the spot tangential view, correlative physical examination and an ultrasound are usually indicated.

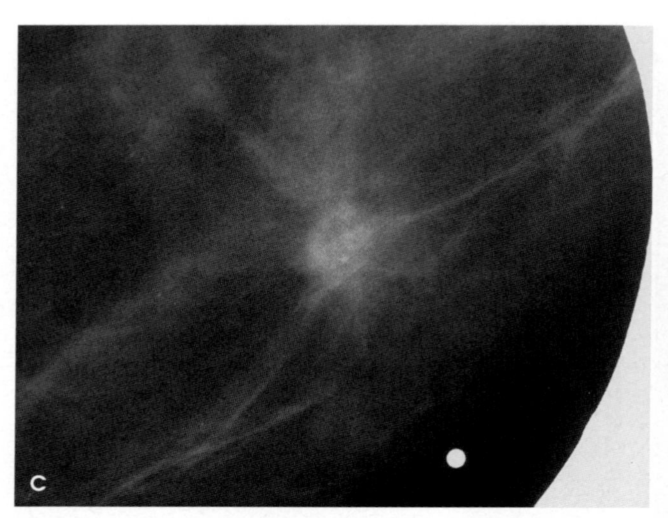

Figure 3.7. Spot tangential **(C)** view of palpable finding in the lower inner quadrant of the left breast.

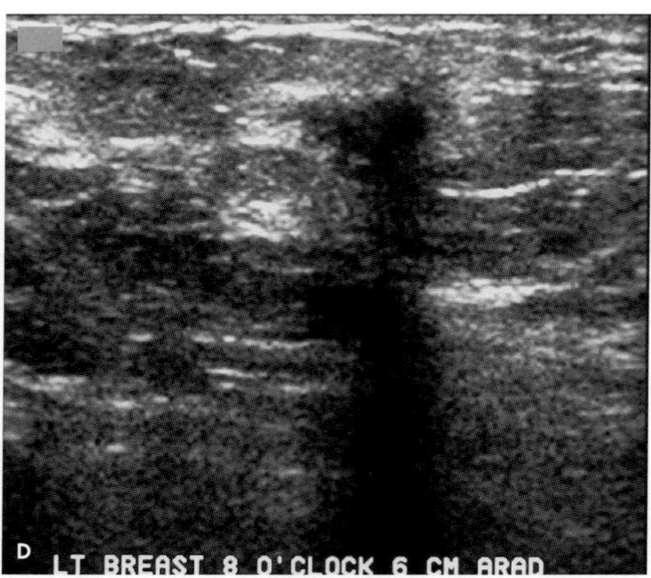

Figure 3.7. Ultrasound image **(D)** of the palpable finding in the lower inner quadrant of the left breast, in the antiradial (ARAD) projection.

How helpful is the tangential view of this patient? At this point, what can you say and with what degree of certainty? What BI-RADS® assessment category would you assign?

For this patient, the tangential view is helpful. A spiculated mass is now readily apparent, corresponding to the palpable finding. Unless the patient has had trauma, or surgery localized specifically to this area, or there are symptoms related to an inflammatory process, a biopsy is indicated and the likelihood of malignancy in an 82-year-old patient is high. The patient has no history of breast-related surgery or trauma.

Is an ultrasound indicated in this patient for the purposes of evaluating the lesion? If not, why do an ultrasound?

Given a spiculated mass and no history of surgery or trauma, or symptoms related to an inflammatory process, corresponding to the site of concern to the patient, a biopsy is indicated regardless of the ultrasound findings. An ultrasound is done to determine if the lesion can be imaged so that the biopsy can be done expeditiously using ultrasound guidance. Ultrasound-guided core biopsies are better tolerated by patients, particularly elderly patients, because the patient is supine as opposed to prone (with her neck turned all the way over to one side) on the dedicated stereotactic table, or sitting, if an add-on device is used. No breast compression or radiation is required when the biopsy is done using ultrasound guidance. Additionally, because orthogonal images of the needle can be obtained following firing of the needle during the biopsy, it is easier to verify that the needle has gone through the mass. This is in contrast to the unidimensional postfire images of needle positioning during a stereotactically guided biopsy.

How would you describe the ultrasound findings? What is your leading diagnosis, and what is your recommendation?

On physical examination, a discrete, hard mass is palpated in the lower inner quadrant of the left breast. There are no findings to suggest an ongoing inflammatory process (e.g., no erythema, tenderness, or warmth over the palpable finding). An irregular, 1.5-cm hypoechoic mass with indistinct and angular margins and shadowing is imaged on ultrasound at the 8 o'clock position, 6 cm from the left nipple, corresponding to the palpable finding. The clinical, mammographic, and ultrasound findings are highly suggestive of a malignancy. Differential considerations include invasive ductal carcinoma not otherwise specified (NOS), tubular carcinoma, or invasive lobular carcinoma. Although it is uncommon, ductal carcinoma in situ can present as a mass, asymmetry density, or distortion in the absence of microcalcifications. If there were a history of trauma or surgery localized specifically to this spot, this could represent an area of fat necrosis. Rarely, in the appropriate clinical setting, this could represent an inflammatory process.

BI-RADS® category 4: suspicious abnormality, biopsy should be considered.

Rather than just consider a biopsy, one is done using ultrasound guidance. An invasive ductal carcinoma (NOS) is diagnosed on the core biopsy. A 1.5-cm grade II invasive ductal carcinoma NOS is confirmed on the lumpectomy specimen. No metastatic disease is diagnosed on the sentinel lymph node [pT1c, pN0(sn) (i−), pMX; Stage I].

What are the clinical and imaging features related to invasive ductal carcinoma NOS?

Invasive ductal carcinoma NOS is the most common breast malignancy diagnosed in approximately 65% of all patients with breast cancer. Depending on tumor size, location, and breast size, the lesion may be palpable, or skin thickening or dimpling may be noted clinically. Subareolar lesions may be associated with nipple retraction, inversion, or displacement. A spiculated mass is the most common mammographic finding in patients with invasive ductal carcinoma NOS. Associated pleomorphic calcifications, reflecting the presence of ductal carcinoma in situ, are sometimes seen in the mass or extending away from it for variable distances. If there are associated calcifications, it is important to characterize them and describe their extent.

A round or oval mass with obscured, indistinct, or ill-defined margins is a less common mammographic presentation for invasive ductal carcinoma NOS. On ultrasound, these lesions are round or oval, solid, hypoechoic masses with well-circumscribed or partially indistinct margins; many have posterior acoustic enhancement. Some may be markedly hypoechoic. Alternatively, a complex cystic mass may be seen. When they present as a round or oval mass, invasive ductal carcinomas NOS are often rapidly growing, poorly differentiated lesions, particularly if the lesion is solid and associated with posterior acoustic enhancement on ultrasound. In lesions with cystic changes on ultrasound, necrosis is commonly present histologically.

What are the more common subtypes of invasive ductal carcinomas, and what are their clinical and imaging features?

Tubular, medullary, mucinous, and papillary carcinomas are some of the more common subtypes of invasive ductal carcinoma. Of these four subtypes, tubular carcinoma is the only one that presents as a small spiculated mass; in some patients, multiple small spiculated masses may be identified. Medullary carcinoma usually presents in premenopausal woman as a round or oval mass and is characterized by rapid growth; many of these patients present with interval cancers (within a year of a normal screening mammogram). Medullary carcinoma can be markedly hypoechoic on ultrasound (simulating a cyst). Mucinous and papillary carcinomas usually present as round or oval masses in older, postmenopausal women and are usually characterized by slower growth patterns. Ultrasound can be helpful in distinguishing among some of the mucinous and papillary carcinomas. Mucinous lesions are commonly iso- to slightly hypo- or hyperechoic and may have posterior acoustic enhancement. Papillary carcinomas, particularly those arising in the subareolar area, are often complex cystic masses with posterior acoustic enhancement.

PATIENT 8

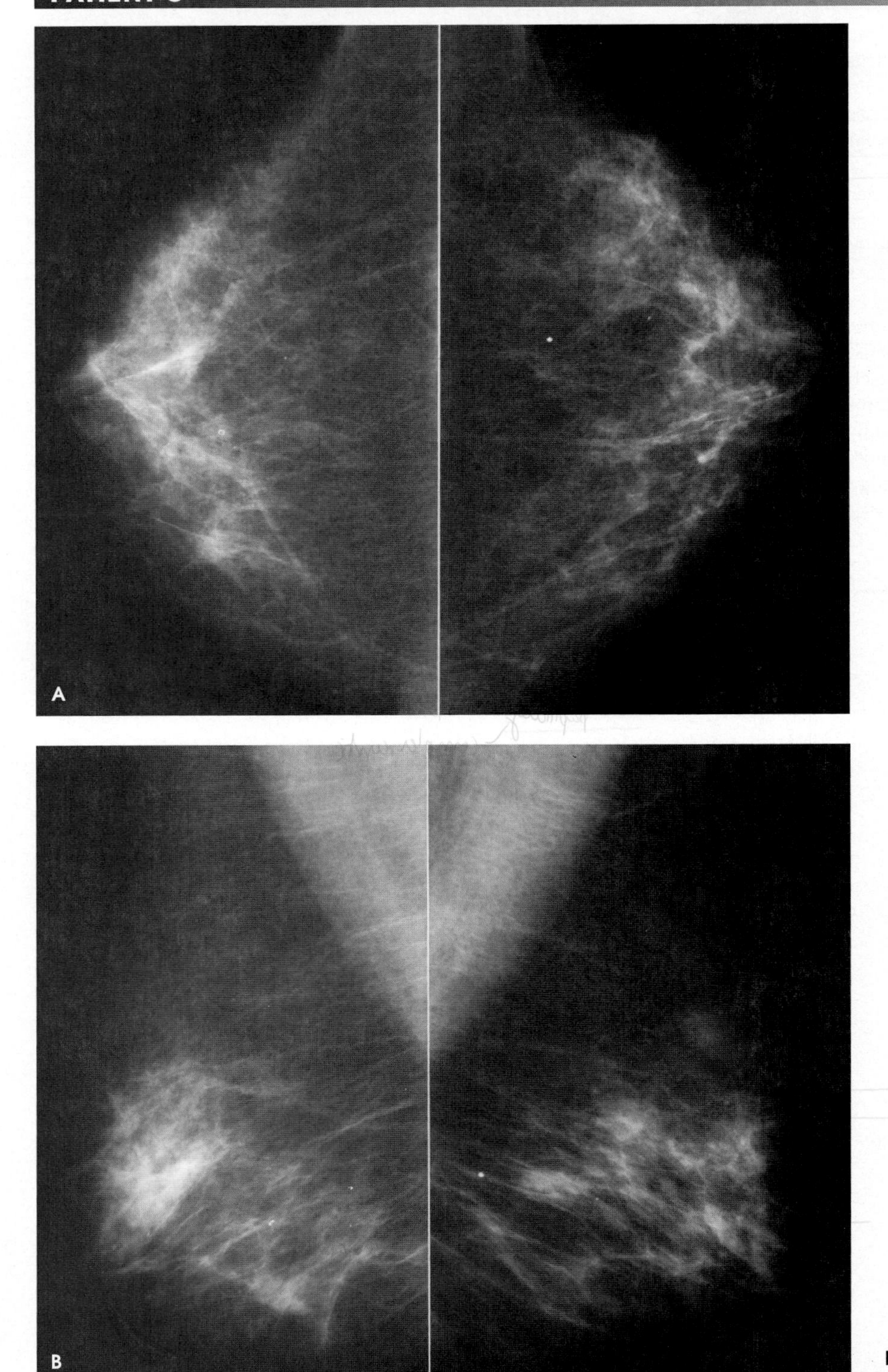

Figure 3.8. Screening study, 67-year-old woman. Craniocaudal **(A)** and mediolateral oblique **(B)** views.

Is this a normal screening mammogram, or do you perceive a potential abnormality?

Remember to focus your attention by splitting the images into thirds. On the oblique views, focus your attention on the lower third of the breasts (Fig. 3.8C); now do you see something? Do you see a corresponding asymmetric area, medially in the right breast (Fig. 3.8D), on the craniocaudal view? What would you do next?

BI-RADS® category 0: need additional imaging evaluation. Spot compression views, correlative physical examination and an ultrasound are indicated.

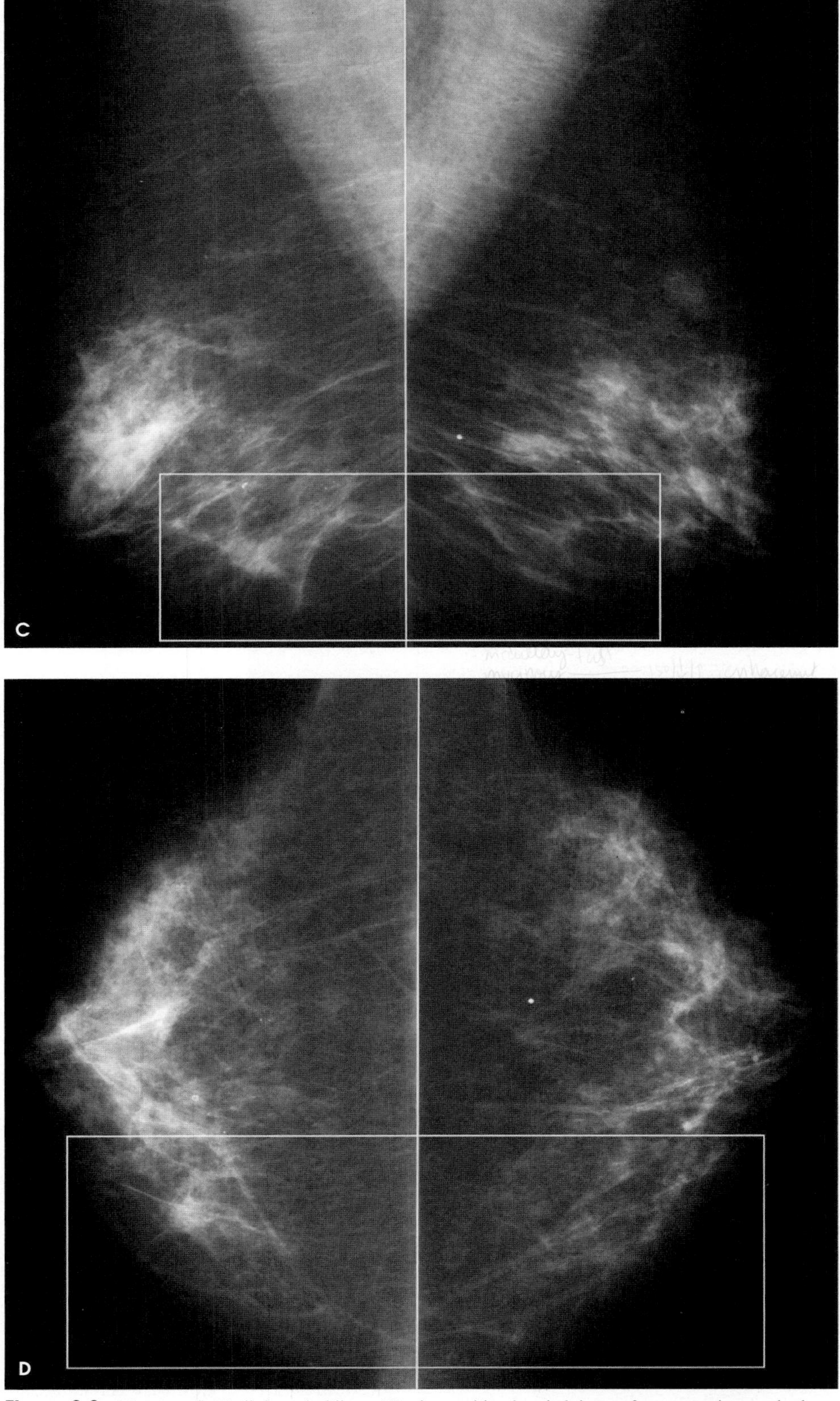

Figure 3.8. (*Continued*) Mediolateral oblique **(C)** views with a box helping to focus attention on the lower thirds of breasts. Craniocaudal **(D)** views with a box to help focus attention on the medial quadrants of the breasts.

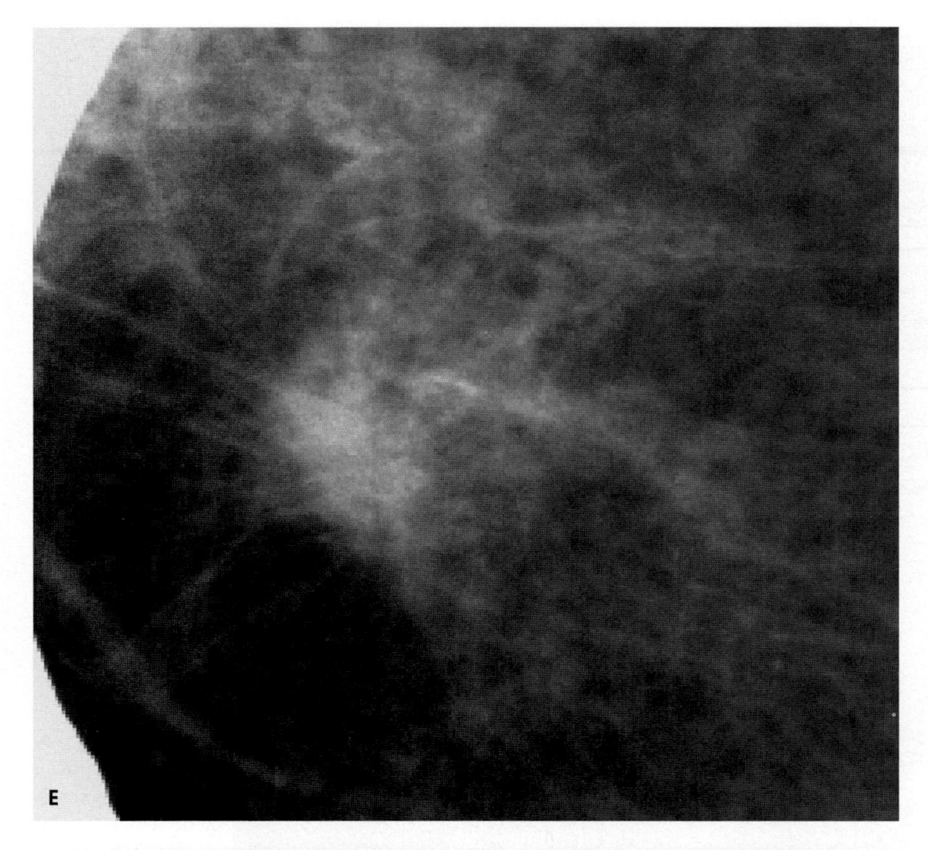

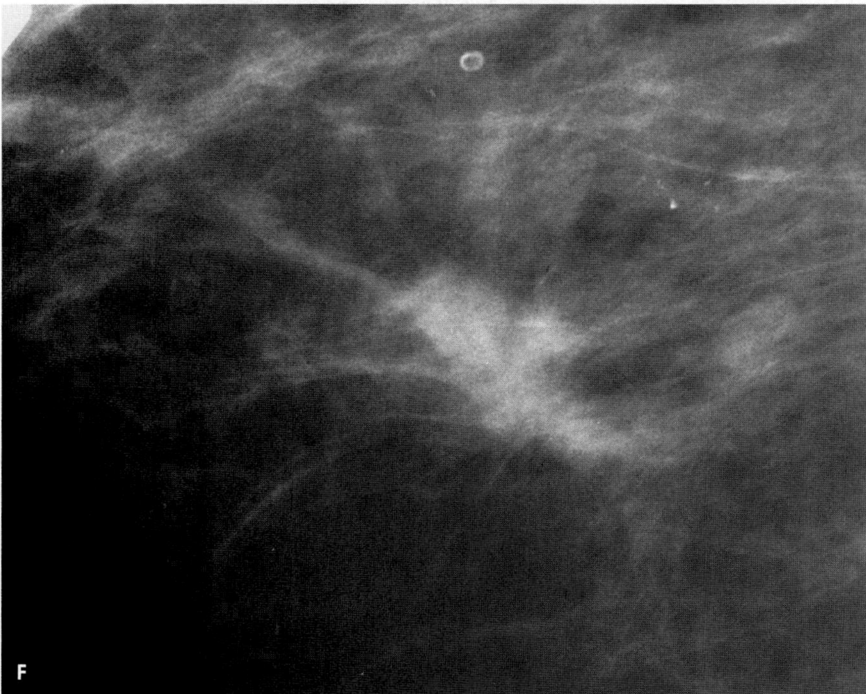

Figure 3.8. (*Continued*) Spot compression views, craniocaudal **(E)** and mediolateral oblique **(F)** projections.

What do you think now?

A 1-cm, irregular, spiculated mass is confirmed on the spot compression views. A small focus of pleomorphic calcifications is also noted in the tissue adjacent to the mass. In the absence of symptoms suggesting an ongoing infection, or a history of surgery or trauma localized to this specific area, this finding requires biopsy. Although a biopsy is indicated on the mammographic findings alone, an ultrasound is done because if the lesion is identified on ultrasound, a core biopsy can be done easily and expeditiously using ultrasound guidance.

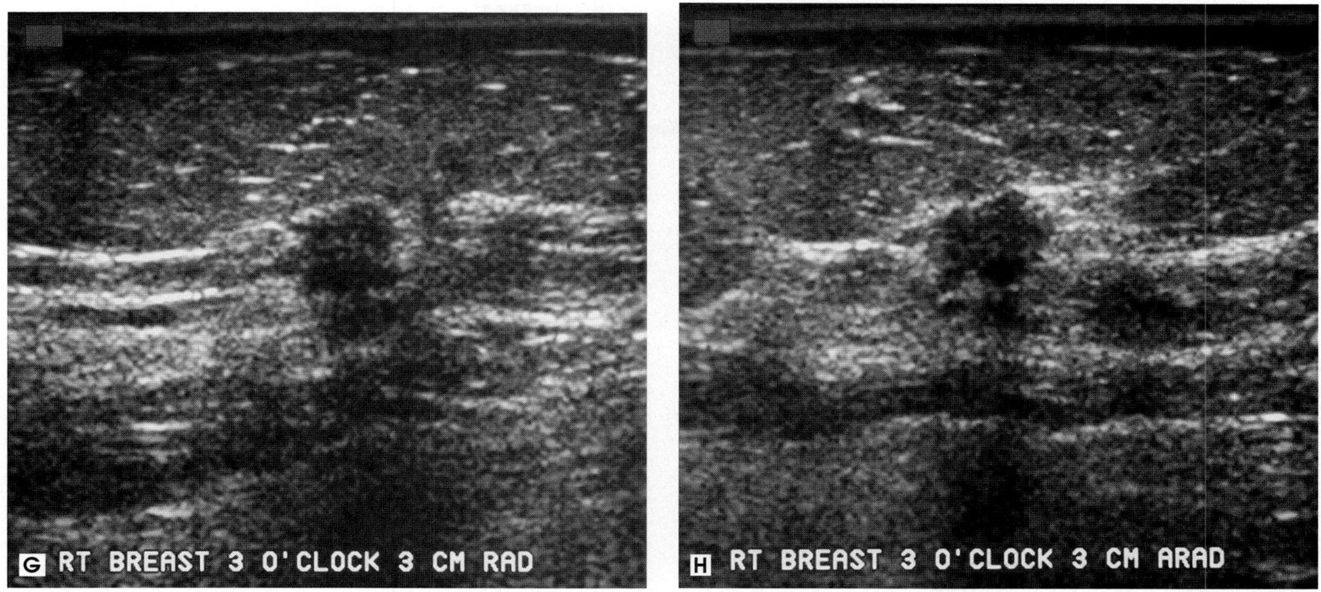

Figure 3.8. (*Continued*) Ultrasound images in the radial (RAD) **(G)** and antiradial (ARAD) **(H)** projections at the 3 o'clock position, 3 cm from the right nipple.

Is this the correct location for the mammographic finding? What is your differential?

A hypoechoic mass with irregular, spiculated, and angular margins, associated shadowing, and disruption of Cooper ligaments is imaged, corresponding to the area of mammographic concern. Although the lesion projects below the level of the nipple on the mediolateral oblique view, the lesion imaged on ultrasound corresponds to the lesion seen mammographically (Fig. 3.8I–K). Differential considerations include fat necrosis if the patient has had surgery or trauma localized specifically to this area, papilloma, sclerosing adenosis, mastitis, granular cell tumor (rare), extra-abdominal desmoid (rare), invasive ductal carcinoma not otherwise specified, tubular carcinoma, or invasive lobular carcinoma. Rarely, ductal carcinoma in situ can present as a mass, asymmetrical density, or distortion in the absence of microcalcifications. Given the imaging features of this lesion (i.e., a spiculated mass with adjacent calcifications), the working diagnosis for this patient is an invasive ductal carcinoma with associated ductal carcinoma in situ.

BI-RADS® category 4: suspicious abnormality, biopsy should be considered.

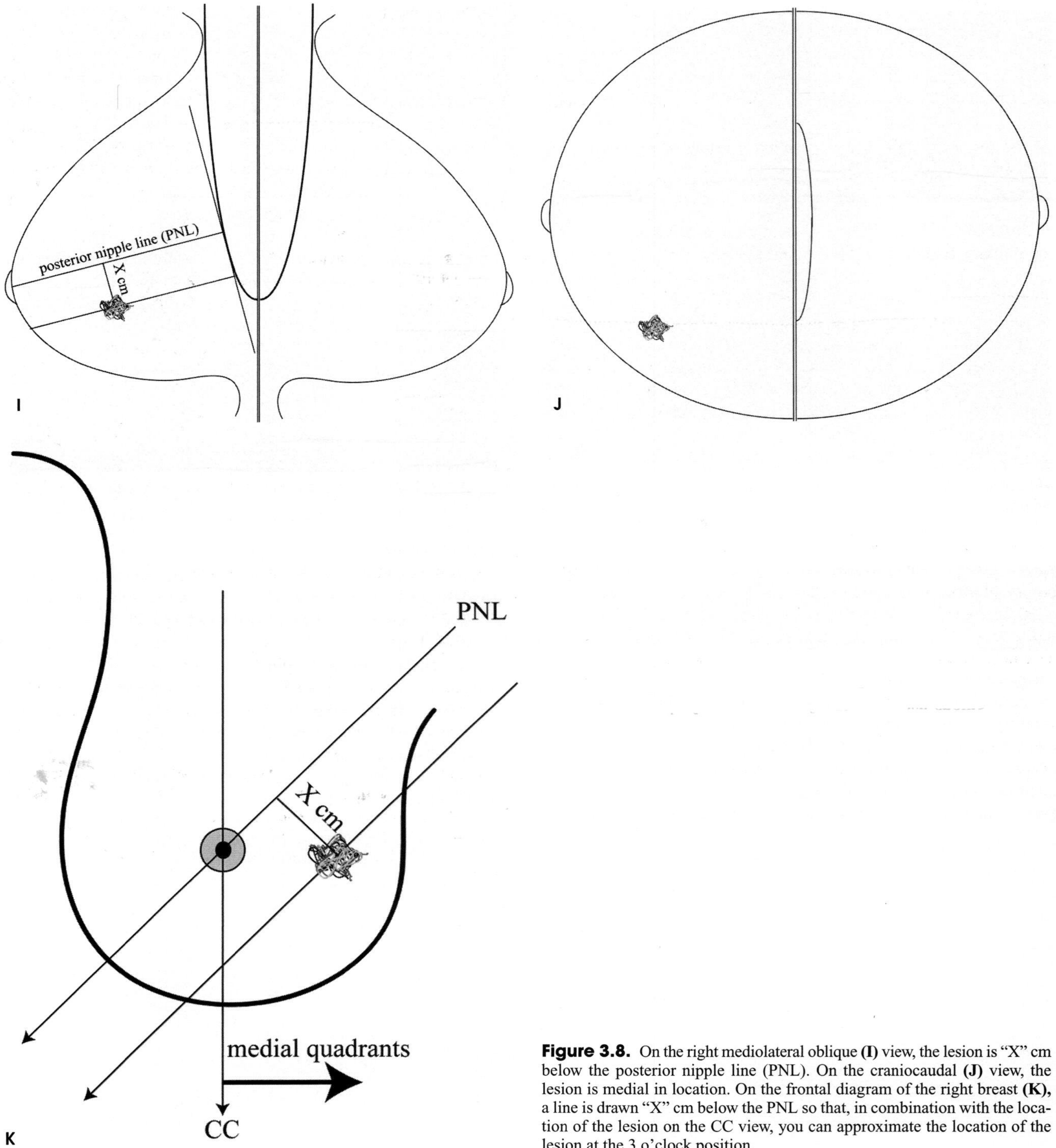

Figure 3.8. On the right mediolateral oblique **(I)** view, the lesion is "X" cm below the posterior nipple line (PNL). On the craniocaudal **(J)** view, the lesion is medial in location. On the frontal diagram of the right breast **(K),** a line is drawn "X" cm below the PNL so that, in combination with the location of the lesion on the CC view, you can approximate the location of the lesion at the 3 o'clock position.

An ultrasound-guided biopsy is undertaken, and an invasive ductal carcinoma is reported on the cores. A 0.9-cm, grade I invasive ductal carcinoma with associated cribriform-type ductal carcinoma in situ is diagnosed on the lumpectomy specimen. Two excised sentinel lymph nodes are normal [pT1b, pN0(sn) (i−), pMX; Stage I].

What is the basic concept underlying sentinel lymph node biopsies?

Traditionally, most patients diagnosed with invasive breast cancer had axillary lymph node dissections (ALND) for staging and as part of the surgical treatment of their breast cancer (i.e., local-regional control). More recently, sentinel lymph node biopsy (SLNB) has been suggested as an alternative to assess the status of the axilla and is being used increasingly to replace ALND for most women diagnosed with breast cancer. It is postulated that the sentinel lymph node(s) is the first node draining a tumor, and that the histologic status of this lymph node accurately predict the status of the regional (axilla) lymphatic basin.

Given some of the complications associated with ALND, sentinel lymph node biopsies are now used routinely at many institutions as an alternative to ALND for patients with clinically normal axillary exams. Axillary lymph node dissections are undertaken if the sentinel lymph node(s) is not identified, metastatic disease is known to be present following fine needle aspiration (FNA), or core biopsy, of ultrasound-detected, abnormal lymph nodes in the axilla, or when abnormal lymph nodes are suspected clinically. Axillary lymph node dissection may also be performed in patients with metastatic disease in the sentinel lymph node(s), to establish the number of axillary lymph nodes involved by tumor.

The methods used to identify the sentinel lymph node are still evolving, undergoing investigation, and vary among institutions. In general, a radioisotope is used alone or in combination with a blue dye (e.g., lymphazurin blue) for lymphatic mapping; these are injected in a peritumoral, intradermal, periareolar, or intratumoral location. The volume used and the interval between injection and surgery vary. If a radioisotope is used, preoperative lymphoscintigraphy can be used to assess the pattern of lymphatic drainage before surgery; this also provides information regarding the internal mammary lymph nodes. Alternatively, a gamma probe is used intraoperatively to identify the "hot spots" in the axillary tail without preoperative lymphoscintigraphy. It has been suggested by many researchers that optimal results are obtained when blue dye and isotope are used in combination. In a review of the literature correlating SLNB with ALND in more than 3,000 patients with breast cancer, Liberman reported technical success rate, sensitivity, and accuracy of 88%, 93%, and 97%, respectively, for SLNB.

The use of SLNB in patients with ductal carcinoma in situ (DCIS) remains controversial. It is probably indicated for women with DCIS and known microinvasion and for patients in whom invasive disease is suspected preoperatively based on the size or imaging features of the DCIS. The alternative approach that can be taken is to excise the DCIS and, if invasive disease is identified on the lumpectomy specimen, have the SLNB done as a second operative procedure.

What is the prognostic significance of isolated tumor cells or micrometastatic disease described following a sentinel lymph node biopsy?

The advent and now widespread use of sentinel lymph node biopsy has resulted in a more meticulous evaluation of excised lymph node(s). This includes serial sectioning of the entire lymph node (as opposed to sample sections from multiple lymph nodes) and a more focused histologic and immunohistochemical (IHC) evaluation of the excised lymph node. Some of the consequences include the observation of isolated tumor cells and micrometastatic disease. Consequently, the significance of these findings (e.g., isolated tumor cells and micrometastases) involving excised sentinel lymph nodes is not yet clear, and there is no consensus on their prognostic significance. Currently, the use of IHC evaluation of sentinel lymph nodes is not encouraged; however, it is done at many institutions. The determination of micrometastatic disease should be based on routine hematoxylin and eosin–stained histologic sections.

PATIENT 9

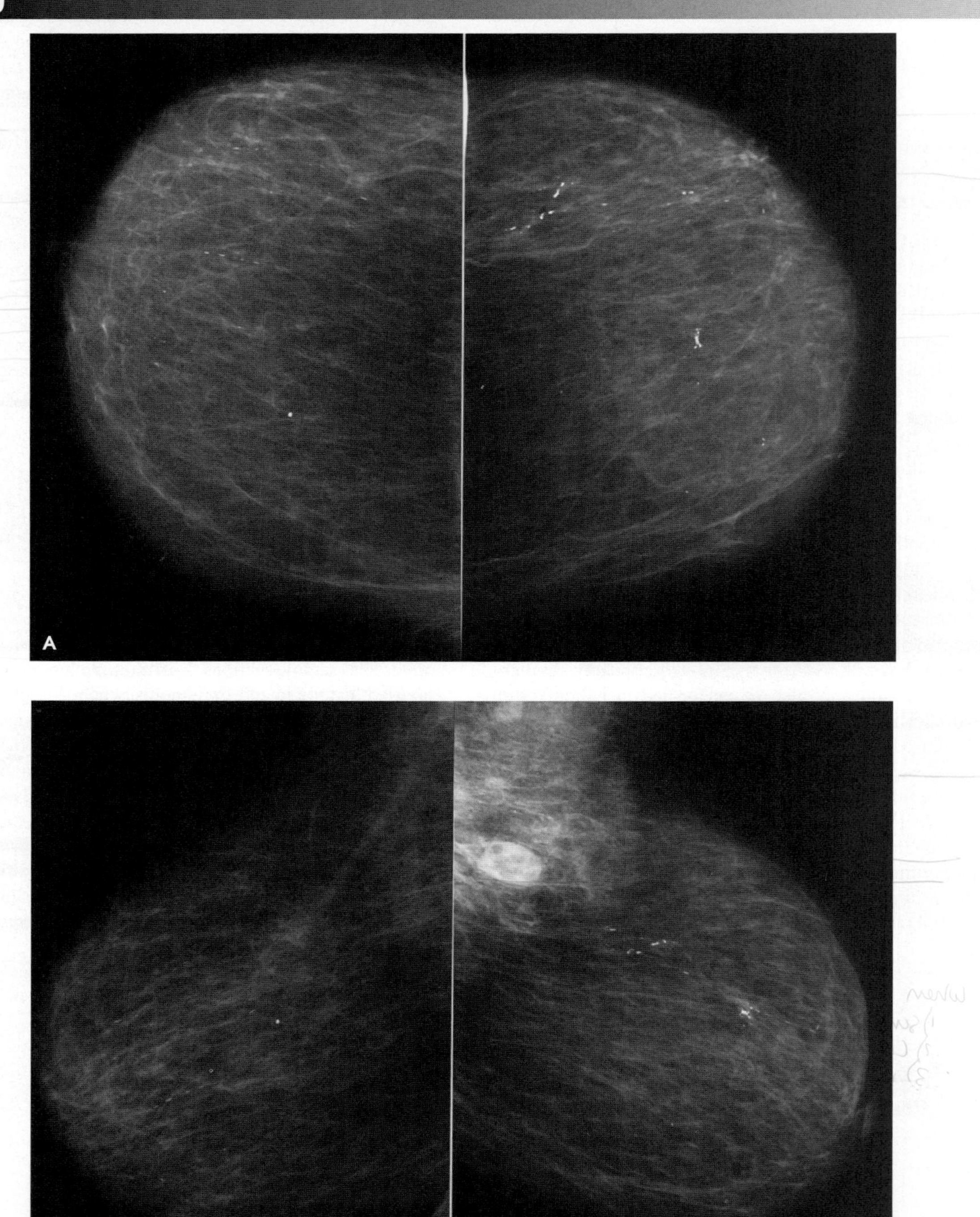

Figure 3.9. Diagnostic evaluation, 79-year-old patient presenting with a "lump" in the mid-axillary region inferior to the left axilla. Craniocaudal **(A)** and mediolateral oblique **(B)** views.

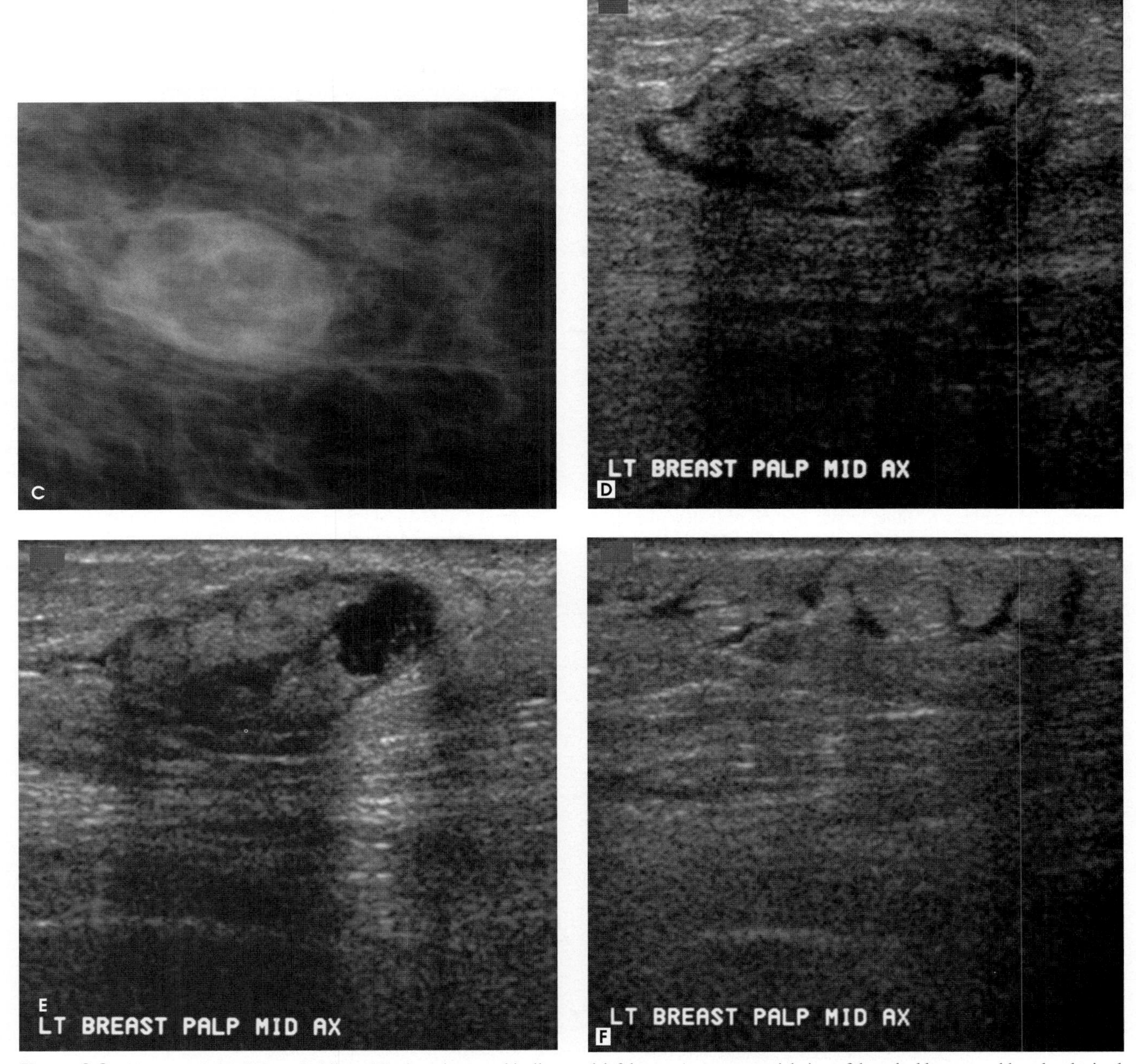

Figure 3.9. (*Continued*) Mediolateral oblique **(C)** view photographically coned, left breast. A spot tangential view of the palpable area could not be obtained. Ultrasound images **(D, E)** of the palpable finding in the left breast. Ultrasound image **(F)** of tissue surrounding the palpable finding. Patient is on coumadin.

How would you describe the findings?

Scattered dystrophic and large rodlike calcifications are present bilaterally. A mixed-density (fat containing) mass is imaged on the left mediolateral oblique view, superimposed on the left pectoral muscle, corresponding to the area of clinical concern. The trabecular markings surrounding the mass are more dense and numerous compared to those in the corresponding area on the right. Given the far lateral and posterior location of the lesion, it is not imaged on the craniocaudal view and a spot tangential view could not be obtained.

What diagnostic considerations would you entertain? Based on the mammographic findings, what BI-RADS® assessment category would you assign, and what would you do next?

The main differential considerations for a mixed-density lesion include lymph node, fibroadenolipoma (hamartoma), fat necrosis, oil cyst, galactocele, postoperative or posttraumatic fluid collection, and abscess. Although malignant lesions may rarely entrap fat, fat-containing lesions should be considered benign; consequently, no malignant lesions are usually included in the differential for a mixed-density lesion. Prior studies in this patient are normal. Specifically, no lymph node or fibroadenolipoma is seen in the upper outer quadrant of the left breast. A galactocele is not a consideration in a 79-year-old patient. Primary considerations at this point include an abscess or a hematoma (particularly because the patient is on coumadin), both of which also help explain the associated prominence of the trabecular markings. Physical findings and additional history may be helpful in sorting through these possibilities.

On physical examination, there is a hard mass just inferior to the left axilla at the mid-axillary line; no associated skin changes or discoloration are noted at this time. The mass is superficial, readily mobile, and nontender. An oval, well-circumscribed mass with a heterogeneous echotexture is imaged on ultrasound at the site of the palpable abnormality. Areas of posterior acoustic enhancement are associated with the cystic areas in the mass, and shadowing is noted with the more solid components. The surrounding tissue is echogenic, consistent with hyperemia, there is disruption of the normal tissue architecture, and lymphatic channels or interstitial fluid collections are seen as thin hypoechoic linear channels subcutaneously. In the absence of significant tenderness or erythema, an abscess is unlikely. On questioning the patient at the time of the ultrasound, she has not had any surgery to either breast, but she does describe having had trauma to this site several weeks before while being lifted from her bed on a Hoyer lift. She states that although at this time there is no skin discoloration, there was a large ecchymotic area at this site immediately following the trauma. The currently palpable mass developed as the ecchymosis resolved.

As hematomas evolve clinically, so do their imaging features. Acutely, there may be a water-density mass. As the hematoma ages, a mixed-density mass is often seen mammographically. This may resolve completely, or an oil cyst may develop eventually, as can dystrophic calcifications. On ultrasound, a complex cystic mass or a solid mass with a heterogeneous echotexture that may include hyperechoic, hypoechoic, and cystic areas can be seen. Increased echogenicity (e.g., reflecting hyperemia) and disruption of the normal tissue architecture is often found in the surrounding tissue.

BI-RADS® category 2: benign finding. Follow-up physical examination and ultrasound in 3 to 4 months is recommended for this patient, to assure resolution. *Note that the BI-RADS® assessment categories should be considered independent of the recommendation.* For this patient, the finding is benign, yet a short-interval follow-up is recommended. For patients in whom I suspect an inflammatory condition or posttraumatic/surgical changes, I recommend a 3- to 4-month follow-up. Under these circumstances, a rapid change (evolution) is expected in the findings. Six months is the usual recommendation for other patients for whom a short-interval follow-up is recommended (e.g., those with assessment category 3—probably benign lesion, such as a well-circumscribed mass in a patient with no prior studies).

PATIENT 10

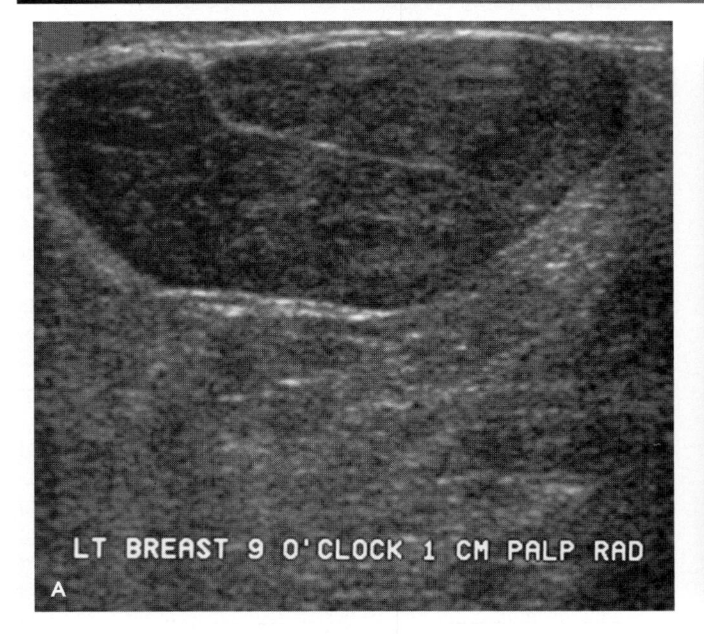

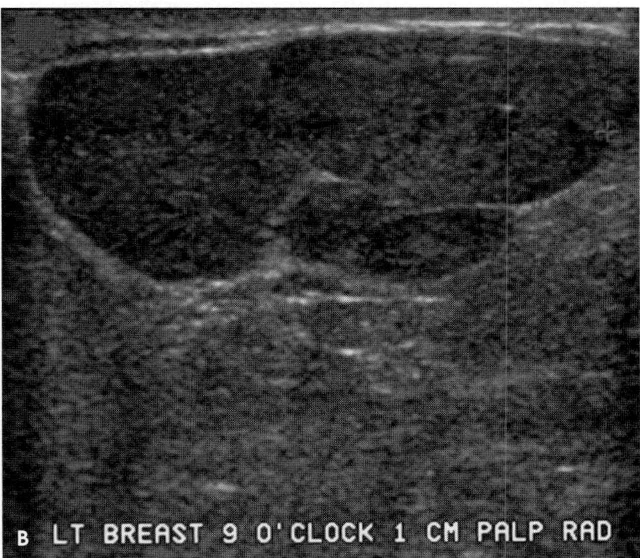

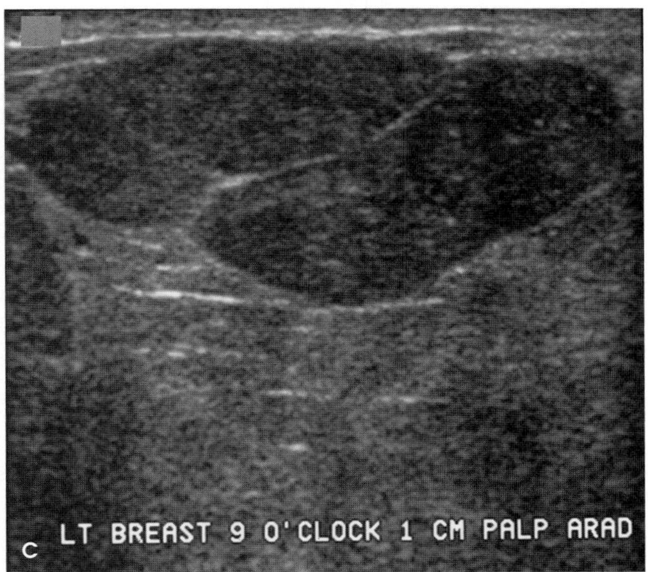

Figure 3.10. Diagnostic evaluation, 24-year-old patient presenting during the third trimester of pregnancy with a "lump" in the left breast. Ultrasound images, radial (RAD) **(A, B)** and antiradial (ARAD) **(C)** projections of the palpable (PALP) mass, laterally in the left breast.

What is your approach to adolescent, pregnant or lactating women, or those under the age of 30 years who present with breast-related symptoms? Under what circumstances would you do a mammogram in this patient population?

Physical examination and an ultrasound are the initial tools used in evaluating adolescent, pregnant or lactating women, or those under the age of 30 years who present with breast-related symptoms. If breast cancer is suspected after the initial evaluation, or diagnosed following a core biopsy, a complete bilateral mammogram is done.

How would you describe the ultrasound findings, and what is the most likely diagnosis?

On physical examination a discrete, readily mobile, nontender mass is palpated at the 9 o'clock position, 1 cm from the left nipple. This corresponds to the site of concern to the patient. A well-circumscribed, 3.7-cm, oval mass with internal septations and some posterior acoustic enhancement is imaged corresponding to the palpable mass. Given the clinical and imaging findings, a lactational adenoma is the most likely diagnosis. An ultrasound-guided core biopsy can be done to confirm this impression; clinical and sonographic follow-up is also discussed with the patient as an acceptable alternative.

What is the typical clinical presentation and course for lactational adenomas, and what are the ultrasound features associated with these lesions?

Although they are termed lactational adenomas, many of these lesions present during the third trimester of pregnancy as a well-circumscribed, mobile mass. Rarely, when these grow rapidly during the second and third trimesters of pregnancy, they outstrip their vascular supply, resulting in areas of infarction so that patients present acutely, describing a rapidly enlarging, tender mass. In most patients, lactational adenomas decrease in size significantly or resolve completely after delivery or following the cessation of lactation. They may recur with subsequent pregnancies. Patients with these lesions can be managed conservatively unless they are anxious or symptomatic (e.g., tenderness) relief is indicated.

The ultrasound features of these lesions suggest a benign etiology in many patients and include oval shape, well-circumscribed margins that may have smooth lobulations, homogenous internal echotexture, and posterior acoustic enhancement. Fibrous bands traversing the lesion and cystic changes may also be noted on ultrasound. However, in some patients, the lesions may demonstrate features more suggestive of malignancy, including irregular, angulated, and ill-defined margins and shadowing, requiring biopsy.

What histologic features characterize lactational adenomas?

It is unclear whether these tumors arise de novo during pregnancy, or whether they reflect the presence of a pre-existing fibroadenoma or tubular adenoma, stimulated by the hormonal changes that occur during pregnancy. Histologically, the features of lactational adenomas vary, depending on the stage of the pregnancy at the time of the diagnosis. Tubules are distended with secretory material and the lining epithelial cells show cytoplasmic vacuoles and variable mitotic activity. Fibrotic bands and areas of infarction can be seen in a small number of the lesions.

Pregnancy and breast cancer

Pregnancy-associated breast carcinoma (PABC) is defined as breast cancer that is diagnosed during pregnancy or in the year following delivery. It is estimated to affect between 1 in 1,500 to 1 in 3,000 pregnant women, and some suggest that this incidence will increase as women delay their child-bearing years. The tumors that occur during pregnancy are similar to those diagnosed in nonpregnant patients. Although some patients have advanced disease at the time of diagnosis, this is attributed to delays in seeking medical attention or masses being followed clinically rather than any inherent aggressive biologic attribute of the tumors developing during gestation or to any pregnancy-related hormonal stimulation of the tumors.

Diagnosis and staging, termination of pregnancy, timing of local and systemic adjuvant therapy and the potential effects of this therapy to the fetus are some of the concerns facing patients diagnosed during pregnancy and the interdisciplinary team of physicians taking care of the patient. If treatment is modified, consideration has to be given to the potential adverse effects to the mother. Even small doses of radiation during the first trimester of pregnancy are associated with significant adverse effects to the developing fetus, such that termination of pregnancy is a serious consideration if radiation therapy is deemed critical during the first trimester. Given the potential adverse effect of radiation to the fetus, some advocate mastectomy for patients diagnosed with breast cancer during the first two trimesters of pregnancy. When patients are diagnosed later in pregnancy, they may be treated conservatively with surgery and radiation therapy can be deferred until after delivery. Alternatively, patients can be induced after 34 weeks with small risk to the fetus, and radiation therapy can then be given following the delivery. Unlike the effects of radiation on a developing fetus, less is known concerning the effects of chemotherapy on pregnancy and the developing fetus; some suggest it can be used safely after the first trimester.

PATIENT 11

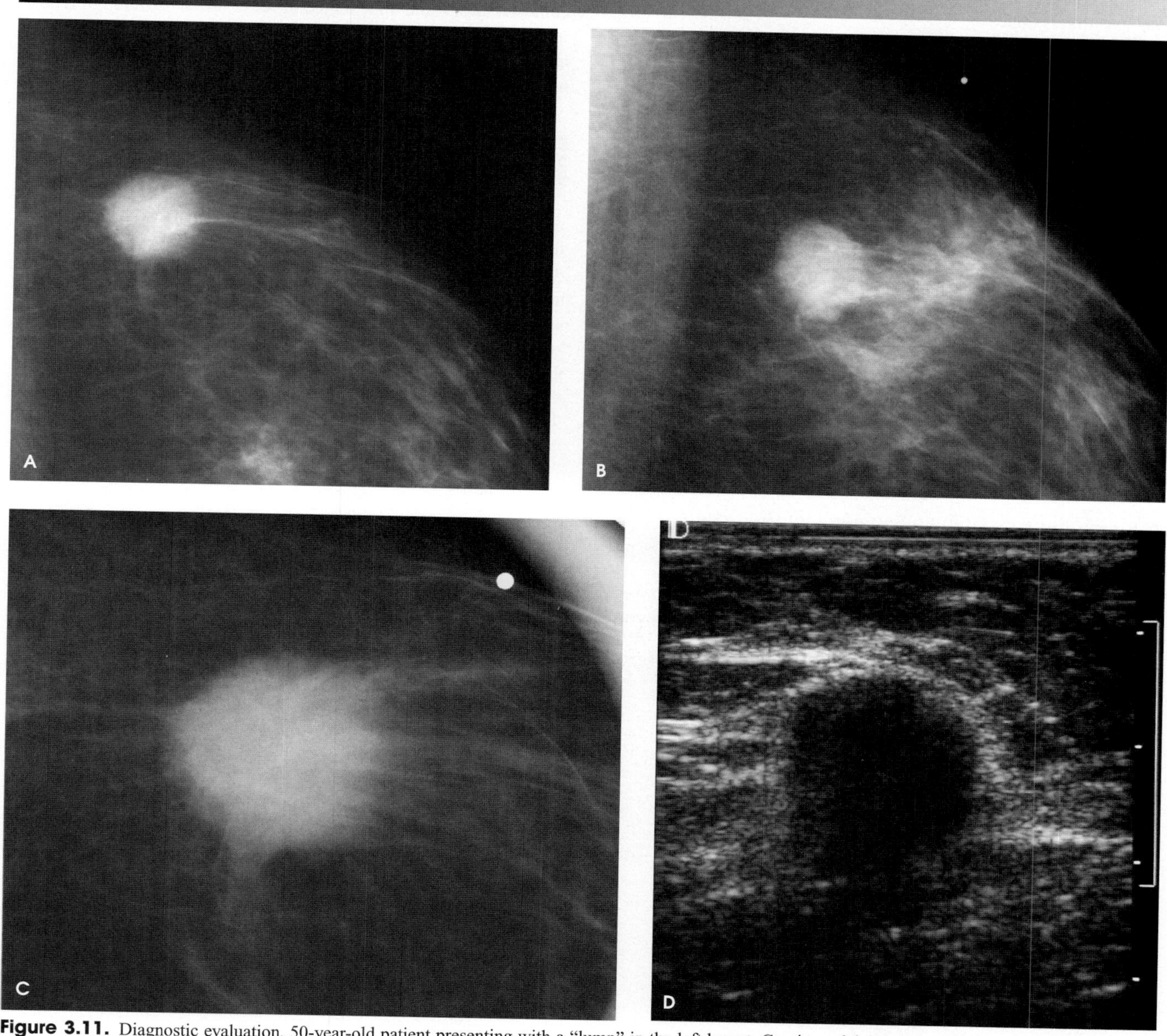

Figure 3.11. Diagnostic evaluation, 50-year-old patient presenting with a "lump" in the left breast. Craniocaudal **(A)** and mediolateral oblique **(B)** views photographically coned to the area of concern in the left breast. Spot compression **(C)** view and ultrasound image **(D)** of the palpable finding. Metallic BB used by the technologist to mark the area of concern to the patient.

How would you describe the finding? What are your differential considerations, and what is your recommendation?

A round, spiculated, 1.5-cm mass is imaged in the upper outer quadrant of the left breast, corresponding to the site of concern to the patient. A solid mass with associated shadowing is seen on ultrasound at the 1 o'clock position, 10 cm from the left nipple. Differential considerations for which history and physical examination may be helpful include fat necrosis if there is a history of recent trauma or surgery localized to this site; an abscess, particularly if there is associated tenderness, erythema, and increased temperature localized to the palpable site; or a galactocele if there is a history of pregnancy within the last several years. A papilloma, focal fibrosis, pseudoangiomatous stromal hyperplasia, phyllodes tumor, sclerosing adenosis, granular cell tumor, or an extra-abdominal desmoid (fibromatosis) are additional benign considerations. Invasive ductal carcinoma not otherwise specified, medullary, mucinous, and papillary carcinomas, lymphoma, or metastatic disease are all malignant considerations. A biopsy is indicated.

BI-RADS® category 4: suspicious abnormality, biopsy should be considered.

A granular cell tumor is reported histologically, and a wide surgical excision is done.

What are the clinical manifestations of granular cell tumors in the breast, and what is the treatment of choice?

Granular cell tumors can occur anywhere in the body but have some predilection for the head and neck, including the oral cavity. Approximately 5% of these tumors occur in the breast, including in male patients. Wide excision is the treatment of choice because less than 1% of these lesions are malignant, but local recurrences have been reported following incomplete excision. Clinically, patients describe a firm, hard, nontender mass. Superficial or subareolar lesions may cause skin retraction or nipple inversion, respectively. Rarely, patients with one granular cell tumor of the breast can be found to have multiple or bilateral breast lesions or granular cell tumors in locations outside the breast. The age of presentation is variable, ranging from 17 to 75 years.

What are the described imaging findings associated with granular cell tumors?

Mammographically, granular cell tumors may be round masses with well-circumscribed to spiculated margins, or they can present as spiculated masses. A solid mass with shadowing is the most common ultrasound appearance of these lesions. Although reports in the literature are scant, it may be that benign granular cell tumors lack the features of malignancy on dynamic sequences with magnetic resonance imaging (e.g., no significant contrast uptake).

What are some of the histologic features associated with granular cell tumors in the breast?

Although the lesions appear well circumscribed grossly, an infiltrative pattern is commonly noted histologically. Nests, or solid sheets, of cells with eosinophilic granules in abundant cytoplasm are characteristic of this tumor. These cells, in contrast to those seen in apocrine carcinomas, which they can resemble, contain glycogen and have a positive immunoreaction for S-100 protein. These tumors may also be positive for carcinoembryonic antigen (CEA), however, they are negative for estrogen and progesterone receptors. Given their positive immunoreaction for S-100 protein, these tumors are thought to have a neural origin (possibly Schwann cells).

PATIENT 12

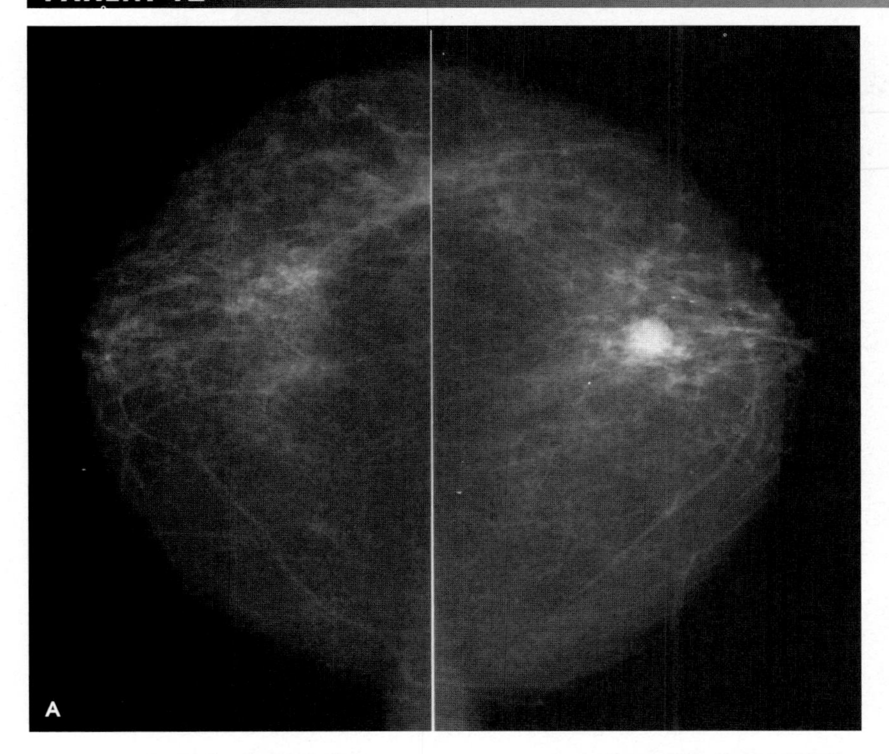

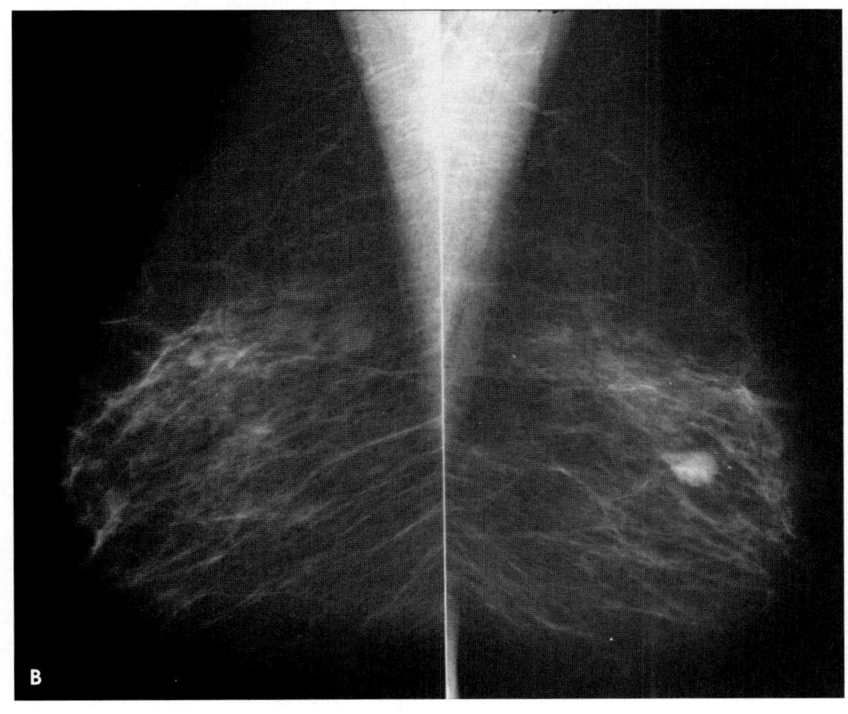

Figure 3.12. Screening study, 78-year-old woman. Craniocaudal **(A)** and mediolateral oblique **(B)** views. Comparison mammogram from 2 years previously (not shown) is normal. The patient is not on hormone replacement therapy.

What is the primary observation and, specifically, what would you do next?

A mass is present in the left breast.

BI-RADS® category 0: additional imaging evaluation is indicated. The patient is called back for additional evaluation. Spot compression views for confirmation and marginal analysis, correlative physical examination and an ultrasound are indicated.

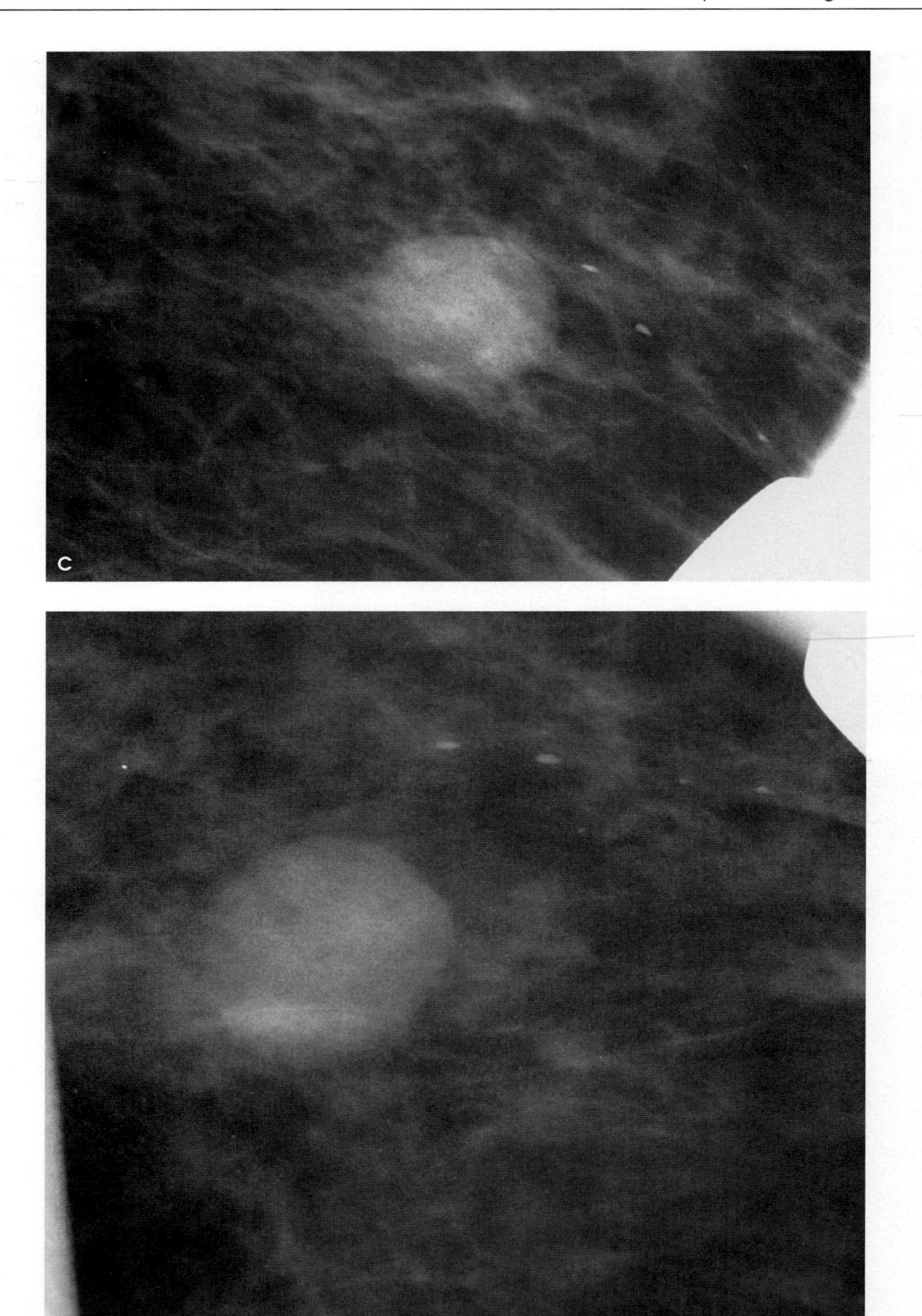

Figure 3.12. (*Continued*) Spot compression views, craniocaudal **(C)** and mediolateral oblique **(D)** projections, left breast mass.

How would you describe the mass, and what is your differential at this point?
What is the next step?

A round 1.5-cm mass with partially indistinct margins is imaged mammographically. Also noted are benign-type calcifications in the adjacent tissue. Differential considerations for a benign water-density mass developing in a 78-year-old woman are limited but include cyst, focal fibrosis, papilloma, abscess, and phyllodes tumor. Although cysts more commonly develop in the perimenopausal years (heralding the beginning of menopausal signs, with symptoms in some women), there is a second, smaller peak of occurrence in older, postmenopausal women. Considerations for malignancy include invasive ductal carcinoma not otherwise specified, mucinous carcinoma, papillary carcinoma, lymphoma, or metastatic disease. A fibroadenoma or focal fibrosis is unlikely to develop in a 78-year-old woman, particularly if she is not on hormone replacement therapy. Although they are more common in older women, invasive lobular carcinomas do not usually present as a round mass.

Next, an ultrasound study is done to evaluate the internal characteristics of this mass. Also, if it is seen on ultrasound and it is solid, a core biopsy can be done. In planning the ultrasound, at what clock position would you expect to find this mass?

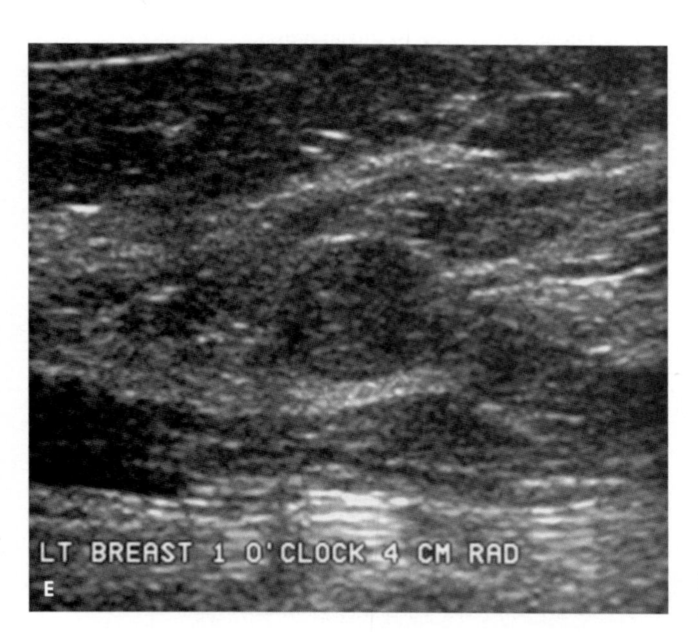

Figure 3.12. *(Continued)* Ultrasound image, radial (RAD) **(E)** projection correlating to the area of mammographic concern, left breast.

How would you describe the ultrasound findings? What do you think is the most likely diagnosis, and what is your recommendation?

A nearly isoechoic, round mass with partially circumscribed and indistinct margins is imaged at the 1 o'clock position, 4 cm from the left nipple. There is some posterior acoustic enhancement. The mass is not palpable, there is no associated skin discoloration, and no tenderness is elicited as gentle pressure is applied directly over the mass. The ultrasound excludes the possibility of a cyst. An abscess is unlikely in the absence of any associated skin change or tenderness, and the ultrasound features are not suggestive of an abscess. A solid mass developing in a 78-year-old woman requires biopsy; given the patient's age, and the imaging features of this lesion (i.e., round, 1.5-cm mass, nearly isoechoic with posterior acoustic enhancement), a mucinous carcinoma is a primary consideration. When doing the core biopsy, evaluate the cores carefully: Cores from mucinous carcinomas have a distinctive gelatinous (Fig. 3.12F, G), almost clear appearance (i.e., not stiff, solid white), and tiny air droplets will develop along the edge of the cores when they are placed in 10% formalin.

BI-RADS® category 4: suspicious abnormality, biopsy should be considered. An ultrasound guided core biopsy is done.

On MR, a small component of the mass centrally demonstrates a high signal on T2-weighted images (Fig. 3.12H). On the T1-weighted dynamic sequence (Fig. 3.12I, K), there is rapid wash-in and wash-out of contrast, with rim enhancement. No additional lesions are identified in either breast.

An invasive mammary carcinoma with mucinous features is reported following the ultrasound-guided core biopsy. A 1.5-cm mucinous carcinoma is diagnosed on the lumpectomy specimen, with no associated ductal carcinoma in situ. No metastatic disease is identified in two sentinel lymph nodes [pT1c, pN0(sn) (i−), pMX; Stage I]. By definition, pure mucinous carcinomas are grade I lesions.

What are the clinical and imaging features associated with mucinous carcinomas?

The imaging features of mucinous carcinomas are well demonstrated in this patient. Characteristically, they develop in older women as round water-density masses with a range of well circumscribed to indistinct margins; some may demonstrate macro- or microlobulation. On ultrasound, the lesions are often iso- to slightly hyperechoic with associated posterior acoustic enhancement; rarely, a complex cystic mass may be seen on ultrasound. Depending on the amount of mucin present, a bright T2-weighted signal can be seen on magnetic resonance imaging. Enhancement following contrast is variable and may be limited to the edge of the lesion (irregular rim enhancement).

What are the histologic findings associated with mucinous carcinomas?

Mucinous carcinomas, also called colloid carcinomas, are a subtype of invasive ductal carcinoma characterized by aggregates of low-grade malignant cells floating in pools of mucin (Fig. 3.12L, M). The mucin-to-cell ratio varies from lesion to lesion, and this may explain some of the imaging variability seen with these lesions. Associated ductal carcinoma in situ may be seen in as many as 75% of patients, usually at the periphery of the lesion. These are usually diploid tumors with estrogen and progesterone receptors. Mucinous carcinomas represent 1% to 2% of all breast cancers.

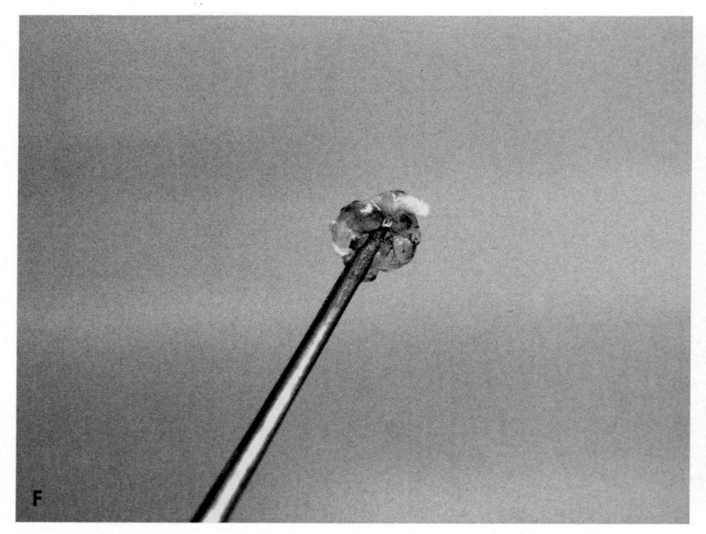

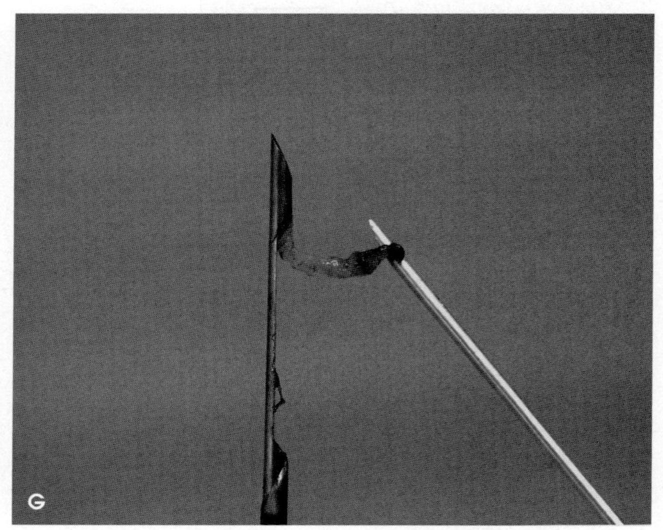

Figure 3.12. (*Continued*) Core samples **(F, G)** demonstrating the typical appearance of a mucinous lesion. The core is gelatinous, with a glassy, glistening appearance. This is in contrast with the stiff, usually white cores obtained through nonmucinous, malignant lesions.

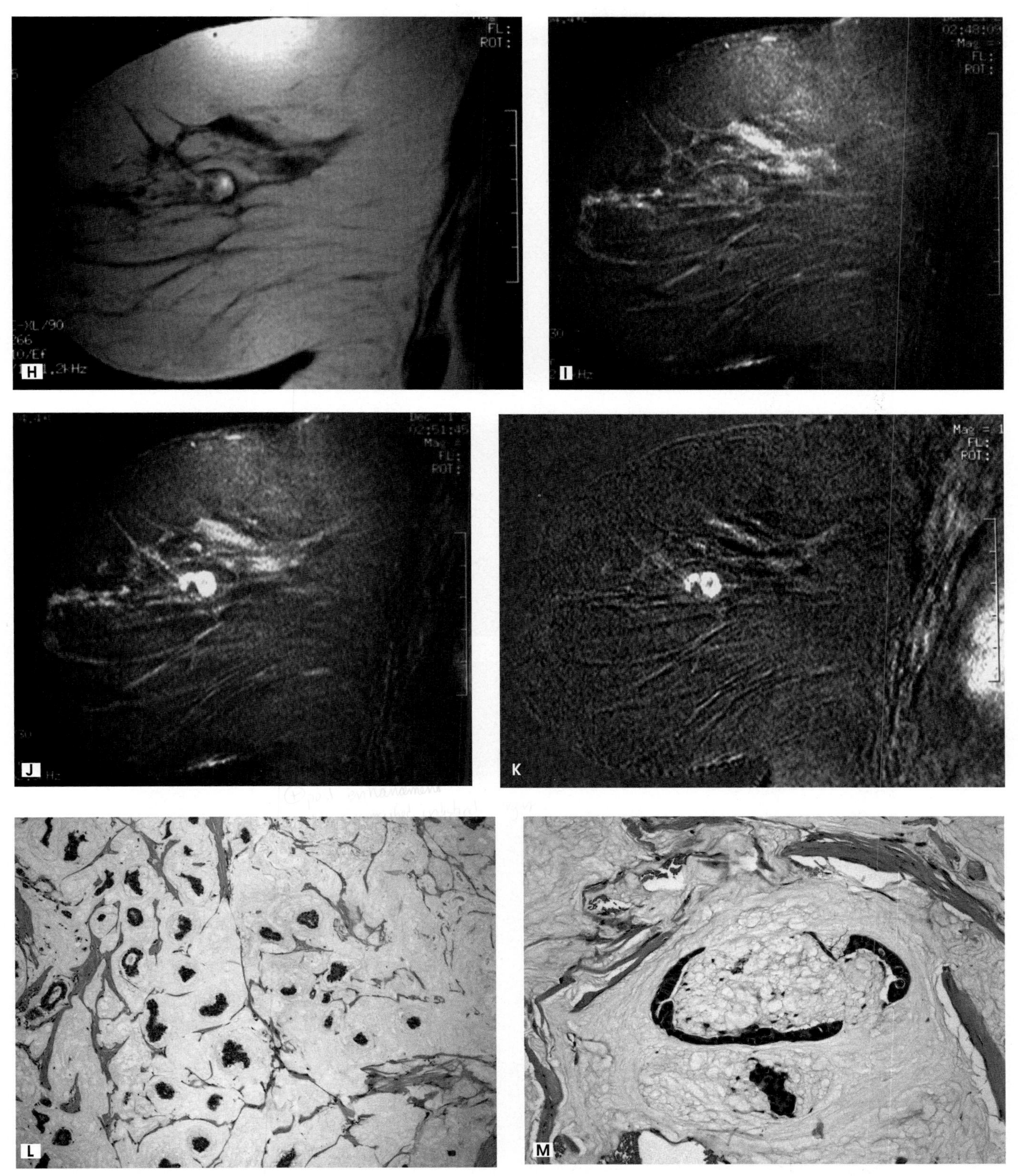

Figure 3.12. (*Continued*) Magnetic resonance imaging, T2-weighted sagittal image **(H)**, right breast. T1-weighted sagittal image **(I)**, right breast, precontrast. T1-weighted sagittal image **(J)**, right breast, 1 minute following an intravenous bolus of contrast, same tabletop position as shown in **(I)**. Subtraction image **(K)**, same tabletop position as **(I)**.Mucinous carcinoma in two different patients **(L, M)**. Clusters of low-grade malignant cells floating in pools of mucin separated by fibrous septa. The cellularity of the aggregates is variable within and among lesions.

PATIENT 13

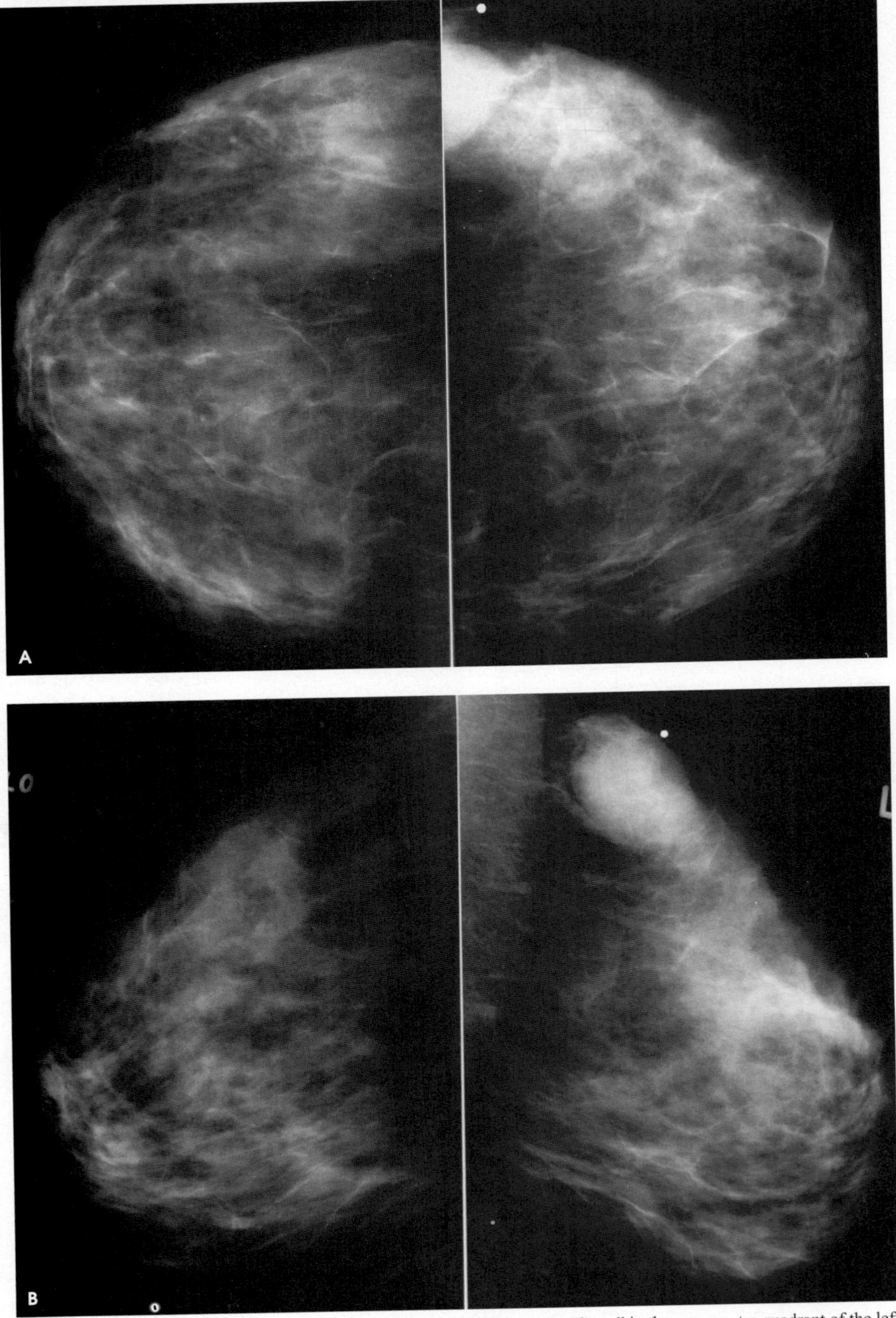

Figure 3.13. Diagnostic evaluation, 52-year-old patient presenting with a "lump" in the upper outer quadrant of the left breast (metallic BB marking "lump"). Craniocaudal **(A),** mediolateral oblique **(B)** views.

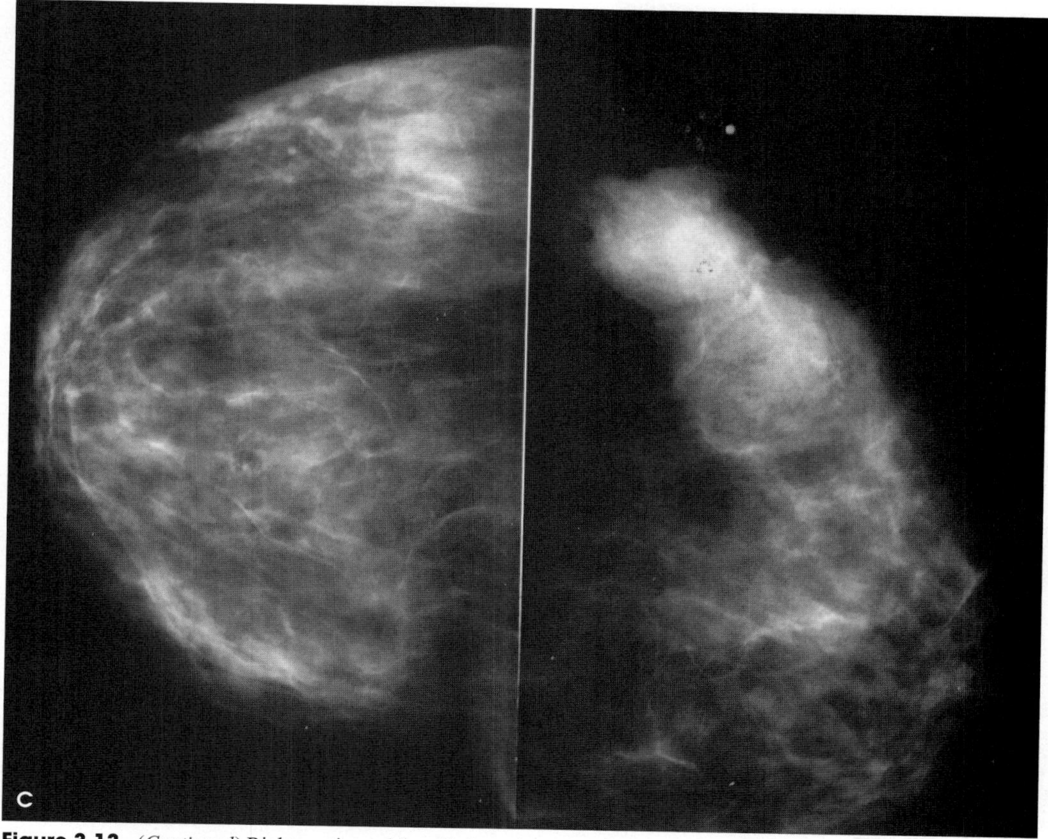

Figure 3.13. (*Continued*) Right craniocaudal and left craniocaudal view exaggerated laterally **(C)** views. Metallic BB is used by the technologist to mark the area of clinical concern.

What is your differential for the mammographic finding, and what would you do next?

An oval, well-circumscribed, 2.5-cm mass is imaged on the mediolateral oblique view, corresponding to the palpable abnormality. This is partially imaged on the routine left craniocaudal view but imaged in its entirety on the craniocaudal view exaggerated laterally. Diagnostic considerations for an oval-round mass in a 52-year-old woman include cyst, fibroadenoma (complex fibroadenoma, tubular adenoma), phyllodes tumor, focal fibrosis, pseudoangiomatous stromal hyperplasia (PASH), papilloma, abscess, postoperative/posttraumatic fluid collection, invasive ductal carcinoma not otherwise specified (NOS), mucinous carcinoma, medullary carcinoma, papillary carcinoma, apocrine carcinoma, adenoid cystic carcinoma, lymphoma, and metastatic carcinoma. A galactocele is unlikely in a 52-year-old woman. Physical examination and an ultrasound are done next to further characterize the mass.

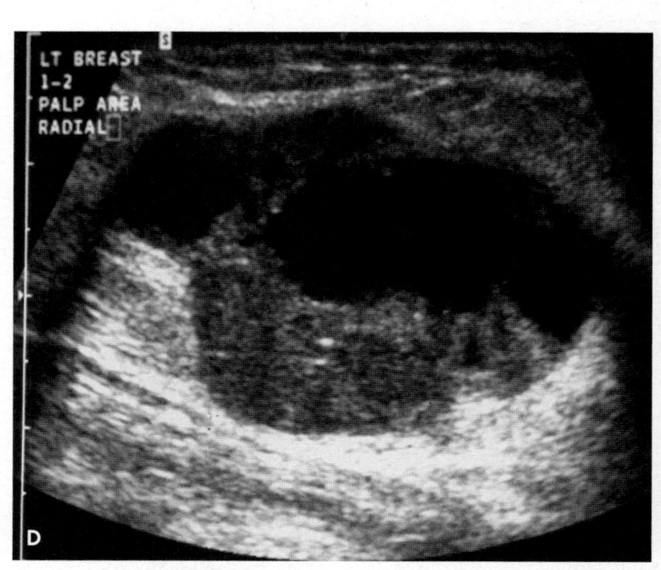

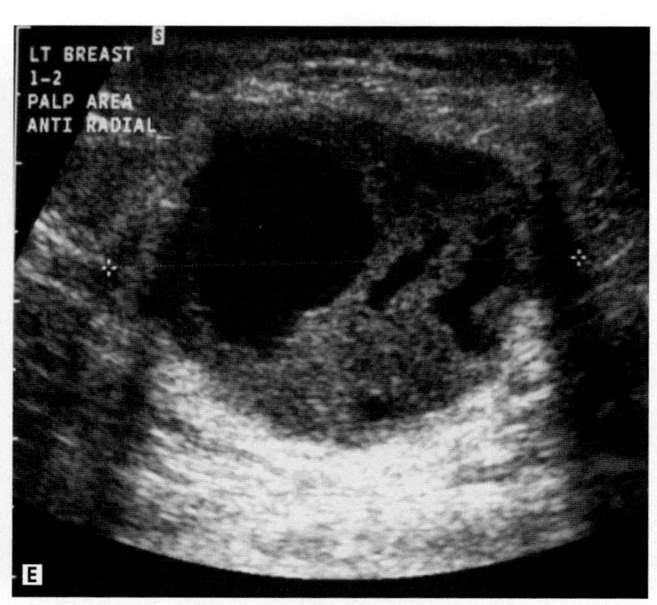

Figure 3.13. (*Continued*) Ultrasound images in radial **(D)** and antiradial **(E)** projections corresponding to the palpable mass in the upper outer quadrant of the left breast.

How would you describe the ultrasound findings in this patient?
What are your primary considerations now, and what is your recommendation for this patient?

On physical examination, a discrete, readily mobile, hard mass is palpated in the upper outer quadrant of the left breast. There is no skin discoloration. On ultrasound, a well-circumscribed complex cystic mass with posterior acoustic enhancement is imaged at the 1- to 2-o'clock position in the left breast. No history of surgery or trauma is elicited from the patient, and there is no associated tenderness when this area is palpated. The ultrasound eliminates the possibility of a simple cyst. With no history of surgery or trauma, this is unlikely to represent postoperative or posttraumatic fluid collection and, in the absence of significant tenderness or erythema, it is unlikely to represent an abscess. Given the age of the patient, the size of the lesion, and its complex appearance on ultrasound, mucinous carcinoma is unlikely. An invasive ductal carcinoma NOS with necrosis (given the complex cystic appearance sonographically) or a papillary lesion is the primary consideration at the time of the ultrasound-guided core biopsy.

BI-RADS® category 4: suspicious abnormality, biopsy should be considered. An invasive papillary carcinoma is diagnosed following the ultrasound-guided needle biopsy.

On MR, variable signal intensities are noted on the T2-weighted images (Fig. 3.13F, G). Following contrast administration, rapid nonuniform enhancement of the mass is noted on the T1-weighted images (Fig. 3.13 H, I).

What are the imaging features that may distinguish central from peripheral papillary carcinomas?

As with papillomas, papillary carcinomas are considered either central (i.e., subareolar) or peripheral. Patients with central papillary carcinomas usually present with a well-circumscribed mass in the subareolar area. The mass may be large enough to cause nipple displacement and overlying skin stretching. Some patients may have associated nipple discharge. A complex cystic mass is commonly seen on ultrasound. Bloody fluid is often obtained on aspiration. Patients with peripheral papillary carcinomas can present with one or multiple masses with well-circumscribed to ill-defined but not usually spiculated margins. Solid, hypoechoic or complex cystic masses are imaged on ultrasound. Papillary carcinomas represent approximately 1% to 2% of all breast cancers and are characterized by in-situ and invasive variants.

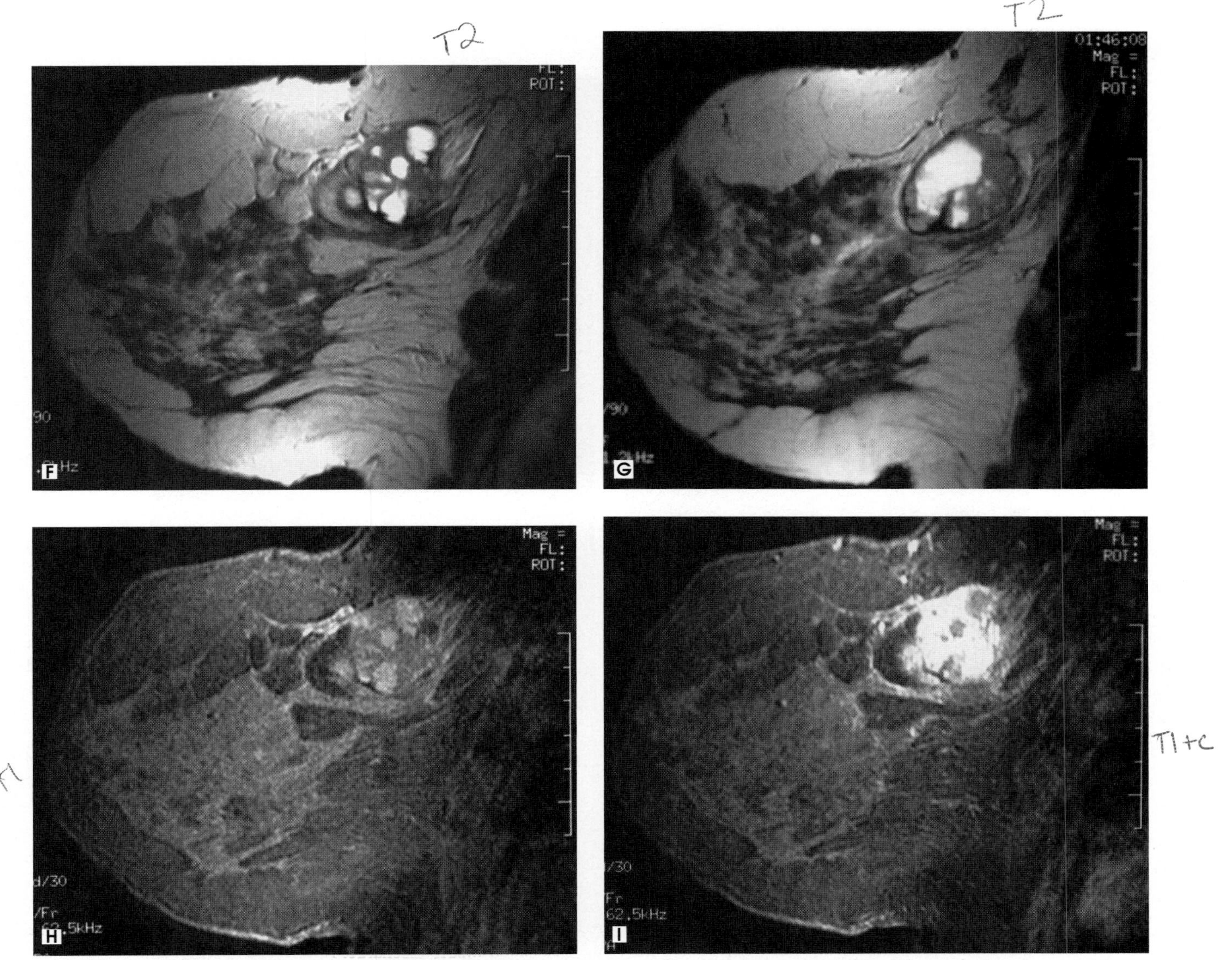

Figure 3.13. Magnetic resonance imaging, T2-weighted sagittal images **(F, G)** at two different tabletop positions. T1-weighted sagittal image **(H),** left breast, precontrast. T1-weighted sagittal image **(I),** left breast, at the same tabletop position as **(H),** 1 minute following bolus intravenous administration of contrast.

PATIENT 14

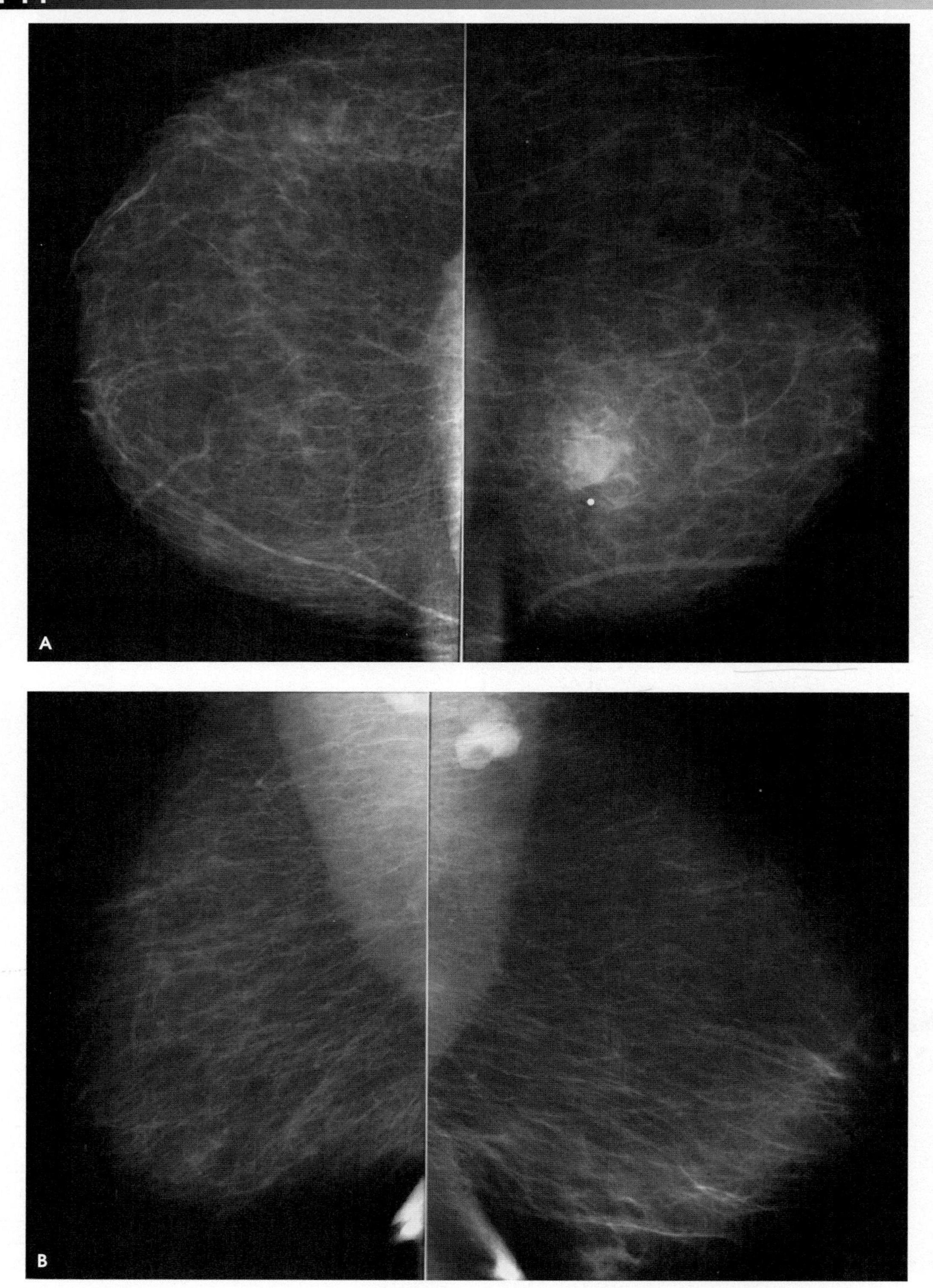

Figure 3.14. Diagnostic evaluation, 51-year-old patient presenting with a "lump" in the left breast. Craniocaudal **(A)** and mediolateral oblique **(B)** views with a metallic BB at the site of concern to the patient.

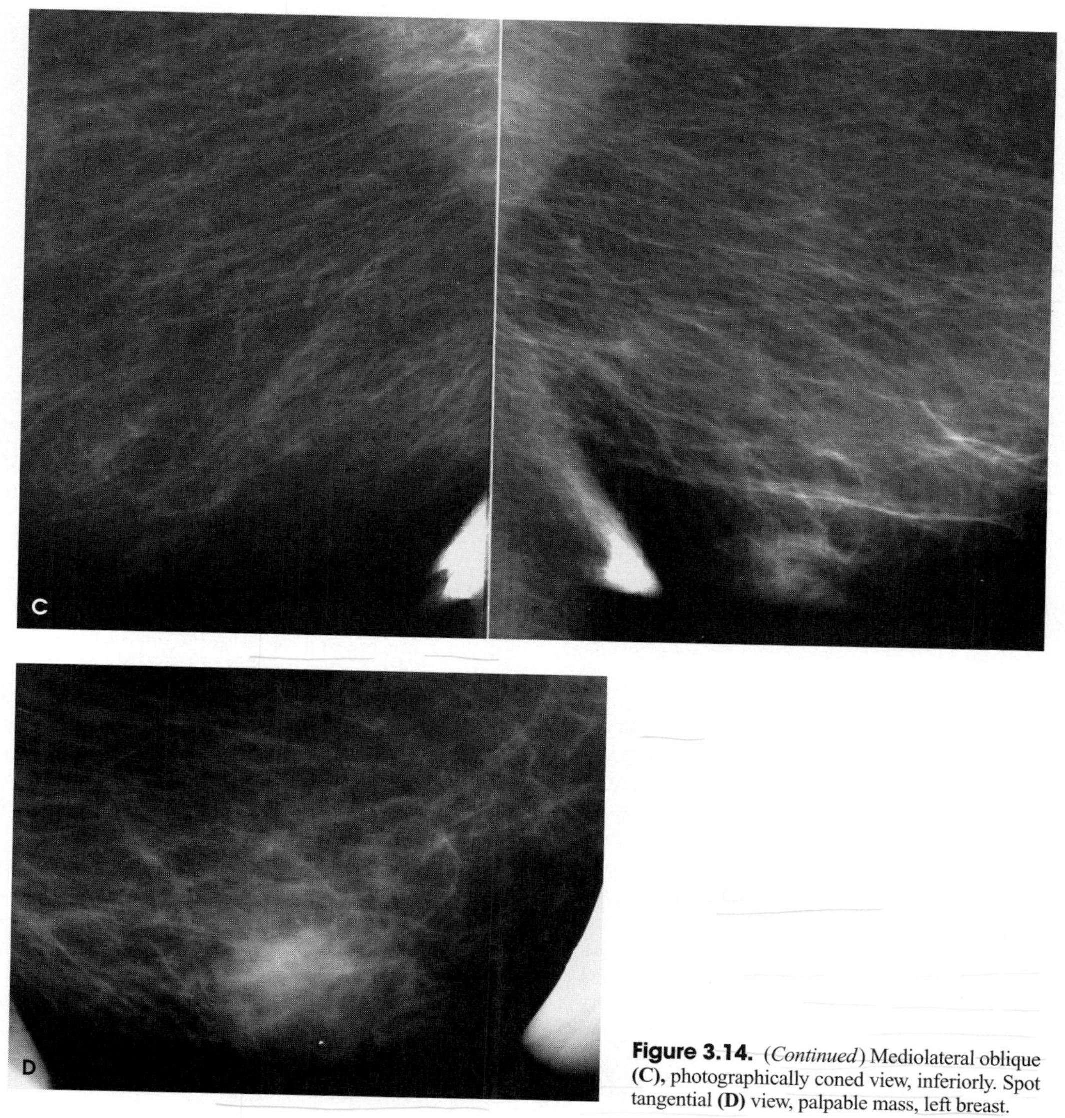

Figure 3.14. (*Continued*) Mediolateral oblique **(C)**, photographically coned view, inferiorly. Spot tangential **(D)** view, palpable mass, left breast.

How would you describe the finding, and what is your differential?
What will you ask the patient, and what will you be looking for when you examine her and do the ultrasound?

A mass with indistinct and ill-defined margins is imaged, corresponding to the area of concern to the patient. Prominence of the surrounding trabecular margins is also noted. A well-circumscribed, dense lymph node is present inferiorly in the left axilla. It retains a fatty hilar region, and comparison with prior studies would be helpful in assessing any change in size and overall density. On the mammographic findings alone, differential considerations include inflamed cyst, abscess, posttraumatic/postoperative fluid collection, invasive ductal carcinoma not otherwise specified, mucinous carcinoma, medullary carcinoma, papillary carcinoma, lymphoma, and metastatic disease. Given its proximity to the skin on the spot tangential view, an inflamed sebaceous cyst is also included in the differential. A galactocele is unlikely in a 51-year-old woman unless there has been a pregnancy with lactation within the last several preceding years. The patient should be asked questions relative to associated symptoms (e.g., "heat" overlying the area, tenderness, general malaise, or recent trauma to this site). Before starting the ultrasound, examine the skin for erythema, ecchymosis, or a prominent skin pore possibly associated with a sebaceous cyst. Compare the skin temperature overlying this area with the corresponding area on the contralateral breast.

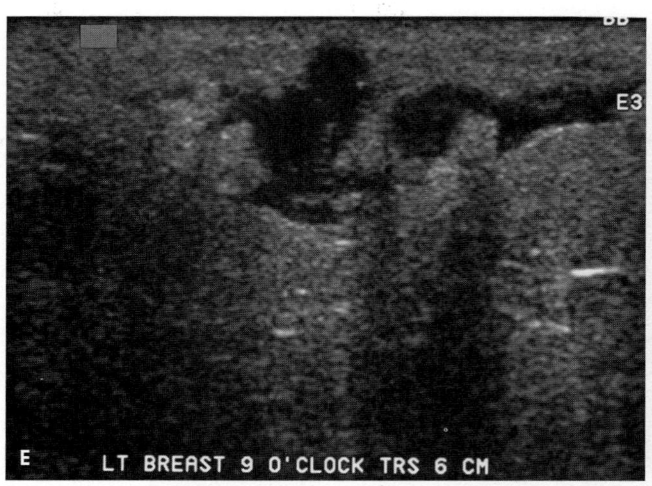

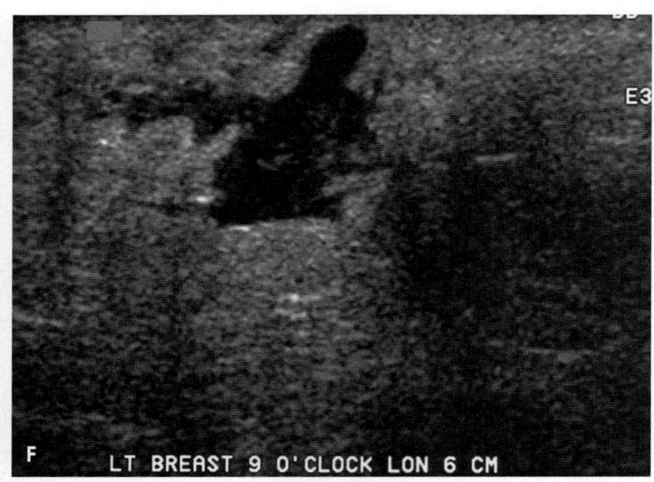

Figure 3.14. Ultrasound images in transverse (TRS) **(E)** and longitudinal (LON) **(F)** projections at the site of concern to the patient, left breast, medially.

How would you describe the ultrasound findings? What is your working diagnosis, and what would you recommend?

On physical examination, there is a small patch of erythema overlying the mass, and this area is warmer than the comparable area on the contralateral breast. The mass is not associated with skin because it can be moved independently of the skin (i.e., it is not a sebaceous cyst). Some tenderness is elicited on deep palpation. There is no history of trauma or surgery. On ultrasound, the tissue is hyperechoic with associated irregular fluid collections at the 9 o'clock position, 6 cm from the left nipple. Normal tissue architecture is disrupted. Given the clinical, mammographic, and ultrasound findings, an abscess with an associated ongoing inflammatory process is the primary consideration. The patient is prescribed a course of antibiotics, with a follow-up ultrasound scheduled after completion of the antibiotic course.

The need for an aspiration for fluid evaluation (i.e., gram stain and culture) and to remove as much of the infected fluid as possible is something to consider in women in whom you suspect an ongoing inflammatory process. Acutely, in some of these patients, aspirations can be quite painful and often yield little fluid (even with an 18G or 16G needle). Nevertheless, depending on the size of individual fluid collections, an aspiration can be done; presumably, removing as much of the fluid as possible will improve the effectiveness of the antibiotics. In this patient, given the relatively small size of the mass and the presence of small fluid locules on ultrasound (as opposed to one single fluid collection), aspiration is not done.

With respect to inflammatory lesions in the breast, what are the two groups of nonlactating patients to consider and how do their clinical courses differ?

Traditionally, mastitis and abscesses are associated with lactating patients. Obstetricians manage this group of patients clinically, and imaging is not usually indicated. It is important to recognize, however, that nonlactating women of all ages can present with mastitis or a breast abscess. For women who are not lactating, consider two groups of patients with different presentations and clinical courses: those with peripheral mastitis or abscess and those with subareolar mastitis or abscess. Peripheral mastitis or abscess is seen in women of all ages and, although some patients may have an underlying condition such as diabetes that may predispose them to the infection, most are otherwise healthy individuals. Patients usually respond well, with complete resolution of symptoms and findings, following one or two courses of antibiotics. Recurrence following treatment is uncommon in these patients. In contrast, patients with subareolar mastitis or abscess are usually young (in their 30s) and heavy smokers. Acutely, some of these patients develop periareolar fistulas (Zuska's disease) that drain purulent material. Patients with subareolar abscesses can be difficult to treat effectively and recurrences following treatment, requiring surgical incision and drainage, are common, as is the development of contralateral subareolar abscess.

BI-RADS® category 2: benign finding. A follow-up ultrasound is scheduled in 3 weeks to confirm complete resolution of symptoms and findings. If symptoms persist and there are residual findings on the ultrasound, a second course of antibiotics is prescribed for some patients. Alternatively, if a larger fluid collection is identified sonographically at the time of the follow-up ultrasound, an aspiration may be done.

PATIENT 15

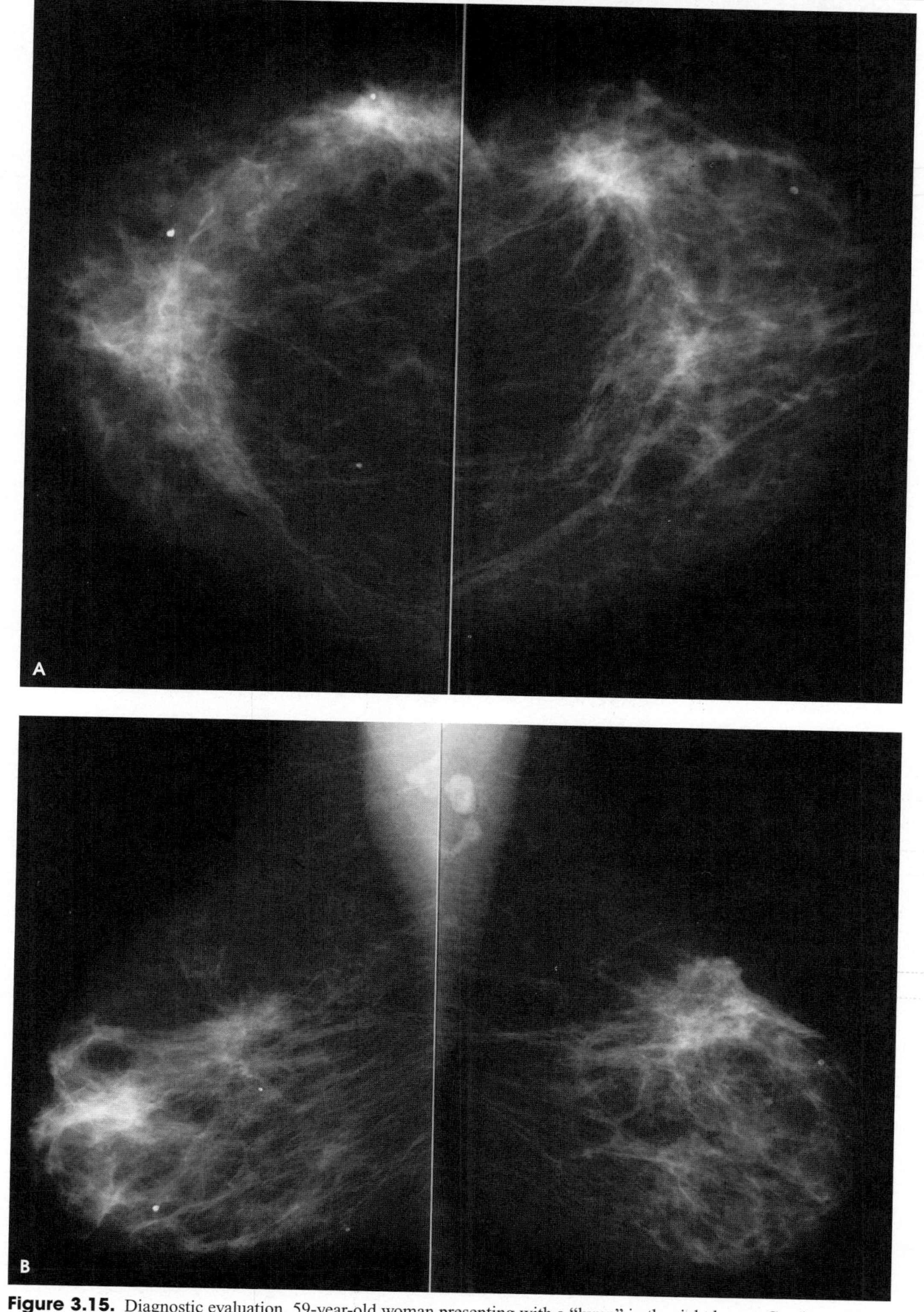

Figure 3.15. Diagnostic evaluation, 59-year-old woman presenting with a "lump" in the right breast. Craniocaudal **(A)** and mediolateral oblique **(B)** views; metallic BB placed at the site of the palpable finding.

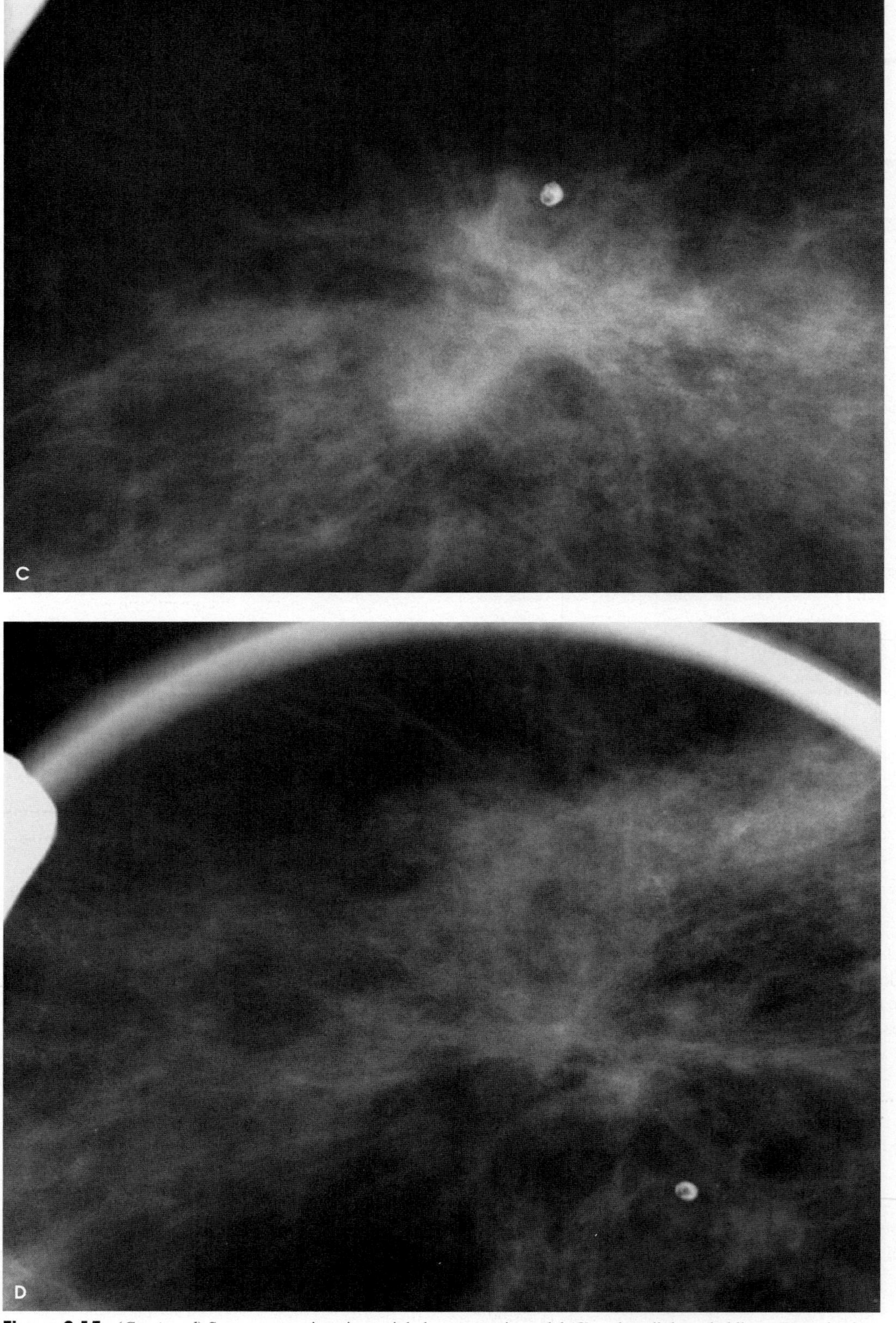

Figure 3.15. (*Continued*) Spot compression views, right breast, craniocaudal **(C)** and mediolateral oblique **(D)** projections.

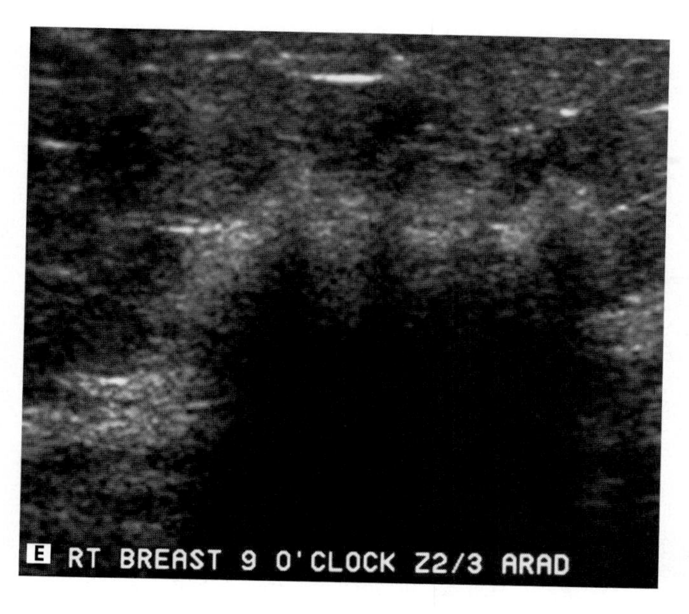

Figure 3.15. (*Continued*) Ultrasound image **(E)** of palpable finding, 9 o'clock position, zone 2/3 (Z2/3), right breast.

How would you describe the findings, and what is your differential?

An irregular mass with spiculation, associated distortion, and scattered punctate calcifications is present in the right breast, corresponding to the area of clinical concern. It is more prominent on the craniocaudal view. On physical examination, no definite mass is palpated; however, the tissue at the 9 o'clock position, 5 to 6 cm from the right nipple, is hard and thickened. On ultrasound, an irregular mass with an echogenic rim and significant shadowing measuring at least 4 cm is imaged, corresponding to the area of clinical concern. Given the lack of a discrete mass on physical examination, a more prominent appearance on the craniocaudal view, and the amount of shadowing seen on ultrasound, an invasive lobular carcinoma is a more likely diagnosis; however, invasive ductal carcinoma can present with similar findings. Possible benign considerations are limited but include an inflammatory process or diabetic fibrous mastopathy if the patient has a history of long-standing, insulin-dependent diabetes.

A biopsy is indicated. In planning for the biopsy, consider needle placement carefully. In my experience, these types of lesions with significant shadowing can be hard and often yield little or no tissue on one or more of the passes. Sometimes the inner portion of the needle advances into the mass but the outer sheath does not follow because it cannot cut through the tissue adequately. In targeting these lesions, I aim for the edges of the lesion as opposed to trying to advance the needle into the area of shadowing and, depending on the appearance of the tissue obtained, I will make extra passes as needed to obtain one or two solid tissue cores.

So, are we done with this patient? Do you have any additional observations? How about the left breast?

Remember, when presented with obvious clinical and mammographic findings, focus away from them and evaluate the remainder of the mammogram. Did you notice the irregular mass with associated spiculation and distortion in the left breast (comparable location to that on the right)? The patient has bilateral lesions, requiring biopsy (this information is also factored in when considering invasive lobular carcinoma as the likely diagnosis).

Following ultrasound-guided core biopsies, invasive lobular carcinomas are diagnosed bilaterally. Multicentric (5.5-cm and 3-cm foci) invasive lobular carcinoma with associated lymphovascular space involvement is diagnosed following a right simple mastectomy. Metastatic disease is identified in one excised right axillary lymph node [pT3, pN1, pMX; Stage IIIA]. A 4.5-cm invasive lobular carcinoma with associated lymphovascular space involvement is diagnosed in the left breast following a simple mastectomy. Metastatic disease is diagnosed in 8 of 14 excised left axillary lymph nodes [pT2, pN2, pMX; Stage IIIA].

What are the clinical, mammographic, and sonographic findings associated with invasive lobular carcinoma?

Invasive lobular carcinoma is the second most common type of breast cancer, with a reported incidence of 5% to 15%. The incidence of this tumor type varies with patient age: It is uncommon in premenopausal women and increases in frequency with advancing age. Multifocality and bilaterality (synchronous or metachronous) should be considered in patients diagnosed with invasive lobular carcinoma. Clinically, a discrete mass may be palpated; however, it is more common to palpate an area of thickening (described by some as "induration"), which in some patients can be subtle.

A spiculated mass is the most common mammographic finding in women with invasive lobular carcinoma, occurring in close to 40% of patients. Parenchymal asymmetry and distortion are the next most common mammographic findings. These changes may be more apparent in one projection, commonly the craniocaudal view. Diffuse changes include a progressive shrinkage of the involved breast or, alternatively, diffuse enlargement and reduced compressibility of the involved breast may be seen. Invasive lobular carcinoma rarely presents as a round or oval mass. Likewise, when an invasive lobular carcinoma is diagnosed following biopsies done for microcalcifications, the calcifications are usually not found in association with the invasive lesion. The calcifications are found in benign changes such as fibrocystic changes, fibroadenoma, and sclerosing adenosis, and the invasive lobular carcinoma is an incidental finding.

Solid masses with irregular, spiculated, and angular margins are seen on ultrasound. Subtle distortion may be the only finding on ultrasound. In some lesions (such as the one presented here), significant shadowing is seen associated with the lesion. In our experience, some of the most striking shadowing seen is associated with invasive lobular carcinomas.

How accurately does mammography predict tumor extent in patients with invasive lobular carcinoma?

Having described the imaging presentation of invasive lobular carcinoma, it is important to emphasize that invasive lobular carcinoma can be subtle clinically, mammographically, sonographically, and pathologically (I refer to it as the "sleaze disease"). The extent of disease is often underestimated clinically, mammographically, and sonographically. In our own patients, metastatic disease to the axilla is seen in as many as 60% of patients at the time of presentation.

What are the distinguishing histologic features of these lesions?

Histologically, small monomorphic cells infiltrating the stroma in single files characterize these lesions. The cells infiltrate the tissue insidiously, invoking little or no desmoplastic reaction (this likely reflects the subtle imaging changes associated with some of these lesions). In a significant number of patients, lobular neoplasia (i.e., lobular carcinoma in situ), although not considered as a precursor or premalignant lesion, is seen in the tissue surrounding invasive lobular carcinoma. Invasive lobular carcinomas often express estrogen and progesterone receptors; rarely, the HER-2/neu oncoprotein is expressed.

PATIENT 16

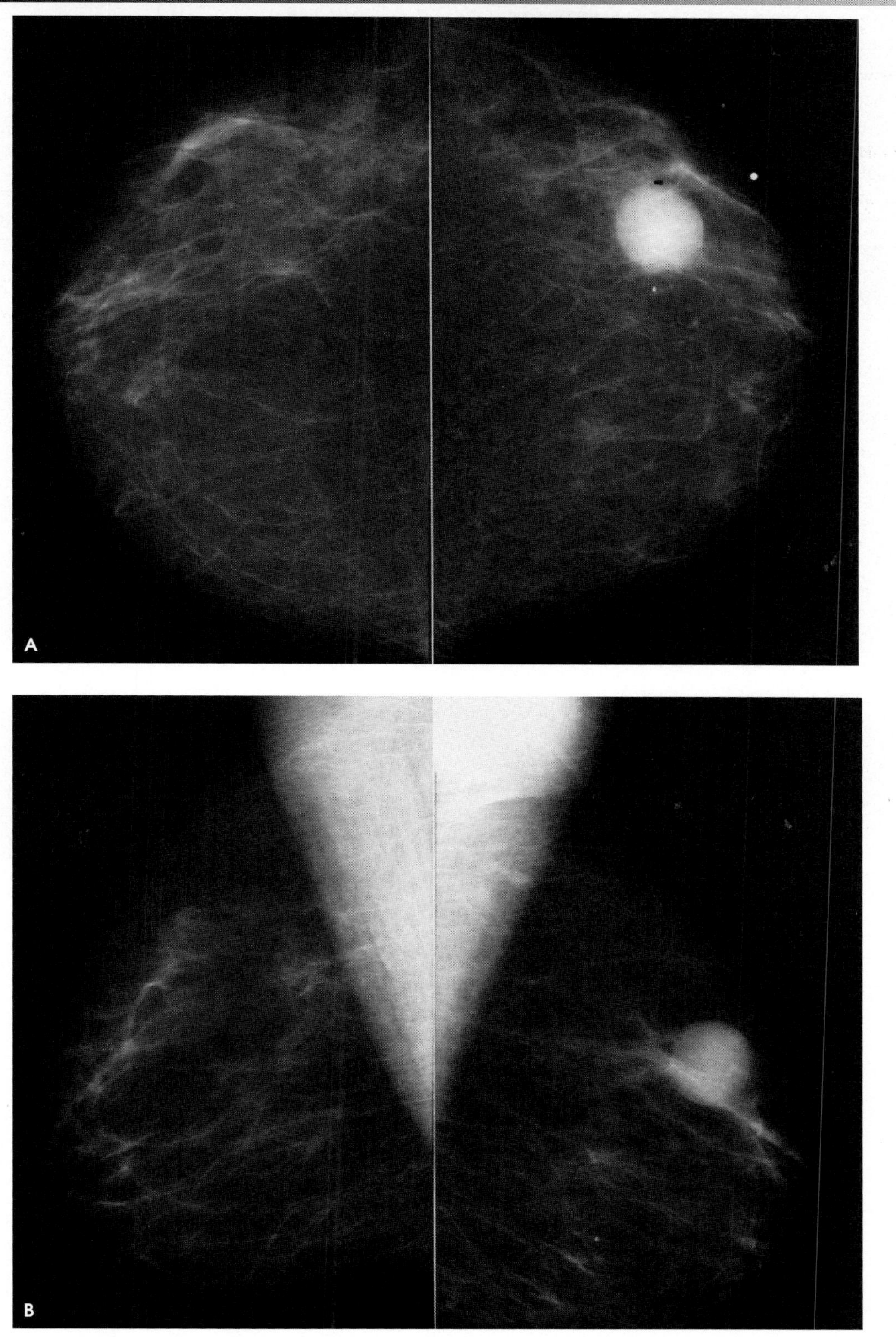

Figure 3.16. Diagnostic evaluation, 53-year-old patient presenting with a "lump" in the left breast. Craniocaudal **(A)** and mediolateral oblique **(B)** views, metallic BB at site of "lump," left craniocaudal view.

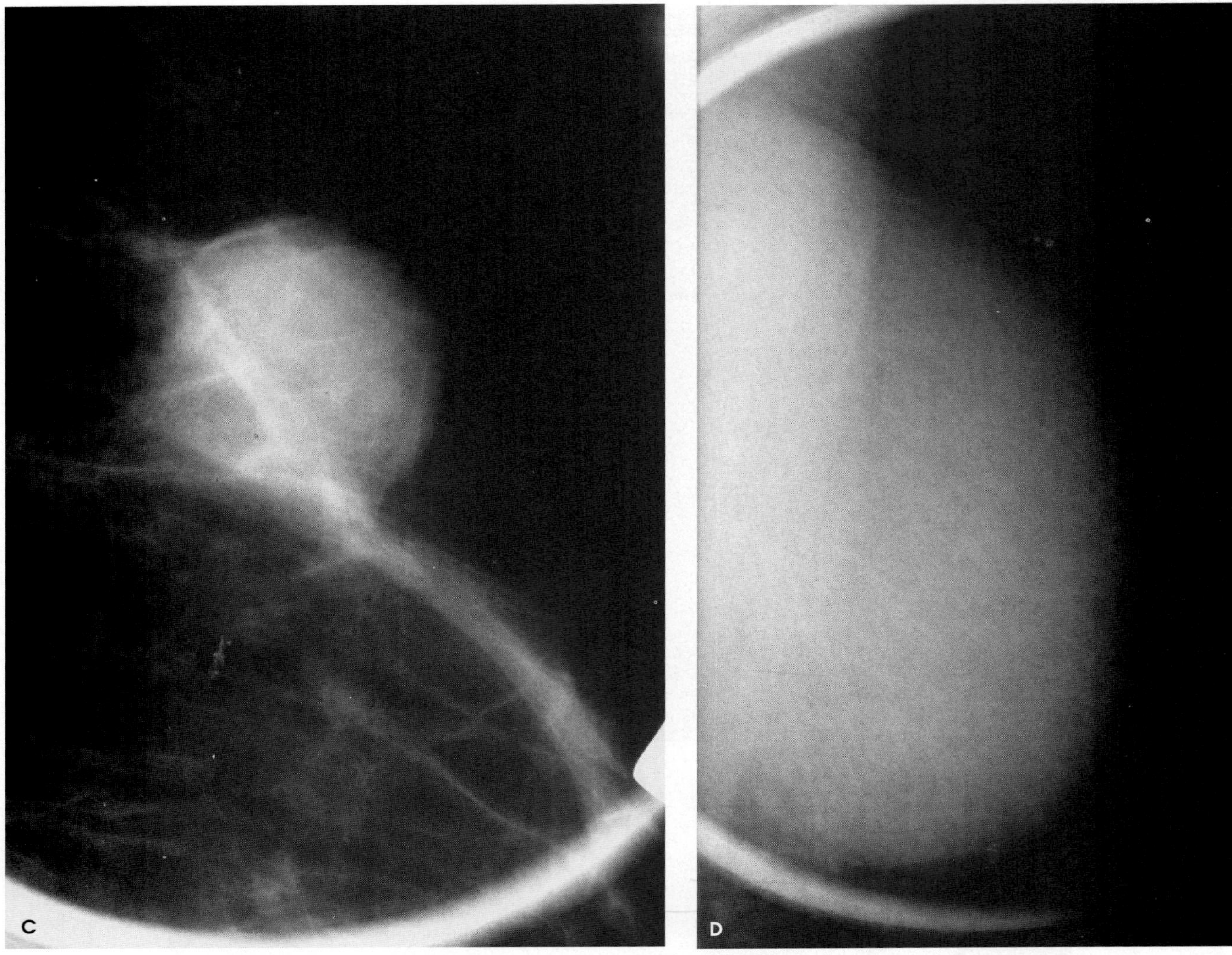

Figure 3.16. (*Continued*) Spot tangential **(C)** view, left breast mass. Axillary **(D)** view, left axilla.

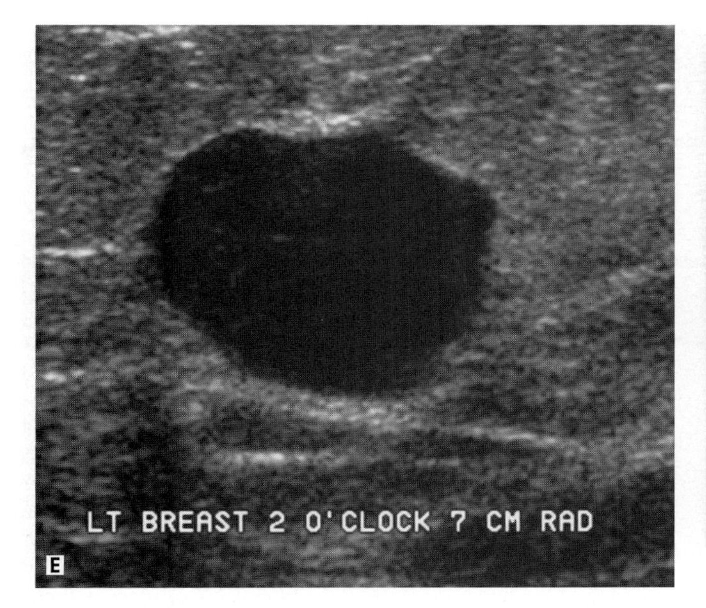

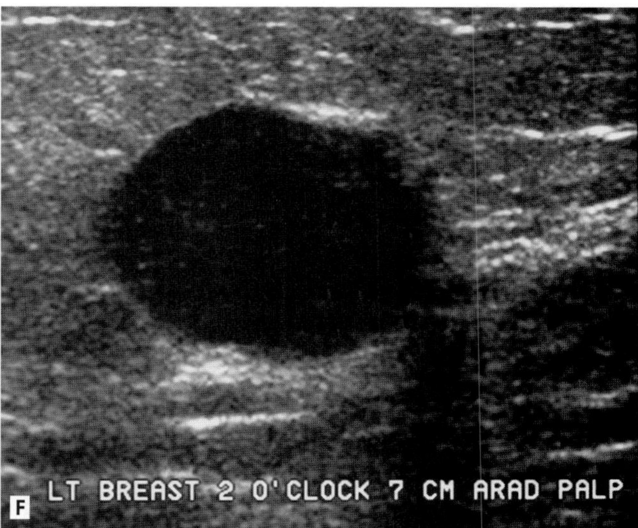

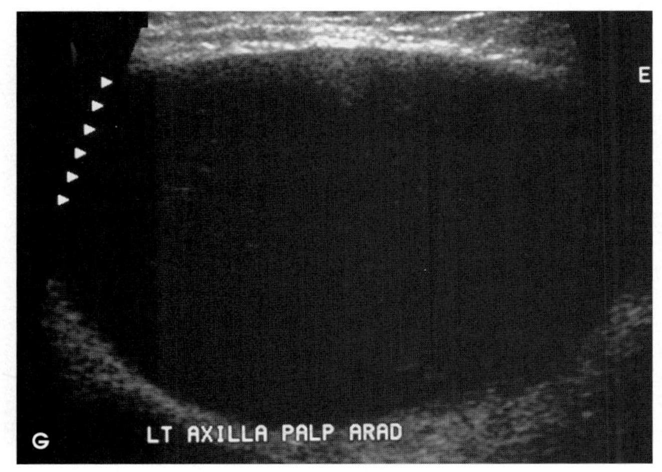

Figure 3.16. Ultrasound images in radial (RAD) **(E)** and antiradial (ARAD) **(F)** projections of the mass in the left breast. Ultrasound image **(G)** of the mass in the left axilla.

How would you describe the findings, and what is your differential?

A round 1.5-cm mass with partially circumscribed and indistinct margins is imaged in the left breast, corresponding to the area of concern to the patient. An additional mass measuring at least 3 cm is partially imaged in the left axilla. Given this constellation of findings, the differential is limited. Malignant possibilities include an invasive ductal carcinoma not otherwise specified, with metastatic disease to the axilla. Given the margins and shape of the breast mass and the presence of axillary adenopathy, this is likely to be poorly differentiated. In premenopausal women with a round mass, medullary carcinoma is the primary subtype of invasive ductal carcinoma to consider. Papillary and mucinous carcinomas also present as round masses, but they are more common in older, postmenopausal women. Alternatively, this could represent lymphoma. An inflammatory process with abscess formation in the breast and reactive adenopathy in the axilla is a possible benign diagnostic consideration. Physical examination and an ultrasound are indicated.

How would you describe the findings? Do you think this could be a cyst?

On physical examination, a hard mass is palpated at the 2 o'clock position, 7 cm from the left nipple; a hard, fixed mass is also palpated in the left axilla. No skin changes are noted, and no tenderness is elicited on palpation. A round, well-circumscribed, markedly hypoechoic mass with some posterior acoustic enhancement is imaged corresponding to the palpable finding in the breast, and a 4-cm, well-circumscribed, markedly hypoechoic (nearly anechoic) mass is imaged in the left axilla. Although you might be tempted to say that the mass in the axilla could be a cyst, it is important to recognize that abnormal, enlarged axillary lymph nodes can be nearly anechoic in some patients.

What is your recommendation?

A malignant process has to be the leading consideration in this patient, so biopsies of the left breast and axillary masses are indicated.

BI-RADS® category 5: highly suggestive of malignancy—appropriate action should be taken.

Appropriate action is taken, and a medullary carcinoma with metastatic disease to the left axilla is diagnosed following core biopsies of the breast and axillary masses. The patient is treated with neoadjuvant therapy.

What are the clinical and imaging findings associated with medullary carcinoma?

Medullary carcinomas are a described subtype of invasive ductal carcinoma. When strict histologic criteria are used to classify these lesions, they represent <2% of all breast cancers. Clinically, they present most commonly as a palpable mass that is often described by the patient as developing rapidly. Mammographically, these are commonly round or oval masses with margins that can range from well circumscribed to ill-defined; however, they are not usually spiculated. On ultrasound, they are moderately to markedly hypoechoic (they may simulate a cyst) and may demonstrate some posterior acoustic enhancement. Because these tumors may have areas of necrosis, you may obtain bloody material if you attempt an aspiration; however, a residual solid component will remain, so a core biopsy can be also be done.

What histologic findings are described for medullary carcinoma?

These tumors are described as having nests of large, high-nuclear-grade epithelial cells forming a syncytial pattern and lacking a significant amount of surrounding stroma. The nuclei are pleomorphic, and a high number of mitotic figures are present. The tumors are surrounded by a significant infiltrate of lymphocytes and plasma cells. Ductal carcinoma in situ is not usually an associated finding. Given the locally aggressive nature of these lesions, areas of necrotic tumor may be present histologically. Presumably, the vascular supply is outstripped by the rapid growth of the tumor. Many of these tumors are estrogen and progesterone receptor negative.

PATIENT 17

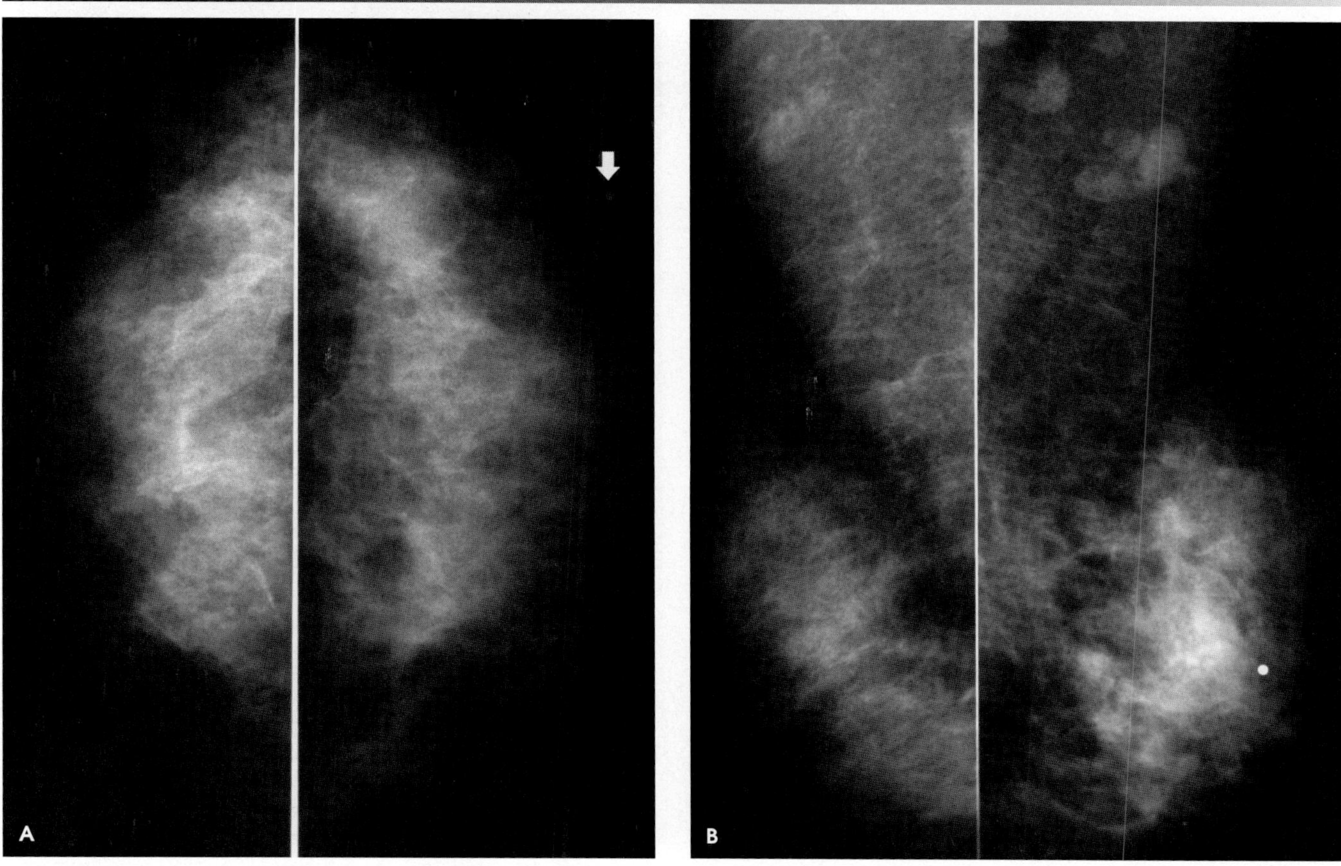

Figure 3.17. Diagnostic evaluation, 51-year-old patient presenting with a "lump" and thickening of the left breast. Craniocaudal **(A)** and mediolateral oblique **(B)** views with a metallic BB (*arrow* on CC view) used at the site of concern to the patient. Technical factors used for the exposures are as follows:

Factor	RTCC	LTCC	RTMLO	LTMLO
kV	26	31	26	27
mAs	296	293	269	439
Comp (mm)	63	76	60	68

What do you think, and how would you describe the findings?

The overall density of the left breast is increased and the breast appears larger than the right. As evidenced by the millimeters of compression used, the left breast is less compressible than the right. These observations are confirmed and supported by the technical factors used for adequate exposures. Although the kilovoltage used for the left mediolateral oblique (MLO) view is increased by one compared to that used for the right breast, the resulting milliamperage is much higher on the left MLO. In comparison, when the kilovoltage is increased to 31 kV for the left craniocaudal (CC) view, the resulting milliamperage is comparable to that noted for the CC and MLO views of the right breast. Also noted are slightly more prominent axillary lymph nodes in the left axilla compared to those in the right axilla.

What diagnostic possibilities are you considering at this point?
What would you recommend?

Differential considerations for usually unilateral, although rarely bilateral, diffuse changes include radiation therapy effect, inflammatory changes (e.g., mastitis), trauma, ipsilateral axillary adenopathy with lymphatic obstruction, dialysis shunt in the ipsilateral arm with fluid overload, invasive ductal carcinoma not otherwise specified, inflammatory carcinoma, invasive lobular carcinoma, or lymphoma. Invasive lobular carcinoma can lead to increases in breast density and size or a decrease in breast size (the shrinking breast). Differential considerations for usually bilateral, although sometimes unilateral, diffuse changes include hormone replacement therapy (e.g., estrogen), weight changes, congestive heart failure, renal failure with fluid overload, and superior vena cava syndrome. Additional rare benign causes include granulomatous mastitis, coumadin necrosis, arteritis, and autoimmune disorders (e.g., scleroderma). Obtaining a thorough history, examining the patient, and doing an ultrasound are often helpful in sorting through the differential considerations.

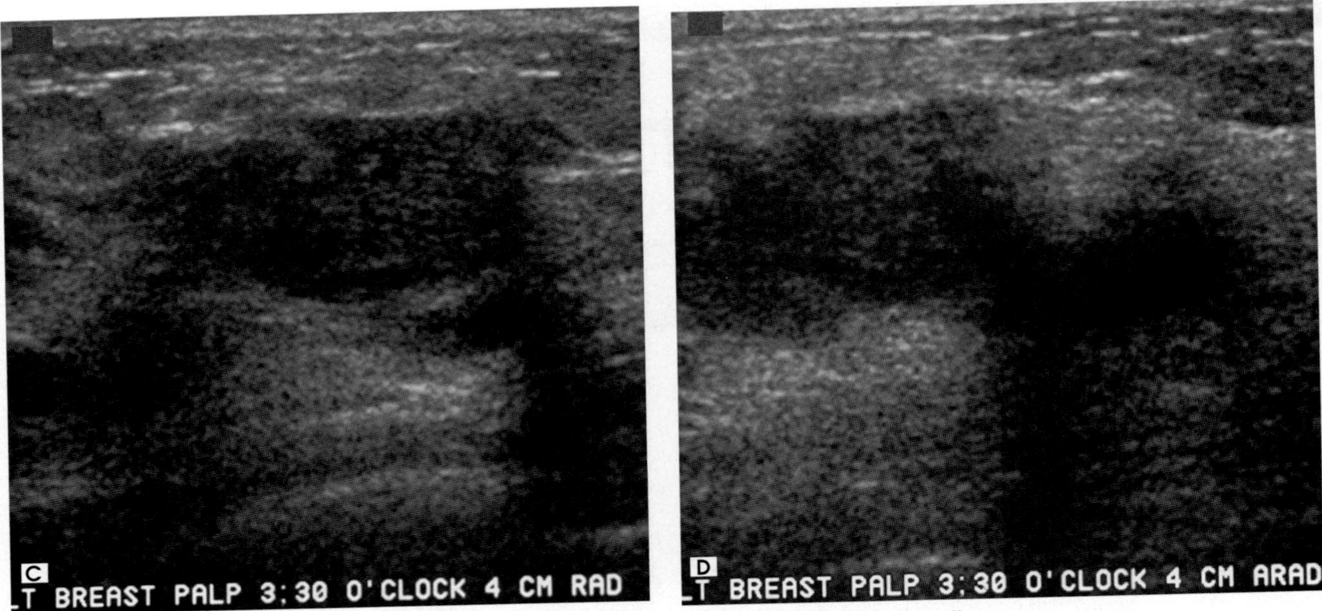

Figure 3.17. Ultrasound images, radial (RAD) **(C)** and antiradial (ARAD) **(D)** projections, left breast laterally.

How would you describe the ultrasound findings?

An irregular area of hypoechogenicity, with associated areas of enhancement and shadowing, is imaged at the 3:30 o'clock position 4 cm from the left nipple. Some tenderness is elicited during the ultrasound study, but there is no erythema, increased warmth, or *peau d'orange* change. No other relevant clinical history is elicited (no history of trauma, radiation therapy, or other known medical problems). The clinical and imaging findings do not provide a definite benign etiology; rather they are of concern for a possible malignancy.

BI-RADS® category 4: suspicious abnormality—biopsy should be considered.

An ultrasound-guided core biopsy is done. A severe mastitis with features suggestive of abscess formation is diagnosed on the core biopsy. Surgical incision and drainage is undertaken following incomplete resolution of symptoms and findings after two courses of antibiotics. No malignancy is diagnosed on excised tissue taken at the time of the surgical drainage, and the patient had an uncomplicated post-operative course with complete resolution of symptoms.

What diagnosis has to be pursued aggressively in patients with this type of presentation?

Given the clinical and mammographic presentation of this patient, inflammatory carcinoma is the main diagnostic consideration. Inflammatory carcinoma represents $<1\%$ of all breast cancers, and patients usually present acutely with rapidly developing symptoms that simulate those of an inflammatory process. Inflammatory carcinoma is primarily a clinical diagnosis considered in patients who present describing the rapid development of diffuse breast changes including warmth, heaviness, thickening, skin changes consistent with edema (*peau d'orange*) and redness of the breast. Although there may be some tenderness, this is not usually a significant component. Axillary adenopathy is present in $>50\%$ of patients with inflammatory carcinoma at the time of presentation. The diagnosis of inflammatory carcinoma can sometimes be delayed as patients are treated repeatedly with antibiotics. If symptoms do not resolve, or worsen, on antibiotics, the diagnosis of an inflammatory carcinoma needs to be pursued aggressively. A skin biopsy is often done to establish the diagnosis. However, if focal findings are identified on ultrasound, an ultrasound-guided biopsy can also be helpful in establishing the diagnosis. Because adenopathy reflecting metastatic disease is common in women with inflammatory carcinoma, the axilla should be scanned, and either a fine-needle aspiration or a core biopsy can be done if a potentially abnormal lymph node is identified.

In patients with inflammatory carcinoma, the compressibility of the breast is significantly decreased, the density of the parenchyma is increased, and associated skin thickening leads to significant difficulties in obtaining an adequate exposure mammographically (two layers of thickened skin now need to be penetrated for adequate exposure of the parenchyma). On ultrasound, skin thickening, disruption of the normal tissue architecture, increased echogenicity of the tissue (consistent with hyperemia), and dilated subcutaneous lymphatic vessels can be seen. In a small number of women, one or more masses may be identified in the involved breast. A poorly differentiated invasive ductal carcinoma, with associated tumor emboli in dilated dermal lymphatics, is the most common finding in women with inflammatory carcinoma. The presence of tumor in dilated lymphatics is identified in approximately 80% of women with clinical signs and symptoms of inflammatory carcinoma.

PATIENT 18

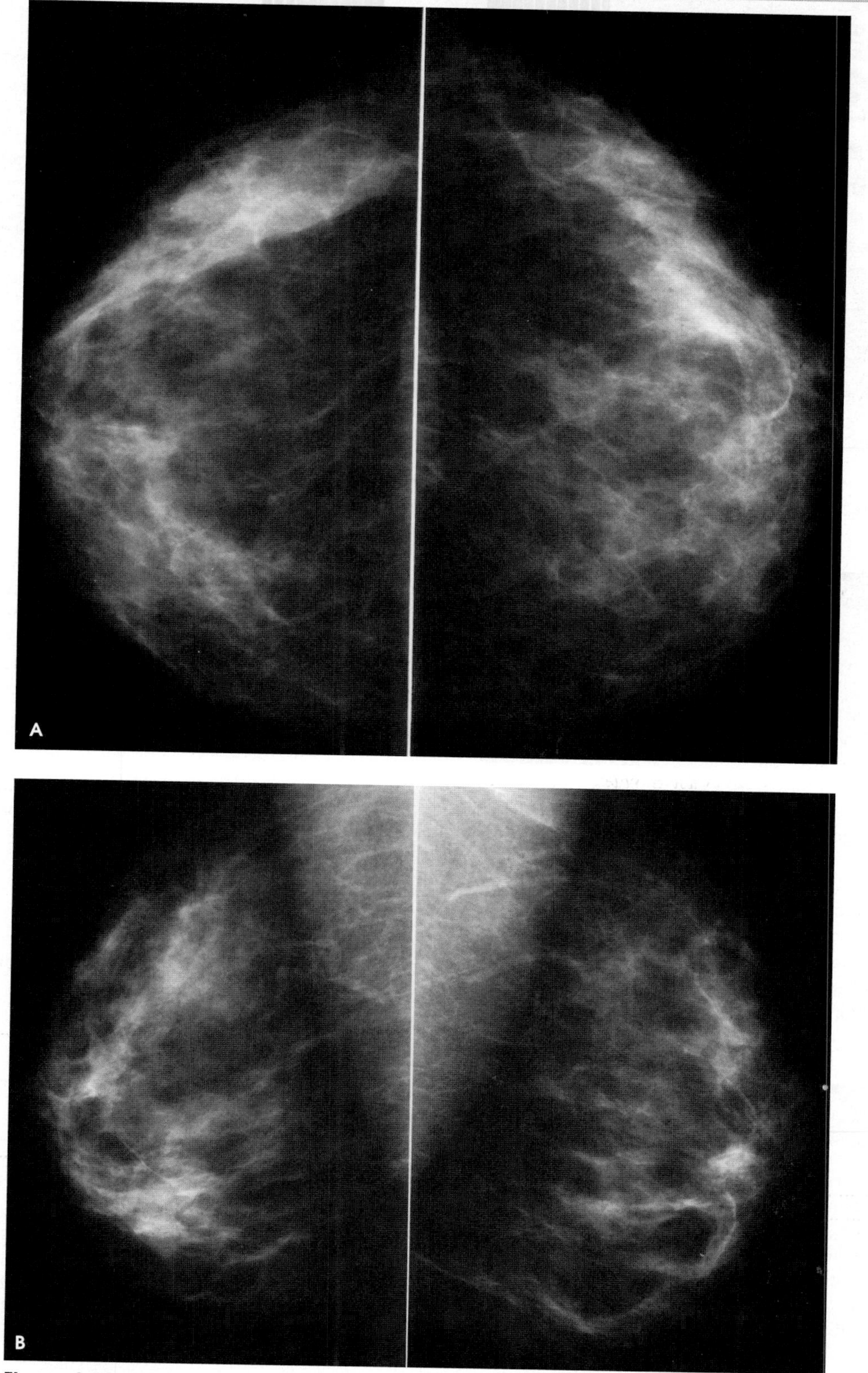

Figure 3.18. Diagnostic evaluation, 37-year-old patient presenting with a "lump" in the left breast. Craniocaudal **(A)** and mediolateral oblique **(B)** views.

At this point, what can you say and with what degree of certainty?
What else would you tell the technologist to do?

No abnormality is apparent on the craniocaudal (CC) and mediolateral oblique (MLO) views. In women over the age of 30 years who present with a "lump" or other focal symptom (focal pain, skin changes, etc.), a metallic BB is placed at the site of focal concern and CC and MLO views, as well as a spot tangential view at the site of the focal abnormality, are done. A unilateral study of the symptomatic breast is done, if the patient has had a mammogram within the last 6 months. Based on these initial images, additional spot compression or double spot compression magnification views may be done. Depending on the location of the focal finding, and the appearance of this area on the spot tangential view, correlative physical examination and an ultrasound are usually indicated. The ultrasound may be deferred in patients in whom there is no chance the lesion has been excluded from the field of view and completely fatty tissue or a benign lesion (e.g., an oil cyst) is imaged, corresponding to the area of concern.

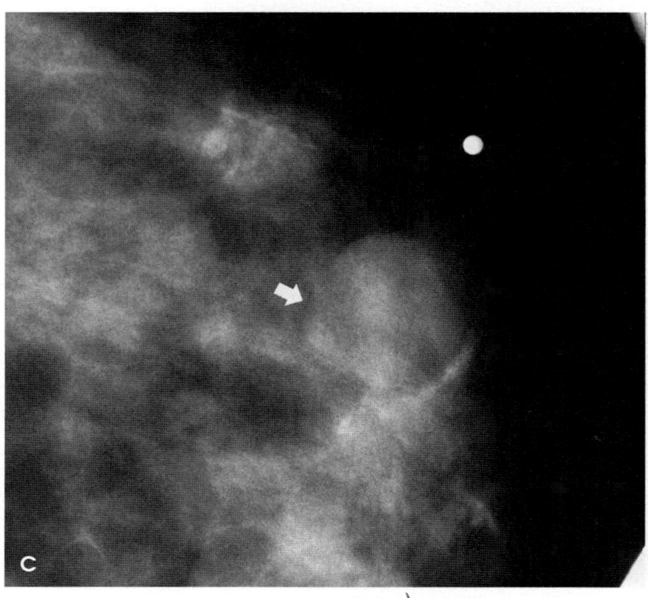

Figure 3.18. (*Continued*) Spot tangential **(C)** view done at the site of the palpable finding in the upper outer quadrant of the left breast.

At this point, what can you say and what is your differential?

A 1-cm, round mass with well-circumscribed margins is demonstrated on the spot tangential view. A partial halo sign is seen (arrow, Fig. 3.18C). The halo sign, defined as a 1- to 2-mm sharp radiolucency partially or completely outlining a mass, is a good sign that a lesion is benign. The halo sign is as good a sign that a lesion is benign as spiculation is a sign of malignancy. Some lesions demonstrating a halo sign turn out to be malignant, but most are not; some spiculated masses turn out to be benign, but most are not. The halo sign is thought to reflect a rapidly growing lesion, most commonly a cyst or a fibroadenoma (consequently, it can be seen with the more rapidly growing malignant lesions). Other benign considerations in this patient include tubular adenoma, papilloma, pseudoangiomatous stromal hyperplasia (PASH), focal fibrosis, galactocele, phyllodes tumor, posttraumatic fluid collection, or an abscess. Invasive ductal carcinoma not otherwise specified and medullary carcinoma are the primary malignant considerations for a patient this age. Mucinous carcinomas are typically smaller and more common in older, postmenopausal women, as are papillary carcinomas. Invasive lobular carcinomas do not typically present as a round mass and are more common in older, postmenopausal women.

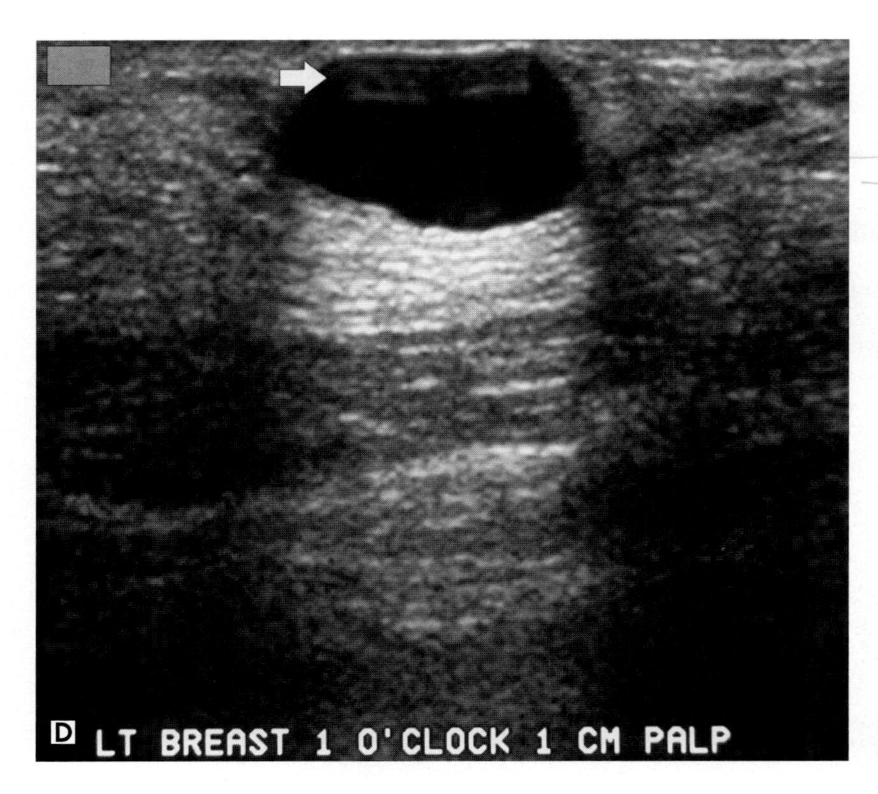

Figure 3.18. (*Continued*) Ultrasound image **(D)** of the palpable mass in the upper outer quadrant of the left breast.

What is your diagnosis?
What BI-RAD® category would you assign?
Would you do anything else?

On physical examination, a superficial, discrete, hard, readily mobile mass is palpated at the 1 o'clock position, 1 cm from the left nipple. A well-circumscribed, 1.3-cm, anechoic mass with posterior acoustic enhancement is imaged, corresponding to the palpable finding. This is a simple cyst. Reverberation artifact (arrow, Fig. 3.18D) is present superficially. In this patient, no further intervention is warranted unless there is significant tenderness or the patient requests an aspiration. Part of our job is to educate women. So, it is important to tell women that cysts are common (i.e., most women have them at some point in their life), often multiple, and may fluctuate in size and associated tenderness. But what are these patients waiting specifically to hear from you? They are hanging on your every word, waiting for you to tell them with confidence that what they are feeling is *not* breast cancer. So I make it a point of looking them in the eye when I specifically tell them: "The lump you are feeling is not breast cancer, it is a cyst, a fluid pocket in your breast, and it will not turn into cancer." However, you still have to assess every patient individually for her response to this information. If I sense continued concern, I will discuss doing an aspiration. Included in this discussion is the likelihood of recurrence following aspiration and the small risk of causing bleeding or infection.

Aspirated fluid may be variable in appearance. The fluid may be free-flowing and range from clear or opaque serous to green to almost black. In some women the fluid is thick and gelatinous; in these patients, aspiration may be incomplete even with an 18G needle. I do not routinely submit the fluid for cytology unless I obtain grossly bloody fluid after an atraumatic tap.

BI-RADS® category 2: benign finding. Annual screening mammography is recommended starting at age 40 years unless there are intervening or persistent clinical concerns requiring earlier evaluation.

PATIENT 19

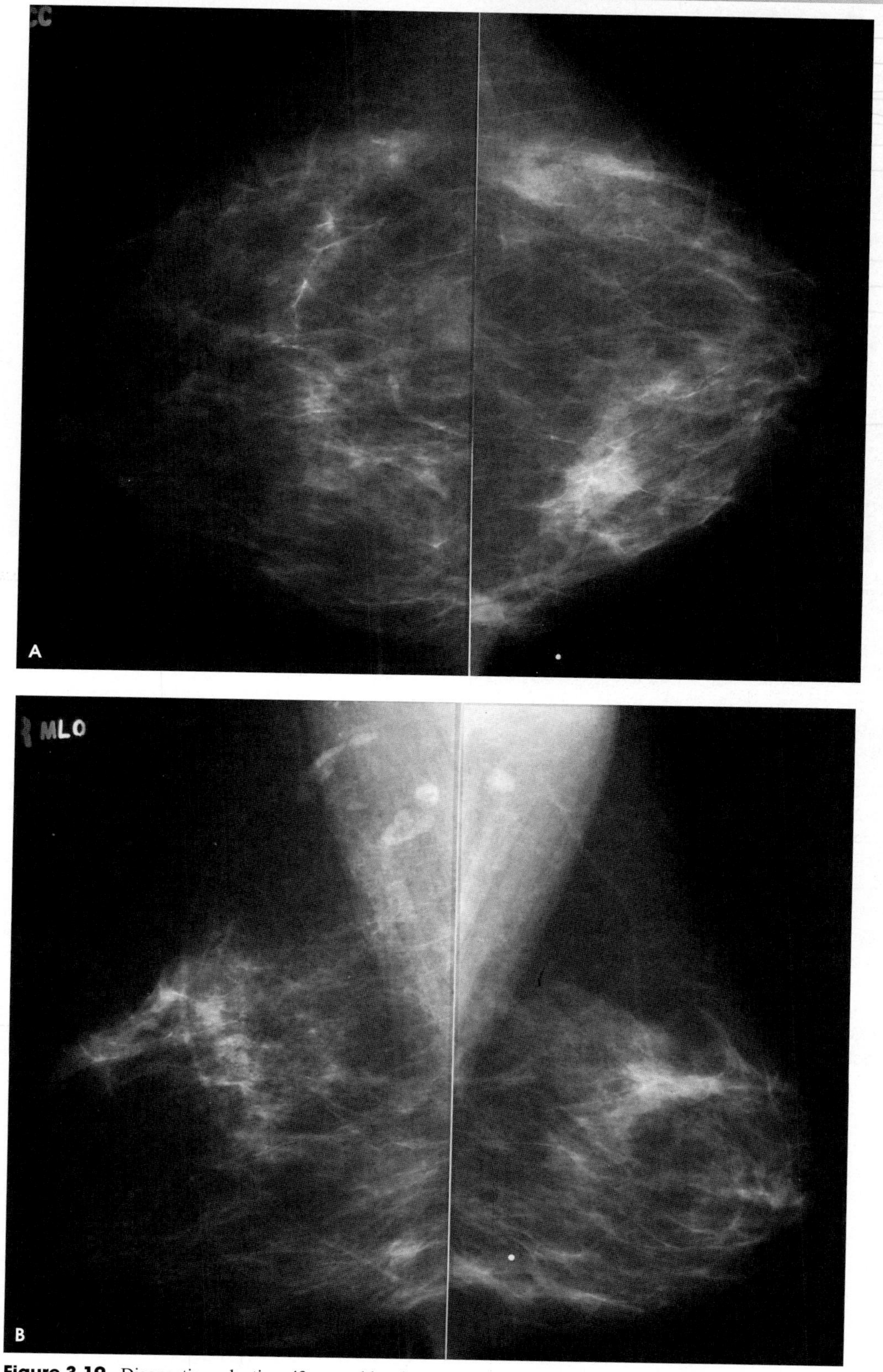

Figure 3.19. Diagnostic evaluation, 42-year-old patient presenting with a "lump" in the left breast. Craniocaudal **(A)** and mediolateral oblique **(B)** views, with a metallic BB on the palpable abnormality.

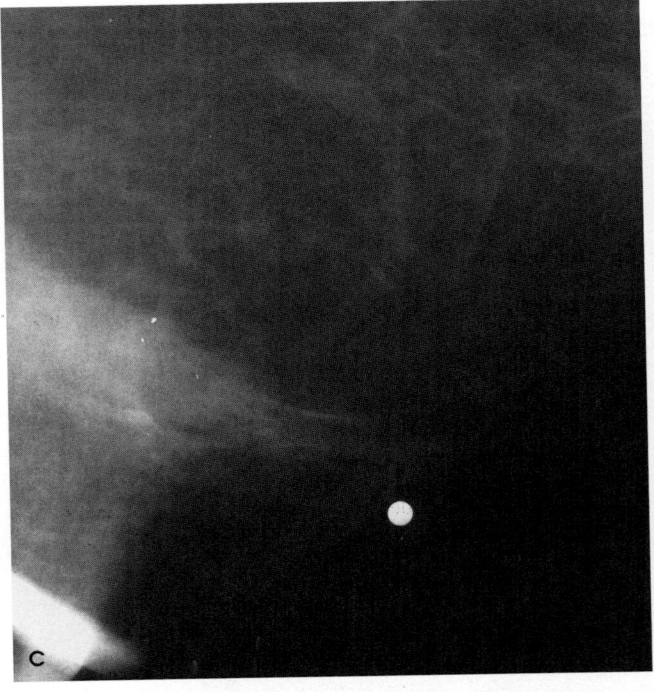

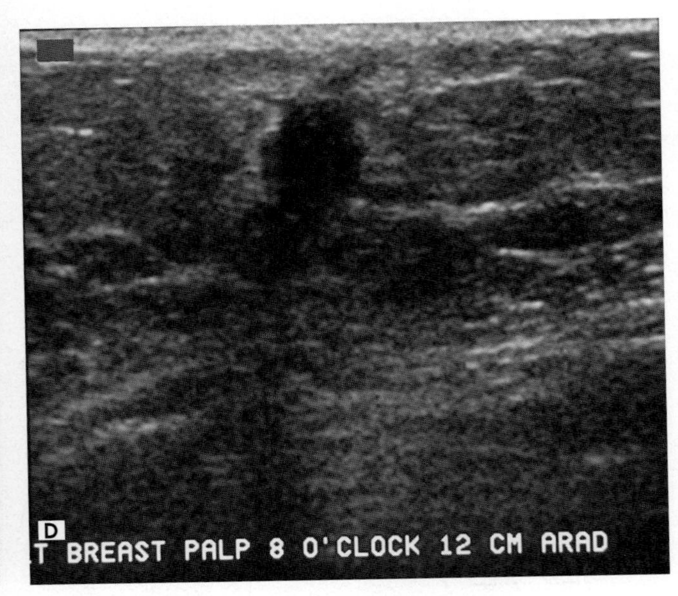

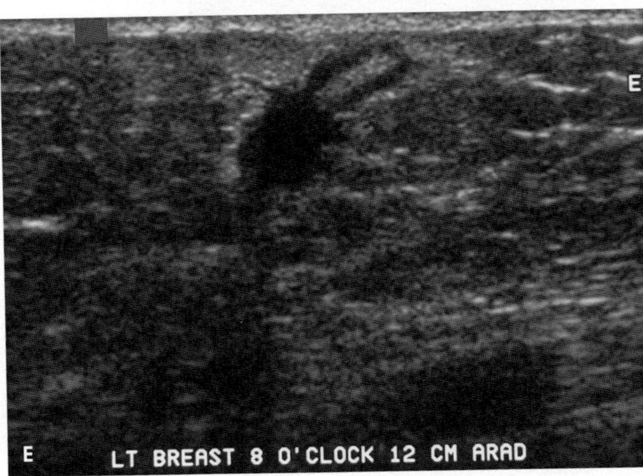

Figure 3.19. (*Continued*) Spot tangential **(C)** view of palpable finding. Ultrasound images **(D, E),** antiradial (ARAD) projections taken through two different areas of the palpable (PALP) mass.

How would you describe the imaging findings?

Scattered lymph nodes are noted bilaterally, superimposed on the pectoral muscles. Focal parenchymal asymmetry is incompletely imaged at the site of concern to the patient, inferomedially in the left breast. On physical examination, a tender, hard, fixed mass is palpated just above the medial-most extent of the inframammary fold on the left. This is associated with some dimpling of the overlying skin. A vertically oriented mass, with spiculated and angular margins and some shadowing, is imaged corresponding to the palpable finding at the 8 o'clock position, 12 cm from the left nipple.

42

What is your differential, and what is your recommendation to the patient?

More common diagnostic considerations include an inflammatory process or posttraumatic changes; rare benign lesions to consider include a papilloma, sclerosing adenosis, granular cell tumor, or fibromatosis (particularly with a lesion in close proximity to or associated with the pectoral muscle). Invasive ductal carcinoma not otherwise specified and invasive lobular carcinoma are the primary malignant considerations. Rarely, ductal carcinoma in situ can present as a mass, asymmetric density, or distortion in the absence of microcalcifications. Given the described clinical and imaging findings, a biopsy is indicated.

BI-RADS® category 4: suspicious abnormality—biopsy should be considered.

Fibromatosis (extra-abdominal desmoid) is reported histologically on the cores. The diagnosis is confirmed following excisional biopsy.

What are the imaging features of fibromatosis?

Mammographically, a spiculated, irregular, noncalcified mass is the most common finding in women with fibromatosis. Less commonly, focal parenchymal asymmetry that may have associated distortion can be seen. On ultrasound, the lesions are usually hypoechoic, round, oval or irregular masses with an echogenic rim, posterior acoustic shadowing, and margins that are not well circumscribed. Less commonly, well-circumscribed margins and posterior acoustic enhancement may be seen. In a limited number of case reports, these lesions described as heterogeneous on MR imaging, with low to high signal intensity on T2-weighted images, isointense on T1-weighted images, with moderate to strong enhancement following contrast administration. In our experience, the enhancement of these lesions is variable, and some may not enhance significantly on MR.

What is fibromatosis (extra-abdominal desmoid), and what is critical in the management of patients diagnosed with fibromatosis?

Fibromatosis is an uncommon tumor accounting for <0.2% of all primary breast tumors and is indistinguishable from fibromatosis occurring elsewhere in the body. The tumor is composed primarily of spindle cells lacking significant atypia, low to moderate cellularity, rare mitotic figures and collagen. They do not typically metastasize, but they can recur locally and be fairly aggressive, particularly if the lesion is inadequately excised. Wide surgical excision is therefore critical in the management of these patients. Fibromatosis can occur anywhere in the breast, but is often noted in close proximity to the pectoral muscle. Nipple retraction has been reported in lesions close to the nipple. In some patients, this lesion is associated with Gardner syndrome. An association with trauma and silicone implants has also been reported. Although they are typically painless, they can be tender, as in this patient. Histologically, it is important to distinguish these lesions from fibrosarcomas that can metastasize.

PATIENT 20

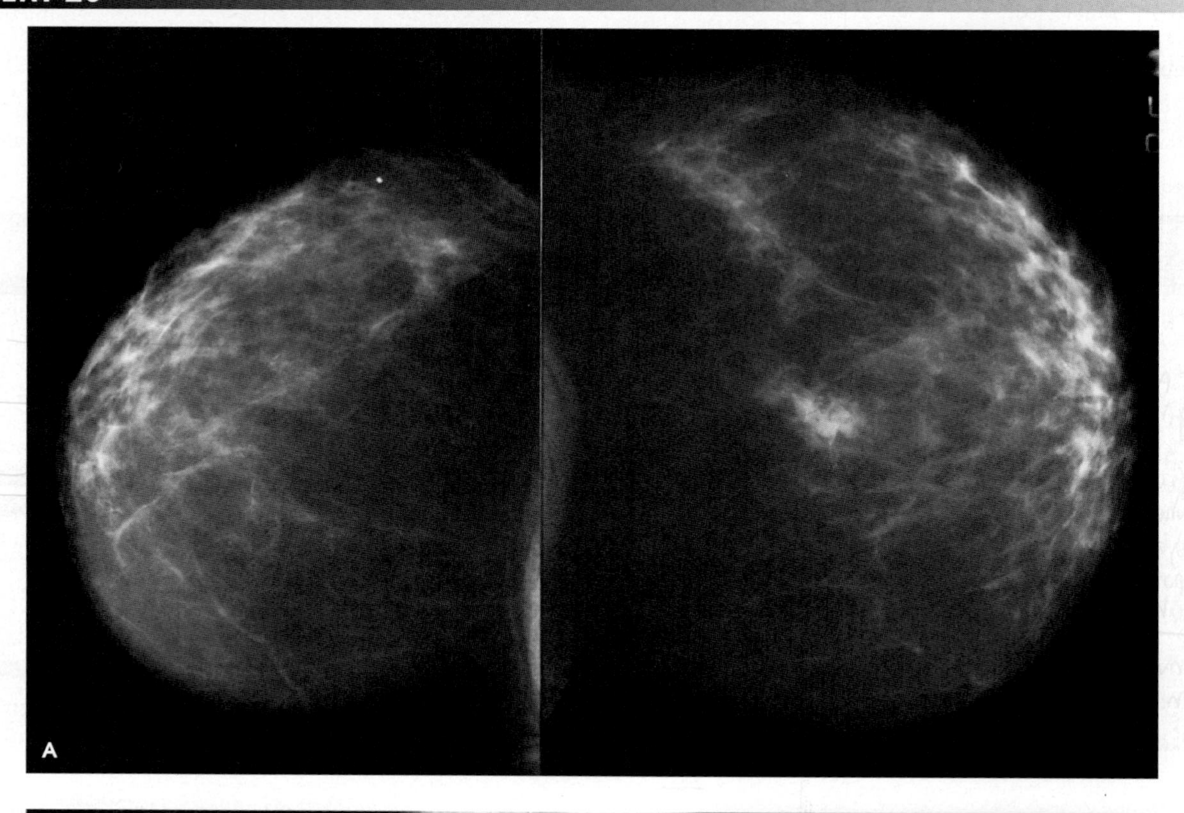

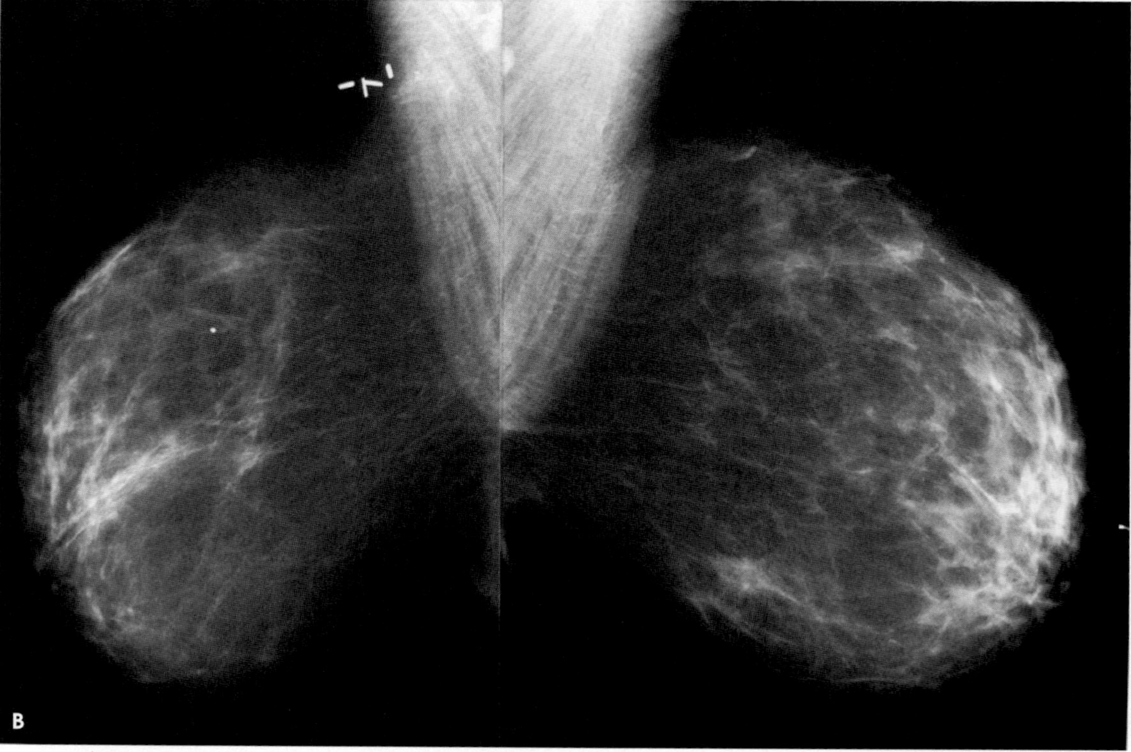

Figure 3.20. Diagnostic evaluation, 42-year-old patient with a history of Ewing sarcoma of the spine 15 years ago, previously treated with radiation therapy, and right breast cancer treated with lumpectomy and radiation therapy 3 years prior to this mammogram. Craniocaudal **(A)** and mediolateral oblique **(B)** views.

What do you think?
What recommendations would you make to this patient?

The right breast is smaller compared to the left, and surgical clips are present on the mediolateral oblique view, anterior to the pectoral muscle, consistent with the history of a right breast cancer 3 years that was previously treated conservatively. Do you see a potential abnormality in the left breast? How about additional evaluation before making any recommendations?

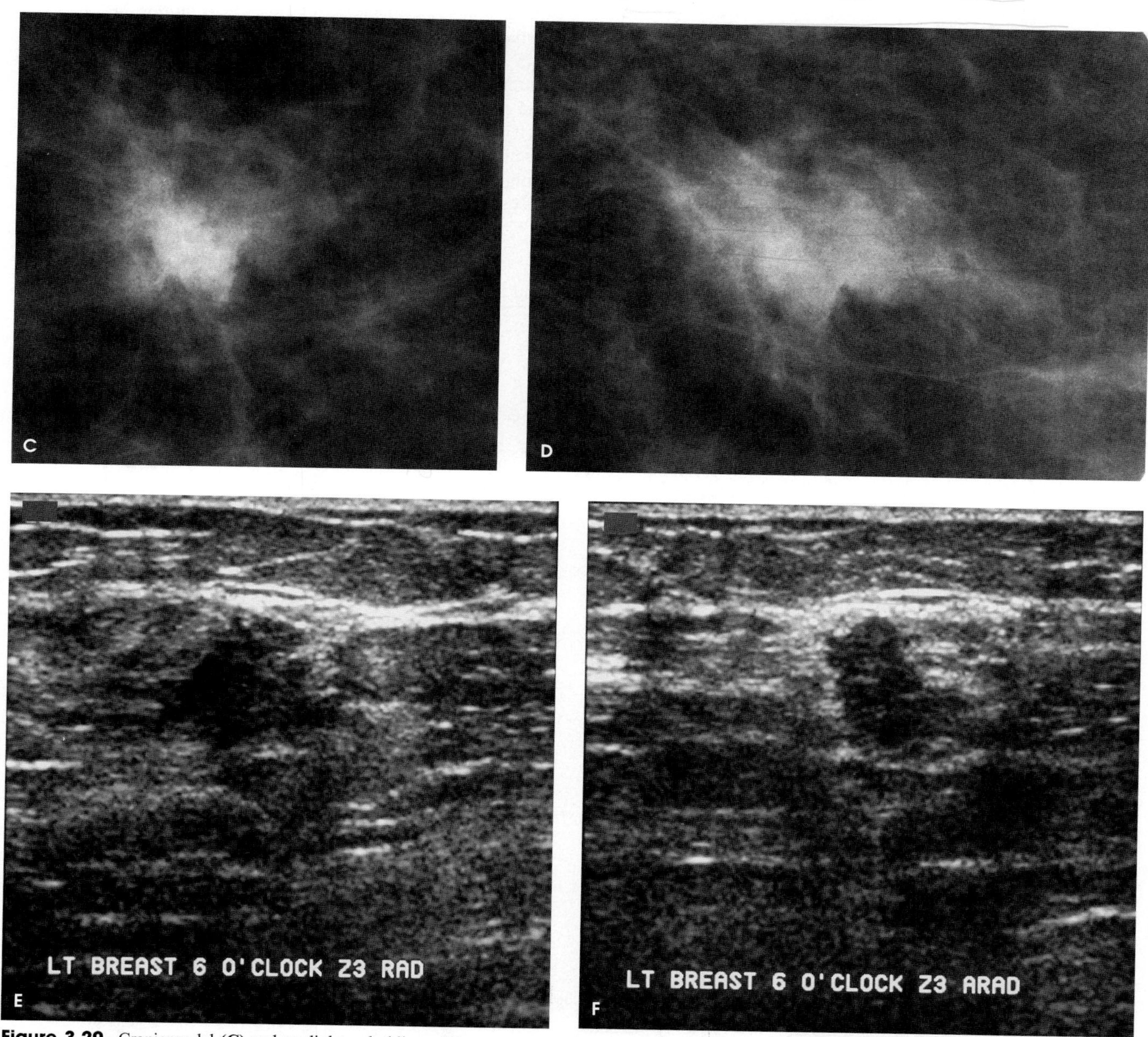

Figure 3.20. Craniocaudal **(C)** and mediolateral oblique **(D)** spot compression views, left breast. Ultrasound images, in radial (RAD) **(E)** and antiradial (ARAD) **(F)** projections of the lesion at 6 o'clock in zone 3 (Z3).

How would you describe the finding, and what differential considerations would you entertain? What is your recommendation?

A 1.2-cm irregular mass with areas of lobulation, as well as indistinct and ill-defined margins, is confirmed on the spot compression views. This is a vertically oriented hypoechoic mass with indistinct, partially microlobulated, spiculated, and angular margins on ultrasound. The mammographic and sonographic findings are suggestive of an ongoing malignant process, particularly in a patient with a personal history of breast cancer. Differential considerations include a metachronous invasive ductal carcinoma not otherwise specified, invasive lobular carcinoma, lymphoma, or a metastatic lesion. Rarely, ductal carcinoma in situ can present as a mass, asymmetric density, or distortion in the absence of microcalcifications. Benign considerations include an inflammatory process or posttraumatic changes, focal fibrosis, a papilloma, sclerosing adenosis, granular cell tumor, and an extra-abdominal desmoid. A biopsy is indicated.

BI-RADS® category 4: suspicious abnormality—biopsy should be considered. An ultrasound-guided biopsy is undertaken. A complex ductal carcinoma in situ (DCIS) is reported on the core samples. A complex DCIS measuring 1.1 cm is confirmed on the lumpectomy specimen. No invasion is reported. Two excised sentinel lymph nodes are normal [pTis(DCIS), pN0(sn) (i−), pMX; Stage 0].

Pleomorphic calcifications, particularly when individual calcifications are linear, or when linear, round, and punctate calcifications demonstrate linear orientation (distribution), are the most common mammographic findings associated with DCIS. Rarely, DCIS can be detected mammographically as a mass (well circumscribed to spiculated, and in some patients macrolobulated), focal parenchymal asymmetry, or distortion in the absence of calcifications. Clinically, some patients diagnosed with DCIS present with a palpable mass, spontaneous nipple discharge (which can be clear or serous, negative for occult blood) or Paget's disease of the nipple.

PATIENT 21

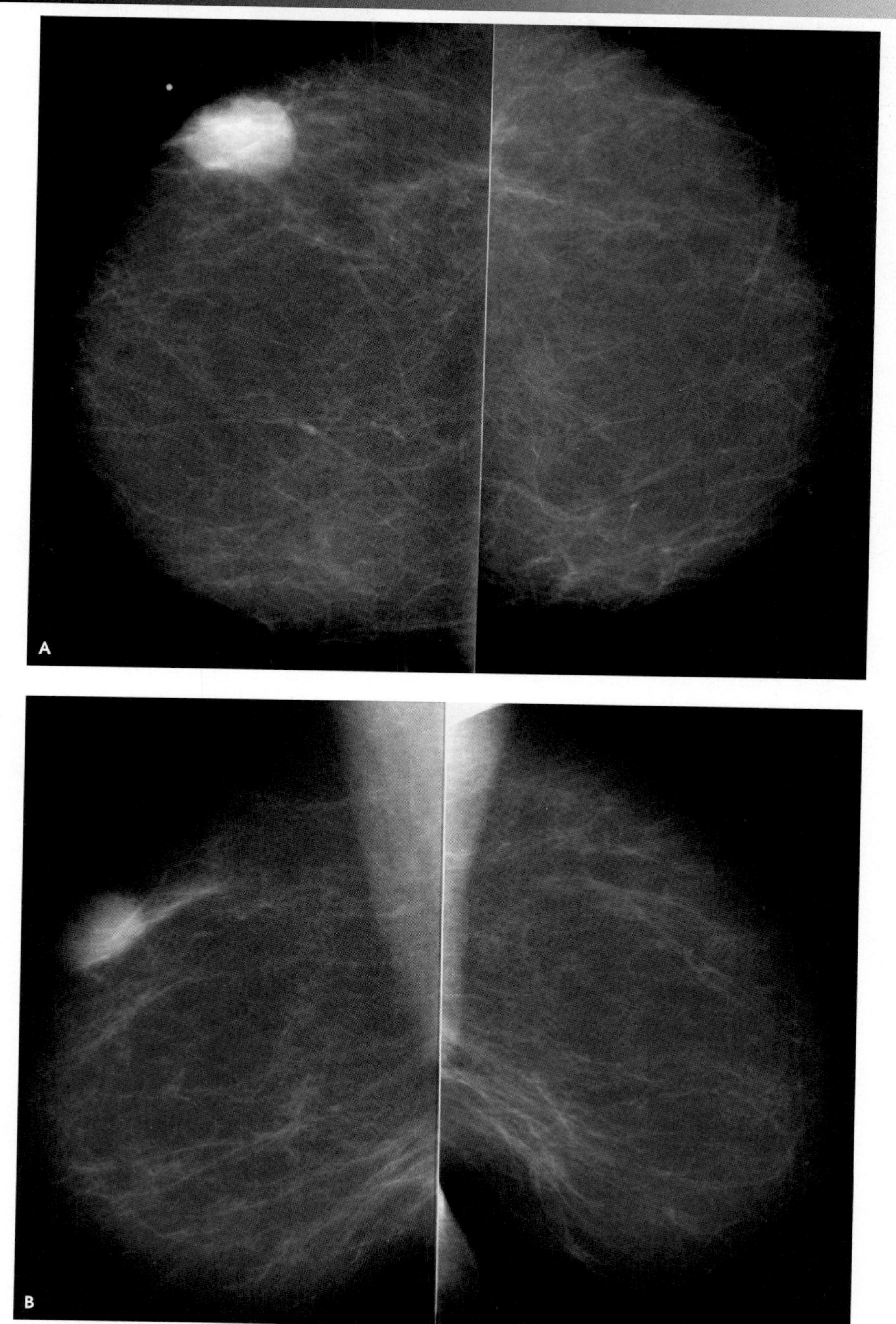

Figure 3.21. Diagnostic evaluation, 64-year-old patient presenting with a "lump" in the right breast. Craniocaudal **(A)** and mediolateral oblique **(B)** views, metallic BB at site of clinical concern.

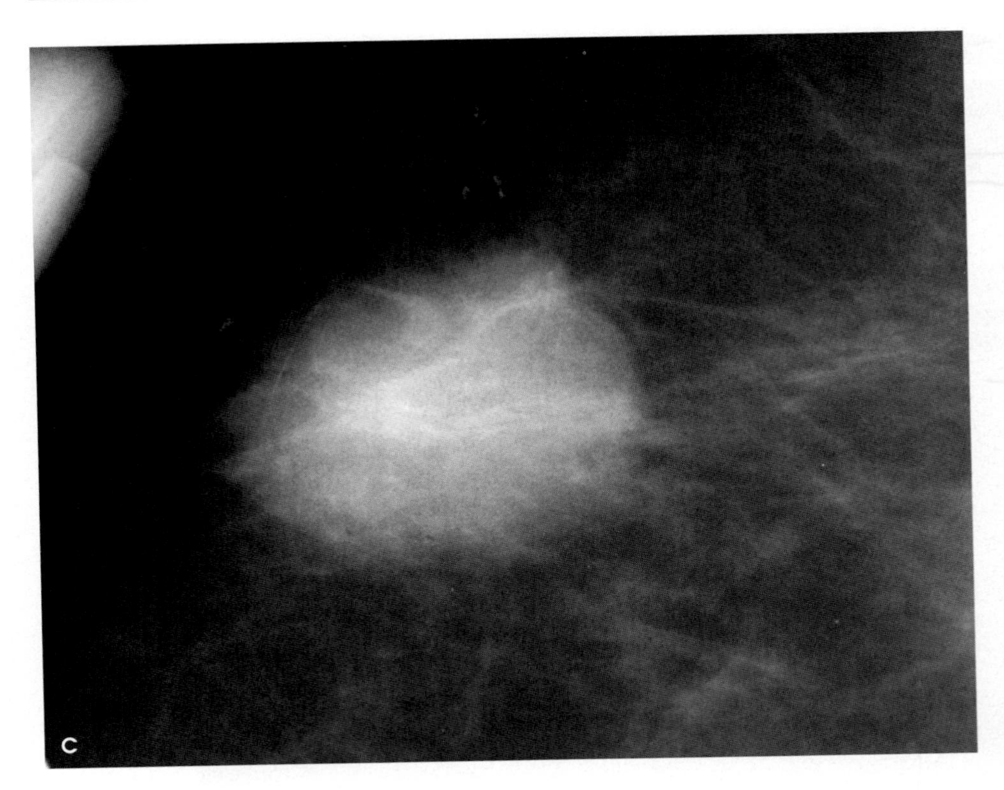

Figure 3.21. (*Continued*) Spot tangential (C) view, right breast mass.

64

What is your differential, and what is the next appropriate step in the evaluation of this patient?

A 2.5-cm oval mass with indistinct margins is imaged at the site of concern to the patient, laterally in the right breast. Benign differential considerations based on the mammographic finding include a cyst (a galactocele is unlikely in a 64-year-old woman), fibroadenoma (complex fibroadenoma, tubular adenoma), phyllodes tumor, papilloma, nodular adenosis, pseudoangiomatous stromal hyperplasia (PASH), focal fibrosis, posttraumatic fluid collection, and abscess. Malignant considerations include invasive ductal carcinoma not otherwise specified, mucinous carcinoma, papillary carcinoma, and lymphoma. A metastatic lesion is also a consideration, particularly if there is a history of an underlying malignancy (melanoma, lung, renal, colon, etc.), although, in the differential for a round, well-circumscribed mass, medullary carcinoma is less likely given the patient's age. Invasive lobular carcinomas do not usually present as round or oval masses. Correlative physical examination and an ultrasound are undertaken.

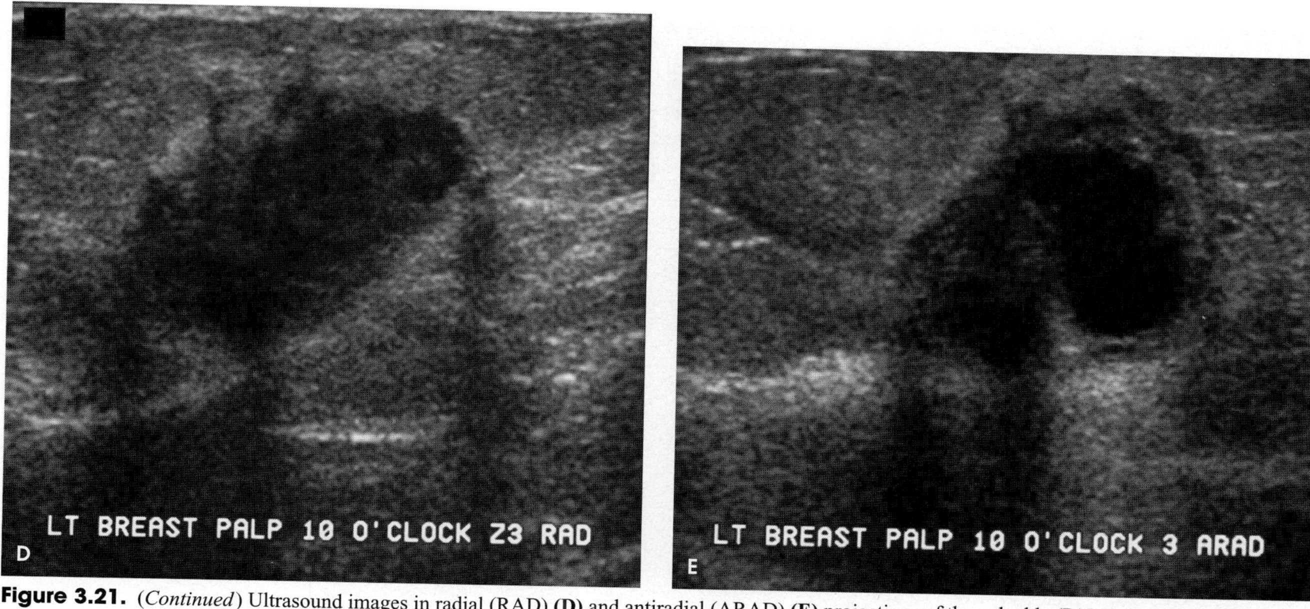

Figure 3.21. (*Continued*) Ultrasound images in radial (RAD) **(D)** and antiradial (ARAD) **(E)** projections of the palpable (PALP) finding, right breast.

How would you describe the findings and further evaluate this patient?

A hard mass is palpated at the 10 o'clock position, posteriorly (Z3) in the right breast. A complex cystic mass with indistinct, microlobulated, spiculated, and angular margins is imaged corresponding to the palpable mass. Given the mammographic and sonographic findings, a poorly differentiated, invasive ductal carcinoma with necrosis is the leading diagnostic consideration. A stepwise approach is taken in the evaluation of this patient. The first step is to attempt an aspiration. If no fluid is obtained, or there is a residual abnormality after the aspiration, an ultrasound-guided core biopsy is done. Although it is unlikely, if nonbloody fluid is aspirated and no residual abnormality is seen on ultrasound, a pneumocystogram can be done to evaluate for the presence of mural abnormalities. Only a small amount of bloody fluid is aspirated in this patient. A core biopsy is done.

BI-RADS® category 4: suspicious abnormality—biopsy should be considered. An invasive ductal carcinoma with necrosis is reported on the core samples. A 3.2-cm, grade III invasive ductal carcinoma is diagnosed on the lumpectomy specimen. Lymphovascular space involvement is present. Malignant cells are described on the imprints from one of two sentinel lymph nodes; a full axillary dissection is completed at the time of the lumpectomy. Metastatic disease with extracapsular extension is described involving the sentinel lymph node. No metastatic disease is diagnosed in 14 additional excised lymph nodes [pT2, pN1a, pMX; Stage IIB]. The tumor is aneuploid and negative for estrogen and progesterone receptor expression.

Poorly differentiated, necrotic, invasive ductal carcinomas often present as round or oval, circumscribed (as opposed to spiculated), solid masses with posterior acoustic enhancement and associated cystic changes (reflecting the necrotic tumor). A rim of poorly differentiated invasive ductal carcinoma is commonly present. It has been suggested that extensive necrosis may be a poor prognostic factor, particularly because nearly 50% of patients with necrotic tumors have axillary nodal metastases and the tumors are aneuploid and typically lack estrogen and progesterone receptors, as described for this patient. It may be that these tumors are proliferating so rapidly that they are outstripping their vascular (angiogenetic) supply.

Lymphovascular space involvement is described in approximately 15% of patients with invasive ductal carcinoma. It has been described as an unfavorable prognostic finding, particularly in node-negative patients treated with either mastectomy or lumpectomy. The significance in patients with positive axillary lymph nodes (such as our current patient) is not clear. Extracapsular tumor extension in involved lymph nodes has also been described as an unfavorable prognostic factor, and some consider this finding an indication for axillary irradiation, particularly in patients who have not had an axillary dissection. The presence of metastatic disease in axillary lymph nodes, however, is the single most important prognostic factor, and there is a direct correlation between the number of positive lymph nodes and disease-free survival as well as mortality.

PATIENT 22

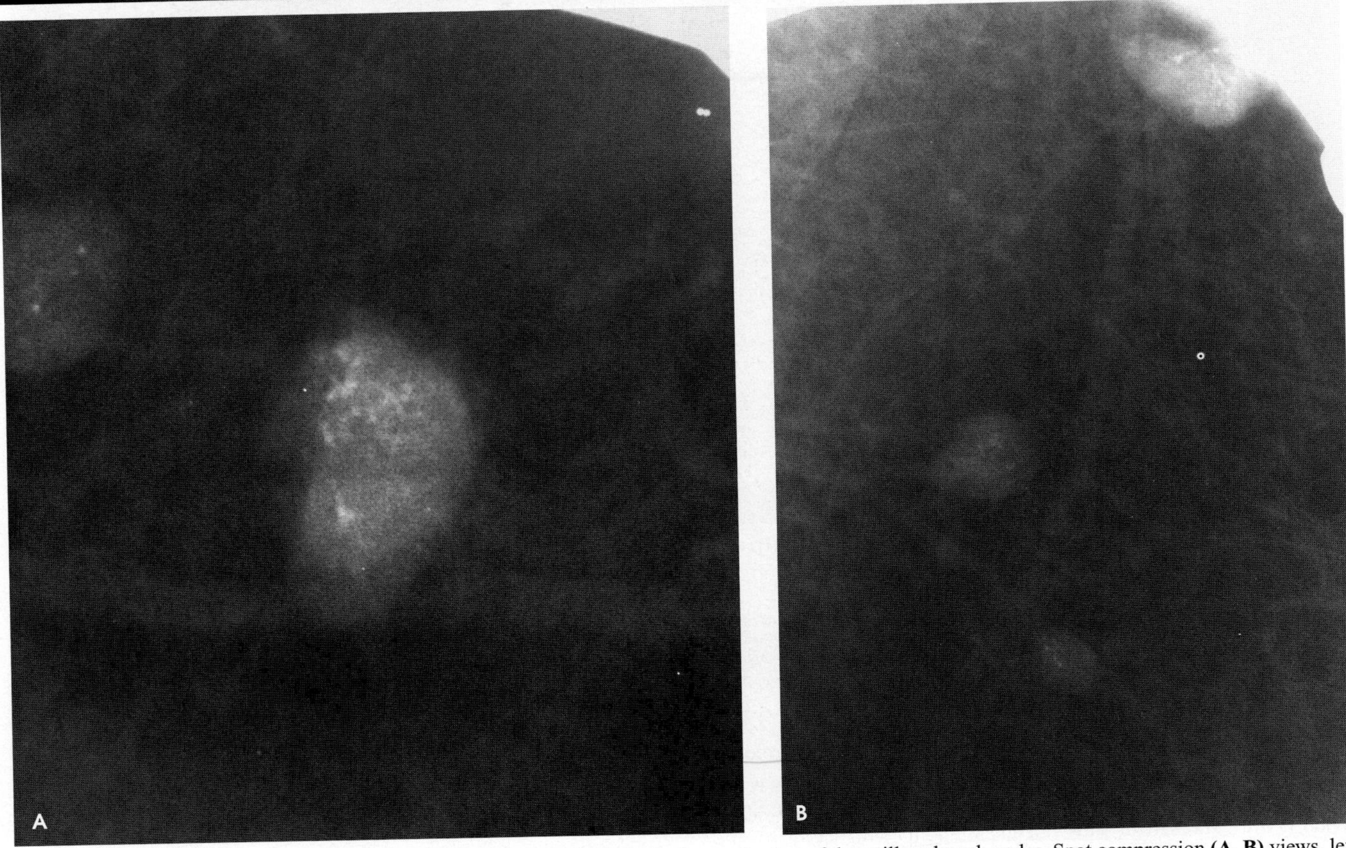

Figure 3.22. Diagnostic evaluation, 76-year-old woman called back for further evaluation of the axillary lymph nodes. Spot compression **(A, B)** views, left axilla. Similar findings are noted in the right axilla (not shown).

How would you describe the findings, and what is your differential?

Several axillary lymph nodes present with punctate, round, and amorphous forms of a high-density material (lacelike in appearance). Although they are somewhat high in density, these may reflect calcifications. Granulomatous diseases including histoplasmosis, tuberculosis, and sarcoid involving axillary lymph nodes may calcify; however, calcifications reflecting granulomatous changes are usually coarse, dense, and larger that what is seen in this patient. Metastatic disease from ovarian or thyroid papillary-type primaries can present with round, punctate, and amorphous calcifications involving one or several axillary lymph nodes. In these diseases the calcifications usually reflect psammoma body formation in the tumor. Lastly, calcifications may be seen in the lymph nodes involved with metastatic disease from a breast primary. These typically represent calcifications developing in a necrotic tumor. Although there have been reports of ductal carcinoma in situ with associated calcifications in the axillary lymph nodes, this is exceedingly rare (i.e., one would not expect metastatic disease to an axillary lymph node to reflect an intraductal, noninvasive process).

Is there any other possibility to consider?

The alternative possibility is that this material is not calcium and, given the high density of the material, this should be suspected. In the past, patients with rheumatoid arthritis have been treated with systemic gold. Mammographically, the gold can be seen deposited bilaterally in all of the visualized intramammary and axillary lymph nodes. Given the bilateral involvement of all lymph nodes in this patient, the next appropriate step is to talk to the patient and ask her if she has rheumatoid arthritis and if she has been treated with gold. The answer is yes, she has rheumatoid arthritis and she has been treated with systemic gold. No further intervention or follow-up indicated.

BI-RADS® category 2: benign finding. Annual screening mammography is recommended.

PATIENT 23

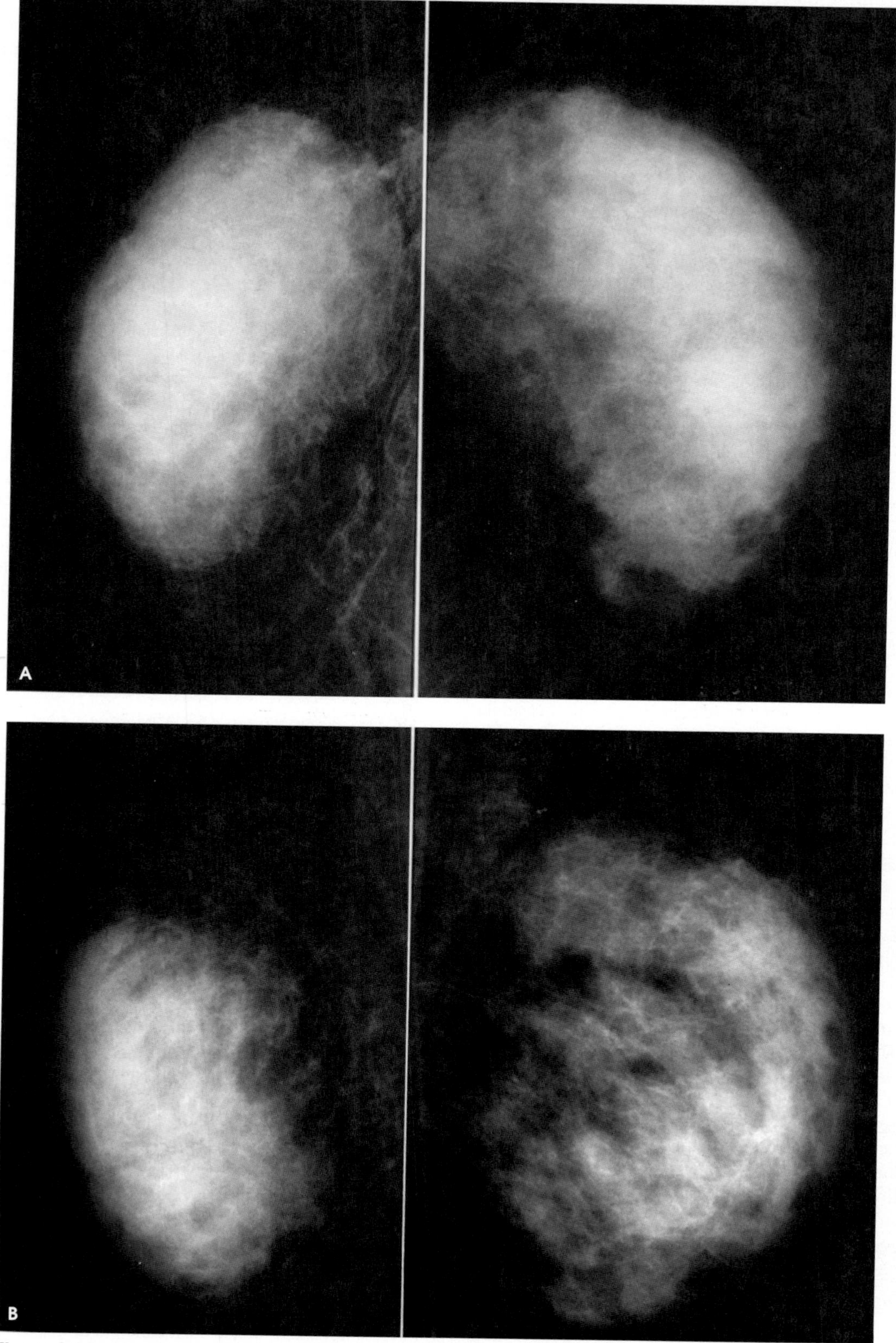

Figure 3.23. Diagnostic evaluation, 88-year-old patient presenting with tender "lumps" bilaterally. Craniocaudal **(A)** and mediolateral oblique **(B)** views.

What do you think? In reviewing films, what information do you look at?

There is a dense fibroglandular pattern. No focal abnormality is apparent. In reviewing films you should routinely review the name of the patient, date of birth, and the technical factors used to obtain the image (e.g., kilovoltage, milliamperage, centimeters of compression, angle of obliquity used for the mediolateral oblique view). *Remember: Make no assumptions.* Although most patients who present with a breast-related problem are women, not all are. By verifying the name of the patient (and talking with the technologist), you can establish that this is a male patient presenting with tender, bilateral "lumps." The lumps the patient is describing reflect the presence of breast tissue. He has developed gynecomastia and requires no additional imaging evaluation or follow-up.

BI-RADS® category 2: benign finding.

Male patients who present for breast imaging are usually symptomatic and describe uni- or bilateral breast enlargement, a mass, or focal tenderness. Our role with these patients is to exclude an underlying malignancy. Depending on the underlying process, mammographic findings will vary. In men with gynecomastia, glandular tissue is imaged centered on the subareolar area. The amount of tissue can vary from a few trabecular strands to dense tissue indistinguishable from that seen in some women. The findings may be uni- or bilateral, symmetric or asymmetric in appearance. The diagnosis of gynecomastia is established mammographically; sonography is not usually indicated. On ultrasound, gynecomastia has a variable appearance. It is often an irregular area of hypoechogenicity centered in the subareolar area. Pseudogynecomastia may be seen in obese men as breast enlargement characterized by adipose tissue with no associated glandular tissue.

The mammographic presentation of male breast cancer is similar to that described in women and includes a spiculated or round mass that may have associated pleomorphic microcalcifications. Less commonly, distortion or asymmetry may be seen. The lesions may be subareolar, or more eccentric in location.

What is gynecomastia, and is it considered a risk factor or a precursor for the subsequent development of male breast cancer? Do these patients require mammographic follow-up?

Gynecomastia reflects the proliferation of ductal and stromal tissue in male patients. It can present as unilateral or bilateral (simultaneously or at different times) diffuse breast enlargement that may be associated with tenderness or as a "mass" centered in the subareolar area. Gynecomastia is not considered to be a risk factor or a precursor lesion for the development of male breast cancer. If the clinical and mammographic findings are consistent with gynecomastia, I do not recommend any additional imaging studies or follow-up.

In what groups of males can gynecomastia be seen as a "physiologic" change?

Physiologic gynecomastia related to hormonal imbalances can occur during three different phases in male patients. In newborn males, rapidly regressing gynecomastia is common and reflects the effect of placental estrogens. As many as 60% to 70% of pubertal boys (ages 12 to 15) present 1 to 2 years after testicular enlargement begins with gynecomastia that typically regresses within 2 years of onset. Lastly, in older males, as testosterone levels decrease, and particularly in those with a body mass index greater than 25 kg/m^2, breast enlargement may be seen.

What are some of the conditions that should be considered in a male presenting with gynecomastia who does not fall into one of the three categories of physiologic gynecomastia?

Pathophysiologic causes of gynecomastia can be considered in several major categories, including (1) estrogen excess (tumors including Leydig, Sertoli, and granulosa-theca cell tumors, choriocarcinoma, seminoma, teratoma, embryonal cell, hepatoma, and pituitary and feminizing adrenal tumors), (2) androgen deficiency (primary testicular failure—e.g. Klinefelter's syndrome—secondary testicular failure from trauma, orchitis, cryptorchidism, irradiation, hydrocele, or varicocele), (3) drug related (anabolic steroids, diethylstilbestrol, digitalis, estrogen, heroin, marijuana, cimetidine, diazepam, ketoconazole, phenytoin, spironolactone, amiodarone, bumetanide, busulfan, calcitonin, furosemide, isoniazid, methyldopa, nifedipine, reserpine, theophylline, tricyclic antidepressants, verapamil, finasteride), (4) systemic diseases (hyperparathyroidism, cirrhosis, chronic renal failure, chronic pulmonary disease, acquired immunodeficiency syndrome [AIDS] and human immunodeficiency virus [HIV] infection, and chest wall trauma) and (5) idiopathic.

What histologic features are associated with the two main phases of gynecomastia?

Gynecomastia is characterized histologically by an active, florid proliferative phase of ducts and an inactive fibrous phase. Epithelial proliferation with papillary and cribriform-like patterns, associated myoepithelial cell hyperplasia, and increased cellularity of the periductal stroma with increased vascularity is described in the florid proliferative phase. Within 1 to 2 years of onset, the epithelial proliferation becomes much less prominent and dense fibrous stroma with sparse cellularity and decreased vascularity are present. Pseudogynecomastia is characterized by adipose tissue with no ductal or stromal proliferation.

What component of female breast tissue is not typically seen in men who develop gynecomastia (consequently, what group of pathologic processes is rare in men)?

Lobule formation is not typically seen in otherwise normal men. Consequently, lobular processes such as fibroadenomas, cysts, sclerosing adenosis, and invasive lobular carcinoma are rare in men. Ductal and stromal processes such as papillomas, duct ectasia, pseudoangiomatous stromal hyperplasia, apocrine metaplasia, and squamous metaplasia have been reported in men and in association with gynecomastia. Inflammatory processes, epidermal inclusion cysts, lipomas, intramammary lymph nodes, granular cell tumors, and fat necrosis related to trauma can also affect male patients, with presentations similar to those described in women.

What management options are available for men with gynecomastia?

At the time of presentation, it is important to exclude a serious underlying cause of gynecomastia (e.g., an estrogen-secreting tumor). Treating (or removing) the underlying cause is appropriate for those men in whom the cause of the gynecomastia is identified. In considering treatment for those patients in whom no definite cause for the gynecomastia is identified, it is important to recognize that in most men, a conservative approach is appropriate because spontaneous regression is common. Reassurance that the process is benign may be all that is needed. However, several medical treatments have been reported, with variable responses (and associated, sometimes, with significant side effects), including the use of dihydrotestosterone, danazol, and tamoxifen. The surgical option of a simple mastectomy is available; however, cosmetic results may not be optimal. More recently, liposuction has been used to treat some men with gynecomastia.

PATIENT 24

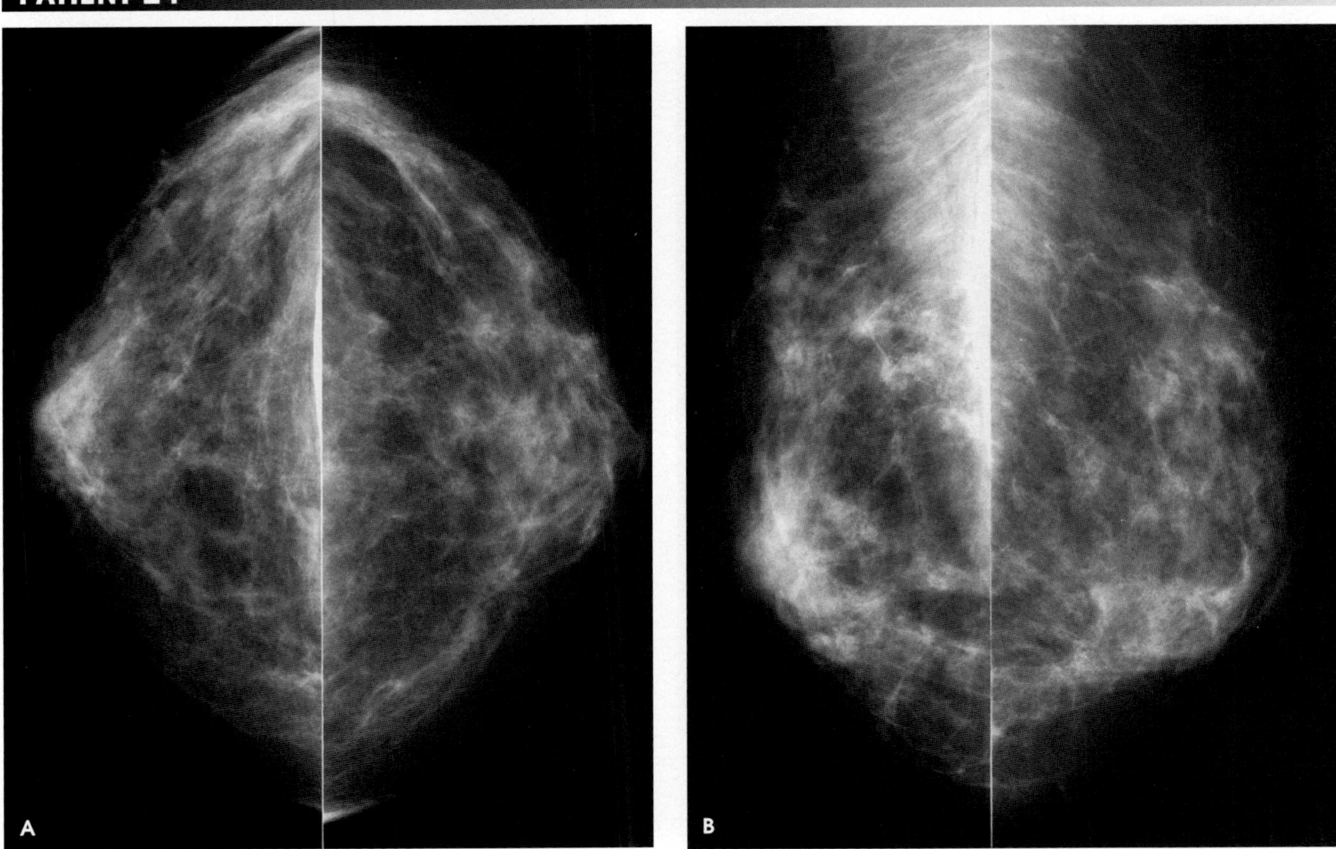

Figure 3.24. Screening study, 55-year-old woman with implants in a subpectoral location. Implant-displaced, craniocaudal **(A)** and mediolateral oblique **(B)** views, left breast.

Is this a normal mammogram, or is there a potential abnormality? If there is an area of concern, where is it?

Review the images systematically. Split the images into thirds such that on the craniocaudal (CC) views you focus your attention on lateral, mid, and medial tissue, and on the mediolateral oblique (MLO) views you review the superior, mid, and inferior aspects of the breasts. Do you see anything? If not, look specifically for possible masses, asymmetry, distortion, or calcifications. Now do you see anything? If you still do not, look in specific places: fat–glandular interfaces, the strip of tissue between the pectoral muscle and glandular tissue on the MLO views, subareolar areas and medial tissue on CC views. In evaluating the medial quadrants on the CC views, do you perceive a subtle asymmetry with possible distortion on the left, anteriorly? In reviewing the left MLO at the approximate distance back from the nipple, there is also a possible area of asymmetry with distortion. The significance of this potential finding on these views is unknown. Additional evaluation will be helpful.

BI-RADS® category 0: need additional imaging evaluation.

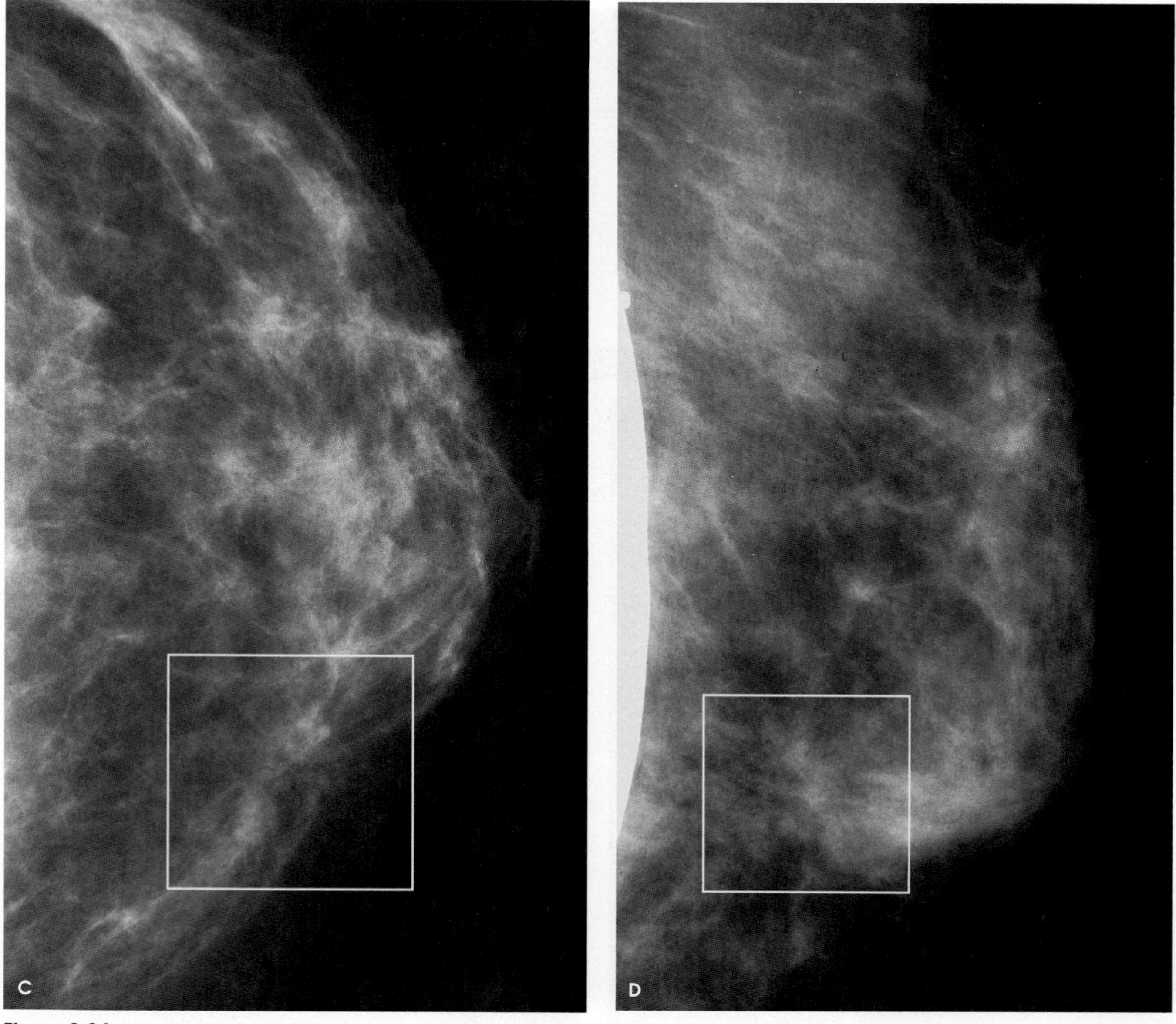

Figure 3.24. (*Continued*) Craniocaudal **(C)** and mediolateral oblique **(D)** views of the left breast, photographically coned. A box is used to enclose the potential abnormality.

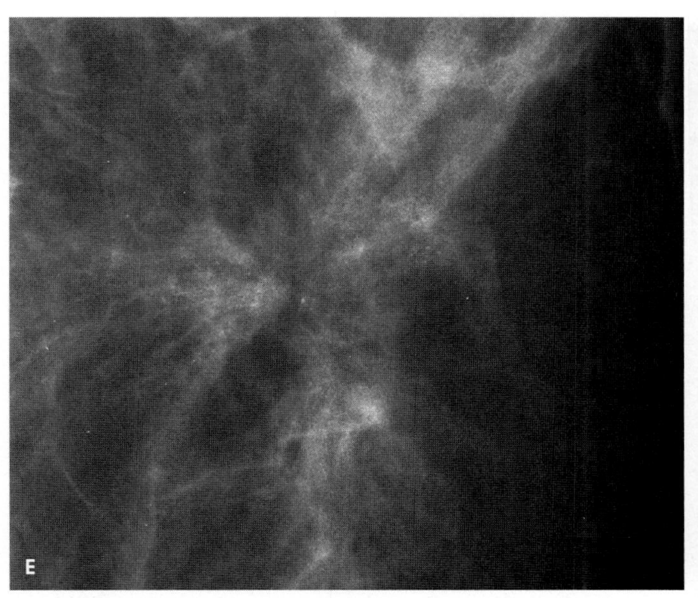

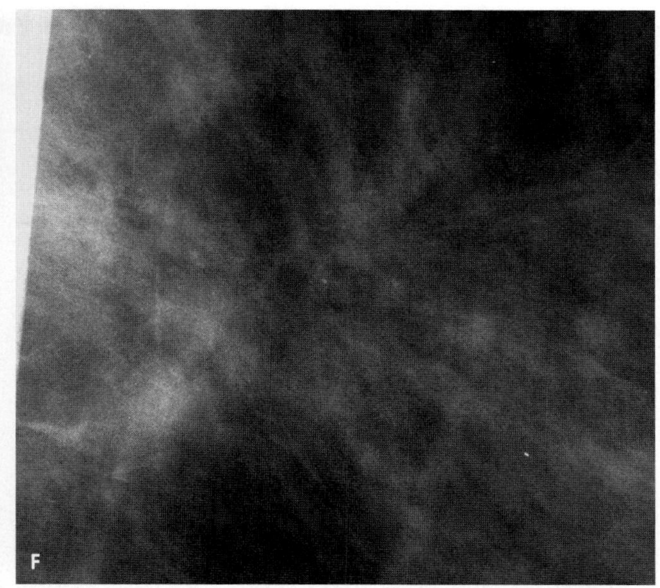

Figure 3.24. (*Continued*) Double spot compression magnification views of the left breast, craniocaudal **(E)** and mediolateral oblique **(F)** projections.

Now how would you describe the findings, and with what degree of certainty can you say that a lesion is present?

The additional views are invaluable in helping us establish the presence of a lesion. An area of distortion with long, curvilinear spicules, central lucency, and associated punctate and round calcifications is confirmed on the additional views. At this point, what are your differential considerations and what would you recommend next? Differential considerations include fat necrosis, particularly if the patient has had a biopsy or trauma that is localized to this site, complex sclerosing lesion (radial scar when less than 1 cm in size), focal fibrosis, sclerosing adenosis, papilloma, an inflammatory process, invasive ductal carcinoma not otherwise specified, and invasive lobular carcinoma. Although it is somewhat larger than most, this could also be a tubular carcinoma.

How can you sort through this differential and narrow the diagnosis?

As a starting point, a good history is helpful. Does the patient have a scar that corresponds to this site? Does she recall any trauma to this site? If there is no scar or trauma localized to this site, fat necrosis is unlikely. Does the patient have any signs or symptoms of inflammation at this site (e.g., erythema, increased warmth, tenderness)? Physical examination is also helpful. Are there any palpable findings? Complex sclerosing lesions are usually not palpable, and normal or subtle findings are seen on ultrasound. In contrast, invasive ductal carcinomas of this size are usually palpable, and on palpation the findings with invasive ductal carcinoma often overestimate the size seen on imaging studies (i.e., they feel larger than what is seen on the images). On ultrasound, a mass that may have associated shadowing is likely with an invasive ductal carcinoma. Invasive lobular carcinoma is unpredictable: Physical findings may be normal, but either an area of thickening without a discrete mass or a mass may be palpable. On ultrasound, a mass with associated shadowing may be seen, but the ultrasound may be normal. This patient has had no surgery or trauma to this site, and her physical examination and ultrasound are normal. This is thought to most likely represent a complex sclerosing lesion.

BI-RADS® category 4: suspicious abnormality—biopsy should be considered.

A complex sclerosing lesion with atypical aprocrine adenosis, columnar alteration with prominent apical snouts and secretions, and florid epithelial hyperplasia without atypia is reported on the excisional biopsy.

Lesions characterized by central sclerosis and surrounding radiating epithelial proliferation are referred to as a radial scar when they are <1 cm in size and as complex sclerosing lesions when they are >1 cm in size. Associated foci of sclerosing adenosis, papilloma formation, cystic changes, and epithelial hyperplasia may be seen in these lesions. Atypical hyperplasia, ductal carcinoma in situ (usually low nuclear grade), lobular neoplasia, and invasive carcinoma have also been reported arising within radial scars but, more commonly, in the larger complex sclerosing lesions. Identified as incidental findings on histology, radial scars (<1 cm in size) are common, multiple, and often bilateral. In contrast, complex sclerosing lesions (>1 cm in size) identified mammographically are less common, presenting as single, unilateral lesions. It has been suggested that infarction occurring in areas of pre-existing proliferative changes may account for the histologic findings. However, these lesions are considered idiopathic and, although the word "scar" is used for the smaller lesions, these lesions do not reflect biopsy changes (i.e., they do not occur at prior biopsy sites).

The mammographic findings that should suggest a complex sclerosing lesion include an area of distortion better seen in one of the two standard projections (usually the craniocaudal view), long curvilinear spicules that contrast with the short stubby spiculation seen with many invasive ductal carcinomas, and central lucency. Approximately 30% of these lesions may have associated round and punctate calcifications. The findings on ultrasound are variable and can be subtle, limited to a small amount of irregular shadowing. Physical examination is often normal or limited to some minimal thickening.

The management of women with complex sclerosing lesions remains controversial. If this entity is suspected based on the clinical and imaging findings, should an imaging-guided biopsy be done, or is an excisional biopsy the appropriate recommendation? If a complex sclerosing lesion is diagnosed following an imaging-guided core biopsy, is excision required or can the lesion be left in the breast? Based on my experience, approximately 30% of patients with complex sclerosing lesions have associated atypical ductal hyperplasia, lobular neoplasia, ductal carcinoma in situ (usually low nuclear grade), or tubular carcinomas. Consequently, if I suspect a complex sclerosing lesion based on the clinical and imaging features of lesion, I recommend an excisional biopsy. If I do a core biopsy on a lesion and a complex sclerosing lesion is reported histologically, I recommend excisional biopsy. Others advocate imaging-guided biopsy of these lesions with no excision required if the biopsy included at least 12 cores, no atypical ductal hyperplasia is reported, and the mammographic findings are reconciled with the histologic findings. It is unclear why there is such confusion in the literature regarding the appropriate management of these lesions. Could it be that, prognostically, the lesions we identify mammographically are not the same as those seen routinely by pathologists as incidental findings in biopsies done for other reasons? The lesions we identify mammographically are not common and almost always measure >1 cm in size; we do not routinely identify the small lesions (i.e., radial scars that measure <1 cm) reported as common, benign incidental findings by the pathologist.

Figure 3.24. Ultrasound image **(G)** demonstrating high specular echoes and subtle shadowing corresponding to the area of mammographic concern in the left breast.

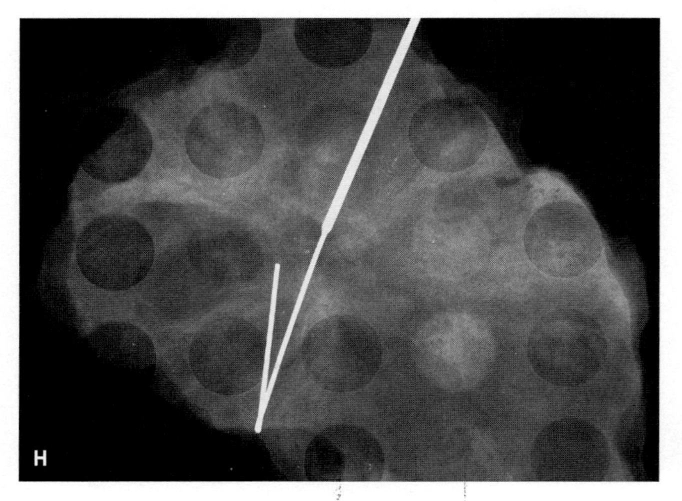

Figure 3.24. Specimen radiograph **(H)** demonstrating distortion and associated punctate calcifications centrally as well as in the surrounding spicules. A portion of the localization wire is also evident.

PATIENT 25

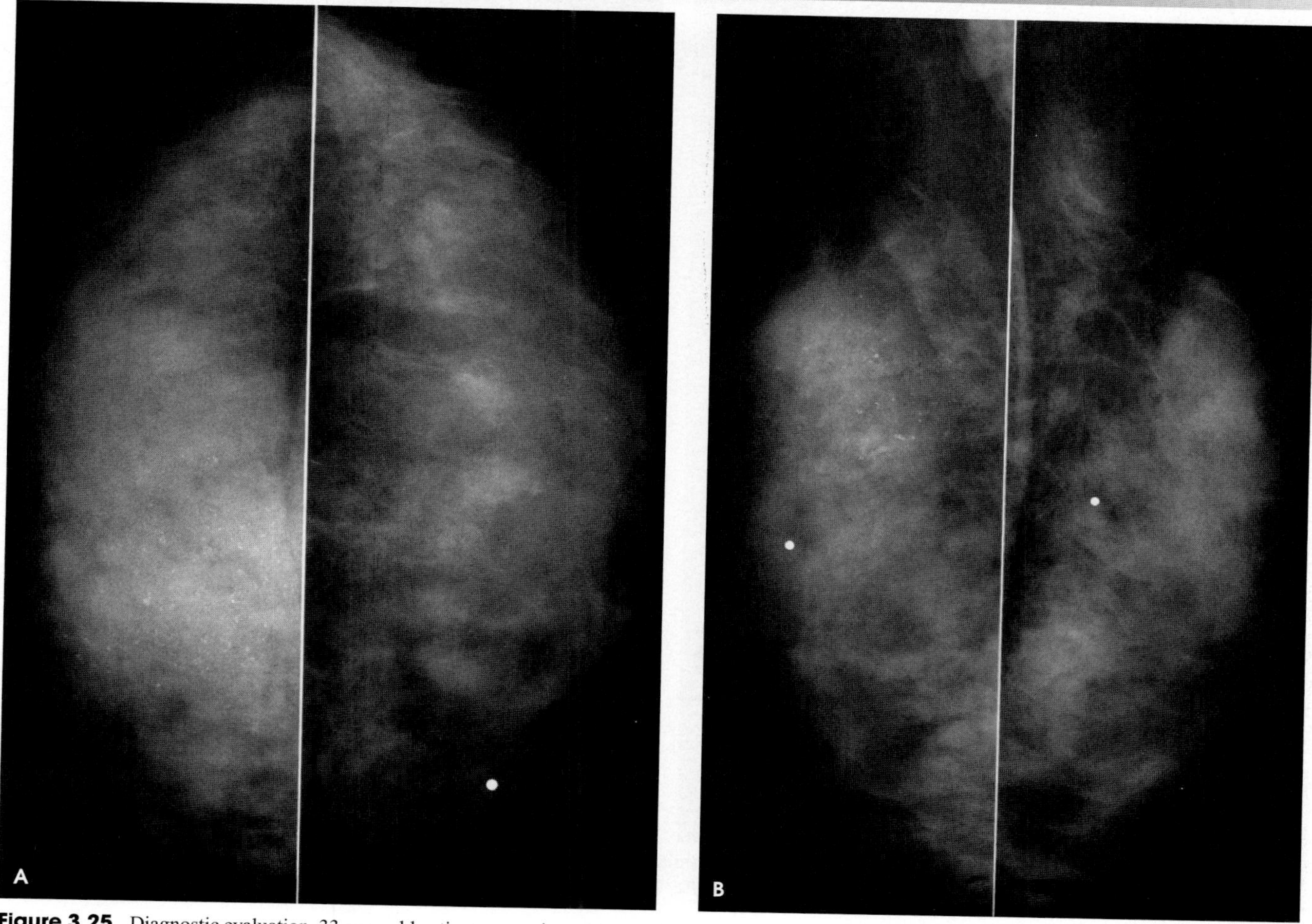

Figure 3.25. Diagnostic evaluation, 33-year-old patient presenting with a "lump" in the upper inner quadrant of the right breast. Craniocaudal **(A)** and mediolateral oblique **(B)** views.

How would you describe the findings?

There is a dense fibroglandular pattern with a regional area of calcification in the upper inner quadrant of the right breast. Did you notice that the appearance of the calcifications is different between craniocaudal (CC) and mediolateral oblique (MLO) views? On the CC view, the calcifications are variable in size, round and not well defined (amorphous); on the MLO view, they are higher in density, better defined, and some demonstrate a curvilinear appearance. This differential appearance between the two views raises the possibility of milk of calcium and, although the diagnosis is established with the current views, a spot compression 90-degree lateral view can be done. In this patient, do we need to do anything else? How about the "lump" she is feeling? Remember not to be lulled by benign findings and forget to look at the rest of the mammogram and evaluate clinical findings.

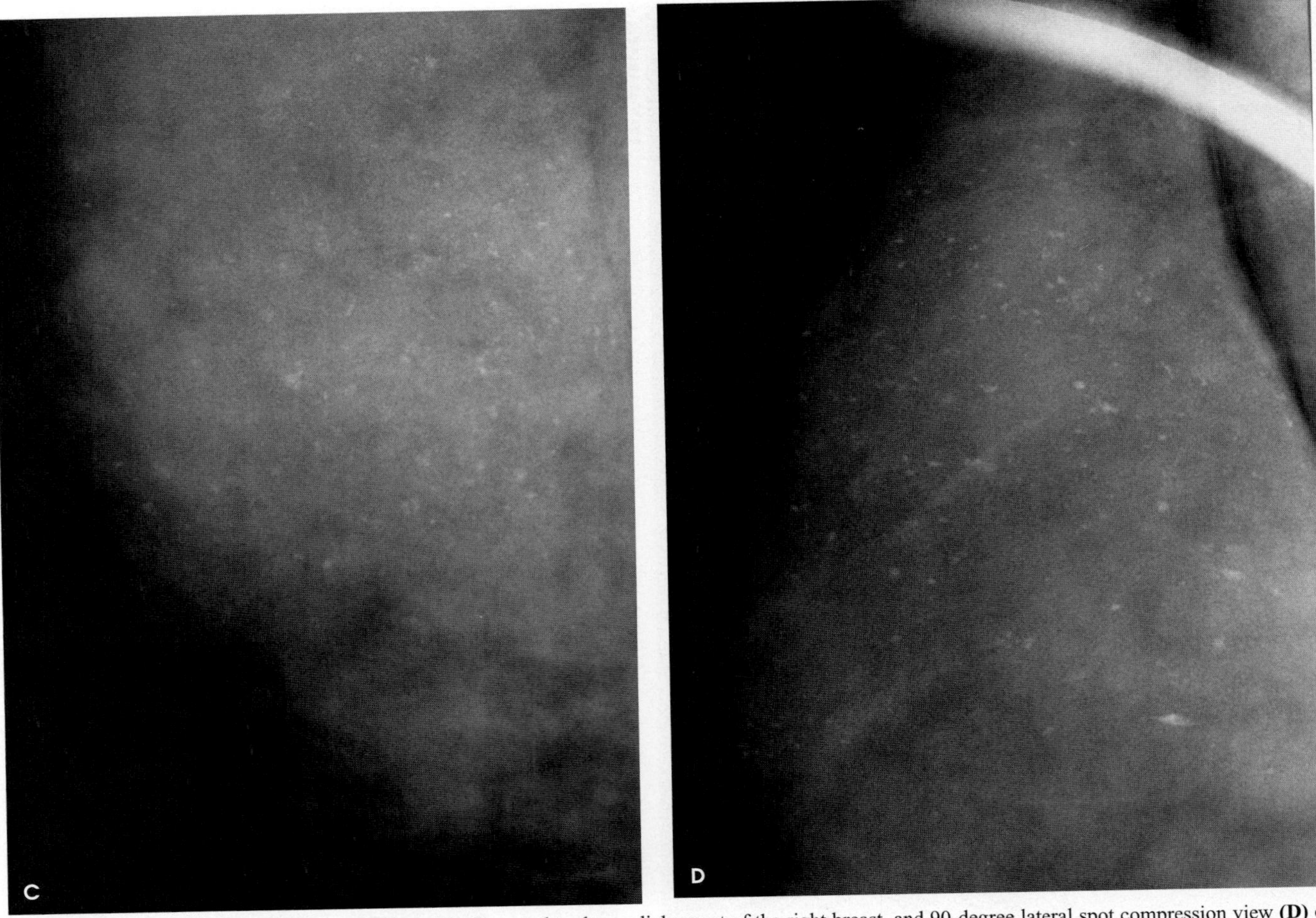

Figure 3.25. Craniocaudal view **(C)**, photographically coned to the medial aspect of the right breast, and 90-degree lateral spot compression view **(D)** of the upper aspect of the right breast, demonstrating the change in appearance of the calcifications on the orthogonal views.

What is indicated next?

Correlative physical examination and an ultrasound of the palpable finding are indicated. On physical examination, a 2- to 3-cm area of globular tissue is palpated, which occupies almost the entire upper outer quadrant of the right breast. It is readily mobile, and tenderness is elicited when gentle compression is applied at this site. No skin changes are present. On ultrasound, cysts of varying sizes are imaged throughout this area. Foci of echogenicity are identified in the dependent portion of many of the cysts. No solid masses are imaged in this quadrant, and there is no distortion or shadowing. This is a palpable fibrocystic complex with associated milk of calcium and corresponds to what the patient is concerned about. I reassure her that what she is feeling is benign and that there are no mammographic or sonographic findings to suggest breast cancer.

BI-RADS® category 2: benign finding.

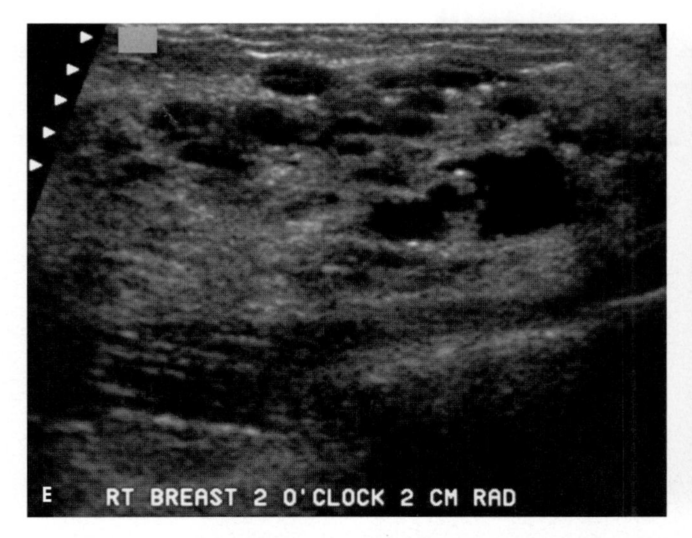

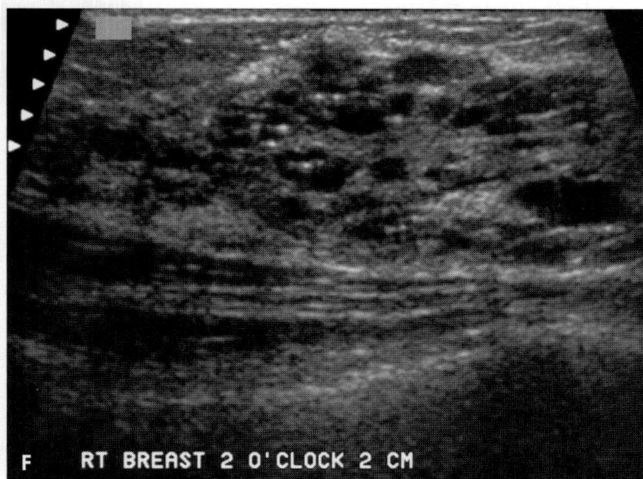

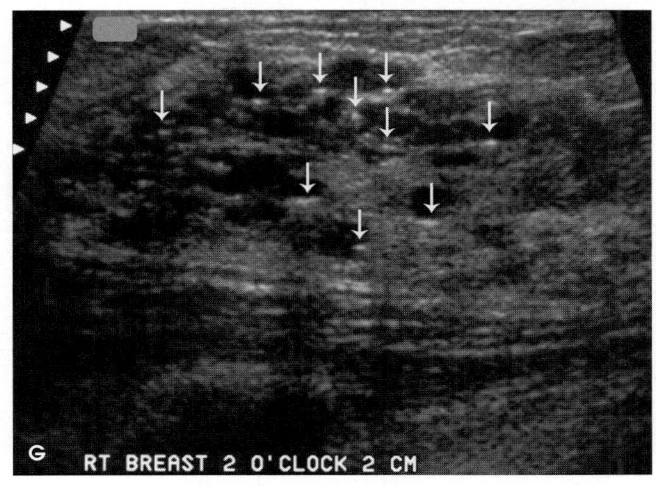

Figure 3.25. (*Continued*) Ultrasound images **(E–G),** upper inner quadrant of the right breast. Cluster of variably sized cysts with associated echogenic foci (*arrows*) corresponding to the calcifications seen mammographically.

PATIENT 26

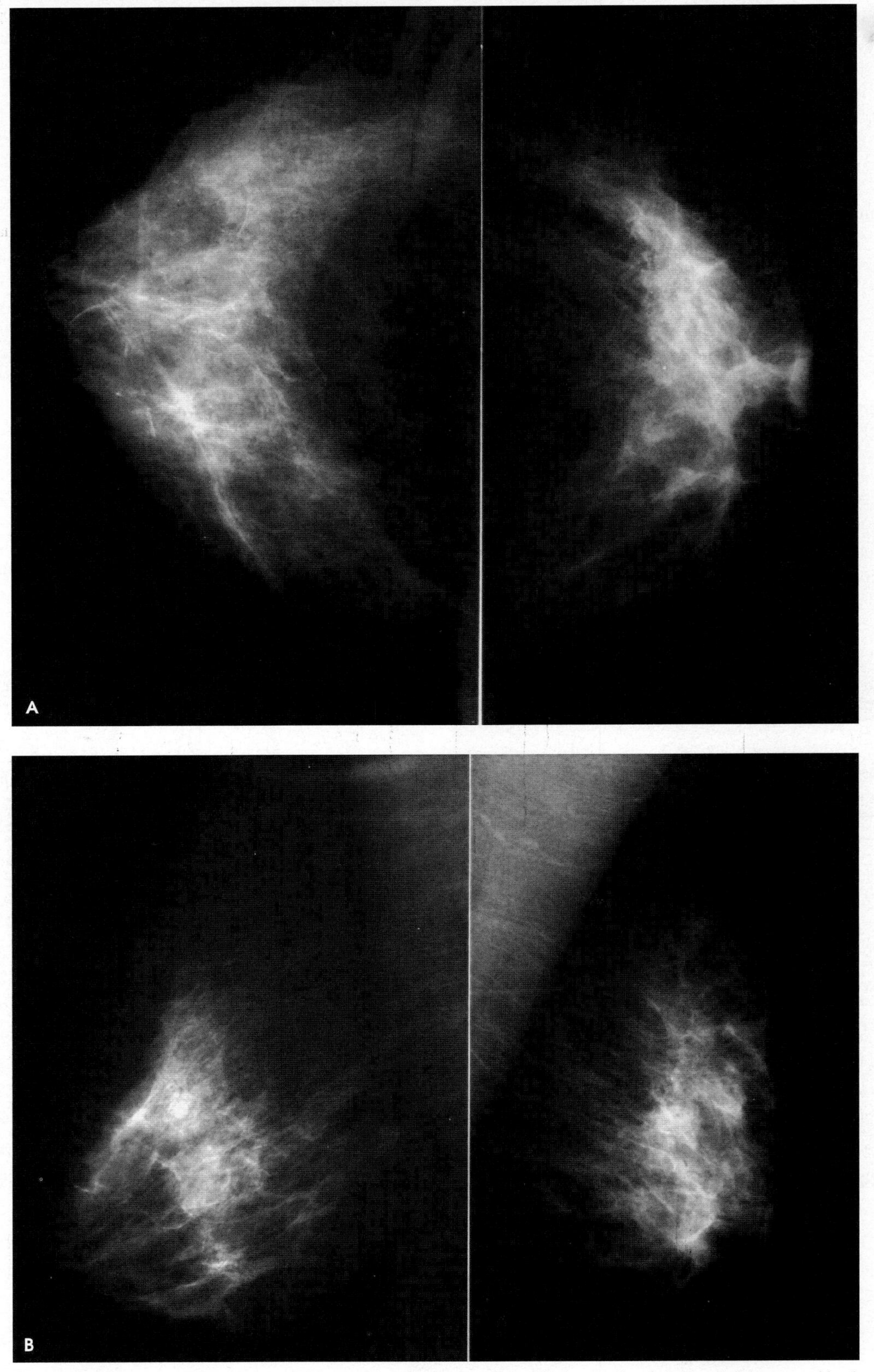

Figure 3.26. Diagnostic evaluation, 73-year-old patient presenting with changes involving her left breast and back pain. Craniocaudal **(A)** and mediolateral oblique **(B)** views.

How would you describe the findings?

The left breast is diffusely abnormal. It is smaller and more dense than the right. Although the appearance is subtle, the tissue on the left has a distorted appearance with associated prominence of the trabecular markings. Diffuse breast changes can be difficult to perceive, particularly if they evolve slowly from one year to the next; however, if you prepare yourself by considering this possibility, they become easier to detect. In some patients, it can be hard to decide which of the breasts is normal. This is why reviewing prior studies and going back to much earlier mammograms can be useful in indicating the progressive change. Also, when you suspect diffuse changes, consider the technical factors used (e.g., centimeters used for compression, kilovoltage, and milliamperage) for the exposure.

Diffuse breast changes can be characterized by increased density of the breast parenchyma, prominence of the trabecular pattern (with a "spidery" appearance), and skin thickening that results in either a progressive decrease (shrinking) or increase in the size of the involved breast. Commonly, the affected breast is less compressible and requires higher kilovoltage and milliamperage for adequate exposure.

On physical examination the left breast is smaller than right (Fig. 3.26 E). There is distortion medially, dimpling inferiorly, and nipple retraction. The left breast is firm compared with the right, but no discrete mass is palpated, no tenderness is elicited, and there are no *peau d'orange* changes. On ultrasound (Fig. 3.26 C, D), the tissue at the 1 o'clock position, 2 cm from the left nipple, is distorted, with significant associated shadowing. Invasive lobular carcinoma is the leading diagnostic consideration in this patient. Less likely considerations include invasive ductal carcinoma, lymphoma, posttraumatic changes, or an ongoing inflammatory process. A biopsy is indicated. An invasive lobular carcinoma is diagnosed following ultrasound-guided core biopsy. The patient is also found to have a positive bone scan with lytic lesions involving the thoracic spine, consistent with metastatic disease.

A spiculated mass is the most common mammographic finding in women with invasive lobular carcinoma, occurring in nearly 40% of patients. Parenchymal asymmetry and distortion are the next most common mammographic findings. These changes may be more apparent in one projection, commonly the craniocaudal view. Diffuse changes include a progressive shrinkage of the involved breast or, alternatively, diffuse enlargement and reduced compressibility of the involved breast may be seen. Invasive lobular carcinoma rarely presents as a round or oval mass. Likewise, when an invasive lobular carcinoma is diagnosed following biopsies done for microcalcifications, the calcifications are usually not found in association with the invasive lesion. The calcifications are found in benign changes such as fibrocystic changes, fibroadenoma, and sclerosing adenosis, and the invasive lobular carcinoma is an incidental finding. It is important to emphasize that invasive lobular carcinoma can be subtle clinically, mammographically, sonographically, and pathologically (I refer to it as the "sleaze disease"). The extent of disease is often underestimated clinically, mammographically, and sonographically. In our own patients, metastatic disease to the axilla is seen in as many as 60% of patients at the time of presentation.

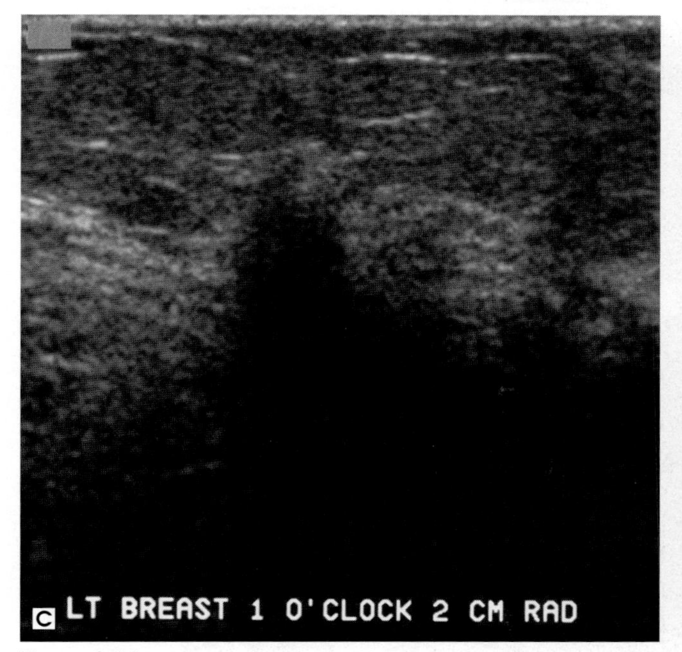

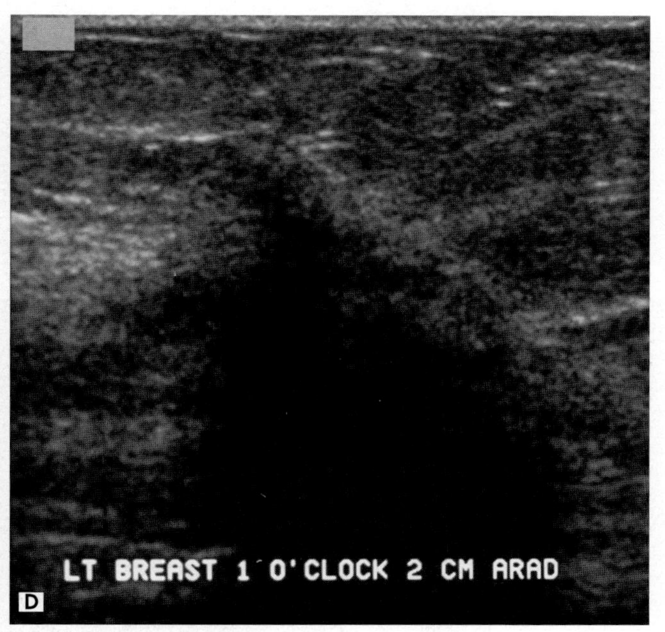

Figure 3.26. (*Continued*) Ultrasound images, radial (RAD) **(C)** and antiradial (ARAD) **(D)** projections.

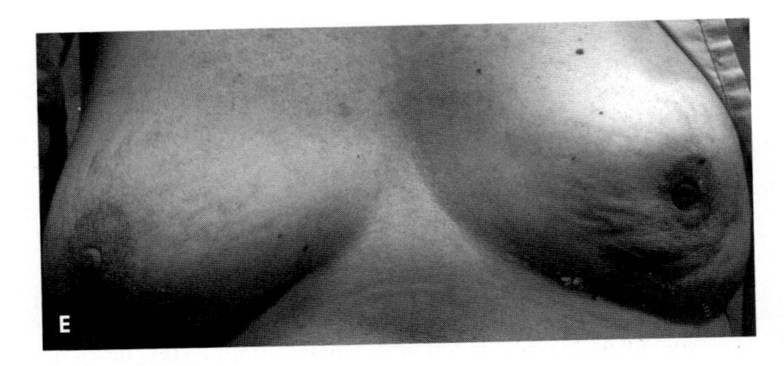

Figure 3.26. (*Continued*) Photograph **(E)** of the breasts in this patient.

PATIENT 27

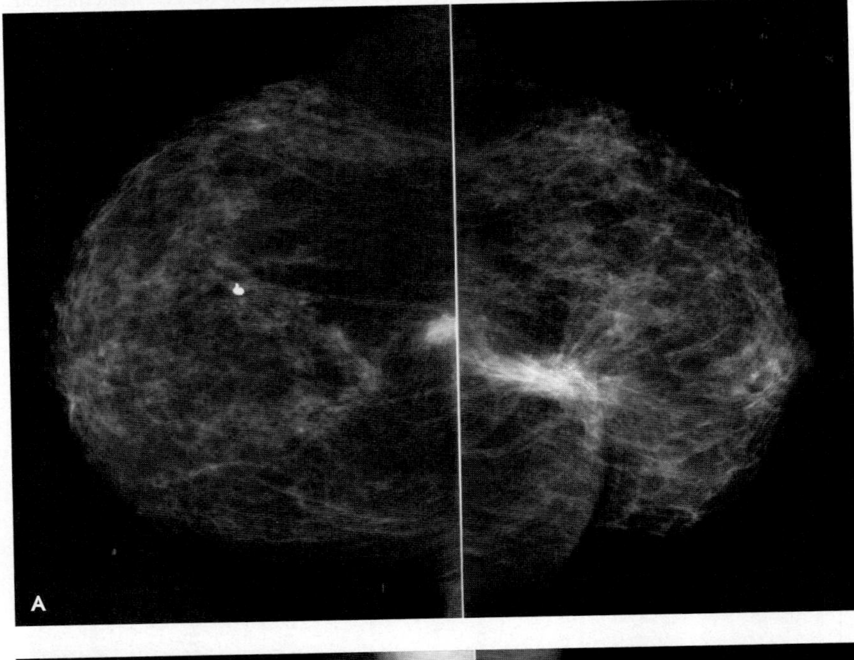

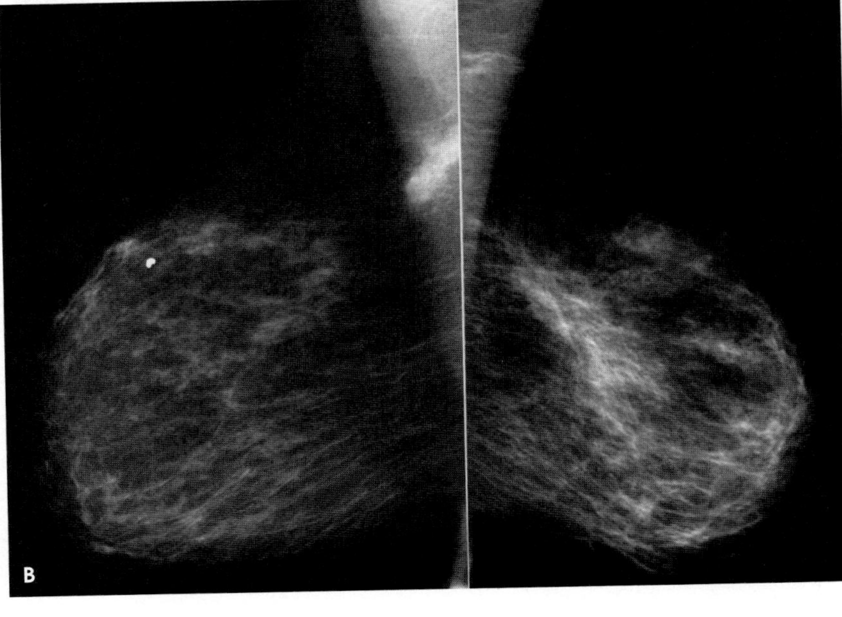

Figure 3.27. Diagnostic evaluation, 57-year-old patient with a history of left breast cancer treated with lumpectomy and radiation therapy. Craniocaudal **(A)** and mediolateral oblique **(B)** views.

How would you describe the findings and what would you do next?

The left breast is smaller compared to the right, there is prominence of the trabecular markings, and parenchymal asymmetry with distortion is seen at the lumpectomy site on the left. These findings are consistent with the history of lumpectomy and radiation therapy on the left. Did you notice the mass on the right? A mass with indistinct margins is present in the upper central to inner aspect of the right breast posteriorly. Although it is of concern, given its location (upper central to inner quadrant), the possibility that this is related to a prior port-a-catheter site should be considered.

On physical examination a healed scar is noted at the site previously occupied by the port-a-catheter in the upper inner quadrant of the right breast. An oval, 1-cm mass with a heterogeneous echotexture, indistinct margins, and a thin tract to the skin is seen corresponding to the scar site and the area of mammographic concern at the 1 o'clock position, 12 cm from the right nipple (Fig. 3.27C). This patient can be managed conservatively. The changes often evolve with complete resolution (Fig. 3.27D, E). Alternatively, the changes stabilize, and in some women calcifications can develop at these sites. Given the number of women with breast cancer who are receiving chemotherapy, you need to be aware of the changes that may be seen following removal of these catheters. These catheters are commonly placed in the upper inner quadrant of the contralateral, normal breast and removed following completion of chemotherapy. If you review prior films, the location of the port-a-catheter can be established and correlated with the appearance of this new finding. The changes we have seen following removal of a catheter include a round mass with well-circumscribed to indistinct margins, a spiculated mass, focal parenchymal asymmetry, and calcifications that can range from punctate, round, and pleomorphic to those with a more dystrophic appearance.

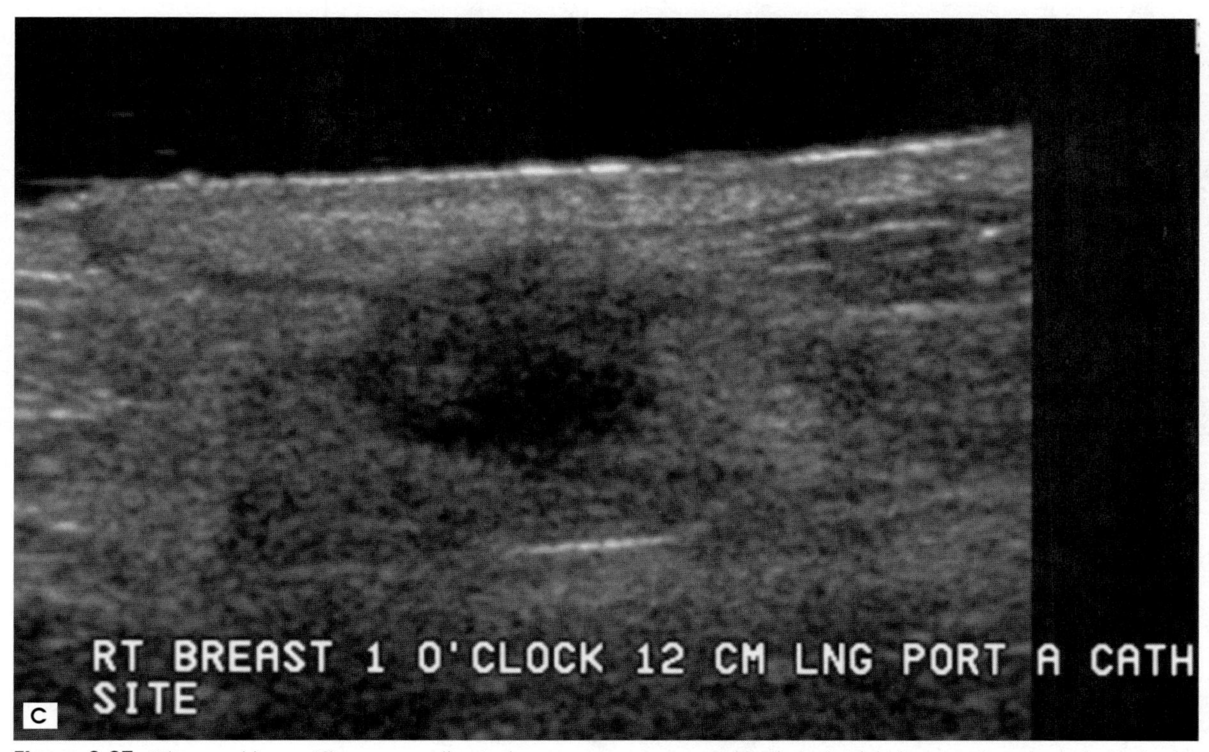

Figure 3.27. Ultrasound image **(C)**, corresponding to the mass seen mammographically in the right breast and on physical examination directly over the location of the port-a-catheter.

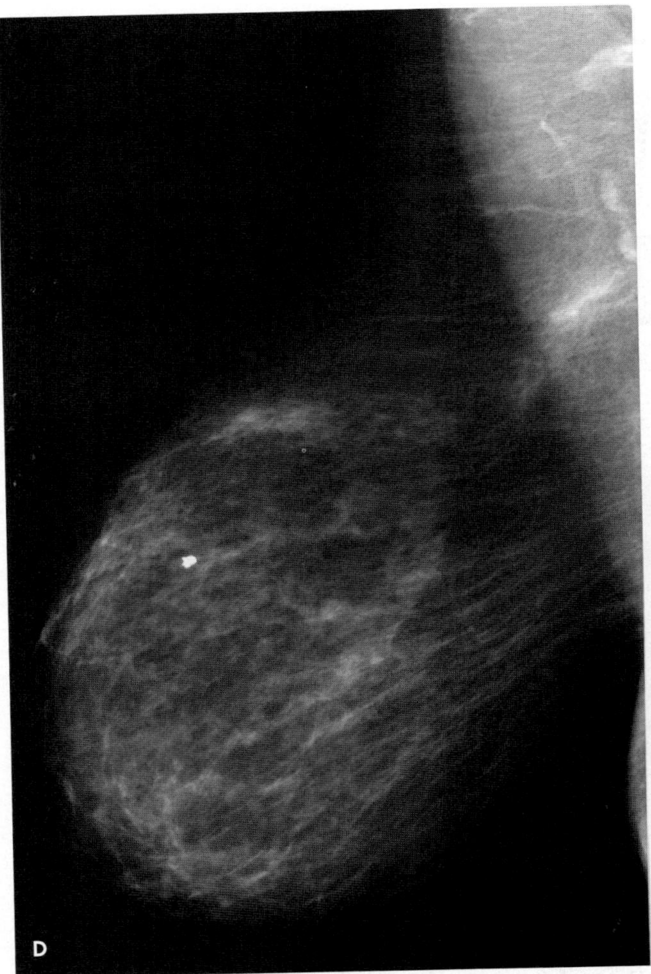

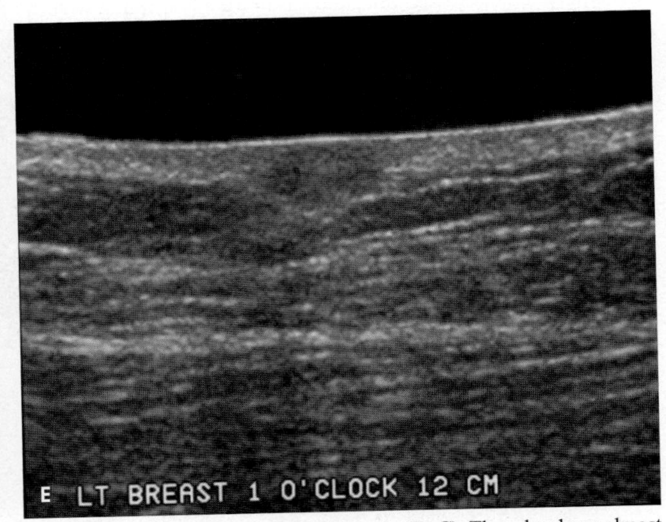

Figure 3.27. Follow-up mediolateral oblique **(D)** view and ultrasound **(E)**, left breast, 6 months following that shown in **(B, C)**. There has been almost complete resolution of the findings noted in **(A–C)**.

PATIENT 28

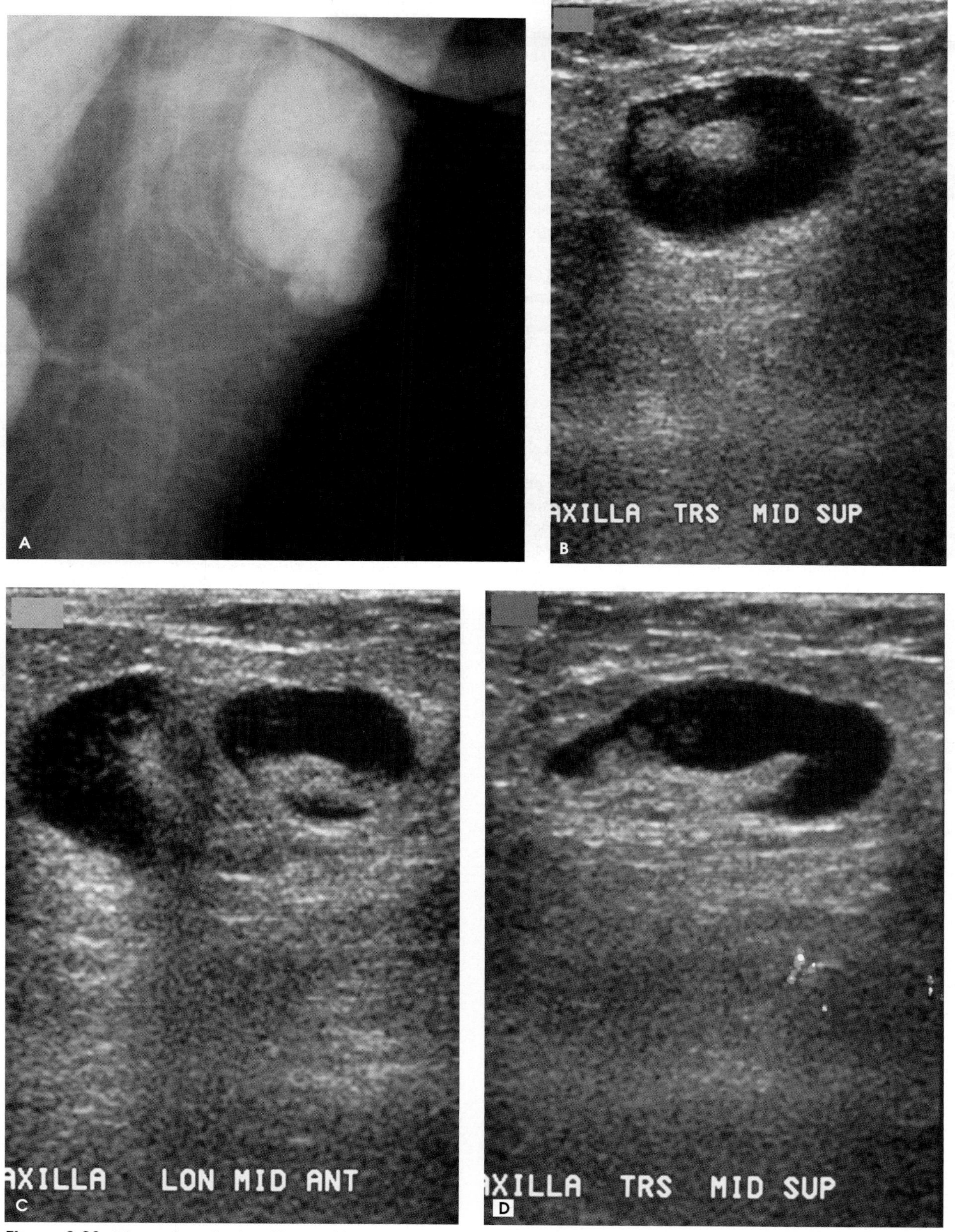

Figure 3.28. Diagnostic evaluation, 39-year-old woman presenting with a tender mass in the left axilla. Axillary view **(A),** left axilla. Ultrasound images **(B–D)** of the left axilla.

How would you describe the findings, and what is your differential?

An oval, well-circumscribed, macrolobulated mass is imaged on the axillary view, corresponding to the area of concern to the patient; a second mass is partially seen at the edge of the film inferiorly. No associated calcifications are present. On physical examination, several hard, movable, exquisitely tender masses are palpated in the left axilla. On ultrasound, well-circumscribed masses with prominent hypoechoic regions and central or eccentrically located areas of hyperechogenicity are imaged corresponding to the palpable findings and consistent with lymph nodes. The findings are nonspecific and the differential is extensive, ranging from reactive adenopathy to lymphoid hyperplasia, collagen vascular disorders (e.g., scleroderma, dermatomyositis), rheumatoid arthritis, granulomatous diseases (sarcoid, tuberculosis, histoplasmosis), human immunodeficiency virus, human immunodeficiency syndrome, dermatopathic, toxoplasmosis, cat scratch disease, metastatic disease (breast or other primary), and lymphoma.

In patients like this, what else might be very helpful in sorting through the differential?

How about obtaining a more extensive history relative to any other underlying systemic diseases, and also examining the patient? During the ultrasound study, as I am examining the patient, I notice several healing scratch marks on her left arm. On questioning her, she describes having recently acquired a kitten, with the scratches having occurred approximately 2 weeks previously. The suspected diagnosis of cat scratch disease is established following serologic testing.

What is cat scratch disease, how do humans contract the disease, and what are the clinical manifestations?

Cat scratch disease is a bacterial infection caused by *Bartonella henselae* and is transmitted to humans following a scratch, lick (on broken skin), or bite from an infected kitten or cat. It is not transmitted from human to human. The infection is more common in the fall and winter months. Within a couple of weeks following the exposure, the patient may develop tender, indurated, erythematous lymphadenopathy in close proximity to the inoculation site, lasting 4 to 6 weeks in most patients, although it can persist for up to a year. The most commonly involved lymph nodes groups include axillary, cervical, submandibular, preauricular, epitrochlear, femoral, and inguinal. Although infections are often mild, some patients can develop systemic symptoms including fever, fatigue, loss of appetite, headache, rash, and sore throat. In some patients the infection can involve the eye (Parinaud oculoglandular syndrome), with a sore on the conjunctiva, redness of the eye, and swollen preauricular lymph nodes. Rarely, with involvement of the central nervous system, encephalitis with high fever, coma, and convulsions can develop within 6 weeks following the development of lymphadenopathy. Optic neuritis with transient blindness has also been reported. Other rare manifestations include osteolytic bone lesions, granulomatous hepatitis, erythema multiforme, thrombocytopenia purpura, and mesenteric lymphadenitis. In most patients, however, this is a self-limited process that resolves on its own and requires no treatment. Although antibiotics are used in some patients, appropriate antibiotic coverage is not established.

What are the imaging features of cat scratch disease?

The intramammary and axillary lymph nodes on the side scratched by the cat can enlarge, increase in density, and lose the fatty hilar region; however, they typically remain well circumscribed. On ultrasound, the involved lymph nodes demonstrate prominence, thickening, and bulging of the hypoechoic cortical region and attenuation, mass effect, or loss of the echogenic focus usually seen in normal lymph nodes.

What are the histologic features of cat scratch disease?

Histologically, necrotizing granulomas surrounded by lymphocytes limited to the lymph nodes are the hallmark of this disease. Gram-negative, branching, Warthin-Starr–positive bacilli may be seen rarely in the necrotic centers. Cultures do not usually yield growth of the causative agent.

PATIENT 29

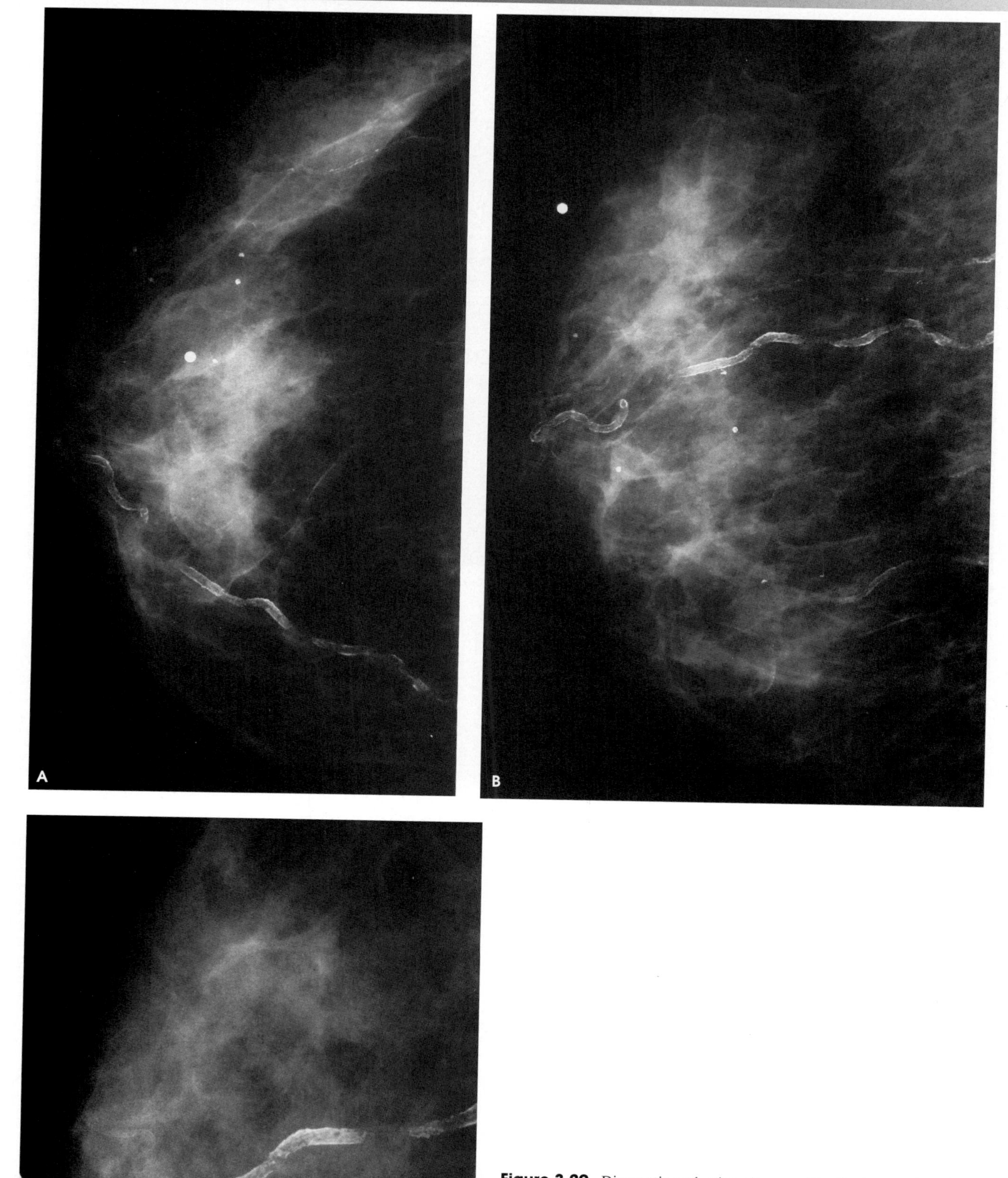

Figure 3.29. Diagnostic evaluation, 64-year-old patient presenting with a "lump" in the right breast. Craniocaudal **(A)** and mediolateral oblique **(B)** views of the right breast. Spot tangential view **(C)** at the site of the palpable finding. The metallic BB is on the palpable finding.

How would you describe the findings, and what would you do next?

Glandular tissue is imaged in the right breast, with no apparent mass or distortion. Scattered dystrophic and arterial calcifications are noted. Correlative physical examination and an ultrasound are indicated.

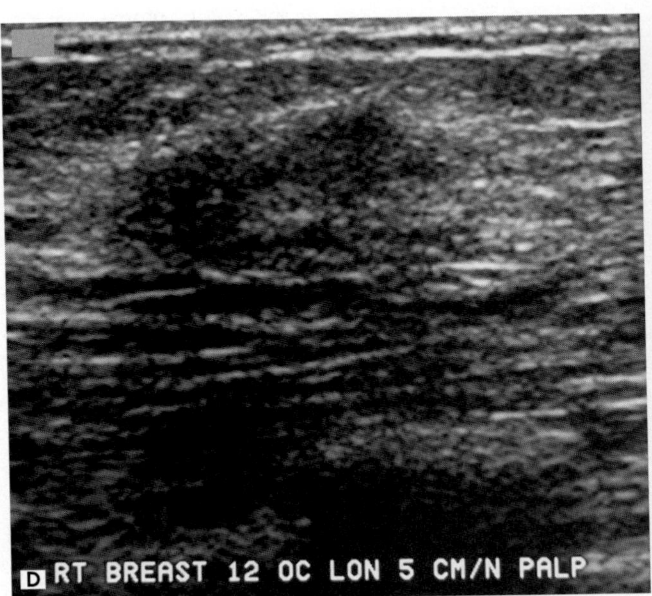

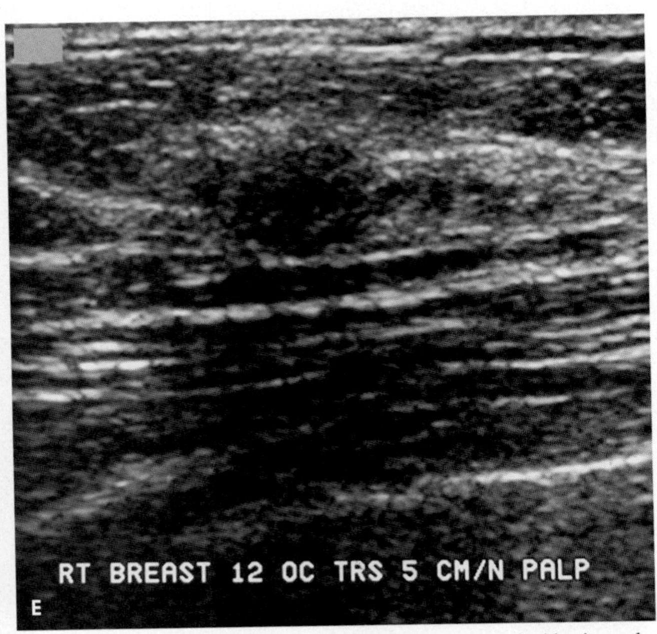

Figure 3.29. (*Continued*) Ultrasound images, in longitudinal (LON) **(D)** and transverse (TRS) **(E)** projections corresponding to the palpable site at the 12 o'clock position, 5 cm from the right nipple.

How would you describe the findings, what is your differential, and what is your recommendation?

On physical examination, a hard mass is palpated at the 12 o'clock position, 5 cm from the right nipple. On ultrasound, a 1.2-cm, irregular mass with a heterogeneous echotexture and some minimal shadowing is imaged corresponding to the palpable finding. Differential considerations include invasive ductal carcinoma not otherwise specified, invasive lobular carcinoma, and lymphoma. Benign considerations are limited but include fibrosis or an inflammatory process. In the absence of focal symptoms, an inflammatory process is unlikely. Biopsy is indicated.

BI-RADS® category 4: suspicious abnormality—biopsy should be considered. Diabetic fibrous mastopathy is diagnosed on the core biopsy. In these patients, an adequate amount of tissue may be difficult to obtain because the dense fibrosis may preclude adequate sampling. If inadequate sampling is a concern, excisional biopsy should be recommended.

How do patients with diabetic fibrous mastopathy present, and in what group of patients is this entity typically diagnosed?

Diabetic fibrous mastopathy is a rare entity affecting long-standing, insulin-dependent diabetic patients who present with one or multiple hard, irregular, readily mobile, discrete, painless palpable masses. Characteristically, dense glandular tissue is imaged mammographically, and an irregular mass with dense shadowing is imaged on ultrasound corresponding to the palpable area. Biopsies through these areas are often difficult because of the resistance encountered and the inability of the needle to cut through the tissue adequately. Given the history of diabetes, vascular calcifications are often seen bilaterally. Multiple lesions may be present, occurring simultaneously or at different times. Many of these patients have other complications associated with diabetes, including nephropathy, retinopathy, and neuropathy.

What histologic findings are reported in patients with diabetic fibrous mastopathy?

The lesions are characterized by dense fibrosis and a predominantly B-cell lymphocytic infiltrate surrounding ducts, lobules, and vessels. An autoimmune etiology has been suggested for this entity.

PATIENT 30

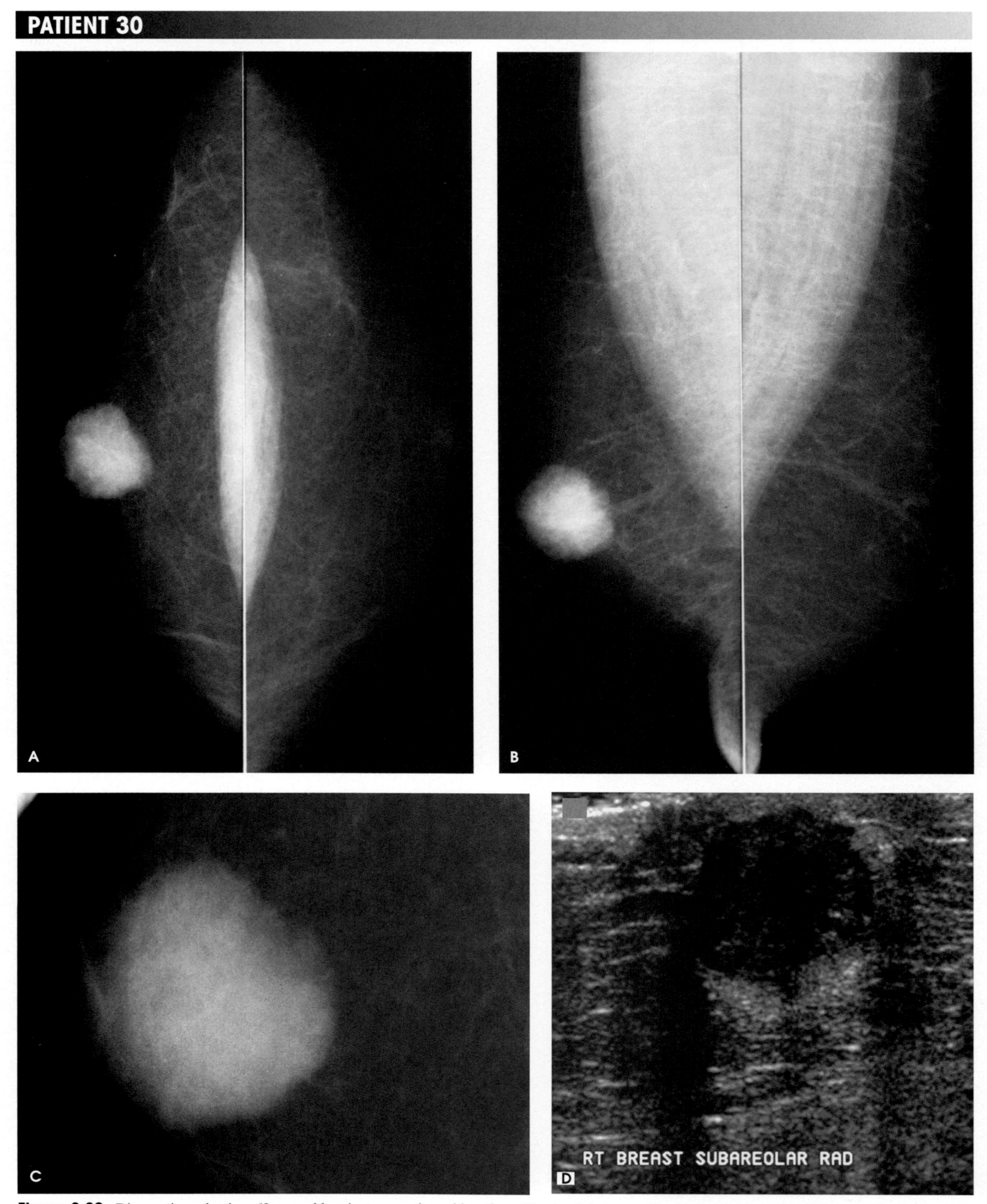

Figure 3.30. Diagnostic evaluation, 62-year-old patient presenting with a "lump" in the right breast. Craniocaudal **(A)** and mediolateral oblique **(B)** views. Spot compression **(C)** view of "lump" in the right breast. Ultrasound image **(D)** in the radial projection of the palpable finding in the right subareolar area.

How would you describe the findings, and what is your differential?

Given the small breast size, prominent pectoral muscles, and the fatty pattern on the left, consider that this may be a male patient. This can be confirmed by looking at the name of the patient on the film. A 2.5-cm round mass, with partially well-circumscribed margins, is present in the right subareolar area. There are no associated calcifications. On physical examination, a hard, nontender mass is palpated in the subareolar area on the right. On ultrasound, a round mass with indistinct and microlobulated margins and associated posterior acoustic enhancement is imaged corresponding to the area of concern to the patient.

The differential in a male patient is limited. The main diagnostic consideration in men presenting with a "lump" is gynecomastia; however, the clinical and imaging findings in this patient are not consistent with gynecomastia. If there is a history of trauma or surgery, this could represent a posttraumatic or surgical fluid collection. An inflammatory process is also in the differential; however, no tenderness is elicited and no skin changes (e.g,. erythema, warmth) are noted on exam. Other benign lesions that can be seen in men include pseudoangiomatous stromal hyperplasia, duct ectasia, papilloma, fat necrosis, epidermal inclusion cyst, and granular cell tumor. In the malignant category, an invasive ductal carcinoma not otherwise specified would be the leading consideration. Papillary carcinoma is reportedly more common in men; other subtypes that may be seen include medullary, mucinous, and adenoid cystic carcinoma. If the patient is known to have a malignancy (prostate, hematopoetic, etc.), this could represent a metastatic lesion. Because men do not usually have lobules, lobular processes such as fibroadenomas, cysts, sclerosing adenosis, and invasive lobular carcinomas are rarely seen in men.

What is your recommendation?

A biopsy is indicated and done. An invasive ductal carcinoma is diagnosed following the core biopsy. A grade III, 2.5-cm invasive ductal carcinoma not otherwise specified, with associated vascular/lymphatic invasion, is confirmed on the mastectomy. Four of eight lymph nodes have metastatic disease, and extracapsular extension is described in one of the positive lymph nodes [pT2, pN2, pMx, Stage IIB].

What are some of the risk factors for male breast cancer?

Male breast cancer is uncommon, accounting for $<1\%$ of all breast cancers. Men with breast cancer present at slightly older ages compared to women and often have longer duration of symptoms. Several risk factors have been postulated for male breast cancer, including increased levels of estradiol and other estrogenic hormones; mumps orchitis (after age 20 years); testicular trauma; undescended testis; traumatic injury to the breast; cirrhosis; history of employment in steel works, blast furnaces, and rolling mills; radiation exposure; Klinefelter's syndrome; the BRCA 2 mutation; and less commonly, but reported, BRCA1. Gynecomastia is not considered a risk factor or a precursor for male breast cancer.

How do men with breast cancer typically present, and what forms of breast cancers are typically diagnosed histologically?

Most male patients present with a painless mass that is either subareolar or more eccentric (e.g., upper outer quadrant) in location or describing nipple discharge. Invasive ductal carcinoma not otherwise specified represents nearly 85% of all breast cancers diagnosed in male patients. An associated intraductal component may be seen in as many as 50% of invasive lesions. About 5% to 10% of patients are diagnosed with intraductal disease in the absence of invasion. Given the absence of lobular tissue in most males, invasive lobular carcinoma is rare. Prostate cancer with metastasis to the breast can sometimes be difficult to distinguish from primary breast cancer, particularly because some prostate cancers are estrogen receptor–positive.

PATIENT 31

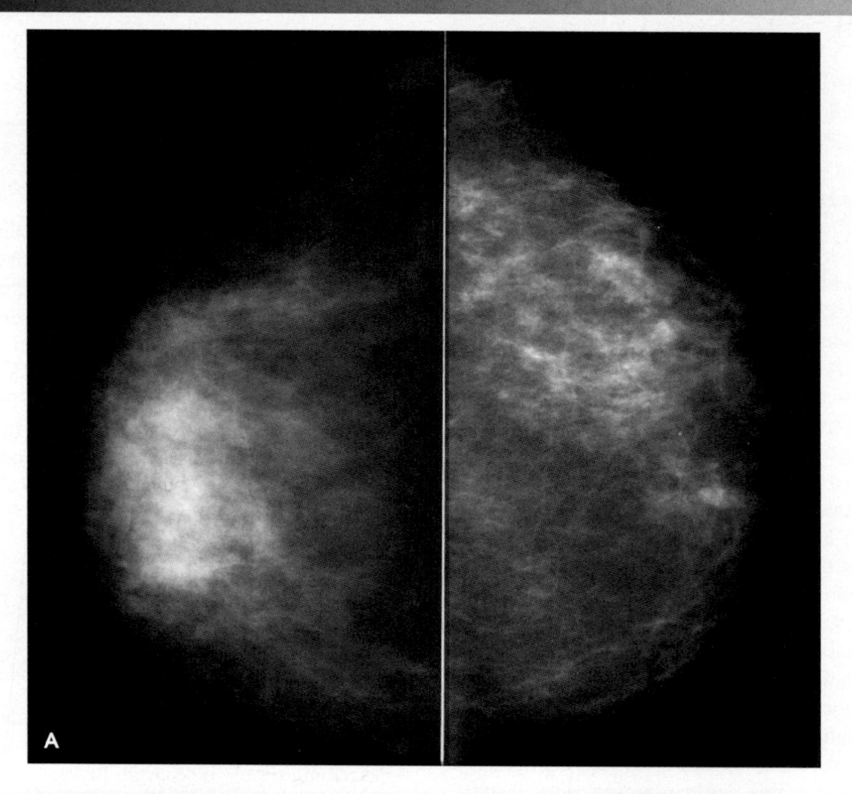

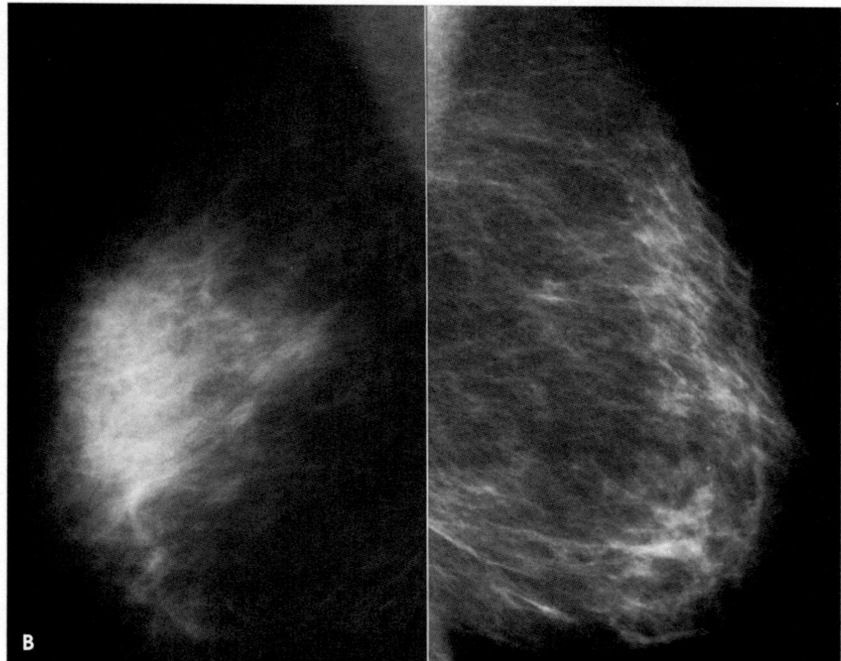

Figure 3.31. Diagnostic evaluation, 66-year-old patient presents describing changes in her right breast. Craniocaudal **(A)** and mediolateral oblique **(B)** views. The technical factors used for the routine views are as follows:

Factor	RTCC	LTCC	RTMLO	LTMLO
kV	35	28	35	28
mAs	201	319	170	341
Comp (mm)	101	79	94	81

What do you think, and what additional information would you like?

The right breast is diffusely abnormal and appears smaller than the left. The decreased compressibility of the right breast is evidenced by the increased number of millimeters required for compression. Also notable is the 35 kV used to obtain adequate exposure of the right breast.

Differential considerations for diffuse changes that are usually unilateral, although rarely can be bilateral, include radiation therapy effect, inflammatory changes (e.g., mastitis), trauma (e.g., hematoma, edema), ipsilateral axillary adenopathy with lymphatic obstruction, dialysis shunt in the ipsilateral arm with fluid overload, invasive ductal carcinoma not otherwise specified, inflammatory carcinoma, invasive lobular carcinoma, or lymphoma. Invasive lobular carcinoma can lead to increases in breast density and size or a decrease in breast size (the shrinking breast). Differential considerations for diffuse changes that are usually bilateral, although they can be unilateral, include hormone replacement therapy (e.g., estrogen), weight changes, congestive heart failure, renal failure with fluid overload, and superior vena cava syndrome. Additional rare benign causes include granulomatous mastitis, coumadin necrosis, arteritis, and autoimmune disorders (e.g., scleroderma). Obtaining a thorough history, examining the patient, and doing an ultrasound are often helpful in sorting through the differential considerations.

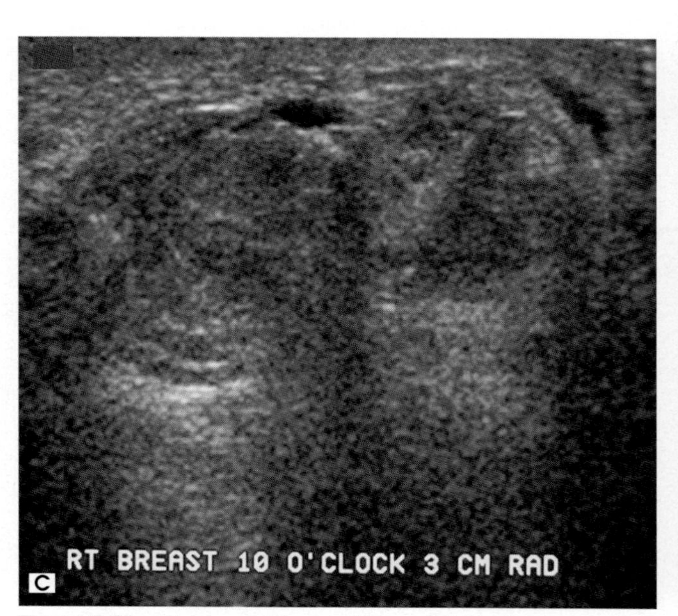

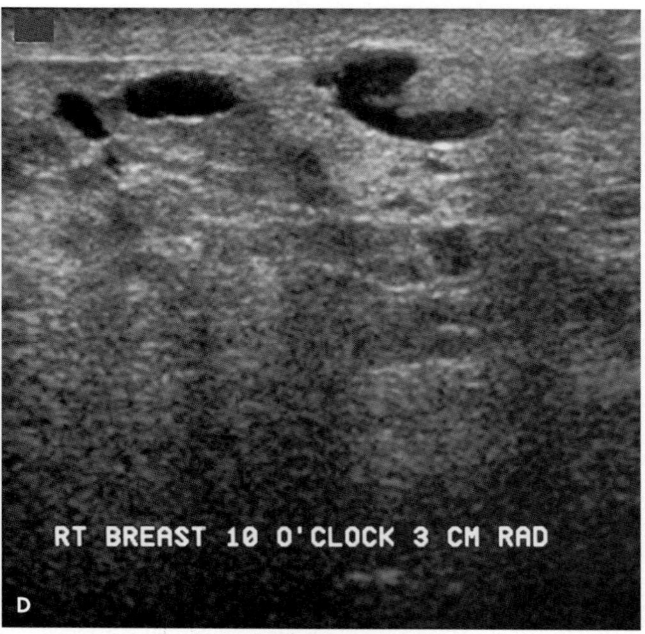

Figure 3.31. (*Continued*) Ultrasound images **(C, D)** taken in the radial projection in the upper outer quadrant of the right breast.

Based on the ultrasound images alone, what is the most likely diagnosis?

Sonographically, the tissue is hyperechoic consistent with hyperemia, and the normal tissue architecture/planes are disrupted with associated scattered fluid collections. The sonographic findings are suggestive of posttraumatic or inflammatory changes. During the mammogram and when doing the ultrasound, no significant tenderness is elicited, as would be expected if this were an ongoing bacterial inflammatory process. In scanning the patient, the radiologist is in a unique position to obtain a thorough, accurate history from the patient. Indeed, in this patient, the history of a car accident with airbag deployment is obtained from the patient as the ultrasound is being done. She describes significant ecchymosis, diffusely involving the breast, following the accident that has now resolved completely. The findings in this patient are likely related to the trauma.

Although a BI-RADS® category 2: benign finding is used, the patient is asked to return in 3 to 4 months for follow-up. As this process resolves, mixed-density masses (fat containing) and oil cysts may develop; alternatively dystrophic calcifications may be seen, or the findings may resolve completely with no intermediate stages.

Note that the assessment categories should be considered independent of the recommendation. In this patient the finding is benign, yet a short-interval follow-up is recommended. In patients in whom I suspect an inflammatory condition or posttraumatic/surgical changes, I recommend a 3- to 4-month follow-up. Under these circumstances, a rapid change in the findings is expected. Six months is the usual recommendation for other patients in whom a short-interval follow-up is recommended (e.g., those with assessment category 3—probably benign lesion—well-circumscribed mass in a woman with no prior films).

PATIENT 32

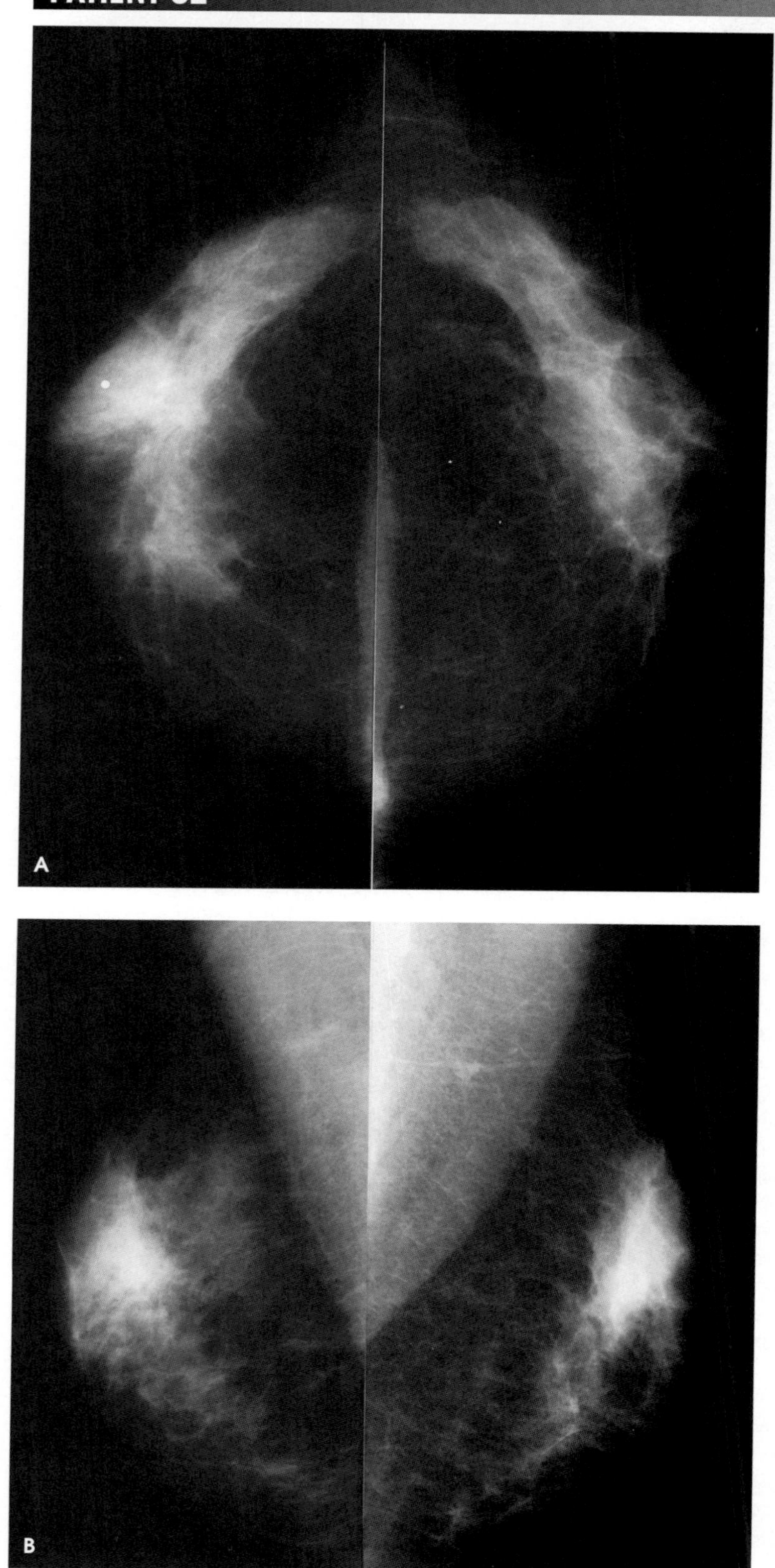

Figure 3.32. Diagnostic evaluation, 42-year-old patient presenting with a "lump" in the right breast. Craniocaudal **(A)** and mediolateral oblique **(B)** views. Metallic BB is seen on the craniocaudal view at the site of concern to the patient.

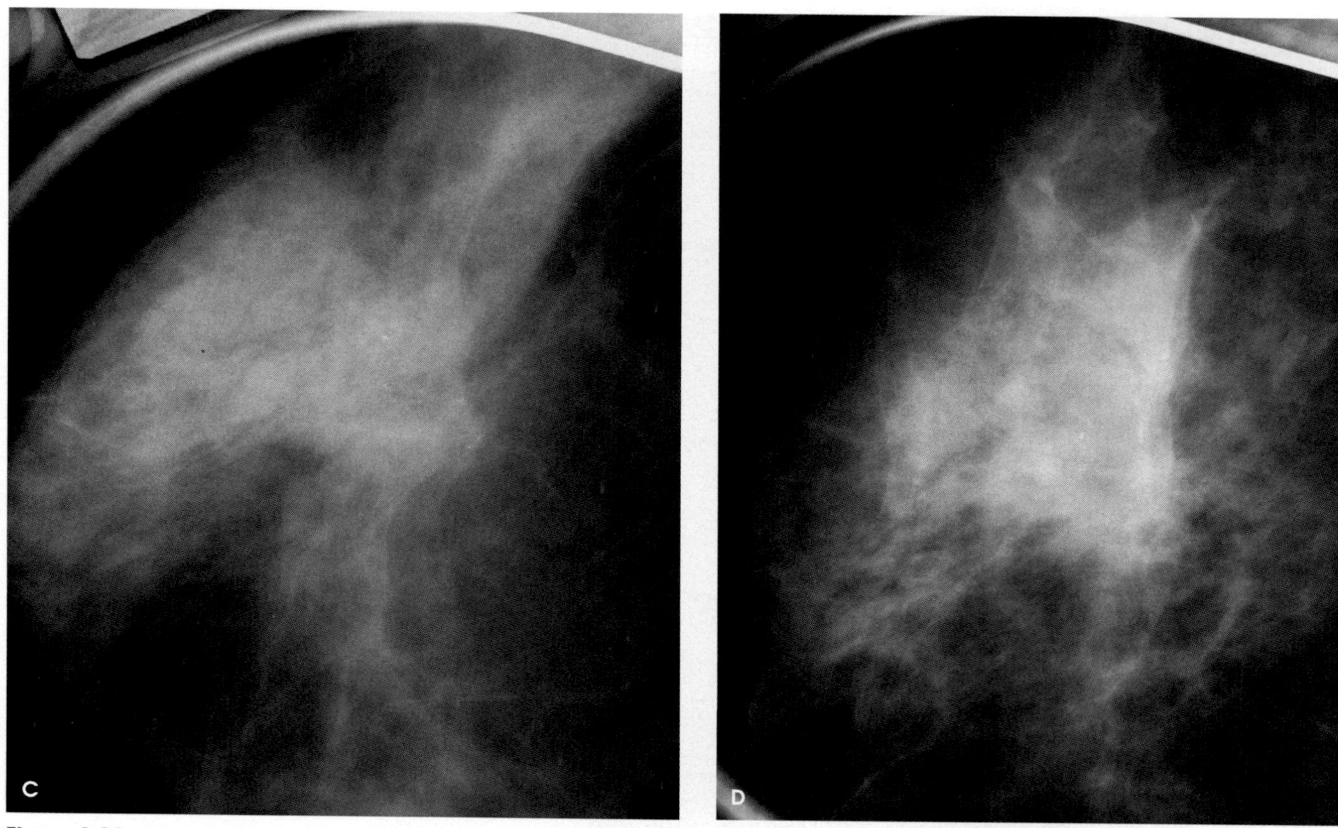

Figure 3.32. (*Continued*) Craniocaudal **(C)** and mediolateral oblique **(D)** spot compression views of palpable abnormality, right breast.

How would you describe the findings, and what are the main differential considerations?

The overall density of the breast parenchyma on the right is increased, and a mass with distortion is noted in the right craniocaudal view at the site of concern to the patient (metallic BB). The right craniocaudal spot compression view confirms the presence of a mass with indistinct and obscured margins, associated distortion, and punctate calcifications. Except for some punctate calcifications, the findings on the mediolateral oblique spot compression view are not striking: No definite mass is seen, there is scalloping of the tissue, and fat seems to be present, intermingled with glandular tissue. Although tumors are usually three-dimensional and readily apparent on all views, there may be times when the findings are more striking in one of the two projections obtained. This is particularly true for invasive lobular carcinoma; however, it can also be seen with invasive ductal carcinoma. Rarely, an inflammatory process might present with this constellation of findings.

On physical examination, a hard fixed mass is palpated, involving the right breast centrally. A 2.5-cm round mass with indistinct, angular, and microlobulated margins is imaged at the 12 o'clock position, 2 cm from the right nipple, corresponding to the palpable finding. Shadowing and enhancement are seen as different areas of the mass are scanned (Fig. 3.32E, F). On magnetic resonance imaging (MRI), the mass demonstrates rapid wash-in and wash-out of contrast, consistent with a malignancy (Fig. 3.32G). No additional lesions are identified in either breast on MRI.

BI-RADS® category 4: suspicious abnormality—biopsy should be considered.

An ultrasound-guided biopsy is done. An invasive ductal carcinoma and ductal carcinoma in situ are diagnosed on the core biopsy. The patient is treated with neoadjuvant chemotherapy followed by lumpectomy and sentinel lymph node biopsy. Residual grade III invasive ductal carcinoma (1.5 cm) and high-grade ductal carcinoma in situ with central necrosis are reported following the lumpectomy. The sentinel lymph node is normal [ypT1c, pN0(sn)(i−), pMX; Stage I].

Traditionally, neoadjuvant therapy (preoperative chemotherapy) has been the treatment of choice in women with inflammatory breast carcinoma. It is being used with increasing frequency, however, in women with locally advanced cancer. Following therapy, as the tumor is downstaged, some of these patients can be treated appropriately with breast-conserving surgery. Patients with a complete histologic remission following neoadjuvant therapy have significantly improved long-term survival compared to those with partial or no response to therapy. Following breast-conserving surgery, radiation therapy is also used to treat these patients.

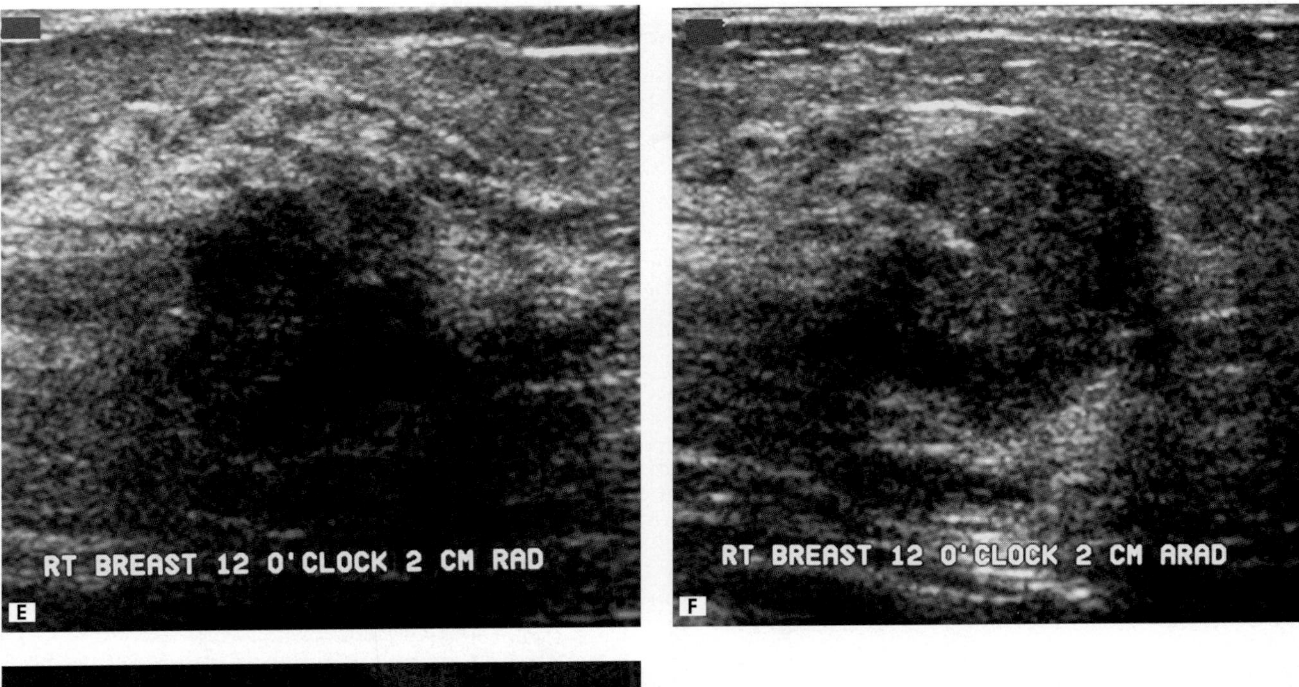

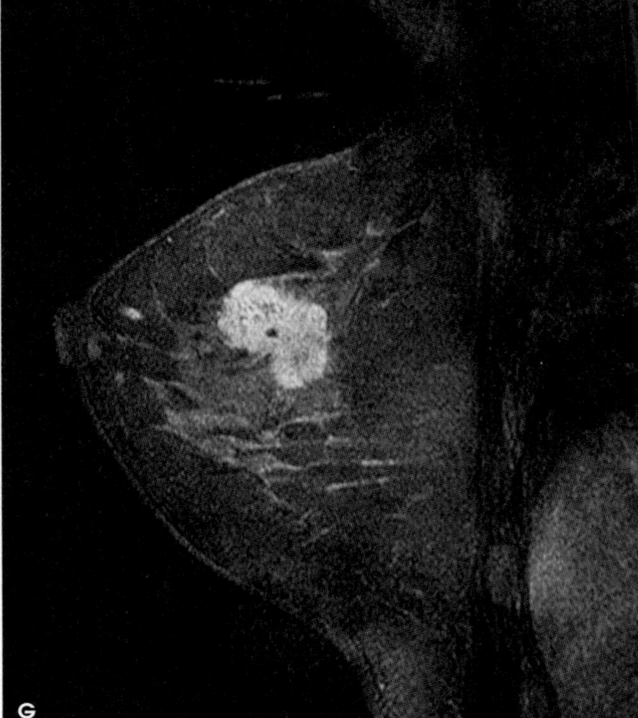

Figure 3.32. *(Continued)* Ultrasound images, in radial (RAD) **(E)** and antiradial (ARAD) **(F)** projections of the palpable finding in the right breast. Magnetic resonance, subtraction image **(G)** of the lesion in the right breast.

PATIENT 33

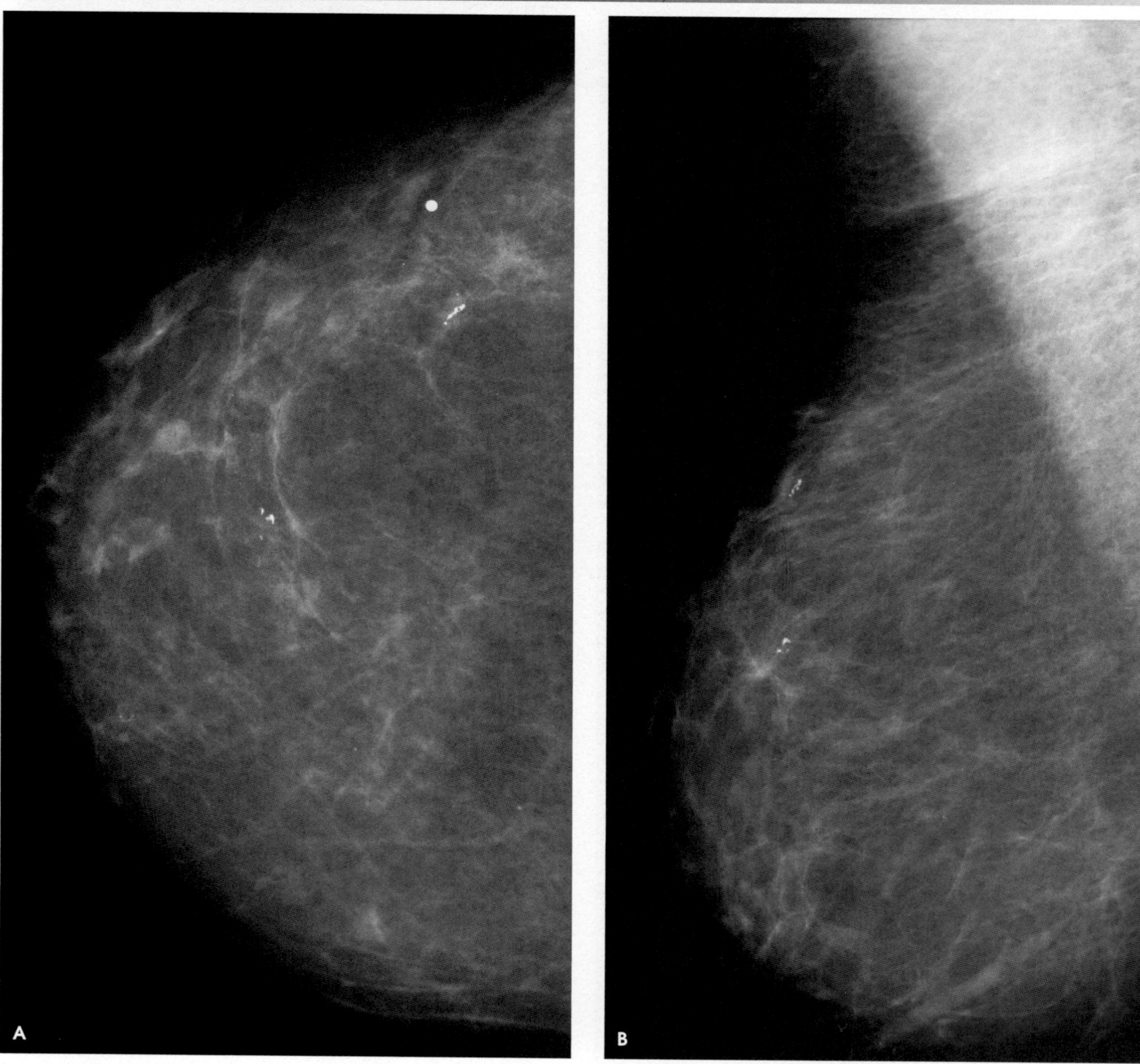

Figure 3.33. Diagnostic evaluation, 77-year-old patient presenting with a "lump" in the right breast. Craniocaudal **(A)** and mediolateral oblique **(B)** views, right breast, with a metallic BB placed at the site of the palpable finding.

What do you think, and with what degree of certainty can you make any recommendations?
What else might be helpful in evaluating women who present with localized findings?

Coarse dystrophic calcifications are present; however, no significant abnormality is apparent on the craniocaudal and mediolateral oblique views of the right breast. A spot tangential view at the site of the palpable finding is done routinely in patients with localized findings. In some patients, the lesion may be partially or completely outlined by fat on the spot tangential view, facilitating detection and characterization of the palpable finding.

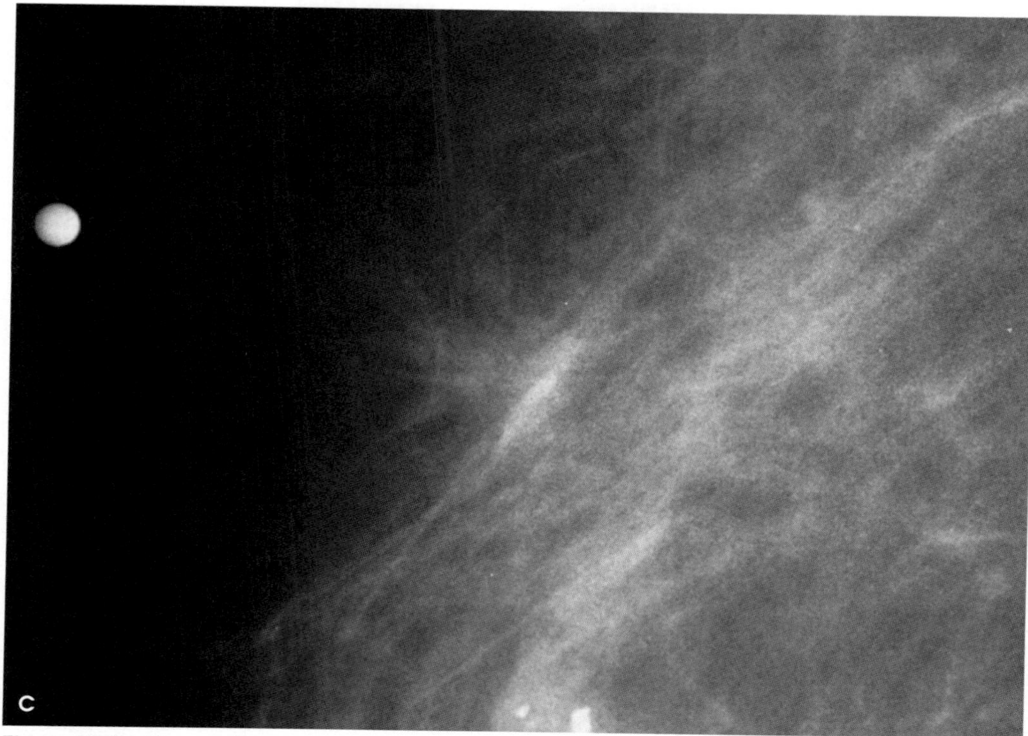

Figure 3.33. (*Continued*) Spot tangential **(C)** view, palpable finding, right breast. Metallic BB used to indicate location of "lump."

Now what can you say, and with what degree of certainty?
What is your differential?

A spiculated mass is imaged on the spot tangential view, corresponding to the palpable finding. Scalloping of sharply defined, thin Cooper ligaments can be seen at the subcutaneous fat–glandular tissue interface in many women. When a ligament is thickened, straightened, or appears irregular and spiculated, as shown here, it is of concern and further evaluation is indicated. Differential considerations include invasive ductal carcinoma not otherwise specified, tubular carcinoma, and invasive lobular carcinoma. Benign considerations include fat necrosis (posttrauma or surgery), sclerosing adenosis, papilloma, complex sclerosing lesion, and inflammatory changes. Rare causes include granular cell tumor or fibromatosis (extra-abdominal desmoid).

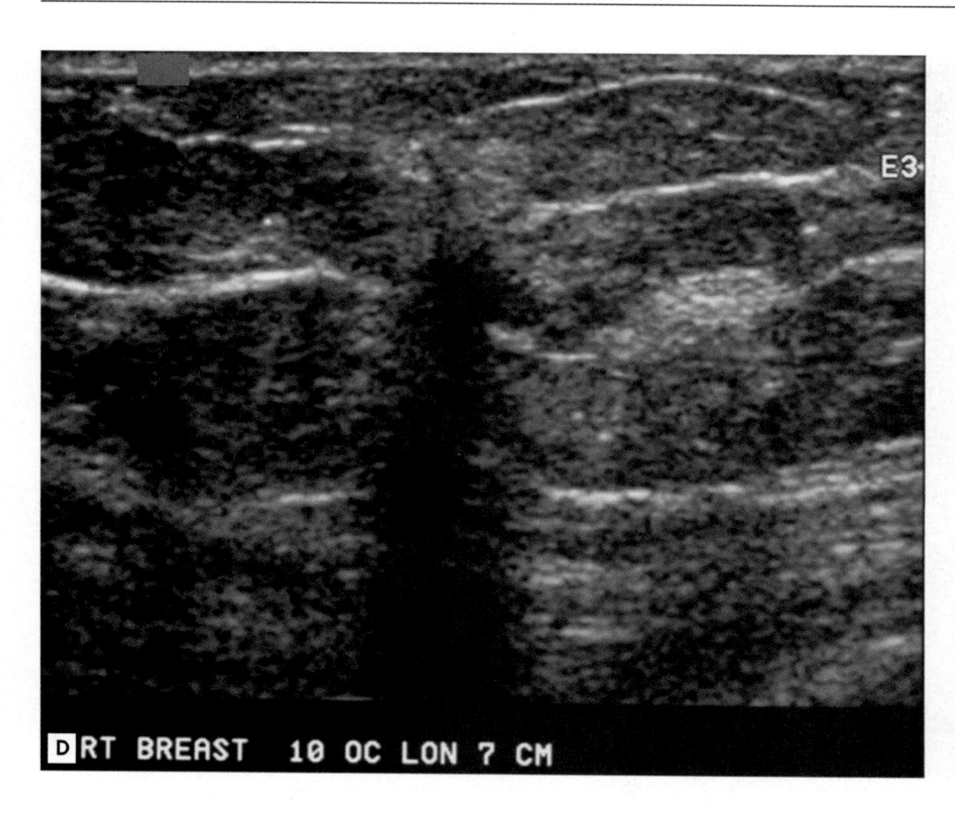

Figure 3.33. (*Continued*) Ultrasound image **(D)** in the longitudinal projection at the site of concern in the upper outer quadrant of the right breast.

How would you describe the findings, and what is indicated next?

On ultrasound, an irregular, hypoechoic, 1-cm mass with spiculated and angular margins and associated shadowing is imaged at the 10 o'clock position, 7 cm from the nipple. This corresponds to the area of concern to the patient and the mammographic finding.

BI-RADS® category 4: suspicious abnormality—biopsy should be considered.

An ultrasound-guided biopsy is done and an invasive mammary carcinoma is reported on the cores. A 1.1-cm grade I invasive mammary carcinoma with tubulolobular features and associated intermediate-nuclear-grade ductal carcinoma in situ is reported on the lumpectomy specimen. Extensive perineural invasion is seen. No metastatic disease is seen in three excised sentinel lymph nodes [pT1c, pN0(sn) (i−), pMX; Stage I].

Tubulolobular carcinomas are classified as a variant of invasive lobular carcinomas, characterized by the presence of small, cohesive cells infiltrating the stroma in single files and the formation of tight tubules (similar to those described for tubular carcinomas but smaller). However, it should be noted that the classification of a lesion with tubules as invasive lobular carcinoma is controversial. Perineural invasion is not a common finding in breast cancers (<10% of invasive carcinomas) and reportedly has no prognostic significance.

PATIENT 34

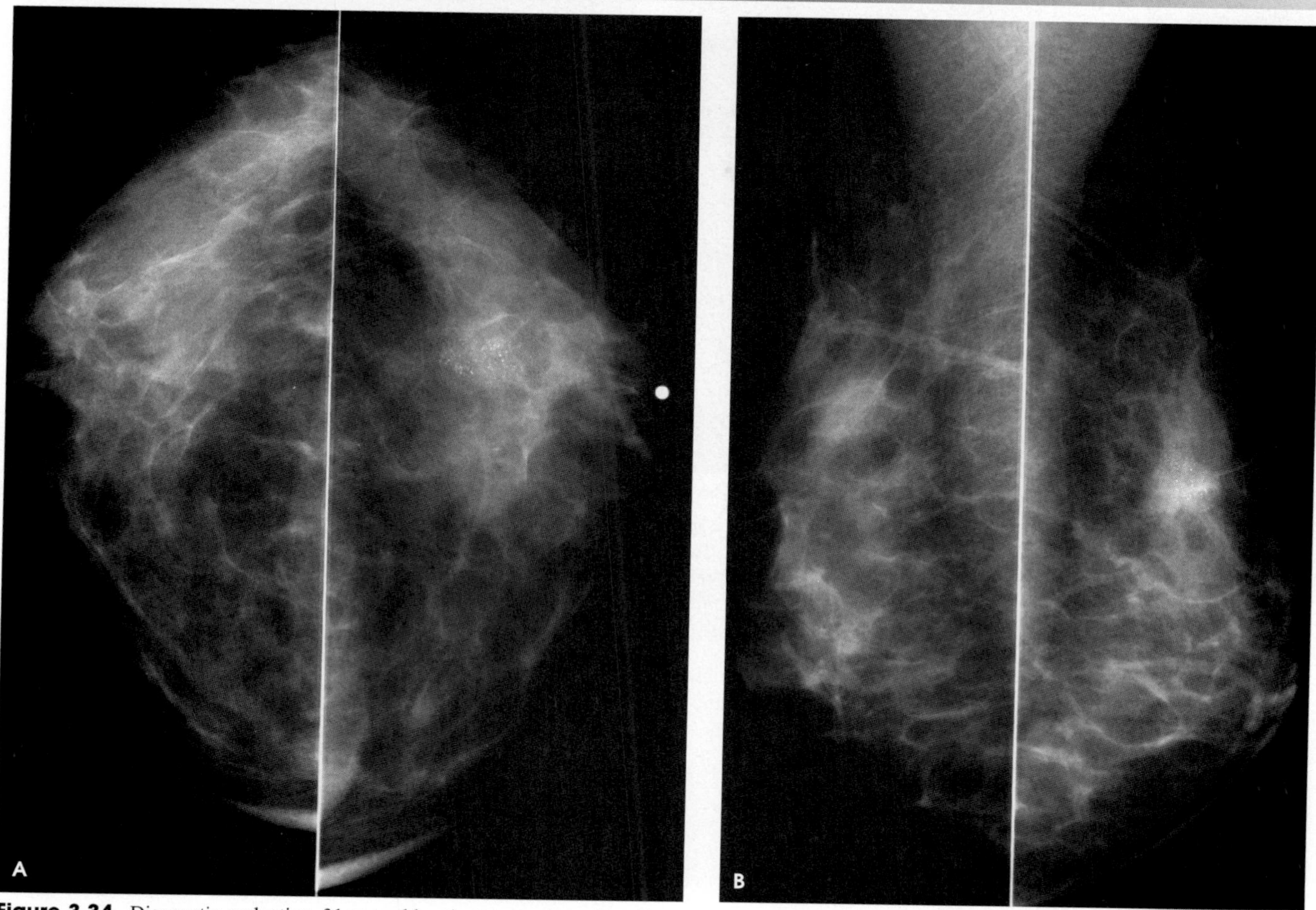

Figure 3.34. Diagnostic evaluation, 31-year-old patient presenting with a "lump" in the left breast. Craniocaudal **(A)** and mediolateral oblique **(B)** views, metallic BB placed at the site of the palpable finding (spot tangential view, not shown).

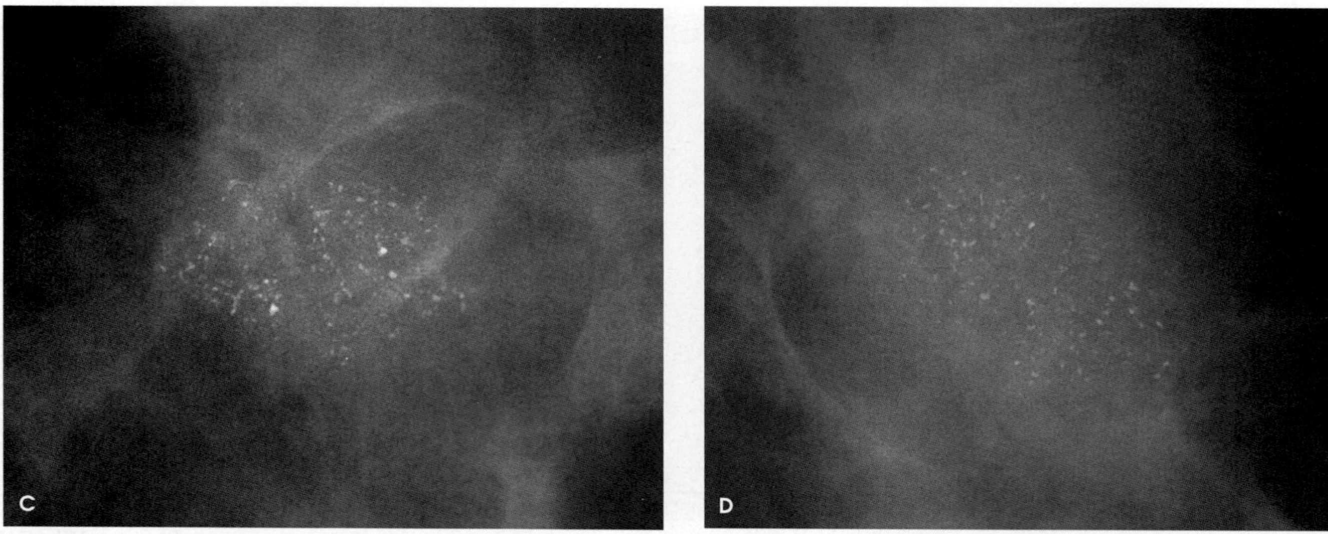

Figure 3.34. (*Continued*) Double spot compression magnification views, craniocaudal **(C)** and mediolateral oblique **(D)** projections.

How would you describe the findings, and what is indicated next?

Given the presence of calcifications on the routine views, double spot compression magnification views are done for further characterization of the calcifications and the extent of disease. A cluster of pleomorphic calcifications is imaged corresponding to the "lump" described by the patient, but no mass is seen mammographically. Correlative physical examination and an ultrasound are undertaken for further evaluation of the palpable findings.

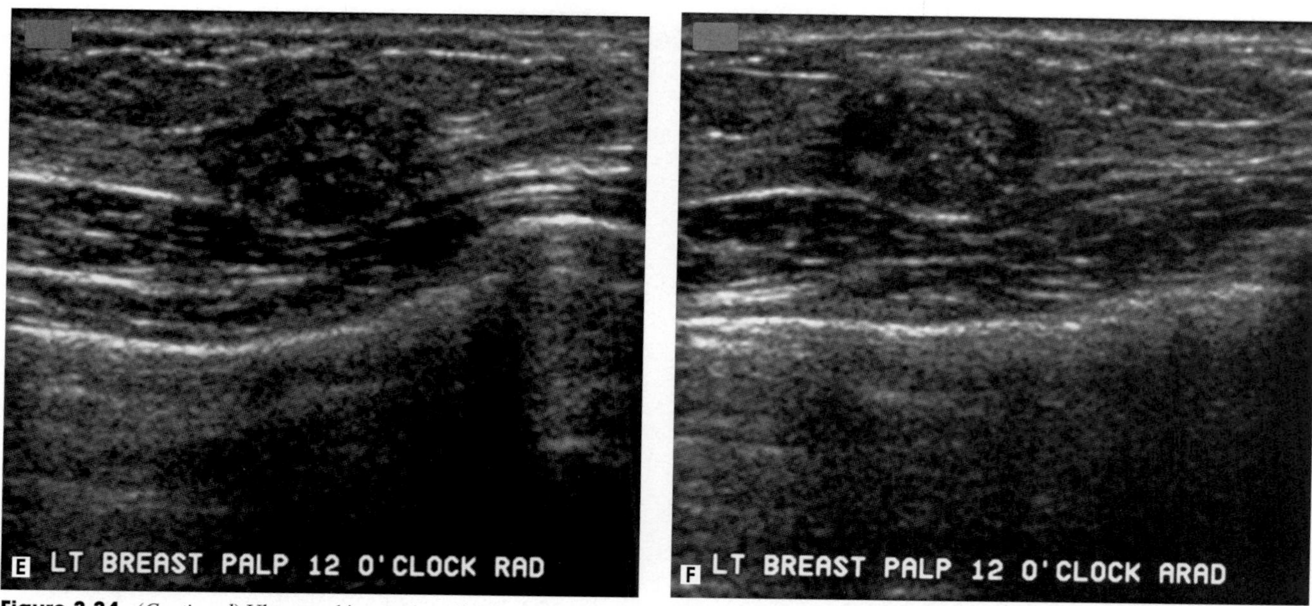

Figure 3.34. (*Continued*) Ultrasound images in radial (RAD) **(E)** and antiradial (ARAD) **(F)** projections of the palpable finding, left breast.

How would you describe the findings, and what is your differential?

A hard mass is palpated on physical examination. A 1.2-cm oval hypoechoic mass with indistinct margins and associated calcifications is imaged on ultrasound at the 12 o'clock position, 3 cm from the left nipple. Cooper ligaments are disrupted and there is mass effect on the deep pectoral fascia. Differential considerations include fibroadenoma (complex fibroadenoma with, because of the associated calcifications, associated sclerosing adenosis; tubular adenoma), sclerosing adenosis, papilloma, phyllodes tumor, pseudoangiomatous stromal hyperplasia, and invasive ductal carcinoma not otherwise specified with associated ductal carcinoma in situ. A ductal carcinoma in situ, with no associated invasive component, is also a possibility, although less likely given the presence of a palpable mass that is confirmed on ultrasound. A biopsy is indicated.

BI-RADS® category 4: suspicious abnormality—biopsy should be considered.

A ductal carcinoma in situ is diagnosed on ultrasound-guided core biopsy. A 1.4-cm, intermediate-nuclear-grade, ductal carcinoma in situ with a cribriform pattern and central necrosis is diagnosed on the lumpectomy specimen. No invasion is reported. No metastatic disease is diagnosed in four excised sentinel lymph nodes [pTis(DCIS), pN0(sn) (i−), pMX; Stage 0].

Patients with ductal carcinoma in situ (DCIS) can present clinically with a palpable mass, spontaneous nipple discharge, or Paget's disease. More commonly, however, DCIS is clinically occult, diagnosed following the mammographic detection of pleomorphic calcifications, particularly when some of these are linear, or when linear, round, and punctate calcifications demonstrate linear orientation. Less commonly, DCIS can be detected mammographically as a mass (well circumscribed to spiculated, in some patients macrolobulated), focal parenchymal asymmetry or distortion in the absence of calcifications.

The use of sentinel lymph node biopsy (SLNB) in patients with DCIS remains controversial. It is probably indicated in women with DCIS and known microinvasion and in those patients in whom invasive disease is suspected preoperatively based on the size or imaging features of the DCIS. An alternative approach that can be taken is to excise the DCIS and, if invasive disease is identified on the lumpectomy specimen, the SLNB is done as a second operative procedure.

PATIENT 35

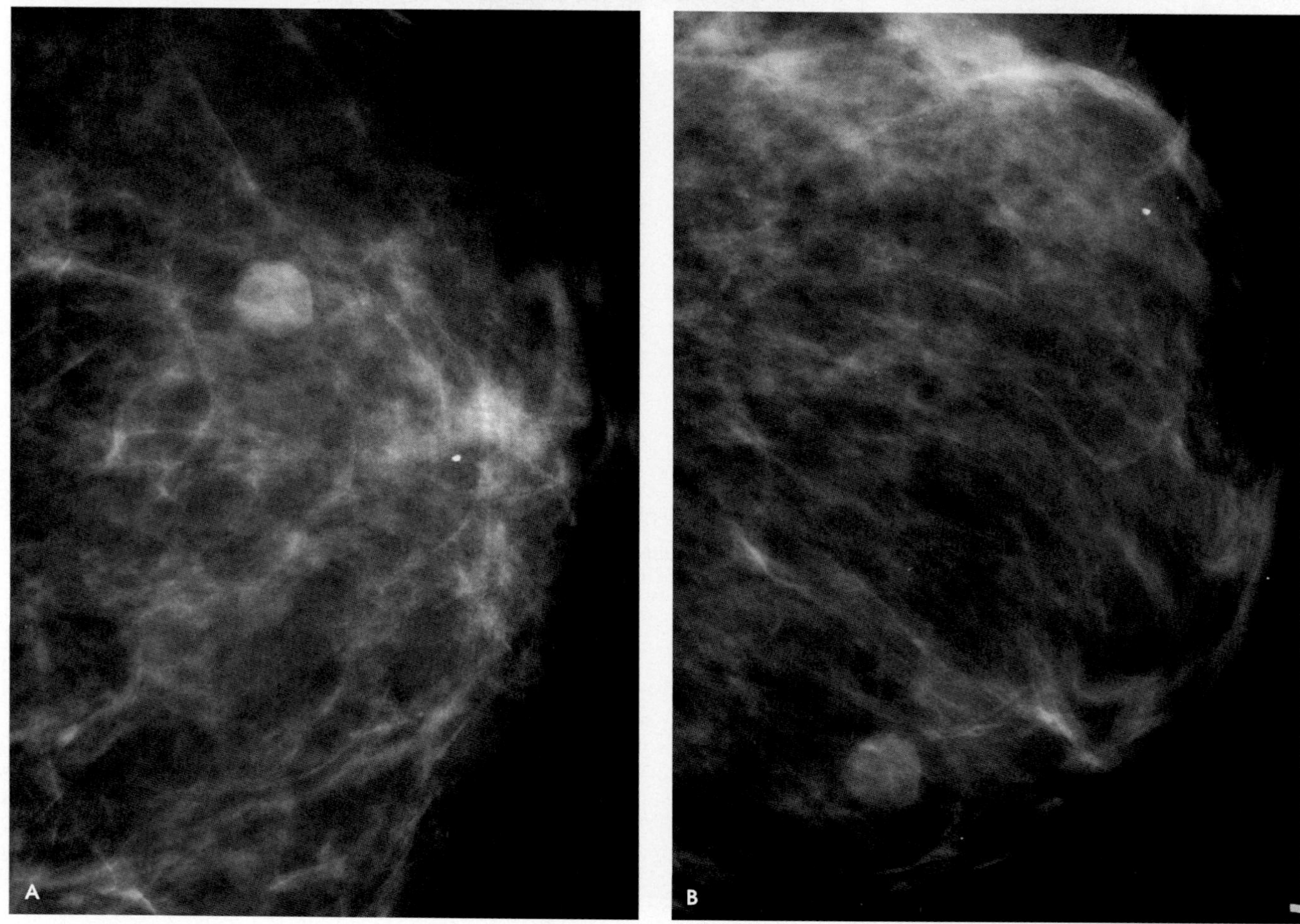

Figure 3.35. Diagnostic evaluation, 40-year-old patient presenting with a "lump" in the left breast. Craniocaudal **(A)** and mediolateral oblique **(B)** views, photographically coned.

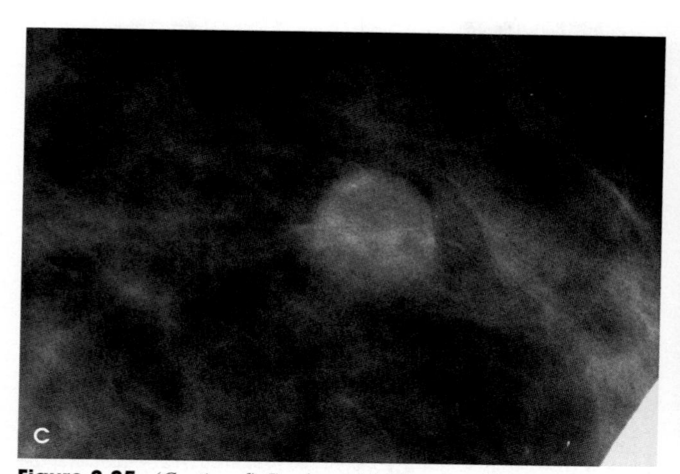

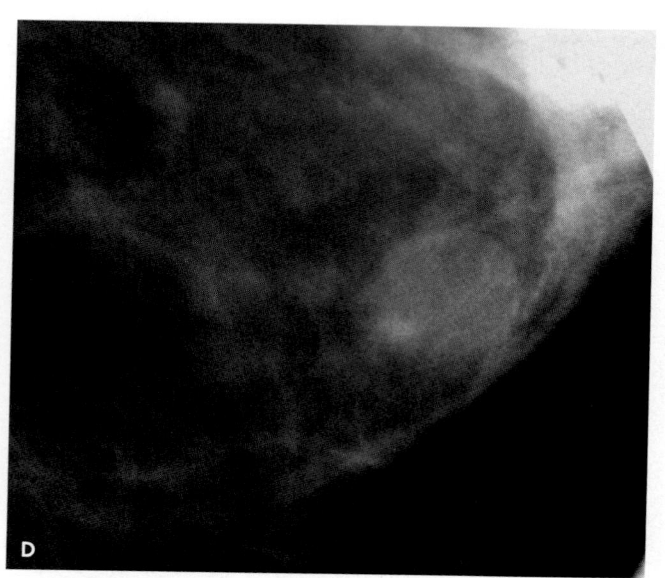

Figure 3.35. (*Continued*) Craniocaudal **(C)** and mediolateral oblique **(D)** spot compression views of palpable finding.

How would you describe the findings, and what differential considerations do you have at this point? What would you do next?

A well-circumscribed, round, water-density mass is imaged corresponding to the "lump" described by the patient. Benign differential considerations based on the mammographic finding include a cyst, galactocele (provided the history supports this), fibroadenoma (complex fibroadenoma, tubular adenoma), phyllodes tumor, papilloma, nodular adenosis, pseudoangiomatous stromal hyperplasia (PASH), focal fibrosis, posttraumatic (or surgical) fluid collection, vascular lesions, granular cell tumor, and abscess. Malignant considerations include invasive ductal carcinoma not otherwise specified, medullary carcinoma, adenoid cystic carcinoma, and lymphoma. Although they are included in the differential for round, well-circumscribed masses, mucinous and papillary carcinomas are unlikely given the patient's age. Correlative physical examination and an ultrasound are indicated for further evaluation.

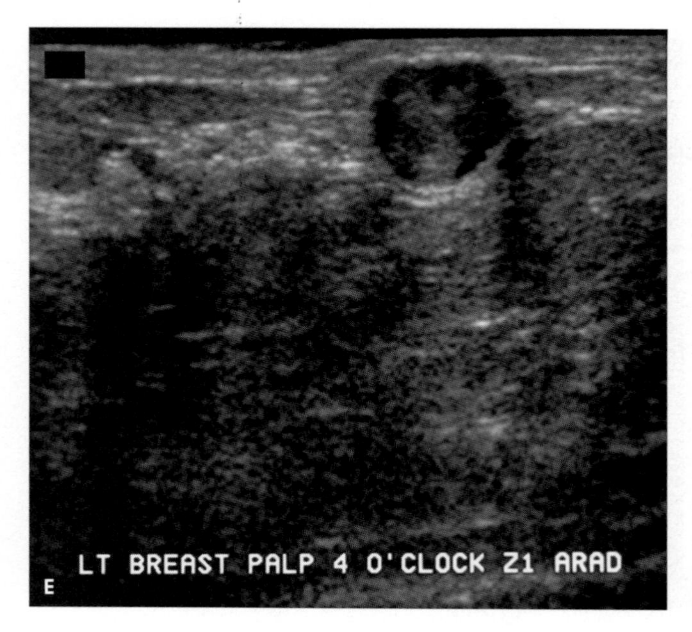

Figure 3.35. Ultrasound image **(E)** of the palpable (PALP) finding at the 4 o'clock position, anteriorly (Z1) in the left breast.

Given the ultrasound findings and the additional history provided, how would you manage the patient?

On physical examination, a superficial, discrete, hard, readily mobile mass is palpated at the site of concern to the patient. A 1-cm, round, well-circumscribed, complex cystic mass with posterior acoustic enhancement is imaged corresponding to the palpable mass. As the ultrasound is being done, the history of a recent pregnancy is elicited from the patient so that a galactocele is a realistic possibility. This patient can be managed in one of two ways. If the patient is otherwise asymptomatic, follow-up in 3 to 4 weeks is a possibility. Alternatively, if this mass is tender, or the patient remains concerned after the discussion of possible etiologies, a stepwise approach is taken for further evaluation. The first step is to attempt an aspiration. If no fluid is obtained, or if a residual abnormality is seen after the aspiration, an ultrasound-guided core biopsy is done. In this patient, thick milky fluid is aspirated and no residual abnormality is seen following the aspiration. No further intervention or follow-up is indicated.

BI-RADS® category 2: benign finding. Next screening mammogram is recommended in 1 year.

What are the imaging findings associated with galactoceles?

Women with galactoceles can present in the third trimester of pregnancy, during lactation, or even several years following the cessation of lactation with a mass that may be tender. Mammographically, galactoceles are often well-circumscribed, round, water- or mixed-density masses but can be characterized by ill-defined and indistinct margins, particularly if they are inflammed. Rarely, a fat/fluid level may be seen. The ultrasound appearance of these lesions is also quite variable, ranging from well-circumscribed solid or cystic masses to complex cystic masses with posterior acoustic enhancement; however, some may be indistinct and associated with significant shadowing. Fluid/fluid levels may be also seen on ultrasound. If they are tender, or the diagnosis cannot be established based on clinical and imaging findings, an aspiration is indicated. If there is a residual abnormality following the aspiration, or concerns persist regarding the diagnosis, a core biopsy can be done.

PATIENT 36

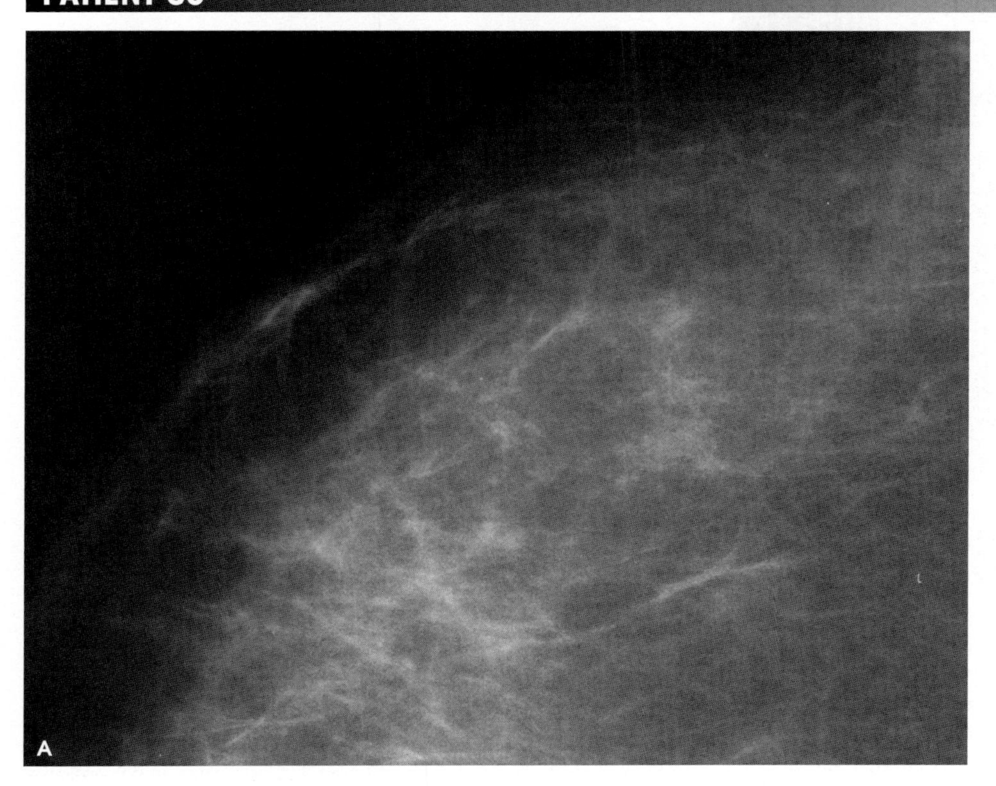

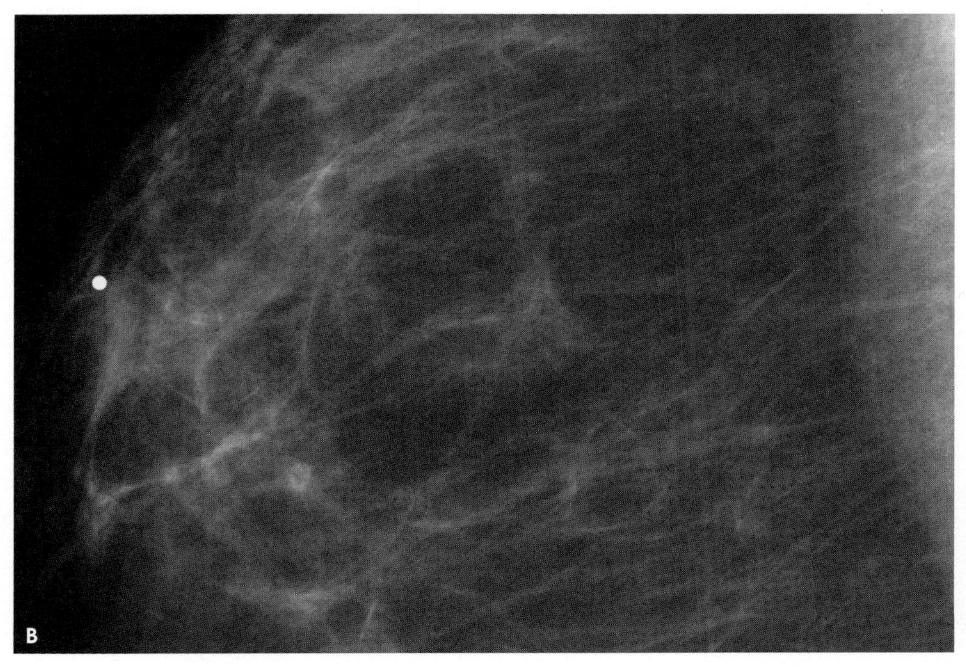

Figure 3.36. Diagnostic evaluation, 47-year-old patient presenting with a "lump" in the right breast. Craniocaudal **(A)** and mediolateral oblique **(B)** views, right breast, photographically coned; metallic BB seen on the mediolateral oblique view at the site of the "lump."

Based on the routine views, what can be said and with what degree of certainty?
What would you do next?

No abnormality is perceived on the routine views. A spot tangential view at the site of the "lump" is helpful in many patients because the lesion may be partially or completely outlined by fat enabling visualization and characterization.

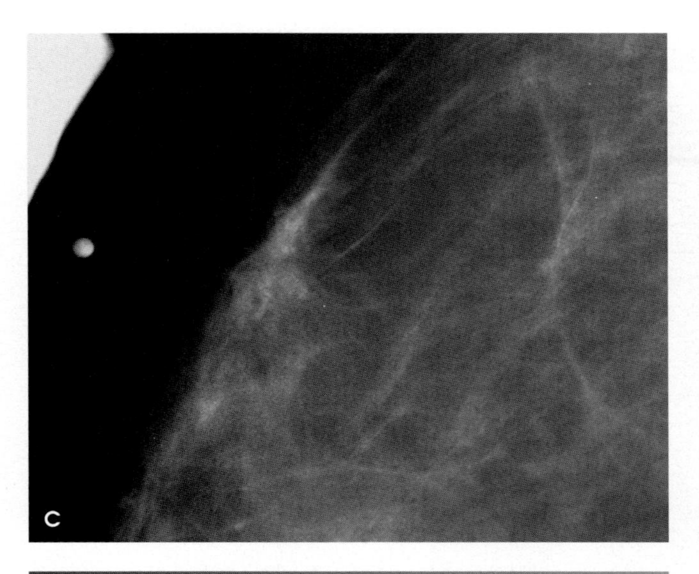

Figure 3.36. (*Continued*) Spot tangential **(C)** view of the palpable finding, right breast.

Now what can you say, and with what degree of certainty?

The spot tangential view demonstrates a spiculated mass corresponding to the area of clinical concern. The differential considerations at this point include invasive ductal carcinoma not otherwise specified (NOS), tubular carcinoma, and invasive lobular carcinoma. Benign considerations include fat necrosis (posttrauma or surgery), sclerosing adenosis, papilloma, focal fibrosis, complex sclerosing lesion, and inflammatory changes (mastitis). Rare causes include granular cell tumor and fibromatosis (extra-abdominal desmoid). Unless there is a direct correlation of this area to a site of prior trauma or surgery, this finding requires biopsy.

A 1-cm hypoechoic, irregular mass with indistinct and angular margins and shadowing is imaged, embedded and disrupting a thickened Cooper's ligament (Fig. 3.36D, E). The clinical, mammographic, and ultrasound findings indicate a biopsy is required.

BI-RADS® category 4: suspicious abnormality—biopsy should be considered.

An ultrasound-guided needle biopsy is done, and an invasive mammary carcinoma is diagnosed on the core samples. A 1.3-cm grade I invasive ductal carcinoma with associated intermediate-grade ductal carcinoma in situ is reported on the lumpectomy. Extensive lymphovascular space involvement is also noted; however, four excised sentinel lymph nodes are normal: [pT1c, pN0(sn)(i−), pMX; Stage I].

Shrinkage artifact can simulate lymphovascular space involvement as artifactual spaces are created around tumor cells during processing. Consequently, the diagnosis of lymphovascular space involvement is sometimes difficult and subjective. Lymphovascular space involvement is described in approximately 15% of patients with invasive ductal carcinoma and in 5% to 10% of patients with no metastatic disease to axillary lymph nodes. It has been described as an unfavorable prognostic finding, particularly in node-negative patients treated with either mastectomy or lumpectomy. The presence of extensive lymphovascular space involvement in patients with otherwise favorable tumors seems to identify a subset of patients with higher systemic recurrences and mortality rates from metastatic breast cancer.

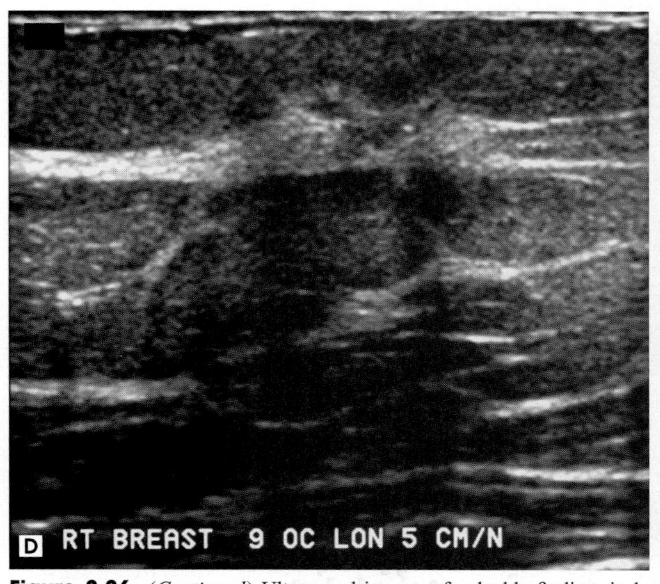

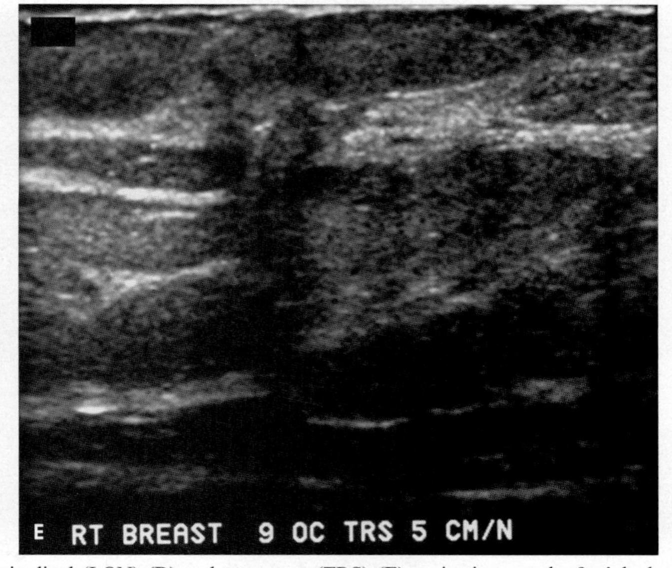

Figure 3.36. (*Continued*) Ultrasound images of palpable finding, in longitudinal (LON) **(D)** and transverse (TRS) **(E)** projections, at the 9 o'clock position, 5 cm from the right nipple.

PATIENT 37

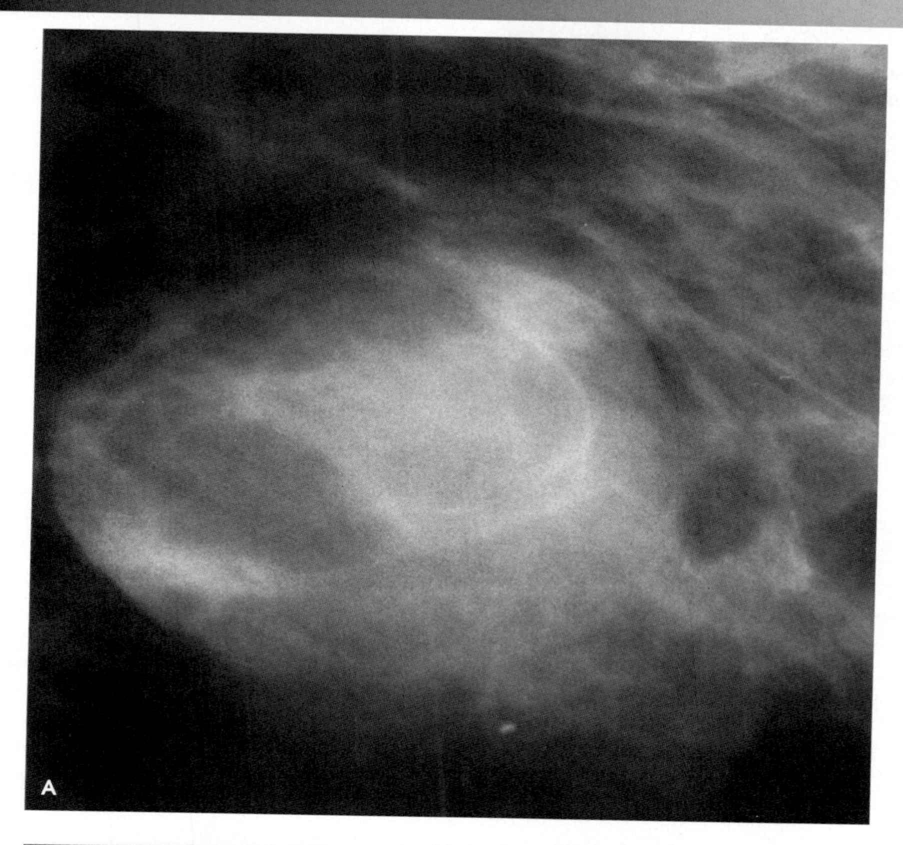

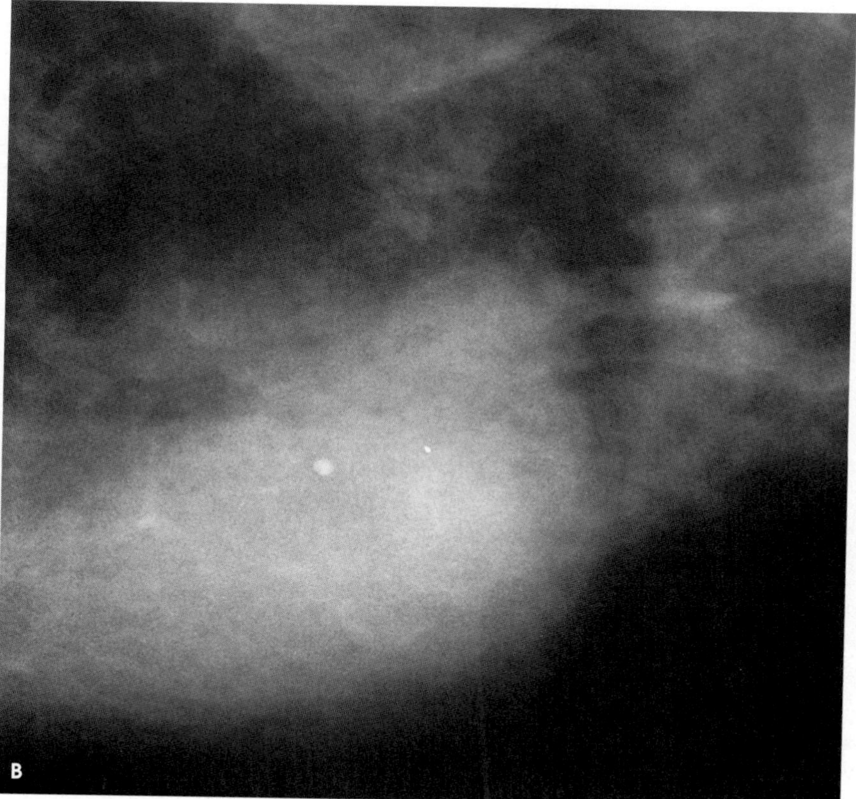

Figure 3.37. Diagnostic evaluation, 44-year-old patient presenting with a "lump" in the left breast. Craniocaudal **(A)** and mediolateral oblique **(B)** spot compression views of a "lump" in the left breast.

How would you describe the findings, and what is your differential?

An oval mass with partially well-circumscribed and obscured margins is imaged corresponding to the palpable finding. Based on the mammographic findings, benign differential considerations include cyst, galactocele, fibroadenoma (tubular adenoma, complex fibroadenoma), phyllodes tumor, focal fibrosis, pseudoangiomatous stromal hyperplasia, abscess, and posttraumatic fluid collection. Malignant considerations include invasive ductal carcinoma not otherwise specified and medullary carcinoma. Mucinous or papillary carcinomas and metastatic lesions usually present as round or oval masses; however, given the patient's age, these are less likely considerations.

A 2.5-cm oval hypoechoic mass with a cystic component is imaged corresponding to the palpable finding at the 9 o'clock position, posteriorly in the left breast (Fig. 3.37C, D). Although the margins are well circumscribed superficially, this is not so for the deep margins.

Would you agree with a BI-RADS® category 3 (probably benign lesion, short-interval follow-up is recommended) designation for this mass? Why not? If not, what would you recommend be done next?

This lesion does not fit the definition of a probably benign lesion, so this designation is not appropriate. The margins are not well circumscribed and the lesion is palpable. A biopsy is indicated and is done. A fibroadenoma is diagnosed. The "probably benign" category should be reserved for mammographically detected and fully evaluated lesions that include nonpalpable, noncalcified, well-circumscribed solid masses, clusters of round or oval calcifications, nonpalpable focal asymmetry with concave margins and interspersed fat, an asymptomatic, single dilated duct and multiple (three or more) similar findings distributed randomly (circumscribed masses, round or oval calcifications in tight clusters or scattered individually throughout both breasts).

If prior films are available, they should be reviewed before assigning BI-RADS® assessment category 3 (probably benign lesion, short-interval follow-up is recommended). If a mass is stable or getting smaller, short-interval follow-up is not indicated. If a mass is solid and enlarging or is new, a biopsy is more appropriate than short-interval follow-up. Also, detected lesions should be evaluated with spot compression views and ultrasound (if a well-circumscribed mass is a cyst, short-interval follow-up is not usually indicated) or, in the case of calcifications, magnification views so that the likely benign features of the lesion can be well documented. In patients with probably benign lesions, it is particularly important to discuss the findings, the low likelihood of malignancy, and available options with the patient. Ultimately, it is the patient's decision, and although most opt for 6-month follow-up, some request that a biopsy be done for histologic confirmation. Other patients in whom a biopsy may be appropriate include those in whom compliance with the follow-up recommendation is a concern.

In my opinion, there is inconsistency in the management of solid, well-circumscribed, noncalcified masses (i.e., probably benign lesions). Why, if a probably benign solid mass is close to the skin or develops in a patient with a small breast and is palpable, do we consider it a surgical disease, yet if that same mass is deep in the breast or develops in a woman with a larger breast and it is not palpable, is it acceptable to recommend a 6-month follow-up for the patient? In my practice, if the clinical, mammographic and ultrasound findings of a mass are consistent with a benign process (e.g., fibroadenoma), and the patient is comfortable with the option, I recommend a 6-month clinical and sonographic follow-up even if the lesion is palpable.

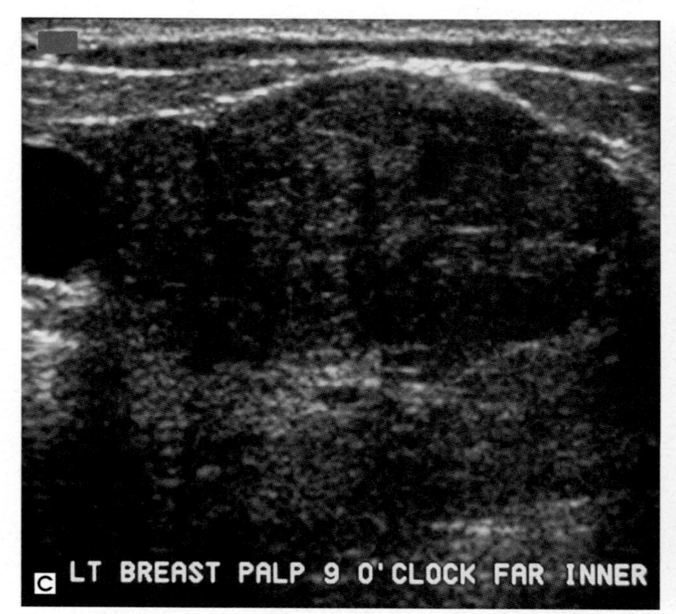

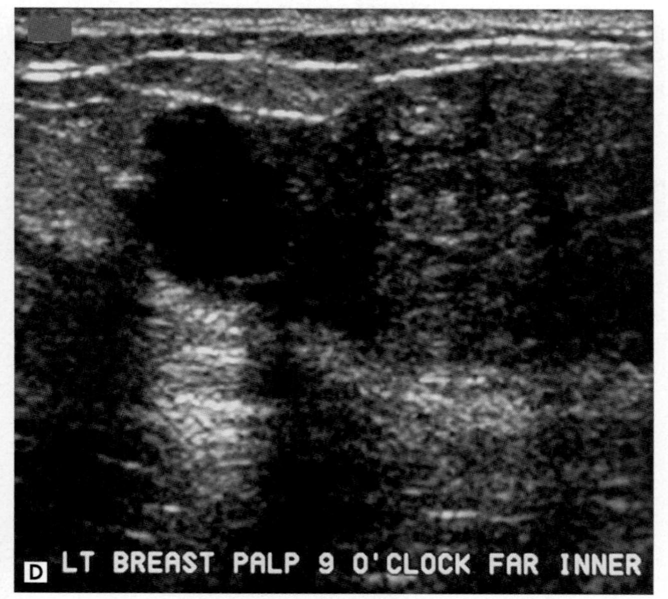

Figure 3.37. (*Continued*) Ultrasound images **(C, D)** of palpable finding, left breast.

PATIENT 38

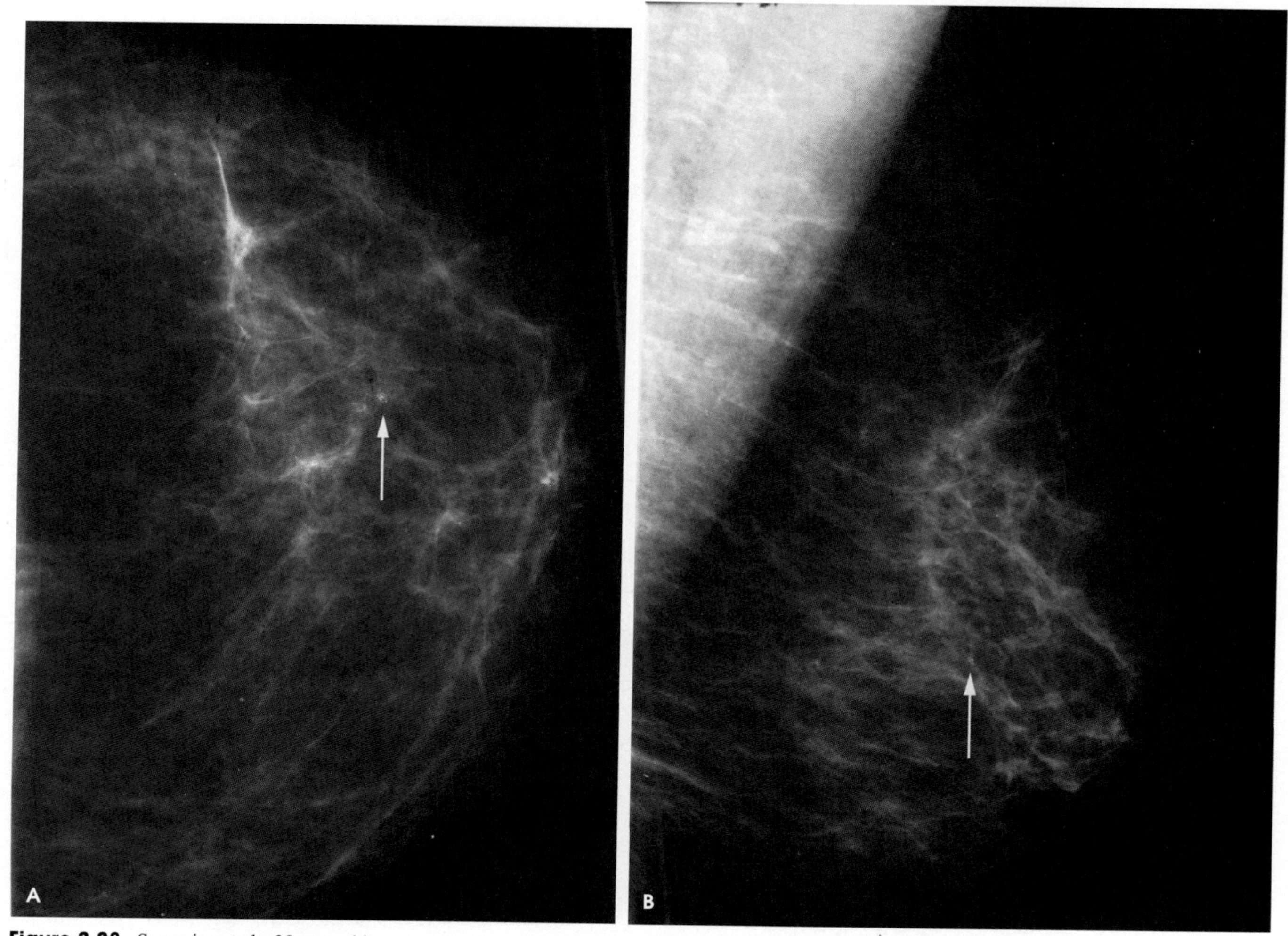

Figure 3.38. Screening study, 38-year-old woman. Craniocaudal **(A)** and mediolateral oblique **(B)** views, left breast.

What should be the next step?

Double spot compression views in two projections are obtained to evaluate calcifications (arrow) detected in the left breast on the screening mammogram.

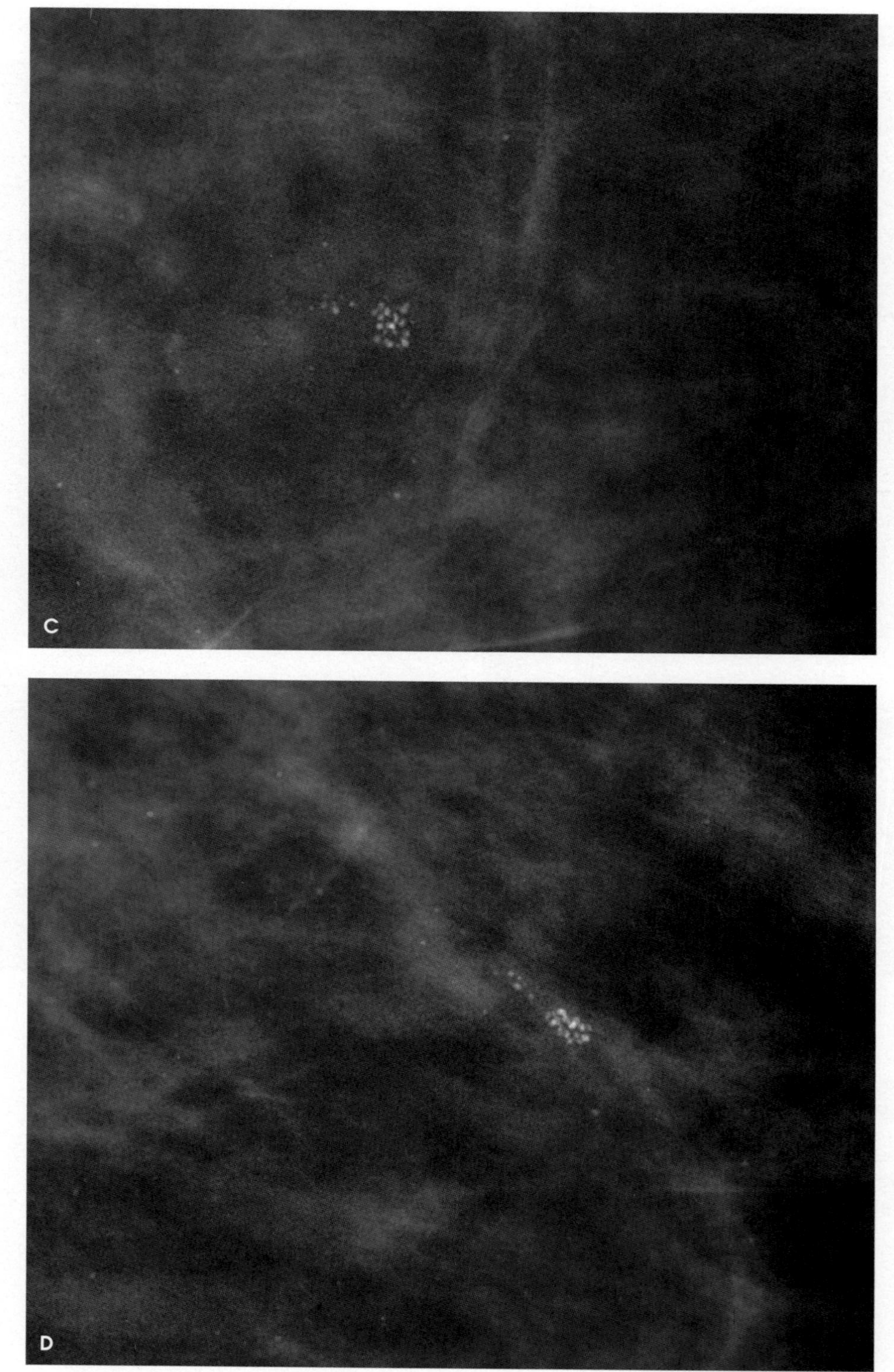

Figure 3.38. Double spot compression magnification views, craniocaudal **(C)** and mediolateral oblique **(D)** projections.

How would you describe the calcifications? What would you do next?

A cluster of calcifications is confirmed on the double spot compression magnification views. The images are well exposed, high in contrast, and demonstrate the calcifications well, with no motion blur. The calcifications are homogenous in density, with no linear forms; however, they are pleomorphic and therefore a stereotactically guided needle biopsy is done. Differential considerations include fibroadenoma, papilloma, fibrocystic changes including ductal hyperplasia, atypical ductal hyperplasia, sclerosing adenosis and columnar alteration with prominent apical snouts (CAPPS), and ductal carcinoma in situ. Sclerosing adenosis with associated calcifications is diagnosed on the core samples. This is congruent with the imaging findings and therefore no further intervention is warranted. Annual screening mammography is recommended starting at age 40 years.

The mammographic presentation of sclerosing adenosis is variable. When a patient presents with calcifications, two distinct patterns for the calcifications can be described: one or multiple clusters of tightly packed, sharply defined but pleomorphic calcifications, some of which may be linear and uni- or bilateral, focal or regionally distributed, amorphous calcifications in dense glandular tissue. Alternatively, a mass with variable marginal characteristics, including spiculation and distortion, may be seen. Some patients may present with a palpable mass, what has been called an "adenosis tumor." Patients who present with an adenosis tumor are typically premenopausal.

Adenosis is qualified by terms that include blunt duct adenosis, microglandular adenosis, and sclerosing adenosis. Histologically, adenosis is a lobulocentric proliferative process with hyperplasia of epithelial and myoepithelial cells and the surrounding intralobular stroma. Specifically, in sclerosing adenosis there is usually some atrophy of the epithelial cell component and prominence of myoepithelial cells. As with fibroadenomas, the glandular component of these lesions is more prominent in premenopausal woman, whereas sclerosis predominates in postmenopausal women. Interestingly, a small percentage of these lesions demonstrate perineural and vascular extension of the proliferating acini.

PATIENT 39

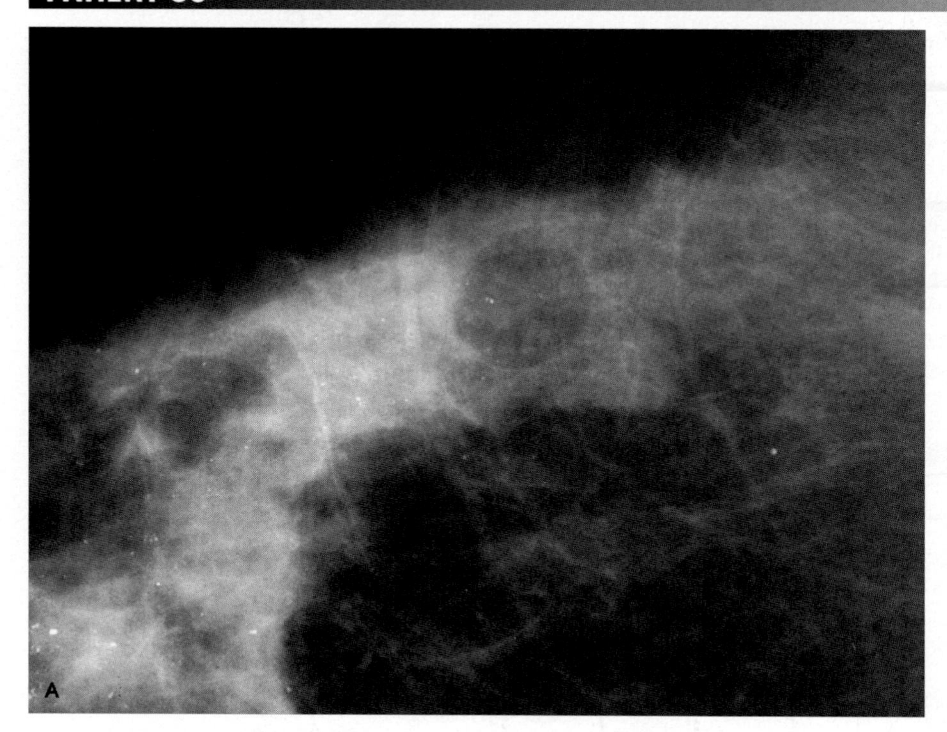

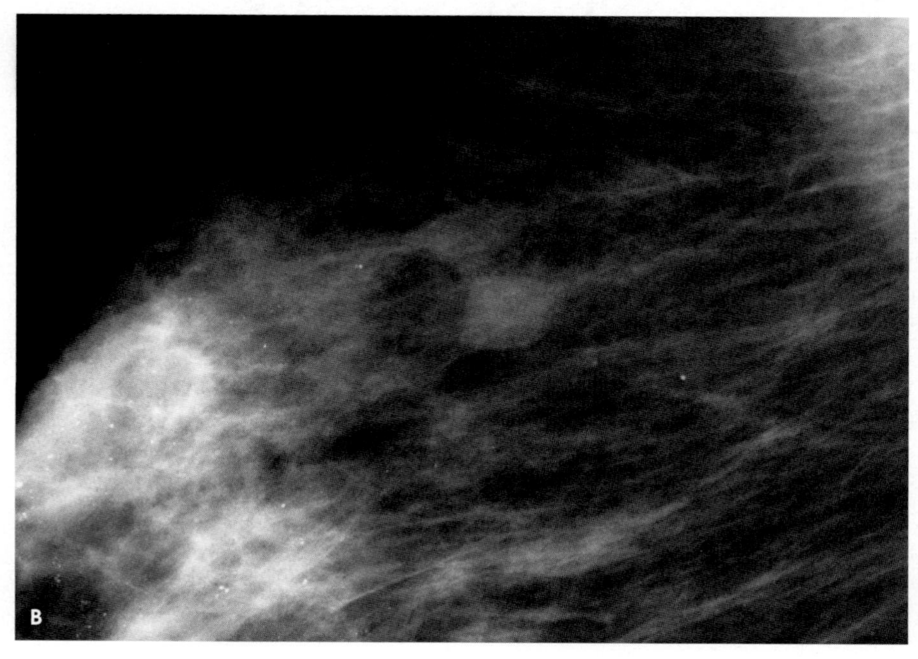

Figure 3.39. Screening study, 60-year-old woman. Craniocaudal **(A)** and mediolateral oblique **(B)** views, right breast, photographically coned.

What are your observations, and what would you do next?

Several observations can be made. There are round and punctate calcifications diffusely scattered in the breast parenchyma. These are benign and do not warrant additional evaluation or intervention. Do you see the round radiolucent mass at the edge of the glandular tissue (Fig. 3.39C, arrow)? What would you recommend for this? Fat-containing masses are benign and do not warrant any additional evaluation. Anything else? Did you notice the water-density mass medial and posterior to the radiolucent mass (Fig. 3.39D, E, arrowheads)? The margins of this mass are indistinct, particularly on the craniocaudal view.

BI-RADS® category 0: Need additional imaging evaluation. Spot compression views (not shown), correlative physical examination, and an ultrasound are done for further evaluation of the water-density mass.

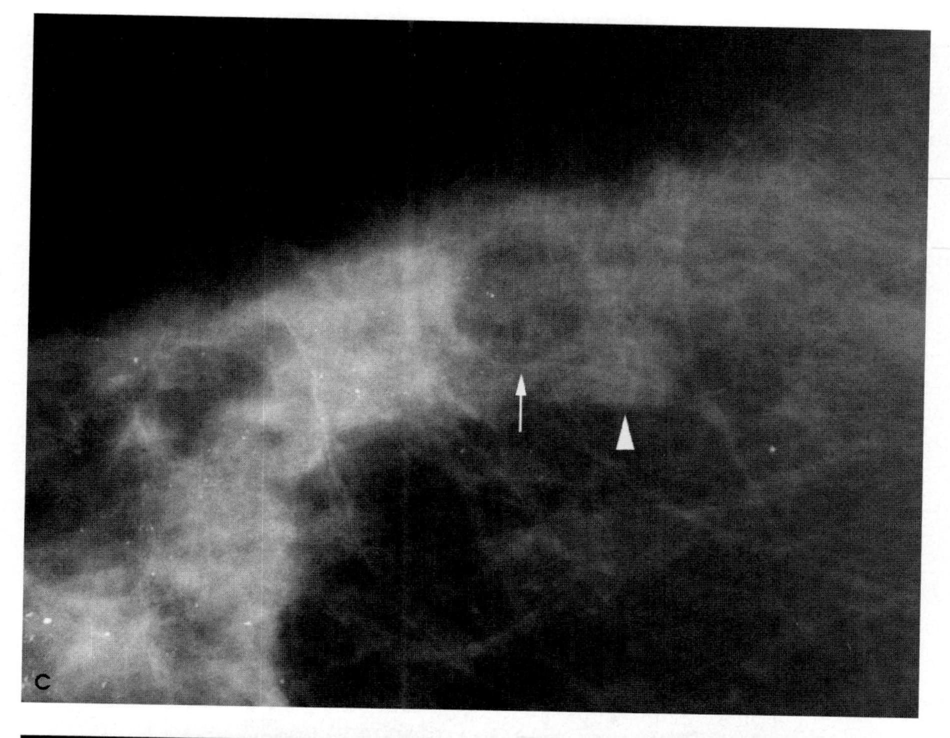

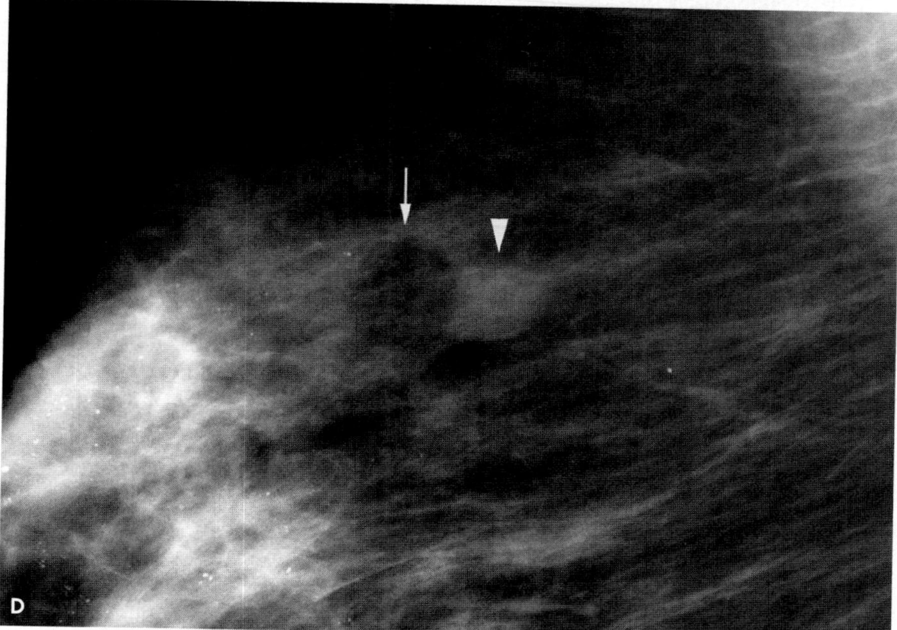

Figure 3.39. (*Continued*) Craniocaudal **(C)** and mediolateral oblique **(D)** views, right breast, photographically coned, demonstrate a round, radiolucent mass (*arrows*) and an adjacent round, water-density mass (*arrowheads*).

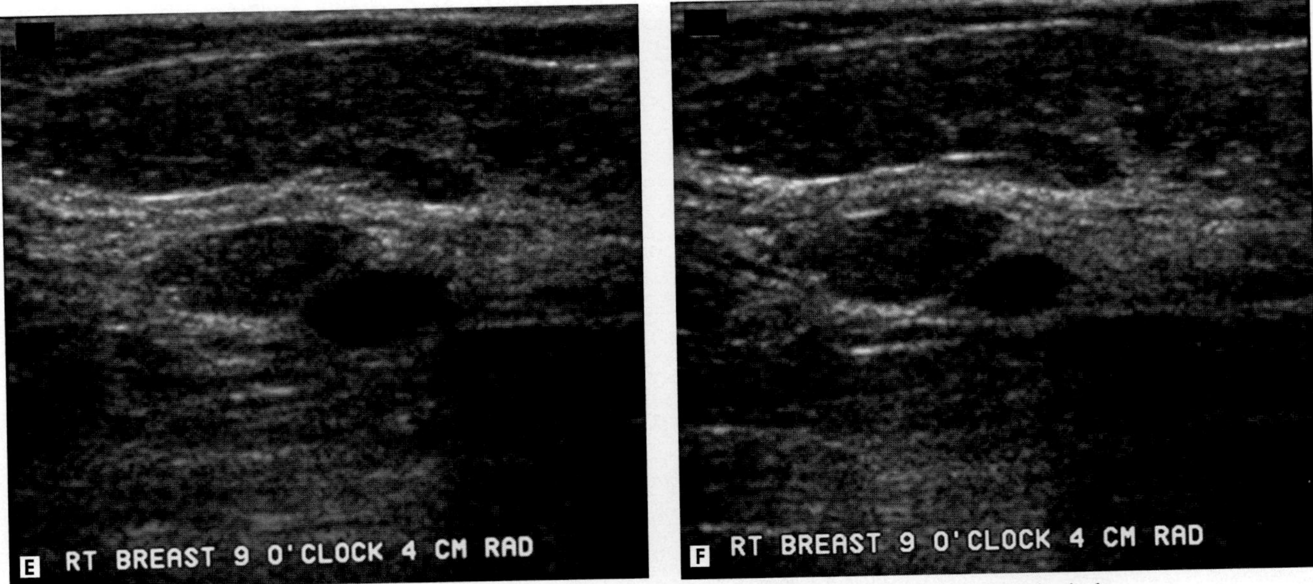

Figure 3.39. (*Continued*) Ultrasound images in the radial (RAD) projection **(E, F)**, 2 o'clock position, 4 cm from the right nipple.

What is your diagnosis based on the imaging findings, and what BI-RADS® category would you use in your report?
What recommendation would you make to the patient?

On ultrasound, two adjacent masses are imaged at the 9 o'clock position, 4 cm from the right nipple. The radiolucent mass, seen mammographically, is a 1.2-cm oval, hypoechoic mass with circumscribed margins and is consistent with a lipoma. A 0.9-cm oval, anechoic mass with circumscribed margins is seen adjacent to the lipoma. Although no posterior acoustic enhancement is seen, this is a simple cyst and requires no further intervention. Posterior acoustic enhancement may not be readily apparent with small cysts or those deep in the breast.

Oil cysts and lipomas may not be distinguishable mammographically, because they are both radiolucent masses. On ultrasound, lipomas are hypo-, iso- to slightly hyperechoic solid masses. In contrast, oil cysts are variable in appearance, ranging from anechoic (indistinguishable from cysts) to complex cystic masses, to irregular solid masses with significant shadowing.

BI-RADS® category 2: benign finding. Next screening mammogram is recommended in 1 year.

PATIENT 40

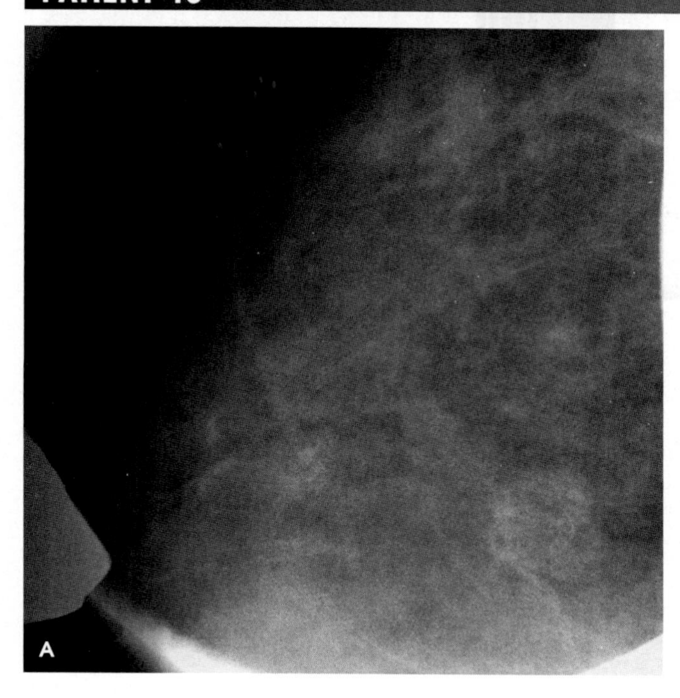

Figure 3.40. Diagnostic evaluation, 42-year-old patient presenting with a "lump" in the right breast. Spot tangential **(A)** view of the "lump" in the right breast. Dense glandular tissue is imaged on the routine views (not shown).

What would you say, based on the tangential view, and what would you do next?

Dense glandular tissue is imaged on the spot tangential view. In this patient, no abnormality is readily apparent on the tangential view. Given the presence of dense glandular tissue on the spot tangential view, correlative physical examination and ultrasound are indicated for further evaluation.

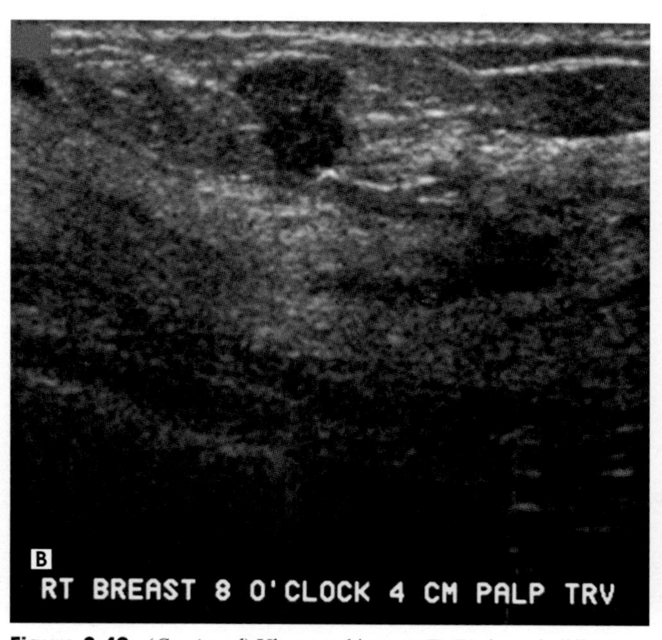

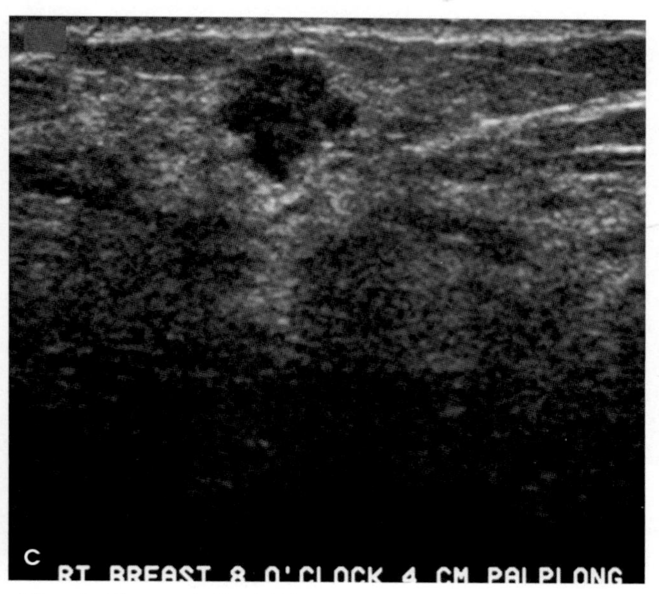

Figure 3.40. (*Continued*) Ultrasound images **(B–D)** through different areas of the palpable mass, in the right breast.

How would you describe the ultrasound findings, and what is your differential? What is indicated next?

On physical examination, a discrete, superficial, hard, readily mobile mass is palpated at the 8 o'clock position, 4 cm from the nipple corresponding to the area of concern to the patient. A vertically oriented, hypoechoic mass with angular and microlobulated margins is seen corresponding to the palpable finding. Ductal extension is noted (Fig. 3.40D, arrows). The clinical and sonographic features of this lesion suggest malignancy; however, differential considerations include fibroadenoma (complex fibroadenoma, tubular adenoma), papilloma, sclerosing adenosis, pseudoangiomatous stromal hyperplasia, invasive ductal carcinoma not otherwise specified, or a medullary carcinoma. Given the patient's age, mucinous and papillary carcinomas are less likely. In the absence of a known malignancy, metastatic disease is also unlikely.

BI-RADS® category 4: suspicious abnormality—biopsy should be considered.

A biopsy is done, and an invasive ductal carcinoma is diagnosed on the core biopsy. Two invasive ductal carcinomas (0.8 cm and 0.6 cm) with high-nuclear-grade ductal carcinoma in situ with central necrosis are reported on the lumpectomy specimen. The sentinel lymph node is negative for metastatic disease [pT1b, pN0(sn) (i−), pMX; Stage I].

Why do spot tangential views in patients who present with localized findings?

In patients who present with focal symptoms, the spot tangential view is sometimes helpful because lesions may be partially (or, less commonly, completely) surrounded by subcutaneous fat, enabling visualization and characterization of a portion of their margin. If a mass or distortion is seen or if, as in this patient, glandular tissue is imaged on the spot tangential, correlative physical examination and an ultrasound are indicated for further evaluation. Sonography may be deferred if completely fatty tissue or a benign finding is imaged on the tangential view corresponding to the area of concern to the patient and there is no chance that the lesion has been excluded from the mammographic images.

What are some of the ultrasound features associated with malignant lesions?

Ultrasound features suggesting a malignant process include a vertical orientation (i.e., taller than wide), microlobulation, spiculation, angular margins, shadowing, duct extension, branch pattern, calcifications, thick echogenic rim, marked hypoechogenicity, and a heterogeneous echotexture. Most malignant masses have multiple features suggestive of malignancy. Tubular structures arising from a mass can be characterized as duct extension or branch pattern, depending on their relationship to the nipple; this is determined during the real-time portion of the study. Duct extension refers to the presence of hypoechoic tubular structures extending from the mass and directed toward the nipple. A branch pattern is present if the tubular structures arising from the mass are directed away from the nipple. In this patient, a branch pattern is present (Fig. 3.40D, arrow).

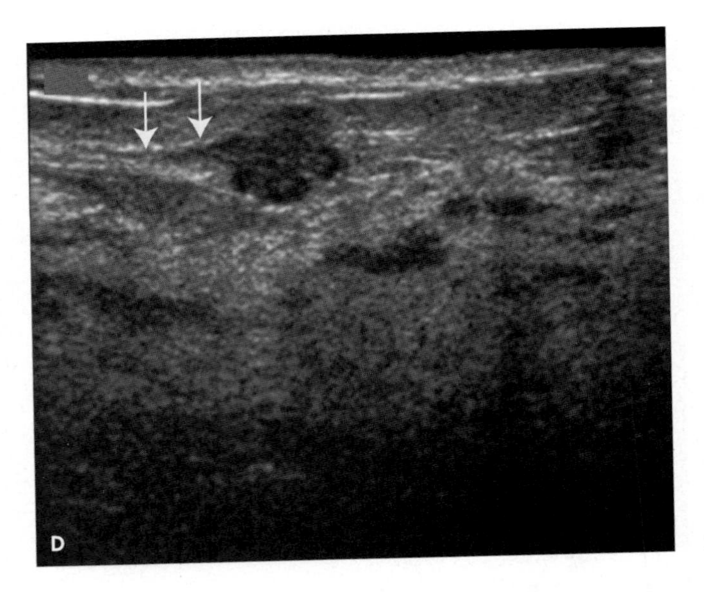

Figure 3.40. *(Continued)*

PATIENT 41

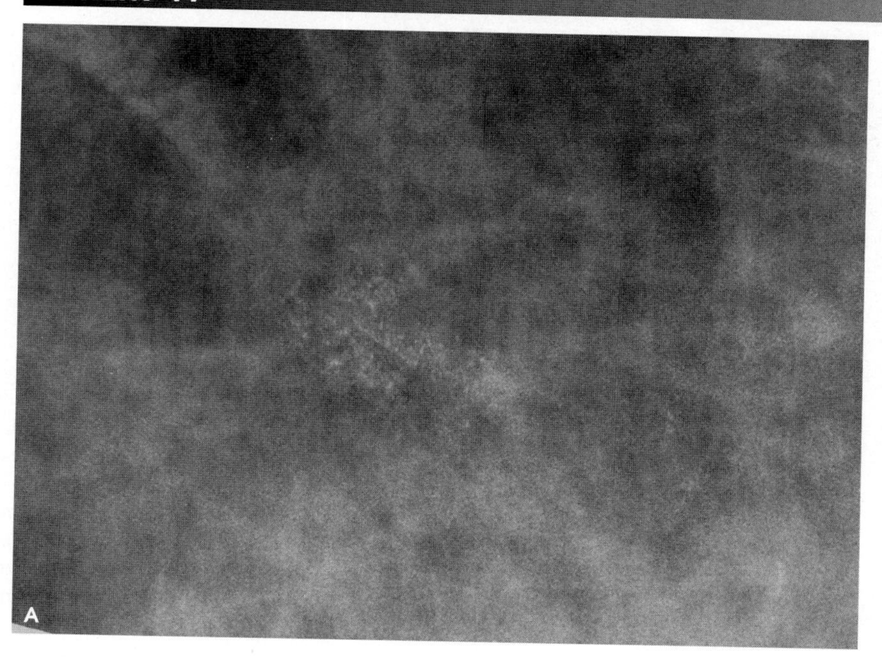

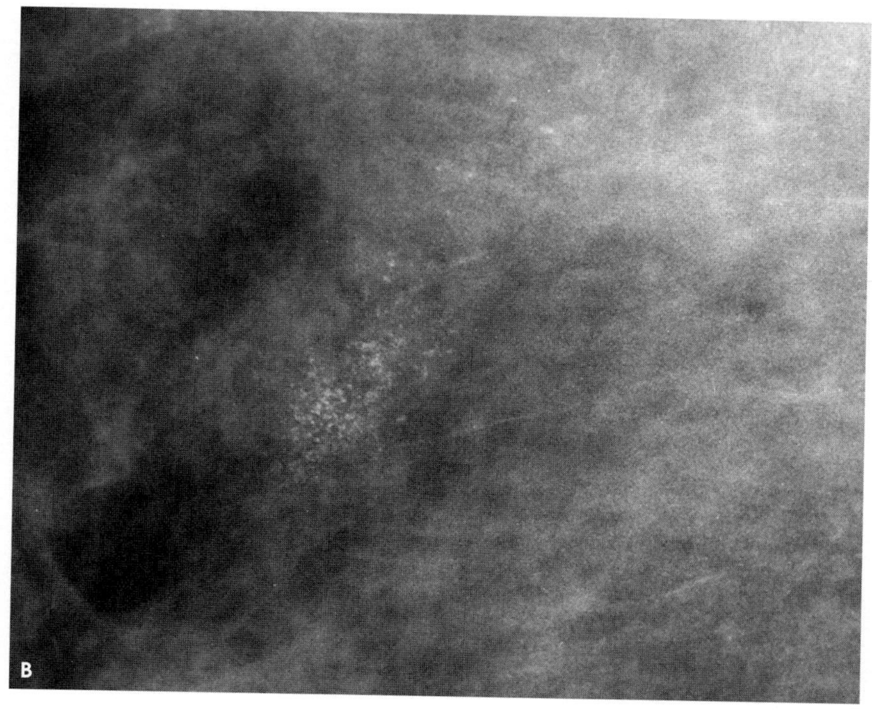

Figure 3.41. Diagnostic evaluation, 62-year-old woman called back for calcifications detected on a screening mammogram. Craniocaudal **(A)** and mediolateral oblique **(B)** double spot compression magnification views.

How would you describe the findings, and what is your recommendation?

A cluster of amorphous ("lacelike") calcifications is demonstrated on the magnification views. Although the term "amorphous" is used to describe these, they actually represent tightly packed, punctate calcifications that are beyond the resolution of the images that can be obtained on a patient. When more magnification is used on specimen radiographs (because exposure length is not an issue with a specimen, more magnification can be obtained), the calcifications can be resolved into punctate calcifications. Differential considerations include fibroadenoma, papilloma, fibrocystic changes including ductal hyperplasia, atypical ductal hyperplasia, sclerosing adenosis and columnar alteration with prominent apical snouts and secretions (CAPSS), and ductal carcinoma in situ (usually a low- or intermediate-nuclear-grade DCIS with no associated central necrosis).

BI-RADS® category 4: suspicious abnormality—biopsy should be considered.

A stereotactically guided core biopsy is done.

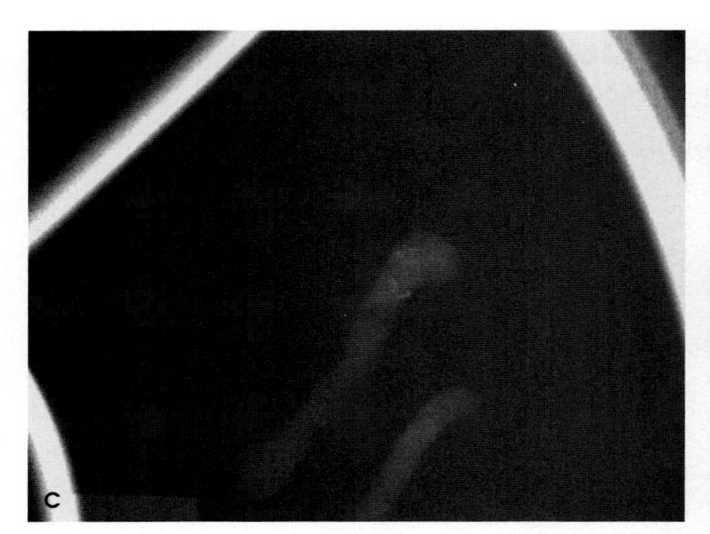

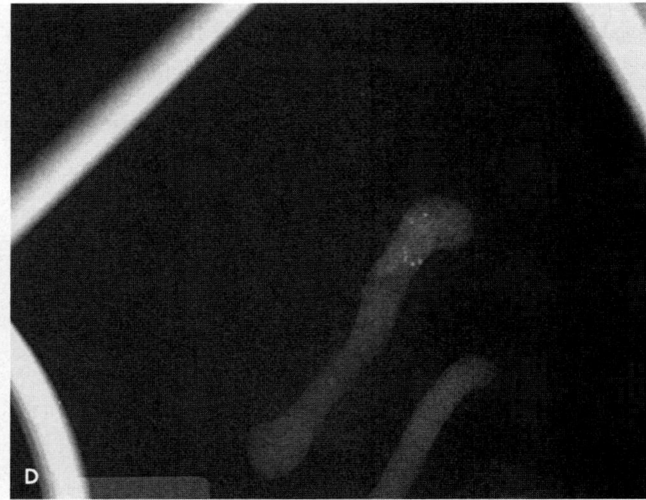

Figure 3.41. (*Continued*) Core radiographs **(C, D),** done as part of the stereotactically guided core biopsy.

What is the difference between these two images, and what caused it?

When a biopsy is done for calcifications, a radiograph of the cores is obtained to make sure that calcifications have been excised for histologic evaluation. We use magnification technique to radiograph the cores. On the first radiograph (Fig. 3.41C), the calcifications are indistinct and difficult to recognize and characterize. When you detect blurry images, you need to consider suboptimal compression, patient motion, or an inappropriate focal spot. Obviously, suboptimal compression and patient motion are not considerations on a core radiograph. The most likely cause is the use of the 0.3-mm focal spot on the magnification views. The repeat image (Fig. 3.41D), done using the 0.1-mm focal spot, demonstrates the calcifications as sharp, distinct structures, while others remain faint and more "amorphous" in appearance. With magnification technique, the focal spot is changed from 0.3 to 0.1 mm to overcome the penumbra effect that results as the object-to-film distance is increased.

CAPSS with associated calcifications but no atypia is diagnosed on the core samples. CAPSS is being reported with increasing frequency in biopsies done for round and punctate or amorphous calcifications identified mammographically. CAPSS involves the terminal duct lobular unit and is characterized by findings that include columnar epithelial cells with prominent apical cytoplasmic snouts, intraluminal secretions, and varying degrees of nuclear atypia and architectural complexity. Some CAPSS lesions can present diagnostic dilemmas for the pathologist because the spectrum of CAPSS ranges from columnar alteration of the epithelial cells with or without atypia to findings suggestive of low-nuclear-grade ductal carcinoma in situ (micropapillary). Excisional biopsy is indicated when CAPSS is associated with atypia or there are concerns regarding an underlying DCIS.

PATIENT 42

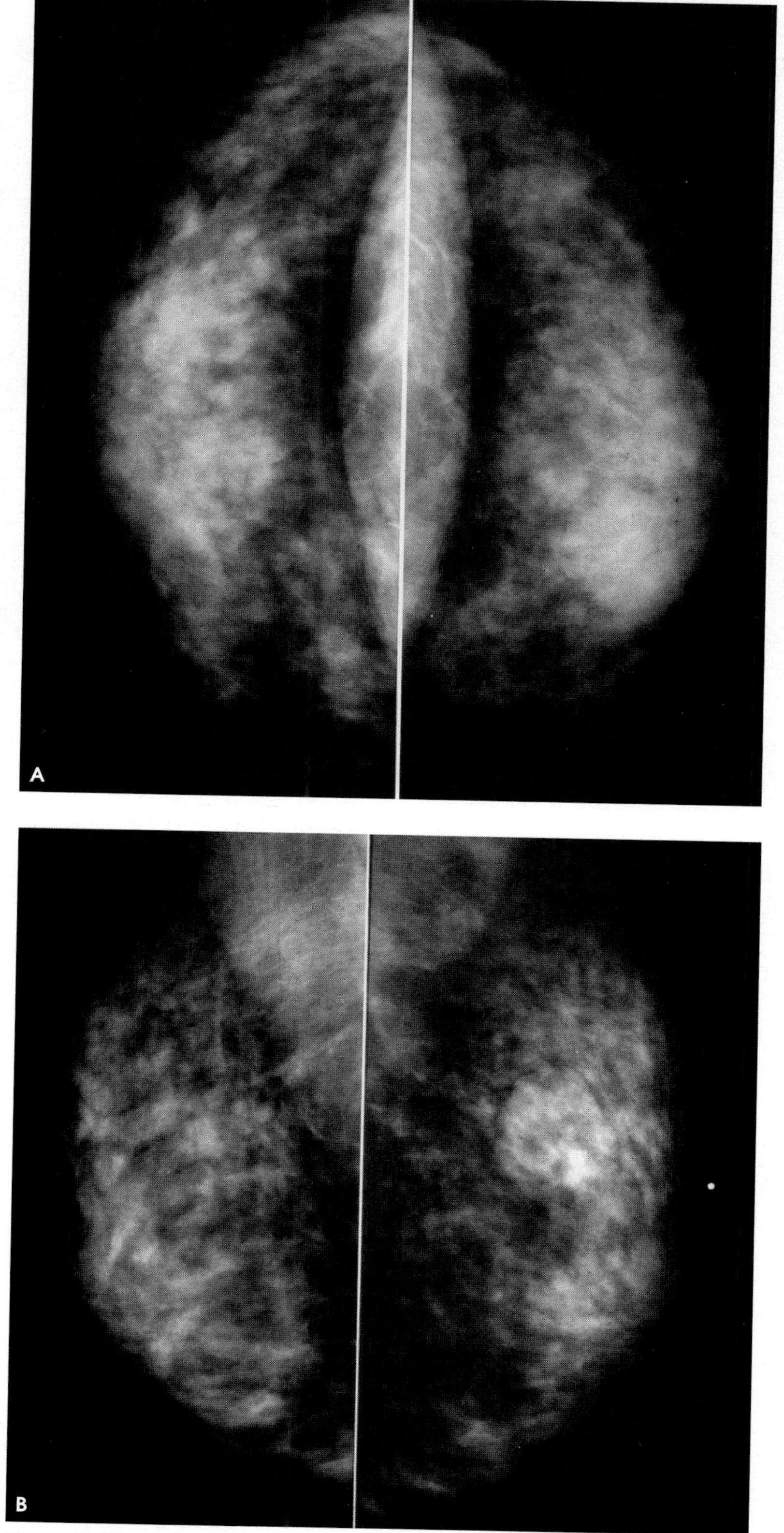

Figure 3.42. Diagnostic evaluation, 41-year-old patient presenting with a "lump" (metallic BB is seen on mediolateral oblique view) in the left breast. Craniocaudal **(A)** and mediolateral oblique **(B)** views.

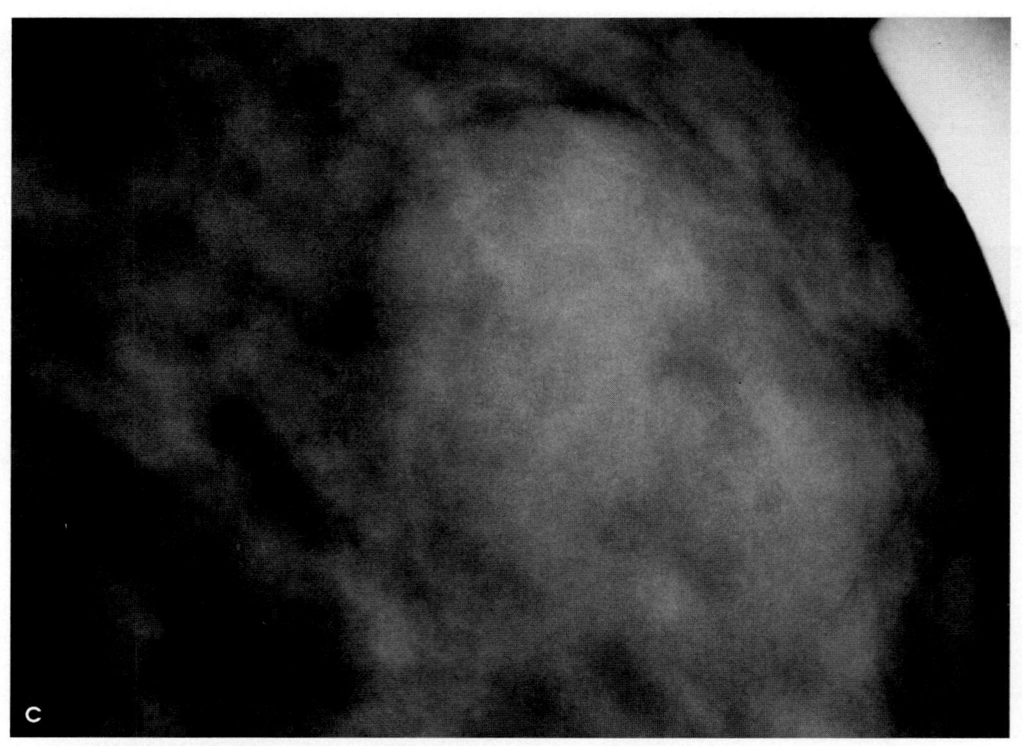

Figure 3.42. (*Continued*) Spot tangential **(C)** view of the "lump", left breast.

How would you describe the findings, and what would you do next?

Dense fibroglandular tissue is present. A round mass with obscured margins is seen in the left breast, corresponding to the "lump" described by the patient. On the tangential view, an oval mass is imaged, with partially well-circumscribed and obscured margins and a "halo" sign associated with a portion of the mass. A hard, readily mobile, nontender mass is palpated in the left breast at the site of concern to the patient.

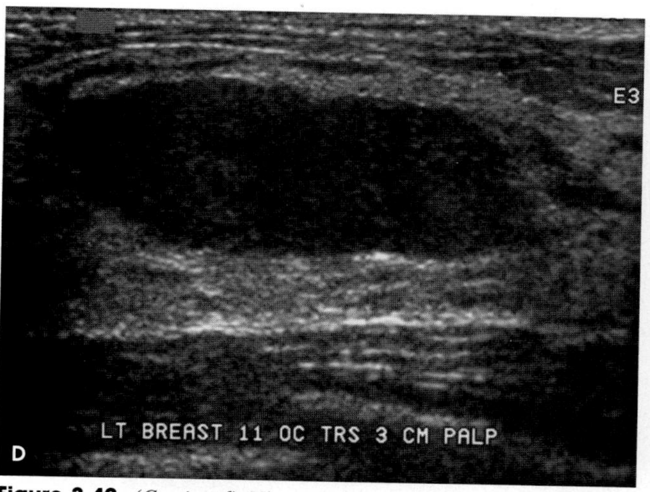

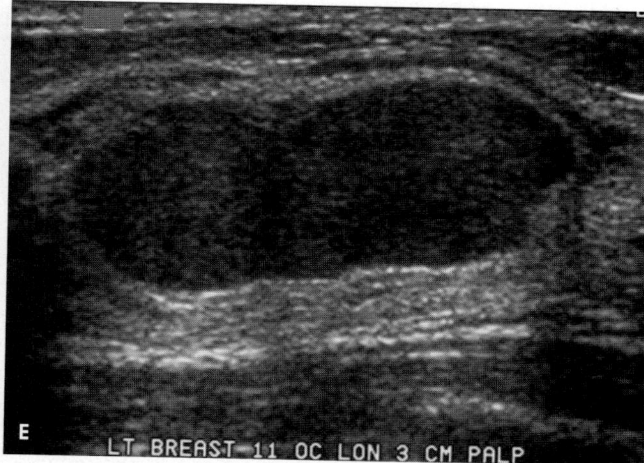

Figure 3.42. (*Continued*) Ultrasound images, transverse (TRS) **(D)** and longitudinal (LON) **(E)** projections of the palpable (PALP) mass, 11 o'clock position, 3 cm from the left nipple.

How would you describe the findings, and what is your differential?

A 2.5-cm, oval, hypoechoic, macrolobulated mass with posterior acoustic enhancement is imaged on ultrasound at the 11 o'clock position, 3 cm from the left nipple, corresponding to site of the palpable abnormality. Although most of the margins are well circumscribed, some nodularity of the margins is noted on the transverse projection. Differential considerations include fibroadenoma (complex fibroadenoma, tubular adenoma), phyllodes tumor, nodular adenosis, pseudoangiomatous stroma hyperplasia (PASH), and focal fibrosis. A papilloma is an additional consideration, but the size of the lesion makes this less probable. Malignant lesions include invasive ductal carcinoma not otherwise specified and medullary carcinoma. Given the patient's age, mucinous and papillary carcinomas are less likely, and without a known malignancy, a metastatic lesion is also unlikely.

What would you recommend and why?

Given some of the margins of this lesion on ultrasound, a biopsy is recommended.

BI-RADS® category 4: suspicious abnormality—biopsy should be considered.

A biopsy is done, and tubular adenoma is diagnosed on the core samples. No further intervention is required unless the patient desires or requests an excisional biopsy. Next screening mammogram is recommended in 1 year.

What are the imaging and histologic features of tubular adenomas?

Tubular adenomas most commonly present as noncalcified, round or oval masses with well-circumscribed or obscured margins mammographically and homogeneously hypoechoic with well-circumscribed margins and possibly posterior acoustic enhancement on ultrasound. The findings are indistinguishable from those associated with some fibroadenomas. In some patients, tightly clustered punctate calcifications, in isolation or with an associated mass, may be seen mammographically.

Tubular adenomas are one of several adenomatous lesion types that include fibroadenomas, complex fibroadenomas, and lactating adenomas. Tightly packed glands (acini), with little surrounding stroma, characterize tubular adenomas histologically. Although they are not common, tightly packed, dense, punctate or irregular calcifications have been reported in tubular adenomas. Histologically, the calcifications reportedly occur within inspissated secretions in dilated glands and not in the stroma.

PATIENT 43

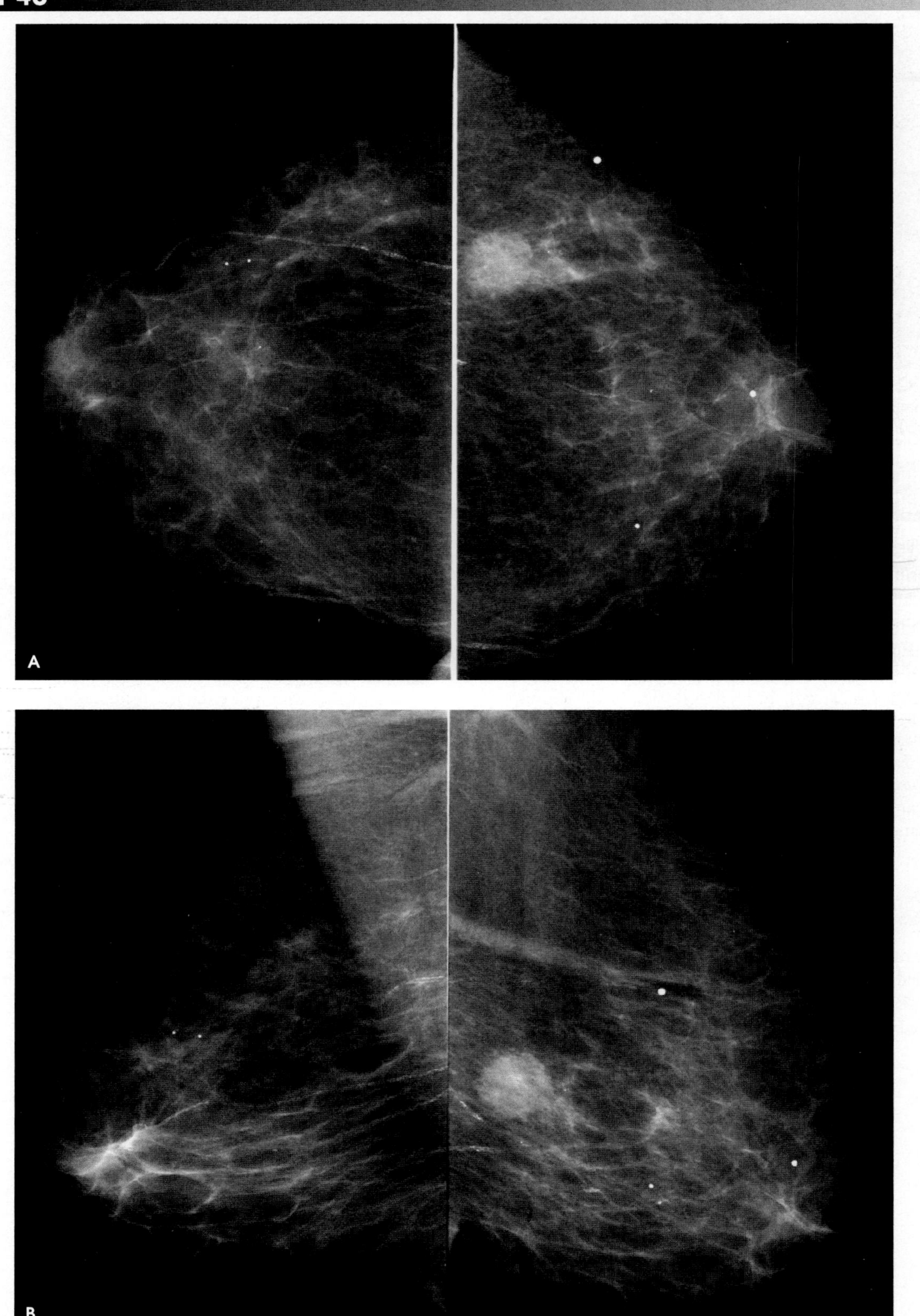

Figure 3.43. Diagnostic evaluation, 84-year-old patient presenting with a "lump" in the left breast. Craniocaudal **(A)** and mediolateral oblique **(B)** views.

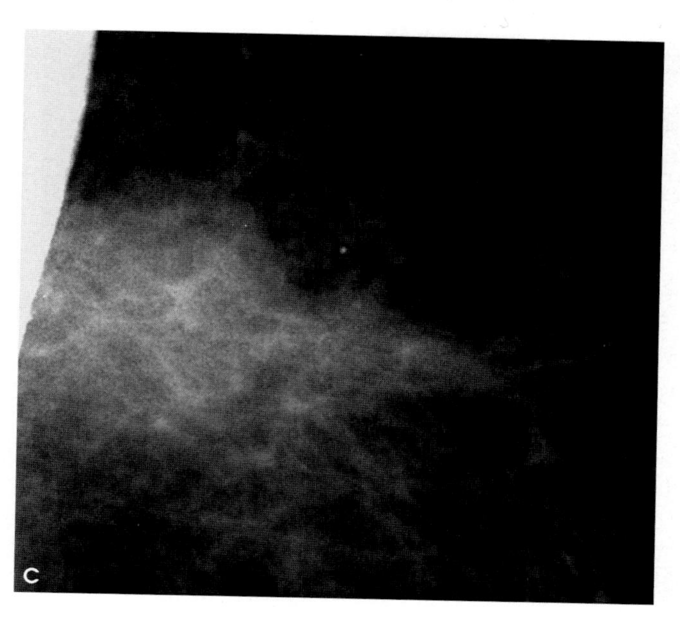

Figure 3.43. (*Continued*) Spot compression **(C)** view, left breast mass.

How would you describe the mammographic findings, and what is your leading diagnostic consideration? What would you do next?

Vascular calcifications are present bilaterally—not an unusual finding given the patient's age. Although there is a patient-related artifact on the spot compression view, a round mass with indistinct and irregular margins is partially imaged in the left breast, corresponding to the area of concern to the patient. In an 84-year-old patient presenting with a palpable mass characterized by indistinct margins, the likelihood of an invasive ductal carcinoma not otherwise specified is high and has to be the leading diagnostic consideration. Other possibilities include metastatic disease (particularly if the patient is known to have an underlying malignancy), papillary carcinoma, mucinous carcinoma, or lymphoma. Although invasive lobular carcinomas are more common in older postmenopausal woman, the round shape of this tumor decreases the likelihood of this diagnosis. Benign considerations include an inflammatory process, particularly if there is associated tenderness, erythema, or warmth at the site of the mass. Posttraumatic or operative fluid collection should be considered if there is a recent history of breast surgery. Lastly, this could represent an atypical presentation for a cyst or papilloma. Cystic changes are most commonly associated with the perimenopausal period; however, there is a second small peak in older postmenopausal women, possibly related to increased estrogen levels from adipose tissue or decreases in liver function.

An ultrasound is done for further characterization of the finding in the left breast. Our routine for patients suspected of a primary breast malignancy is to evaluate the involved breast in its entirety, looking for additional breast lesions. We also scan the ipsilateral axilla. If potentially abnormal lymph nodes are identified, a fine-needle aspiration or a core biopsy is done to establish the presence of metastatic disease. A full axillary dissection (i.e., bypassing the sentinel lymph node biopsy) to establish the number of involved axillary lymph nodes and neoadjuvant therapy is considered for those patients in whom we establish the presence of metastatic disease in the ipsilateral axilla.

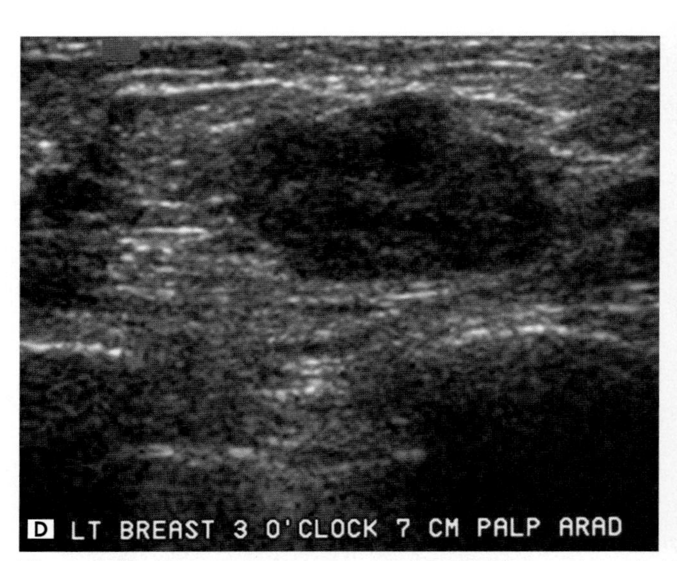

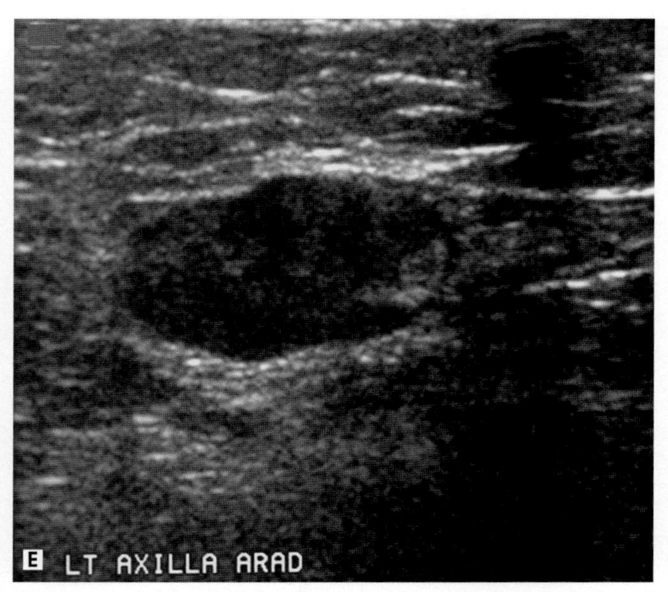

Figure 3.43. Ultrasound image, antiradial (ARAD) **(D)** projection, palpable (PALP) mass, left breast, 3 o'clock position, 7 cm from the left nipple, and ultrasound image, antiradial (ARAD) **(E)** projection, left axilla.

How would you describe the ultrasound findings, and what are your impressions and recommendations?

On physical examination, a hard, fixed mass is palpated laterally in the left breast. There is no associated tenderness, erythema, warmth, or bruising at this site. There is no history of a recent surgical procedure. On ultrasound, an oval, hypoechoic mass with macrolobulated margins is imaged corresponding to the palpable finding in the left breast. An oval, hypoechoic mass with a focus of hyperechogenicity is imaged in the left axilla. The findings support the diagnosis of an invasive lesion, which is likely associated with metastatic disease to at least one axillary lymph node.

An invasive mammary carcinoma with focal squamous differentiation (possibly a metaplastic carcinoma) is reported on the ultrasound-guided core biopsy. Metastatic disease is diagnosed in the axillary lymph node on fine-needle aspiration. A 1.9-cm, grade III invasive mammary carcinoma with squamous differentiation consistent with an adenosquamous or metaplastic carcinoma is diagnosed on the lumpectomy specimen. Because of the patient's age, no lymph nodes are sampled at the time of surgery [pT1c, pNX, pMX; Stage I].

What imaging features in a lymph node suggest the possibility of metastatic disease?

As it relates to the imaging appearance of intramammary and axillary lymph nodes, the overlap between normal and abnormal findings can be significant. Changes and fluctuations in size, density, and a loss of the fatty hilum mammographically can be related to benign reactive changes or metastatic disease, and similarly, normal-appearing lymph nodes with a fatty hilum and no appreciable change in size or density can be found to have significant metastatic deposits when excised. However, based on the clinical presentation and imaging features, metastatic disease in intramammary or axillary lymph nodes can be suspected in some patients and fine-needle aspiration or core biopsy can be done to confirm the diagnostic impression. In patients with a known breast primary, increases in size, density, loss of the fatty hilum, and marginal circumscription (indistinct or spiculated margins) should suggest the possibility of metastatic disease. On ultrasound, prominence, bulging, lobulation, and marked hypoechogenicity of the cortical region are all of concern, particularly if an echogenic hilar region is not identified or it appears attenuated. In some patients, there is apparent mass effect of what is seen of the echogenic hilar region.

If we suspect an abnormal intramammary or axillary lymph node, a fine-needle aspiration or core biopsy (if this can be done safely) of the lymph node is done under ultrasound guidance. In targeting, we avoid the echogenic hilar region because of the theoretical possibility that a needle could disrupt the afferent vessels to the lymph node, potentially having a negative effect on the sentinel lymph node biopsy if one is to be done at a later date.

What are the clinical, imaging, and histologic features associated with metaplastic carcinomas?

Metaplastic carcinomas represent <2% of all breast cancers. They present as a mass described by the patient as having developed rapidly and as a relatively well-circumscribed mass mammographically. In those lesions with osseous metaplasia, dense calcification may be seen mammographically.

These are heterogeneous tumors characterized by metaplasia of the epithelial cells into either squamous or mesenchymal type cells (spindle cell, chondroid, osseous, or myoid). Histologically, these can be broadly divided into those with squamous differentiation and those with heterologous elements such as cartilage, bone, muscle, adipose tissue, vascular elements, melanocytes, and so on.

PATIENT 44

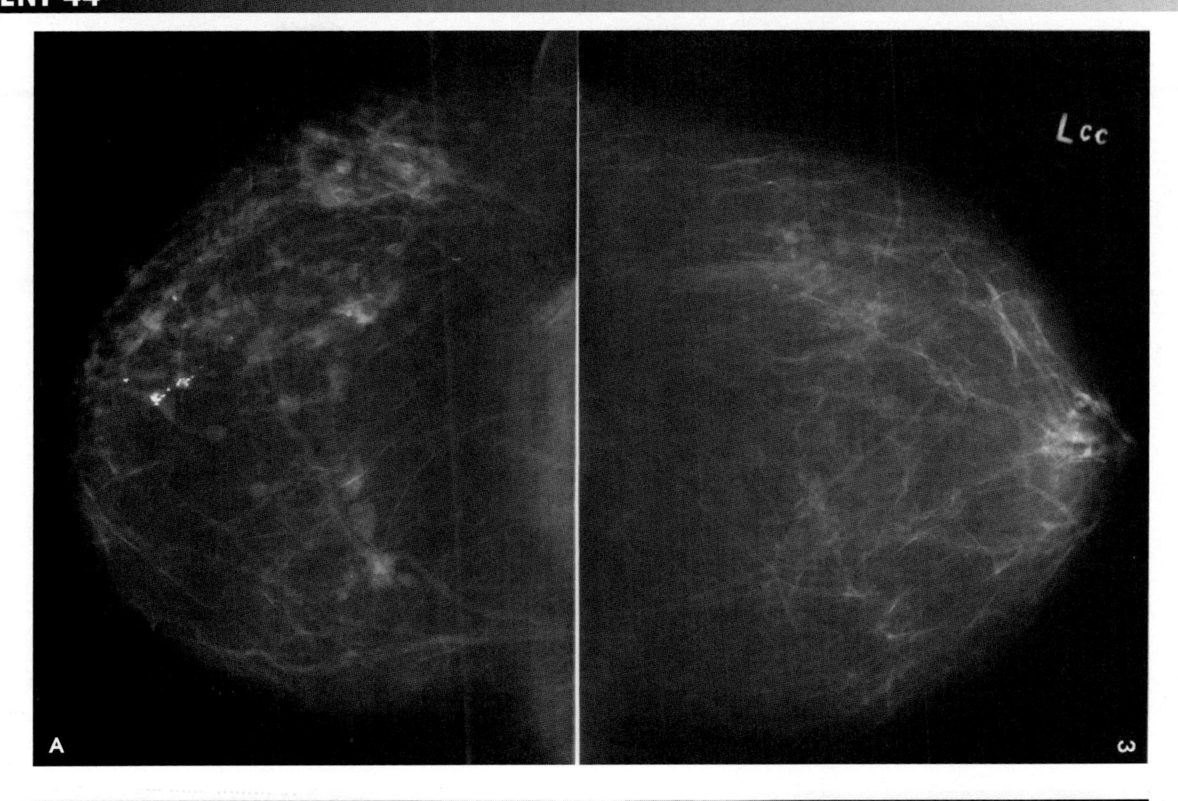

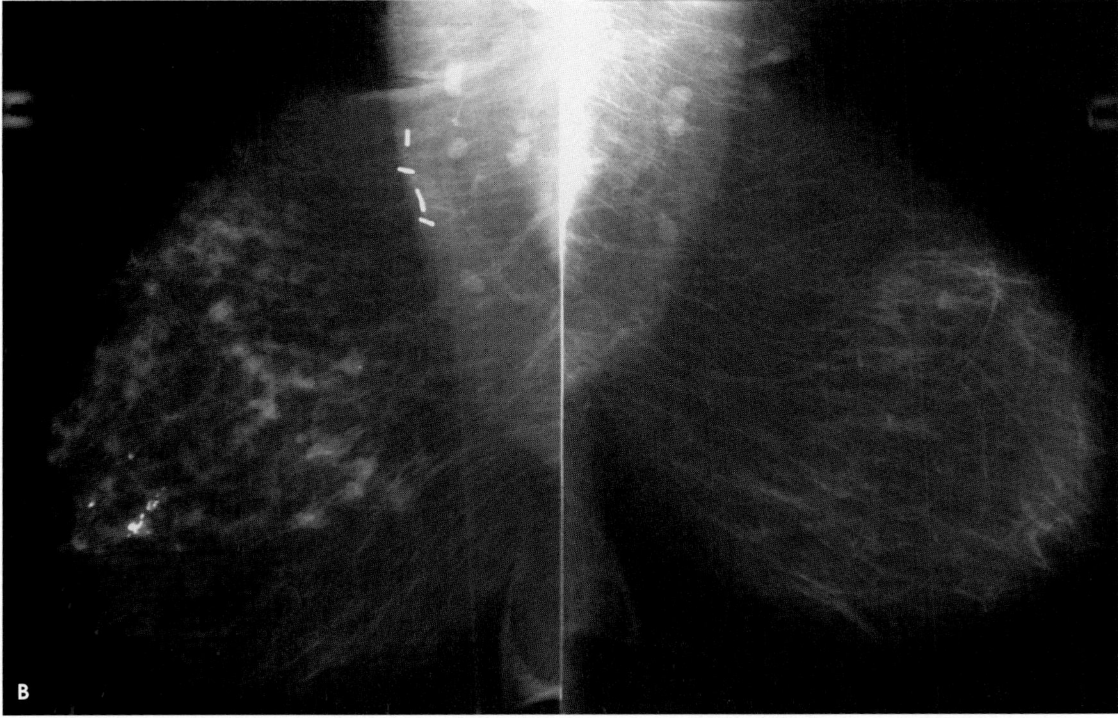

Figure 3.44. Diagnostic evaluation, 61-year-old patient presenting with a "lump" in the right breast. Craniocaudal **(A)** and mediolateral oblique **(B)** views.

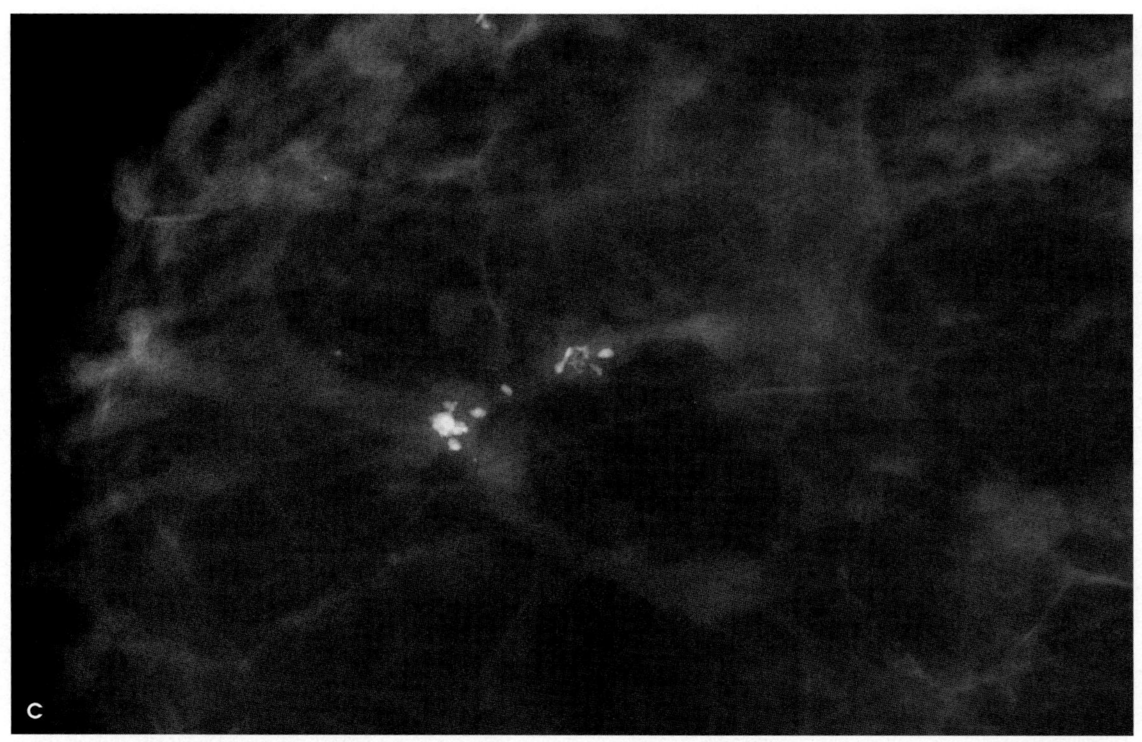

Figure 3.44. (*Continued*) Spot compression **(C)** view, craniocaudal projection, right breast.

How would you describe the findings, what is your differential, and what is your most likely diagnosis? Why?

Multiple subcentimeter-sized masses are present in the right breast, as is a dilated tubular structure within which there are two areas of dense, coarse calcifications. Clips from a prior surgical procedure with a benign diagnosis are also noted in the right mediolateral oblique view.

The left breast is normal. The main benign diagnostic considerations in a patient with multiple masses include cysts, fibroadenomas, and papillomas. Metastatic disease, invasive ductal carcinoma, and lymphoma are the main considerations in the malignant category. In this patient, the additional finding of a prominent tubular structure with associated coarse calcifications makes multiple peripheral papillomas the most likely diagnosis. An ultrasound to evaluate the masses and the "lump" described by the patient is done next.

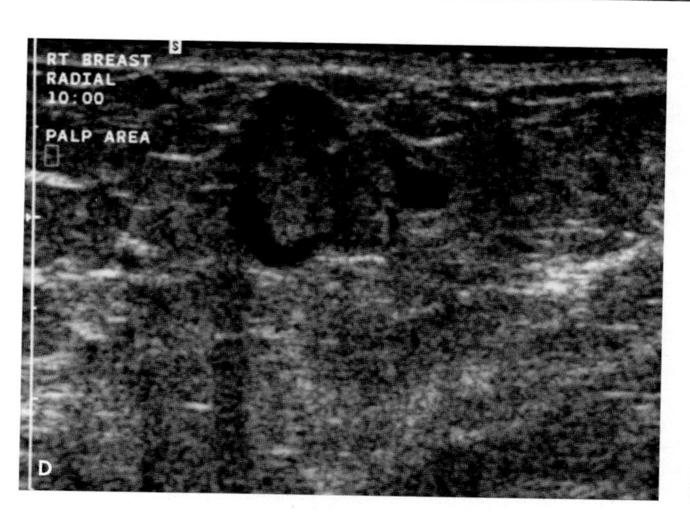

Figure 3.44. Ultrasound image, radial projection **(D)**, palpable finding, right breast, 10 o'clock.

How would you describe the finding corresponding to the area of concern to the patient?

A complex cystic mass is imaged corresponding to the palpable finding in the right breast. This is confirmatory of our initial impression that the mammographic findings represent papillomas. As the remainder of the breast is scanned, additional complex cystic masses and solid hypoechoic masses are seen scattered in the upper outer quadrant of the right breast.

How do solitary and multiple peripheral papillomas contrast, and what is their significance?

Solitary papillomas most commonly occur in the major subareolar ducts and present with spontaneous nipple discharge. They can be identified as a solitary mass or a cluster of round and punctate calcifications (with or without an associated mass) on mammography. Coarse, dense, curvilinear calcifications, noted incidentally within dilated ductal structures, are also likely sclerosed papillomas. Peripheral papillomas are usually multiple and are detected on screening mammograms as multiple masses or multiple clusters of round and punctate calcifications. Their distribution is variable and includes clusters in a small area of tissue, segmental, regional, or diffuse involvement of the breast. In some patients, the findings are bilateral. On ultrasound, the solitary central papillomas may be identified as a solid mass within a dilated duct, a complex cystic mass, or a hypoechoic mass indistinguishable from any other solid mass. Multiple peripheral papillomas are often seen as a combination of complex cystic masses and solid, hypoechoic masses scattered in the breast.

What are the basic histologic features of papillomas?

Papillomas are characterized histologically by the presence of a vascular core and an epithelial lining similar to that seen in the ducts, contiguous epithelial cells, and intermittent basilar myoepithelial cells. Proliferative changes, including hyperplasia, atypical hyperplasia, and ductal carcinoma in situ, have been reported in association with the epithelial lining of papillomas. In contrast to patients with solitary, more centrally occurring papillomas (subareolar), in whom excised surrounding tissue is often bland, patients with multiple peripheral papillomas often have significant proliferative changes in the tissue surrounding the papillomas. The described proliferative changes include areas of atypical ductal hyperplasia, lobular neoplasia, and ductal carcinoma in situ. These changes may be seen in nearly 45% of patients, such that some consider multiple peripheral papillomas as marker lesions. The management of some of these patients can present a dilemma, particularly when the findings are regional or diffuse and bilateral.

Our approach to patients with multiple peripheral papillomas that are localized is to do an excisional biopsy. In women with more regional or diffuse findings, we excise any clinically symptomatic area or any lesion or lesions that change on follow-up mammograms or ultrasounds.

PATIENT 45

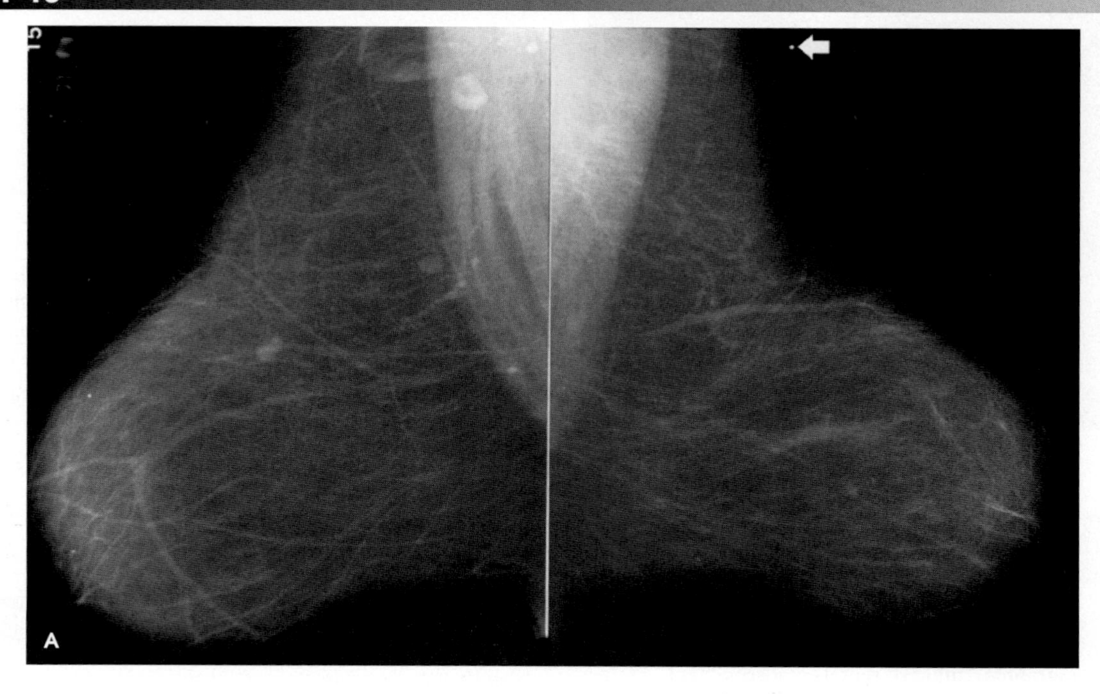

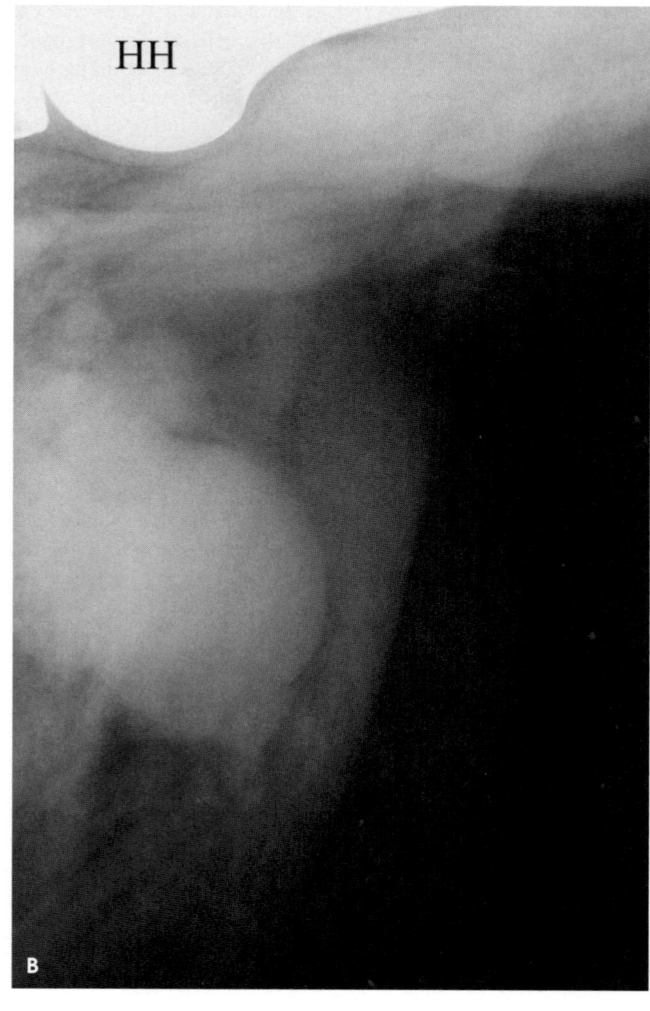

Figure 3.45. Diagnostic evaluation, 36-year-old patient presenting with a tender "lump" in the left axilla. Mediolateral oblique **(A)** views with an arrow denoting position of metallic BB used to mark "lump." Craniocaudal views (not shown) are normal. Left axillary view **(B)**.

How would you describe the findings, what is your differential, and what would you do next?

Predominantly fatty tissue is imaged. Scattered benign-appearing lymph nodes are present on the right. A mass that is at least 3 cm in size is partially imaged on the left axillary view, with associated smaller surrounding masses. As is expected on an axillary view, the humeral head (HH) is also partially seen. The findings in the left axilla most likely represent adenopathy. A detailed history should be elicited from the patient. Specifically, ask about a history of lupus, rheumatoid arthritis, sarcoid, psoriasis, tuberculosis, human immunodeficiency virus (HIV) infection, recent exposure to cats (cat scratch disease), an ongoing infectious process, or known malignancy (lymphoma, breast cancer, melanoma, etc.). Correlative physical examination and an ultrasound are done next.

On physical examination, the patient has significant limitations in the range of motion for her left shoulder and significant tenderness is associated with any movement of the left arm or palpation of the left axilla. A hard mass with satellite nodules is palpated in the left axilla. On ultrasound, a round mass that is markedly hypoechoic is imaged corresponding to the dominant palpable abnormality. During the ultrasound study and following multiple questions, a history of HIV infection is elicited from the patient. Although the findings may be benign and reactive, an ultrasound-guided core biopsy is indicated.

BI-RADS® category 4: suspicious abnormality—biopsy should be considered. A non-Hodgkin B-cell lymphoma is diagnosed on the core biopsy. A CT scan of the chest confirms adenopathy in the left axilla; however, no other adenopathy is identified. Similarly, neck, abdominal, and pelvic CT scans are normal.

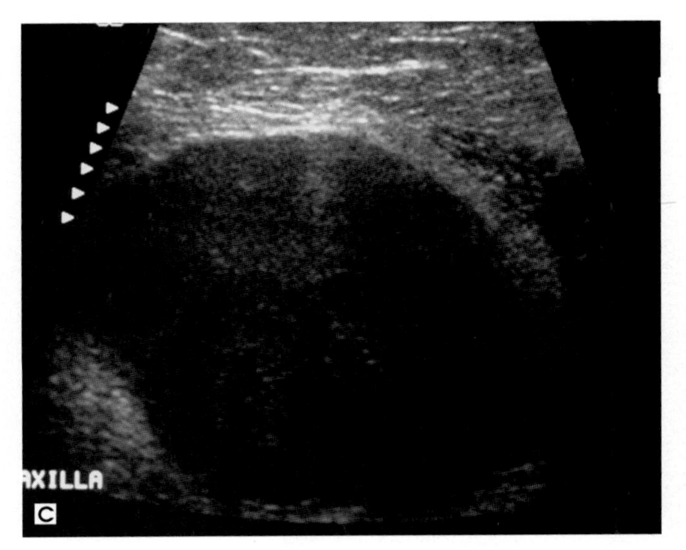

Figure 3.45. Ultrasound image **(C)**, left axilla.

How does primary breast lymphoma present?

Breast lymphoma, classified as an extranodal lymphoma, represents <0.1% of all breast malignancies and is only considered primary when the patient does not have widespread lymphoma or a history of having had lymphoma elsewhere in the body. Patients present with one or multiple masses, more commonly involving one breast, although some present with synchronous (and metachronous) bilateral disease. As many as 20% of patients describe night sweats, fever, and weight loss. Axillary adenopathy is identified in 30% to 40% of patients. Mammographically, one or multiple masses with well- to ill-defined margins are the most common presentation. Rarely, diffuse changes that include increased density, prominence of the trabecular pattern, and skin thickening may be seen. On ultrasound, a solid, hypoechoic mass is the most common finding.

Most patients with primary breast lymphoma have diffuse large-cell lymphoma, B-cell origin, of the immunoglobulin M heavy-chain type. The age of presentation and the course of the disease are variable. Histologic type and stage at the time of diagnosis are the major determinants of prognosis. A second presentation for primary breast lymphoma is that of a Burkitt-type lymphoma with bilateral breast involvement, described in pregnant or lactating patients. This is characterized by a more rapid and aggressive course. Axillary adenopathy is identified in 30% to 40% of patients. Patients are usually treated with lumpectomy followed by radiation therapy.

PATIENT 46

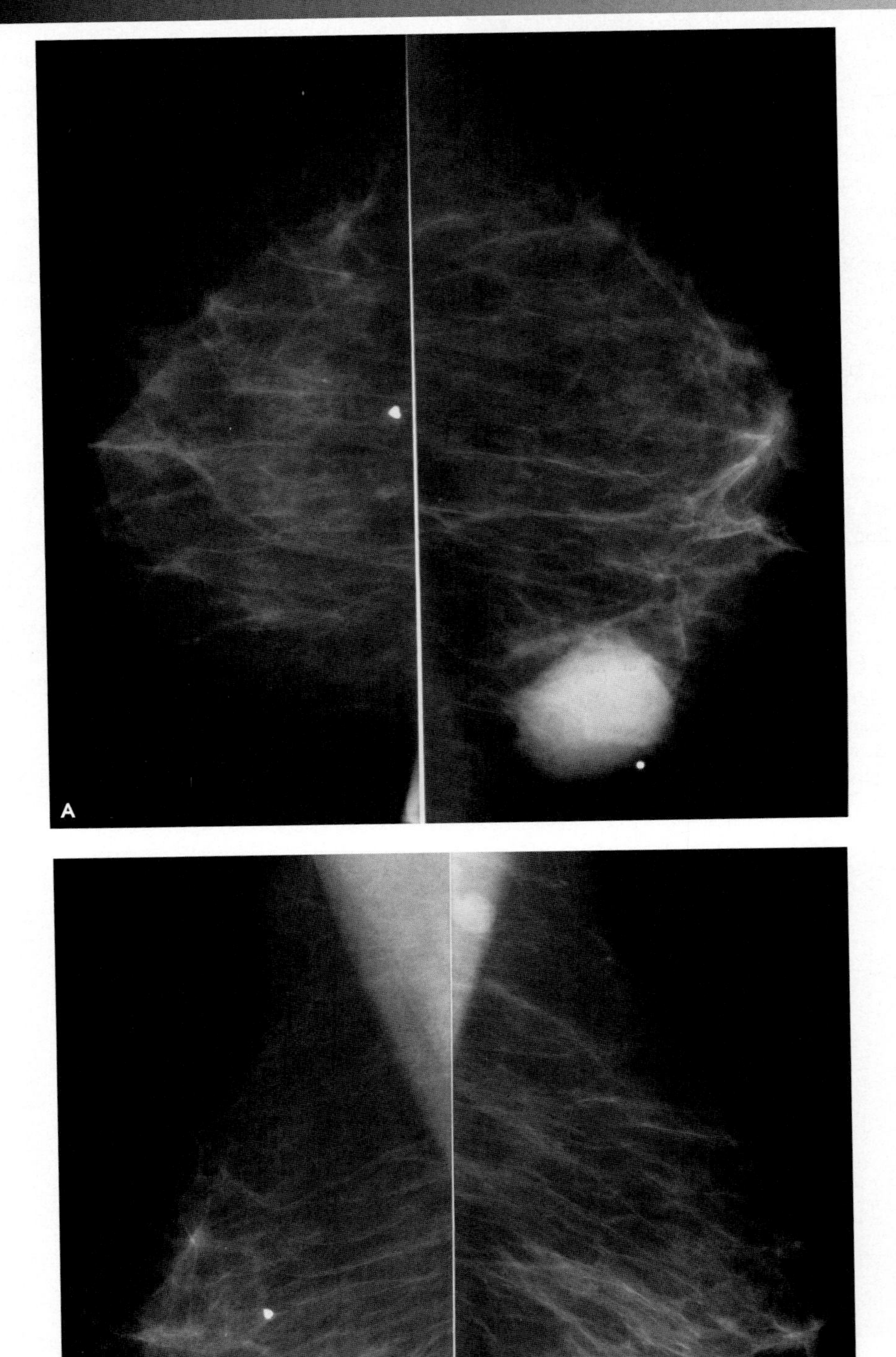

Figure 3.46. Diagnostic evaluation, 74-year-old patient presenting with a "lump" in the left breast. Metallic BB used to mark location of "lump." Craniocaudal **(A)** and mediolateral oblique **(B)** views.

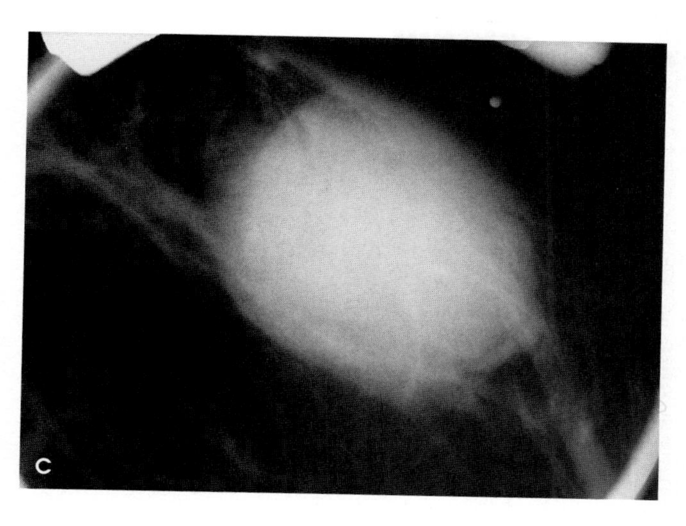

Figure 3.46. (*Continued*) Spot tangential **(C)** view of palpable mass, left breast.

How would you describe the findings, and what is your differential?

A round mass with mostly circumscribed margins and associated skin thickening is present corresponding to the site of concern to the patient. An oval mass is also noted superimposed on the left pectoral muscle inferiorly. The differential for the mass in the left breast includes sebaceous cyst, cyst, and papilloma. A hematoma or abscess would be considerations if there is a history of trauma to this site, or if there are signs and symptoms of an ongoing inflammatory process. Malignant considerations include an invasive ductal carcinoma not otherwise specified, papillary or mucinous carcinoma, or metastatic disease. The mass superimposed on the pectoral muscle is most likely a lymph node.

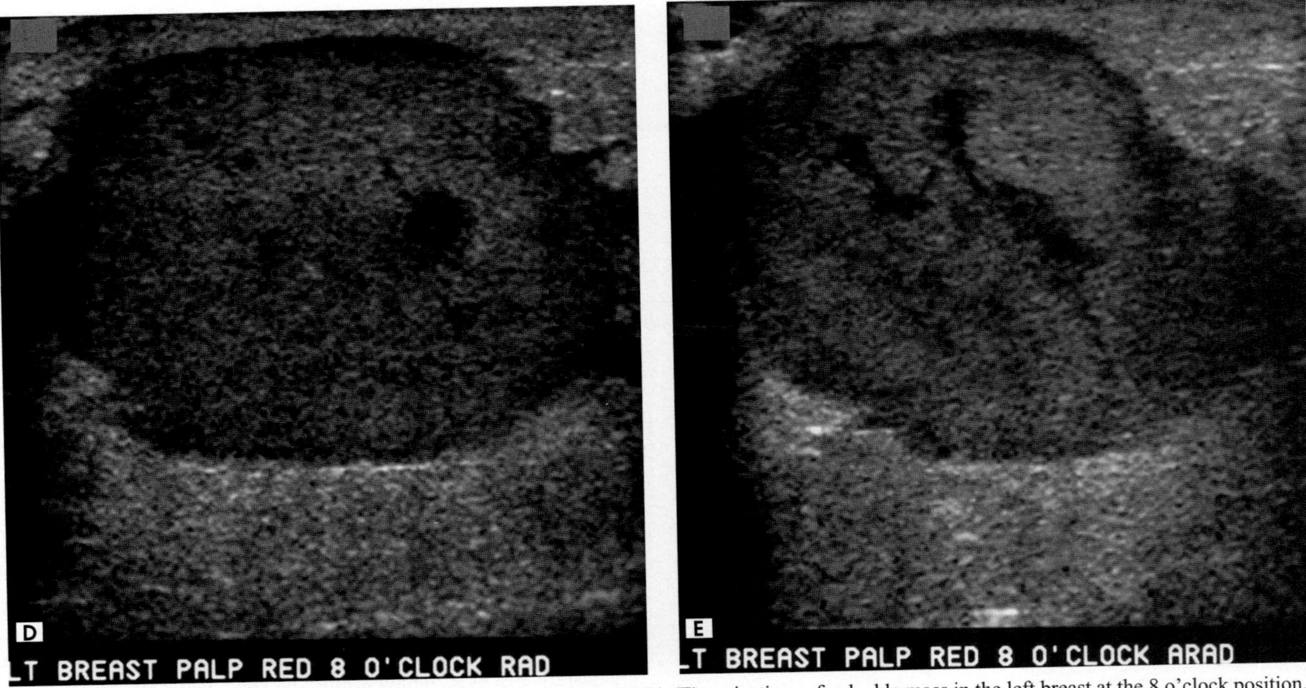

Figure 3.46. Ultrasound images, radial (RAD) **(D)** and antiradial (ARAD) **(E)** projections of palpable mass in the left breast at the 8 o'clock position.

How would you describe the findings, and what is your recommendation?

On physical examination, a hard mass that is fixed to the skin is palpated at the 8 o'clock position of the left breast. The skin is erythematous, but there is no associated tenderness with compression. On ultrasound, a round mass with a heterogenous echotexture and posterior acoustic enhancement is imaged corresponding to the palpable finding in the left breast. Given the erythema, this may represent an inflammatory process, or possibly a hematoma, but a biopsy is warranted.

BI-RADS® category 4: suspicious abnormality—biopsy should be considered.

As a starting point, after infiltrating the skin and breast tissue up to the lesion with lidocaine, you can attempt an aspiration. If no fluid (pus or blood) is obtained, or there is a residual abnormality, core biopsies are done. In this patient, an invasive carcinoma with intra- and extracellular mucin is reported histologically. Although a breast primary is in the differential, the pathologist is concerned about a metastatic lesion to the breast. A lung primary is identified on a CT scan of the chest.

Metastatic disease to the breast is not common, however, it typically presents as one or multiple round masses with variable marginal features that range from well-circumscribed to ill-defined but usually not spiculated. The more common primaries to consider include melanoma, lung, colon and renal; prostate cancer is a consideration in male patients.

PATIENT 47

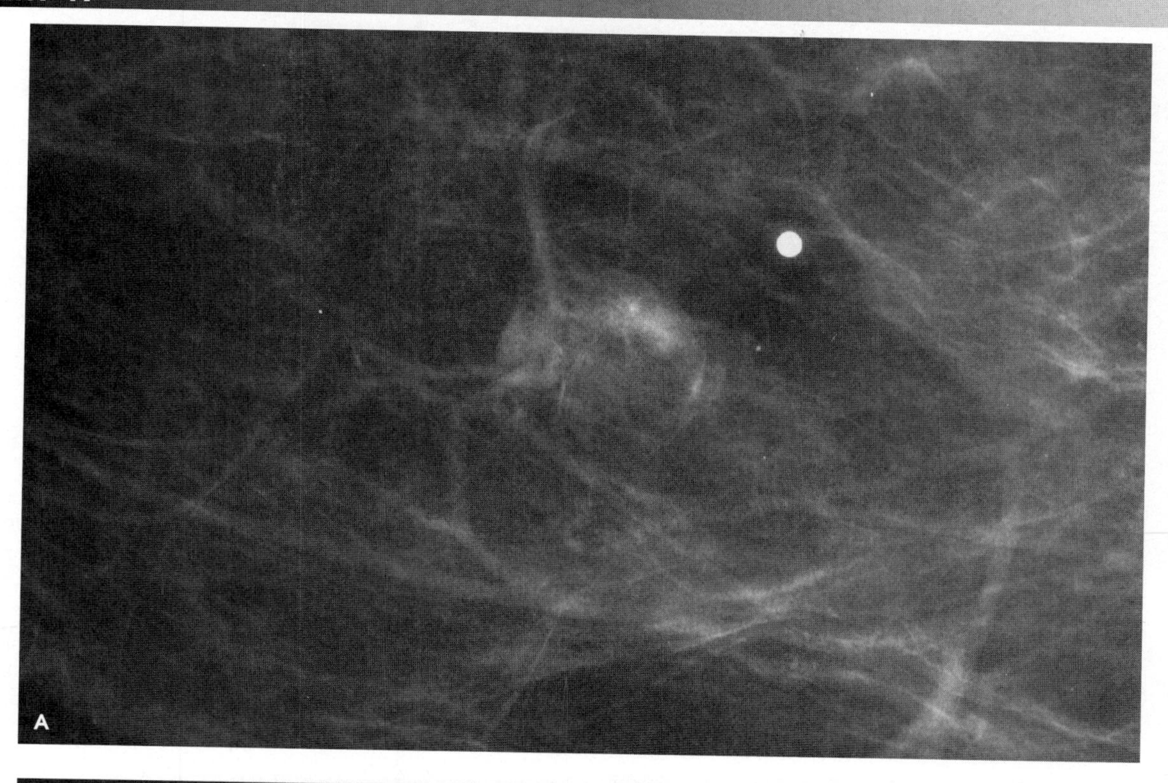

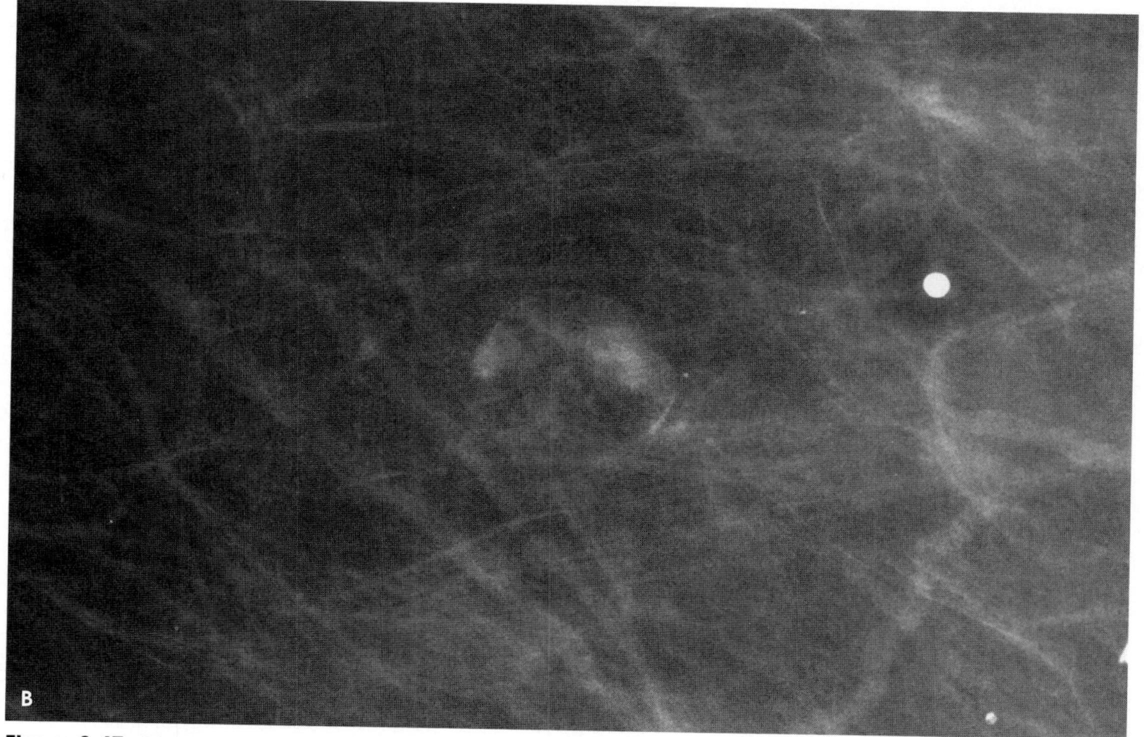

Figure 3.47. Diagnostic evaluation, 55-year-old patient presenting with a "lump" in the left breast. Craniocaudal **(A)** and mediolateral oblique **(B)** views, photographically coned to the area of concern to the patient, left breast.

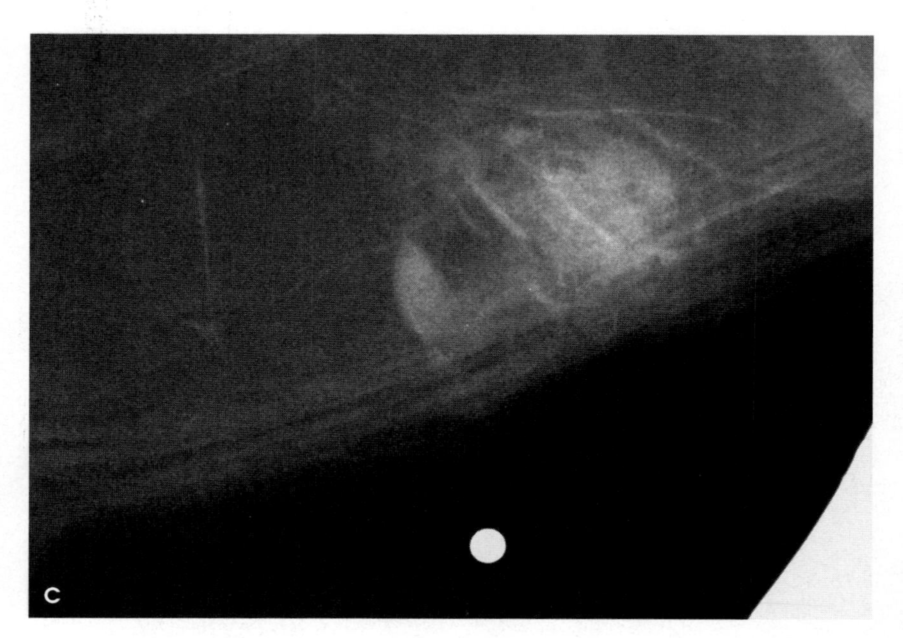

Figure 3.47. (*Continued*) Spot tangential **(C)** view of palpable finding. Metallic BB used to mark the palpable finding.

How would you describe the findings, and what is your differential?

A mixed-density (fat containing) mass is imaged in the upper inner quadrant of the left breast at the site of concern to the patient. Differential considerations include a fibroadenolipoma, fat necrosis related to prior surgery or trauma, oil cyst, galactocele, or an abscess. An intramammary lymph node is also in the differential; however, these are more commonly seen in the lateral quadrants. In establishing an etiology, reviewing prior films and obtaining a history may be helpful. In this patient, a fibroadenolipoma or intramammary lymph node is unlikely because her prior mammogram is normal. In patients with mixed-density lesions, the benign etiology of the finding is established mammographically, and no additional evaluation is indicated.

BI-RADS® category 2: benign finding.

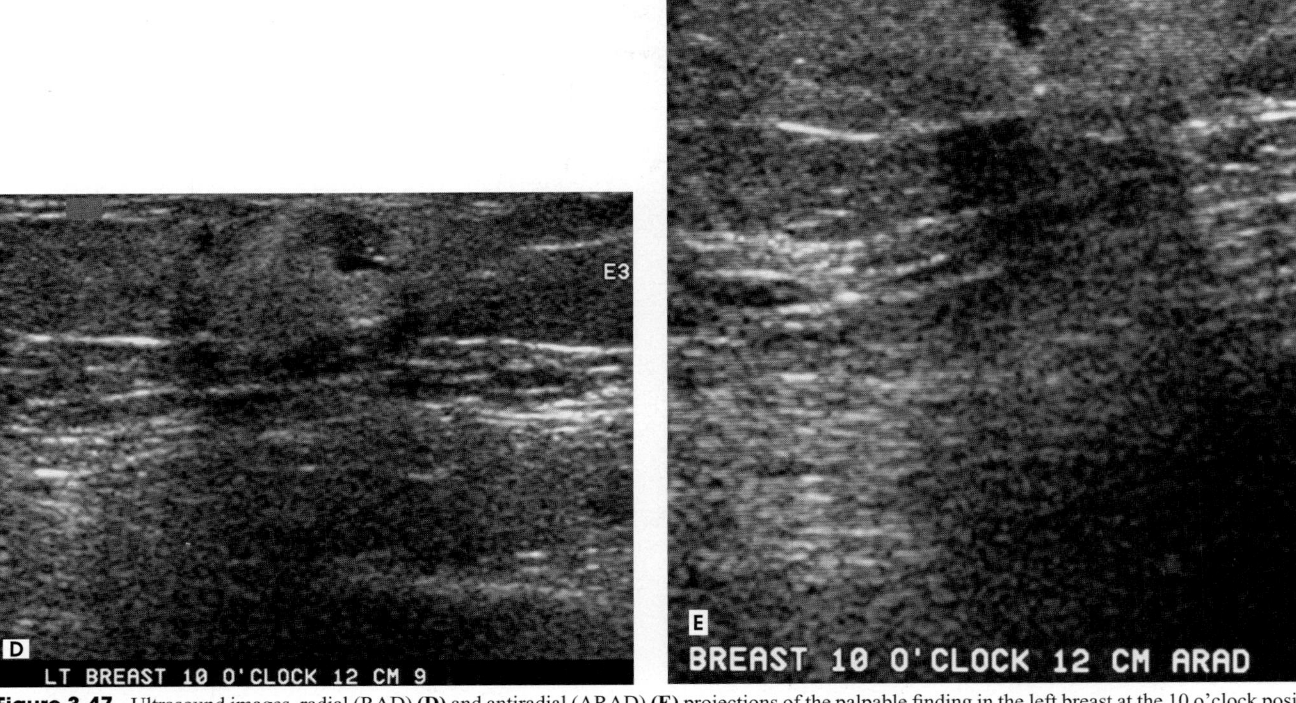

Figure 3.47. Ultrasound images, radial (RAD) **(D)** and antiradial (ARAD) **(E)** projections of the palpable finding in the left breast at the 10 o'clock position, 12 cm from the nipple.

How would you describe the findings, and what is your diagnosis?

An ill-defined round area of slight hyperechogenicity with associated areas of cystic change is imaged corresponding to the palpable finding. No tenderness is elicited as this mass is palpated, making an inflammatory process unlikely. Although on questioning the patient does not recall any trauma to this area, the findings are most suggestive of fat necrosis related to trauma. (I include the ultrasound for completeness, not because an ultrasound is needed to establish the benign etiology of the mammographic finding.)

PATIENT 48

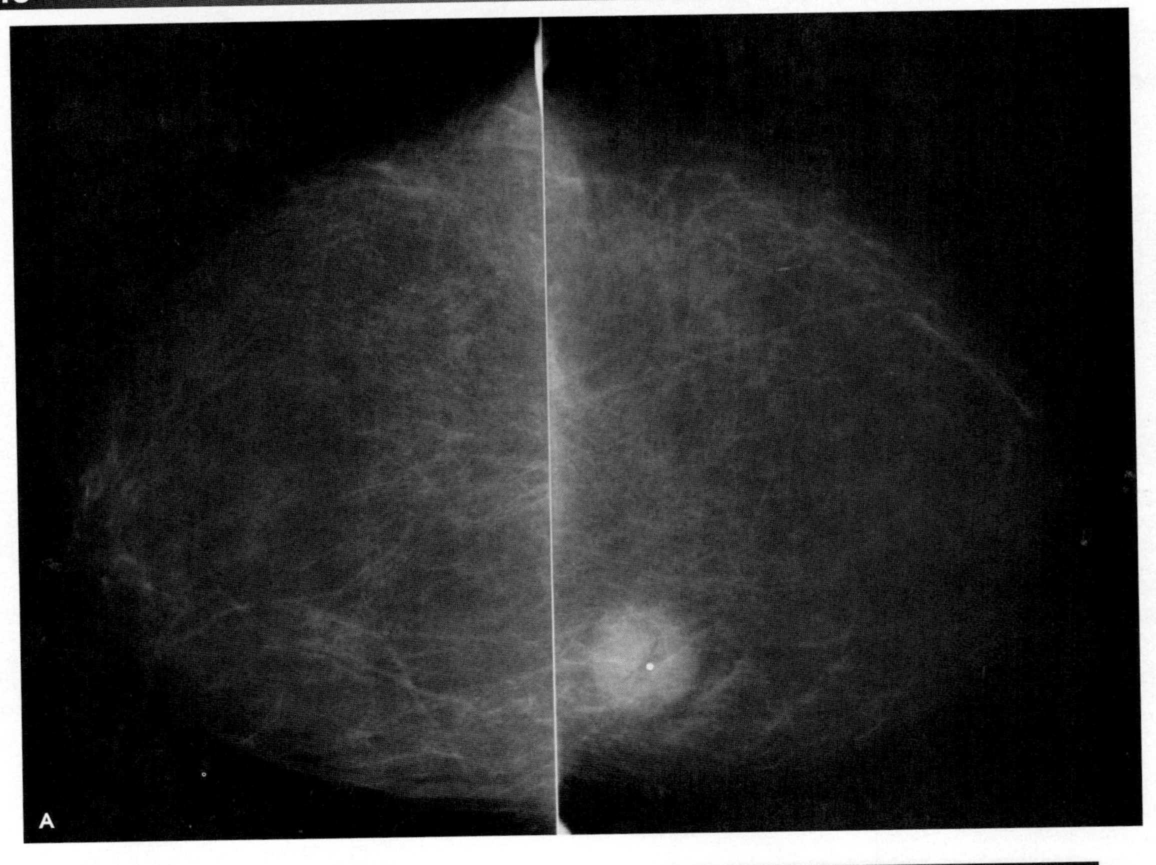

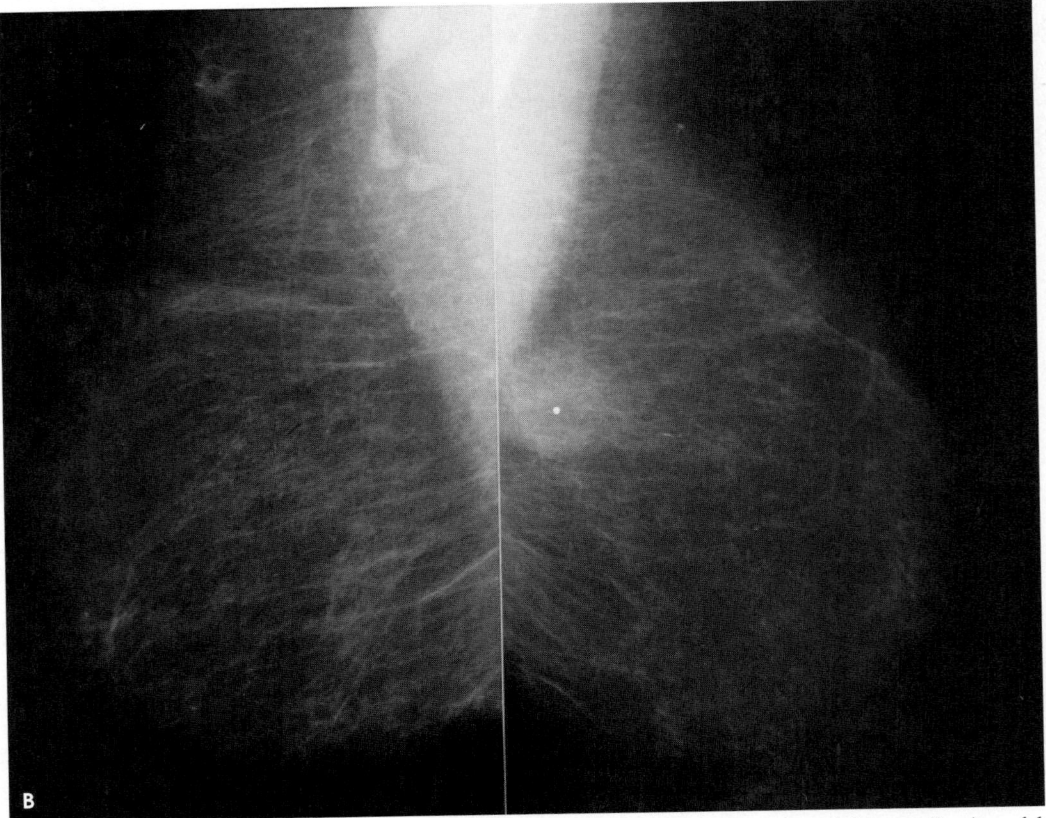

Figure 3.48. Diagnostic evaluation, 78-year-old patient presenting with a tender "lump" in the left breast. Craniocaudal **(A)** and mediolateral oblique **(B)** views with a metallic BB used to mark the palpable finding.

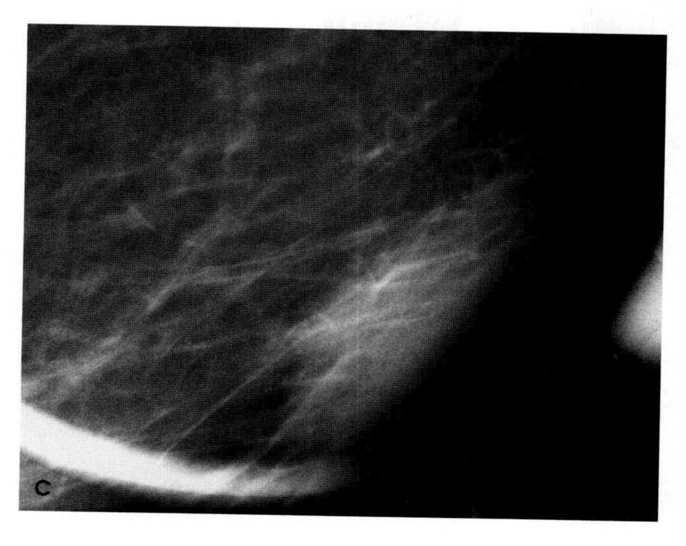

Figure 3.48. (*Continued*) Spot tangential view **(C)** of the palpable finding, left breast.

How would you describe the findings?
What do you think is the likely diagnosis, and how can you confirm your impression?

A round mass with indistinct margins is imaged in the upper inner quadrant of the left breast, corresponding to the "lump" described by the patient. On the spot tangential view this mass is associated with the skin and likely represents a sebaceous cyst. This can be confirmed by examining the patient. On physical examination, a mass that is fixed to the skin (the mass moves with the skin; it cannot be moved independently of the overlying skin) is palpated in the upper inner quadrant of the left breast. On visual inspection, a prominent pore is seen at the center of the palpable finding. With gentle compression, thick white material can be squeezed out of the visualized pore, confirming the impression that the palpable finding is a sebaceous cyst.

BI-RADS® category 2: benign finding.

Sebaceous and epidermal inclusion cysts are clinically, mammographically, and sonographically indistinguishable. Epidermal inclusion cysts have an epidermal cell lining, in contrast to the epithelial cell lining that characterizes sebaceous cysts. These are usually readily palpable, well-defined, cutaneous or subcutaneous masses that can become quite large and may be visible when they cause a smooth bulging of the overlying skin. The orifice of the sebaceous gland may be visible as a dark spot ("blackhead"). In some patients, a thick white cheesy material can be expressed through the orifice of the obstructed sebaceous gland. Mammographically, they are often well-circumscribed masses, commonly in the medial quadrants of the breasts. In some patients the margins are indistinct, particularly if there is associated inflammation. Calcifications may also be seen associated with some sebaceous cysts. On ultrasound, the most common finding is that of a well-circumscribed mass arising in the skin and commonly extending into the subcutaneous tissue. They can be anechoic, hypoechoic, slightly hyperechoic or heterogeneous, and in some patients, a thin hypoechoic tubular (e.g., a track) structure can be seen extending from the mass to the skin surface. Unless the patient is symptomatic, no intervention is required. If the patient is symptomatic surgical excision may be indicated.

BIBLIOGRAPHY

Adeniran A, Al-Ahmadie H, Mahoney MC, Robinson-Smith TM. Granular cell tumor of the breast: a series of 17 cases and a review of the literature. *Breast J.* 2004;10:528–531.

Adler DD, Helvie MA, Oberman HA, et al. Radial sclerosing lesion of the breast: mammographic features. *Radiology*. 1990;176:737–740.

Aguirregengoa K, Benito JR, Montejo M, et al. Cat-scratch disease: series of 14 cases. The diagnostic usefulness of serology. *Enferm Infecc Microbiol Clin.* 1999;17:15–18.

American College of Radiology (ACR). ACR BI-RADS®—magnetic resonance imaging. 4th ed. In: *ACR Breast Imaging Reporting and Data System, Breast Imaging Atlas*. Reston, VA: American College of Radiology; 2003.

American College of Radiology (ACR). ACR BI-RADS®—mammography. 4th ed. In: *ACR Breast Imaging Reporting and Data System, Breast Imaging Atlas.* Reston, VA: American College of Radiology; 2003.

American College of Radiology (ACR). ACR BI-RADS®—ultrasound. 4th ed. In: *ACR Breast Imaging Reporting and Data System, Breast Imaging Atlas.* Reston, VA:. American College of Radiology; 2003.

American College of Radiology. *Mammography Quality Control Manual*. Reston, VA: American College of Radiology, 1999.

American College of Radiology Practice Guideline for the Performance of Diagnostic Mammography. Reston, VA: American College of Radiology; rev. 2002.

Bradley RA, Katner HP, Dale PS. Cat scratch disease presenting as breast mastitis. *Can J Surg.* 2005;48:254–255.

Brenner RJ, Jackman RJ, Parker SH, et al. Percutaneous core needle biopsy of radial scars of the breast: when is excision necessary? *AJR Am J Roentgenol.* 2002;179:1179–1184.

Cohen MA, Sferlazza SJ. Role of sonography in evaluation of radial scars of the breast. *AJR Am J Roentgenol.* 2000; 174: 1075–1078.

Darling ML, Smith DN, Rhei E, et al. Lactating adenoma: sonographic features. *Breast J.* 2000;6:252–256.

Erguvan-Dogan B, Dempsey PJ, Ayyar G, Gilcrease MZ. Primary desmoid tumor (extraabdominal fibromatosis) of the breast. *AJR Am J Roentgenol.* 2005;185:488–489.

Feder JM, de Paredes ES, Hogge JP, Wilken JJ. Unusual breast lesions: radiologic-pathologic correlation. *Radiographics.* 1999; 19:11–26.

Fraser JL, Raza S, Chorny K, et al. Columnar alteration with prominent apical snouts and secretions: spectrum of changes frequently present in breast biopsies performed for microcalcifications. *Am J Surg Pathol* 1998;12:1521–1527.

Frouge C, Tristant H, Guinebretiere JM, et al. Mammographic lesions suggestive of radial scars: microscopic findings in 40 cases. *Radiology.* 1995;195:623.

Garstin WI, Kaufman Z, Mitchell MJ, Baum M. Fibrous mastopathy in insulin dependent diabetics. *Clin Radiol.* 1991;44:89–91.

Godet C, Roblot F, Le Moal G, et al. Cat-scratch disease presenting as a breast mass. *Scand J Infect Dis.* 2004; 36:6–7.

Greenstein-Orel S, Evers K, Yeh IT, et al. Radial scar with microcalcifications: radiologic-pathologic correlation. *Radiology.* 1992;183:479–482.

Harvey JA, Fechner RE, Moore MM. Apparent ipsilateral decrease in breast size at mammography: a sign of infiltrating lobular carcinoma. *Radiology.* 2000;214:883–889.

Ingram DL, Mossler JA, Snowhite J, et al. Granular cell tumors of the breast. Steroid receptor analysis and localization of carcinoembryonic antigen, myoglobin and S100 protein. *Arch Pathol Lab Med.* 1984;108:897–901.

Jacobs TW, Byrne E, Colditz G, et al. Radial scars in benign breast biopsy specimens and the risk of breast cancer. *N Engl J Med.* 1999;340:430–436.

Leibman AJ, Kossoff MB. Sonographic features of fibromatosis of the breast. *J Ultrasound Med.* 1991;10:43–45.

Logan WW, Hoffman NY. Diabetic fibrous breast disease. *Radiology.* 1989;172:667–670.

Markaki S, Sotiropoulou M, Papaspirou P, Lazaris D. Cat-scratch disease presenting as a solitary tumor in the breast: report of three cases. *Eur J Obstet Gynecol Reprod Biol.* 2003;106:175–178.

Miller JA, Karcnik TJ, Karimi S. Granular cell tumor of the breast: definitive diagnosis by sonographically guided percutaneous biopsy. *J Clin Ultrasound.* 2000;28:89–93.

Mitnick JS, Vasquez MF, Harris MN, et al. Differentiation of radial scar from scirrhous carcinoma of the breast: mammographic-pathologic correlation. *Radiology.* 1989;173:697–700.

Murakami K, Tsukahara M, Tsuneoka H, et al. Cat scratch disease: analysis of 130 seropositive cases. *J Infect Chemother.* 2002;8: 349–352.

Nakazono T, Satoh T, Hamamoto T, Kudo S. Dynamic MRI of fibromatosis of the breast. *AJR Am J Roentgenol.* 2003;181:1718–1719.

Nielsen M, Christesen L, Andersen J. Radial scars in women with breast cancer. *Cancer.* 1987;59:1019.

Okada K, Ozeki K, TI, et al. Granular cell tumor of the breast: a case report describing dynamic MR mammography. *Breast Cancer.* 1998;5:179–282.

Povoski SP, Spigos DG, Marsh WL. An unusual case of cat-scratch disease from *Bartonella quintana* mimicking inflammatory breast cancer in a 50-year-old woman. *Breast J.* 2003;9:497–500.

Rosen PP. *Rosen's Breast Pathology.* 2nd ed. Philadelphia: Lippincott Williams & Wilkins; 2001.

Sickles EA. Combining spot-compression and other special views to maximize mammographic information. *Radiology.* 1989;173:571.

Sickles EA. Further experience with microfocal spot magnification mammography in the assessment of clustered breast microcalcifications. *Radiology.* 1980;137:9–14.

Sickles EA. Microfocal spot magnification mammography using xeroradiographic and screen film recording systems. *Radiology.* 1979;131:599–607.

Soler NG, Khardori R. Fibrous disease of the breast, thyroiditis and cheiroarthropathy in type I diagetes mellitus. *Lancet.* 1984;1: 193–195.

Soo MS, Dash N, Bentley R, et al. Tubular adenomas of the breast: imaging findings with histologic correlation. *AJR Am J Roentgenol.* 2000;174:757–761.

Sumkin JH, Perrone AM, Harris KM, et al. Lactating adenoma: US and literature review. *Radiology.* 1998;206:271–274.

Tavassoli FA. *Pathology of the Breast.* 2nd ed. New York: McGraw-Hill; 1999.

Tomaszewski JE, Brooks JS, Hicks D, Livolsi VA. Diabetic mastopathy: a distinctive clinicopathologic entity. *Hum Pathol.* 1992;23:780–786.

Chapter 4

Management

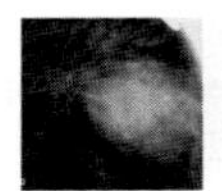
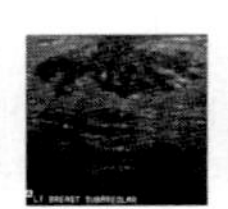
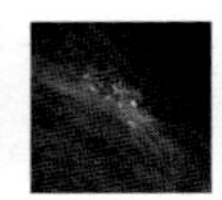
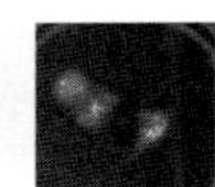

TERMS

Atypical ductal hyperplasia (ADH)
Atypical lobular hyperplasia (ALH)
Columnar alteration with prominent apical snouts and secretions (CAPSS)
Complex sclerosing lesion
Cribriform ductal carcinoma in situ
Ductal carcinoma in situ (DCIS)
Ductography
E-cadherin
False negative (FN)
False positive (FP)
Fibroadenoma
Hyperplasia
Incident cancer detection rate
Intracystic carcinoma
Ipsilateral breast tumor recurrence (IBTR)
Lobular carcinoma in situ (LCIS)
Lobular neoplasia
Local recurrence
Medical audit
Micropapillary ductal carcinoma in situ
Minimal breast cancer
Mucocele-like lesion
Multiple peripheral papillomas
Papilloma
Papillomatosis
Phyllodes tumor
Pneumocystogram
Positive predictive value (PPV)
Prevalent cancer detection rate
Pseudoangiomatous stromal hyperplasia (PASH)
Radial scar
Regional recurrence
Sclerosing adenosis
Secretory carcinoma
Sensitivity
Specificity
True negative (TN)
True positive (TP)

MANAGEMENT

In managing the various situations that arise in breast imaging, it is good to always be thinking not just relative to what the first step should be for your patient's care, but what the second and third steps might be as well. Your patient? Yes, *your* patient. Know and consider the cascade of events you precipitate for patients based on what you say to them, how you word your report, and the recommendations you make. Are you sure enough about what you are saying to justify whatever ensues for the patient? Is your decision motivated by a defensive posture and the recognition, at some level, that the workup is incomplete (substandard) and that you are operating with inadequate or incomplete information, or one that is justifiably based on common sense, a complete workup, and what is good for the patient?

CORRELATION

The need for correlation in every process undertaken is fundamentally important. If an ultrasound is done to evaluate a mammographic or magnetic resonance imaging (MRI) finding, does what you see on ultrasound correlate with the mammographic or MRI finding? If the patient presents with a focal finding, does what you see mammographically correlate with the described clinical finding? When recommending an imaging-guided or excisional biopsy, consider what you will accept as a diagnosis and what you will recommend if the results are different from those expected. Are the imaging and histologic findings concordant? If the imaging and histologic findings are benign and congruent, patients can be returned to annual screening mammography. For patients diagnosed with a malignancy, MRI and surgical consultation are scheduled. If the findings are not concordant, repeat biopsy or excisional biopsy is recommended. For patients with a diagnosis of atypical ductal hyperplasia (ADH), possible phyllodes tumor, multiple peripheral papillomas, fibromatosis, or granular cell tumor, wide surgical excision is indicated following imaging-guided biopsies.

The management of several types of lesions diagnosed on core biopsies remains controversial. Included in this group are solitary papillomas, lobular neoplasia (atypical lobular neoplasia, lobular carcinoma in situ), complex sclerosing lesions, and mucocele-like lesions. The current consensus is that excisional biopsy is appropriate when these lesions are diagnosed on core biopsies because of the reported incidence of associated malignancy and the frequency with which some of these lesions are upgraded to cancer when more tissue is examined histologically.

BREAST IMAGING CONSULTATIONS

As mentioned previously, regardless of the type of study done, the title on the written description of what I do is worded as a "Breast Imaging Consultation" not a "Radiology Report." The comprehensive evaluations that can be undertaken by breast imagers have put us in a consultative role. A general outline used for breast imaging consultative reports includes:

- Type of study (e.g., screening or diagnostic mammogram, ultrasound)
- Reason for study
- Tissue type
- Succinct description and location of findings
- Impression, *with your specific recommendations*
- Assessment category (required under the Mammography Quality Standards Act for all mammographic studies) with wording as provided by the American College of Radiology, Breast Imaging and Reporting Data System (BI-RADS®) for mammography:

Category 1: negative
Category 2: benign finding
Category 3: probably benign finding; short-interval follow-up is recommended
Category 4: suspicious abnormality—biopsy should be considered
Category 5: highly suggestive of malignancy—appropriate action should be taken
Category 6: known biopsy-proven malignancy—appropriate action should be taken
Category 0: need additional imaging evaluation and/or prior mammograms for comparison

Category 4 lesions can be further subdivided at the discretion of the facility for their internal use into:

Category 4A: low suspicion for malignancy
Category 4B: intermediate suspicion for malignancy
Category 4C: moderate concern

I make every effort to generate descriptive but succinct reports that are clinically relevant and that provide specific direction and recommendations. I use no disclaimers in my reports, and I do not abdicate clinical correlation of anything to others. In considering the wording of reports, it is my contention that if, based on complete clinical and imaging evaluations, you have a high degree of certainty relative to the diagnosis, clear consultative reports with specific recommendations can be dictated easily and succinctly (e.g., "a spiculated mass measuring 7 mm is imaged at the 3 o'clock position, 5 cm from the right nipple. Biopsy is indicated. This is undertaken and reported separately."). Make up your mind about what you are going to say before you start dictating. Hedges and disclaimers are used when we are uncomfortable and uncertain about a finding and its significance. In this situation, I would suggest that we need to do whatever it takes to increase our level of certainty so that we can be more definitive.

For potentially abnormal screening mammograms, I state what the potential abnormality is (e.g., mass, calcifications, distortion) and in which breast it is located; I also comment specifically on the other breast. The description and characterization of the lesion is deferred until a thorough evaluation is completed (e.g., for a mass, spot compression views, physical examination, and an ultrasound). The recommendation for a woman with a potentially abnormal screening mammogram is "additional evaluation is indicated and we will contact the patient directly to schedule the additional evaluation" (see the introduction to Chapter 2 for additional discussion). Consequently, the only assessment categories used for screening mammograms are 0, 1, and 2.

In the diagnostic setting, I issue one consultative report that includes the findings for the diagnostic mammogram, physical examination, and ultrasound. Based on the clinical and imaging features of a lesion, the findings are described and an impression with recommendations is generated. The impression is not used to repeat a description of the findings but rather is used to deliver the final, clinically relevant concept with what I think is indicated for the patient.

Read your reports critically. Strive for precision (e.g., give measurements for a lesion and avoid characterizations such as "small" or "large") and eliminate unnecessary words (e.g., "clearly," "appears to be," "very," etc.) that provide no relevant information and may serve to obscure your message. It is important to familiarize yourself with the mammography, ultrasound, and magnetic resonance imaging lexicons provided by the American College of Radiology, Breast Imaging and Reporting Data System (BI-RADS®), as these provide guidelines on what should be described for particular findings and suggests terminology to be used for relevant findings.

MEDICAL AUDIT

In breast imaging, accountability needs to be present every step of the way. Although quality control and data tracking are often relegated to the technologist, radiologists should be actively involved in these processes for their practice. It is only through monitoring results that problems can be addressed and much learning can take place. We need to know how well we are doing, and we want to identify potential problems that can be addressed so that patient care is improved. By tracking data and learning from the results, we can improve patient care. The numbers generated from the audit should be viewed not as one point in time but rather how they change as you gain more experience.

Data that should be collected include:

- Date of audit
- Number of screening studies (first-time study vs. repeat screen)
- Number of diagnostic studies
- Call-back (recall) recommendations (e.g., BI-RADS® category 0: need additional imaging evaluation)
- Biopsy recommendations (BI-RADS® category 4 and 5: suspicious abnormality and highly suggestive of malignancy)
- Biopsy results (e.g., benign vs. malignant; FNA vs. core biopsy vs. excisional biopsy)
- Tumor staging: histologic subtype, grade, size, and nodal status

Data that you can calculate include:

- True positive (TP): cancer diagnosed within 1 year of a biopsy recommendation for an abnormal mammogram

- True negative (TN): no known cancer within 1 year of a normal mammogram
- False negative (FN): cancer diagnosed within 1 year of a normal mammogram; these should be reviewed and analyzed
- False positive (FP):

  FP1 = no known cancer diagnosed within 1 year of an abnormal screening mammogram for which additional imaging or biopsy is recommended
  FP2 = no known cancer diagnosed within 1 year of a recommendation for biopsy or surgical consultation based on an abnormal mammogram
  FP3 = benign disease diagnosed on biopsy within 1 year after recommendation for biopsy or surgical consultation based on an abnormal mammogram

- Positive predictive value:

  PPV1 = percentage of cancers diagnosed following an abnormal screening mammogram
  PPV2 = percentage of cancers diagnosed when a biopsy or surgical consultation is recommended following a screening mammogram
  PPV3 = percentage of cancers diagnosed on the actual number of biopsies done as a result of a screening mammogram

- Cancer detection rate for asymptomatic women (i.e., true screening population)

  Prevalent (rate of cancer detection among women presenting for their first screening mammogram)
  Incident (rate of cancer detection among women with prior screening mammograms)
  By age groups

- Percentage of minimal breast cancers diagnosed
- Percentage of node-negative breast cancers diagnosed
- Call-back (recall) rate
- Sensitivity = TP/(TP + FN), or the probability of detecting a cancer when a cancer is present
- Specificity = TN/(FP + TN), or the probability of a normal mammogram when no cancer is present

Based on reports of audit data, obtainable goals include:

- PPV1 (abnormal screens): 5% to 10%
- PPV2 (biopsy recommendations): 25% to 40%
- Stage 0 or 1 tumors diagnosed: >50%
- Minimal cancers (invasive cancer ≤1 cm or DCIS): >30%
- Node-positive tumors: <25%
- Prevalent cancers/1,000: 6 to 10
- Incident cancers/1,000: 2 to 4
- Call-back (recall) rate: ≤10%
- Sensitivity: >85%
- Specificity: >90%

Published sensitivity rates for mammography range between 85% and 90%. Recognize, however, that this is probably one of the harder statistics to obtain because of the difficulty of establishing an accurate false negative rate. Access to a statewide tumor registry can be helpful; however, if the patient moves (or seeks medical care) out of state, knowledge of a cancer diagnosis may not be readily accessible to the screening facility.

The effect of breast imaging and the role of radiologists in the management of women with breast cancer goes unstated and, in many ways, is often misrepresented. There is continued skepticism and criticisms relative to our contributions to patient care and the significance of what has already been accomplished: the routine identification of lymph node-negative stage 0 and stage I invasive cancers and ductal carcinoma in situ. Recently reported decreases in breast cancer mortality rates are attributed by many to more effective treatment, ignoring or relegating to a secondary role our ability to detect DCIS, stage 0, and stage I lesions in many patients. Is early detection possibly the more important factor, and does not our ability to identify small lesions increase available treatment options and render them more effective for patients?

PATIENT 1

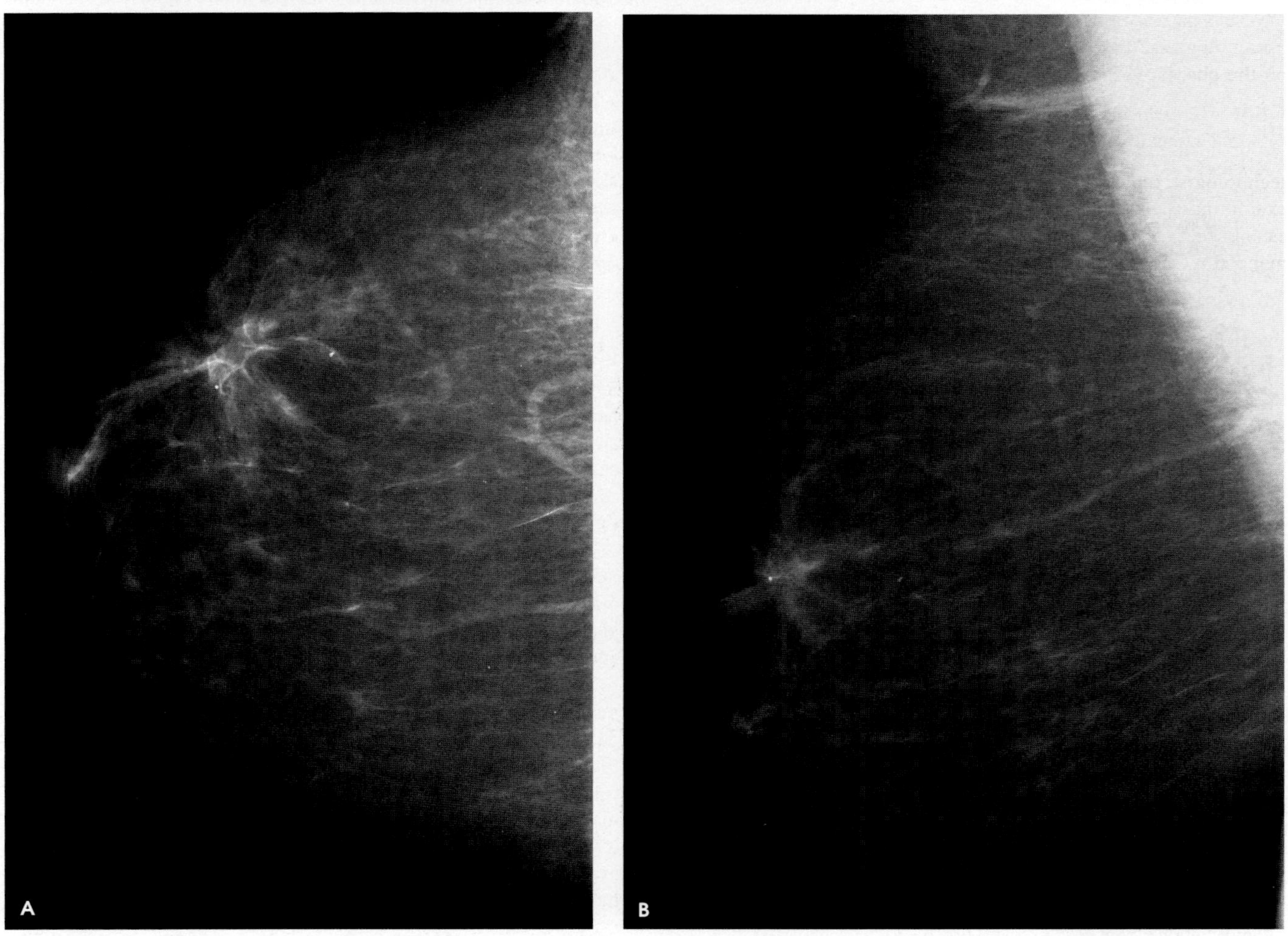

Figure 4.1. Screening study, 60-year-old woman. Craniocaudal **(A)** and mediolateral oblique **(B)** views, right breast.

What do you think? What would you do next?

A mass with a radiolucent center, associated distortion, and long spicules is present anteriorly in the upper outer quadrant of the right breast. Given these features, fat necrosis related to a prior biopsy is one of the main considerations. As a starting point, prior films would be helpful in determining if this finding could be seen previously, and what, if any, evolution has occurred. A review of the patient's history form, looking specifically to see if she has had a biopsy at this site, will also be helpful. Unfortunately, no prior films are available for this patient, and nothing is indicated on the history form relative to a prior biopsy in the right breast. Additional evaluation is indicated.

BI-RADS® category 0: need additional imaging evaluation.

The spot compression views confirm the presence of a mass with a low-density central area, distortion, and long spiculation. The differential for this finding includes fat necrosis related to prior surgery or trauma, complex sclerosing lesion, sclerosing adenosis, papilloma, focal fibrosis, an inflammatory process, invasive ductal carcinoma not otherwise specified, tubular carcinoma, and invasive lobular carcinoma. In discussing the findings with the technologist, she relates not seeing a scar at the site of the spot views. Correlative physical examination and an ultrasound are indicated next.

After introducing myself to the patient and briefly describing what we have seen so far and what I would like to do next, I specifically ask her about prior breast surgery or trauma. She has no recollection of having had surgery or trauma to the right breast. On close inspection of the periareolar region, however, a scar is apparent at the edge of the areola corresponding to the site of the mammographic finding. I palpate no corresponding mass, elicit no tenderness at this site, and the ultrasound is normal throughout the subareolar area extending into the upper outer quadrant of the right breast.

As I approached the patient, I remained open to all diagnostic possibilities; however, I had some skepticism relative to the information provided. In my mind, the mammographic findings (low central density, distortion, and long spiculation), in the absence of a palpable finding, were highly suggestive of fat necrosis or a complex sclerosing lesion. So, rather than totally discard my initial impression, I examine the patient carefully, focusing my attention on the site of the mammographic findings. Although the patient has no recollection of prior surgery (patients do not always recall prior surgical procedures, trauma, or inflammatory processes; some may not even recall a breast cancer diagnosis), and the technologist reported no scars, by spending 2 minutes closely examining the patient, the diagnosis of postoperative change is established and no additional intervention or follow-up is recommended.

Given our total fascination with technology and images, we often dismiss or underestimate simple and inexpensive tools such as physical examination, and yet this often provides the correct answer expeditiously. I cannot emphasize enough how many times direct communication with the patient and a thorough physical examination provide an efficient means of arriving at the correct answer for a given patient. As clinical breast imagers, we are in a unique position to integrate clinical, physical, imaging, and histologic findings to provide accurate, optimal patient care. Do not sell yourself or your patients short by passing up an opportunity to examine and talk to the patient directly. Do not relegate physical examination and the performance of ultrasound studies to others.

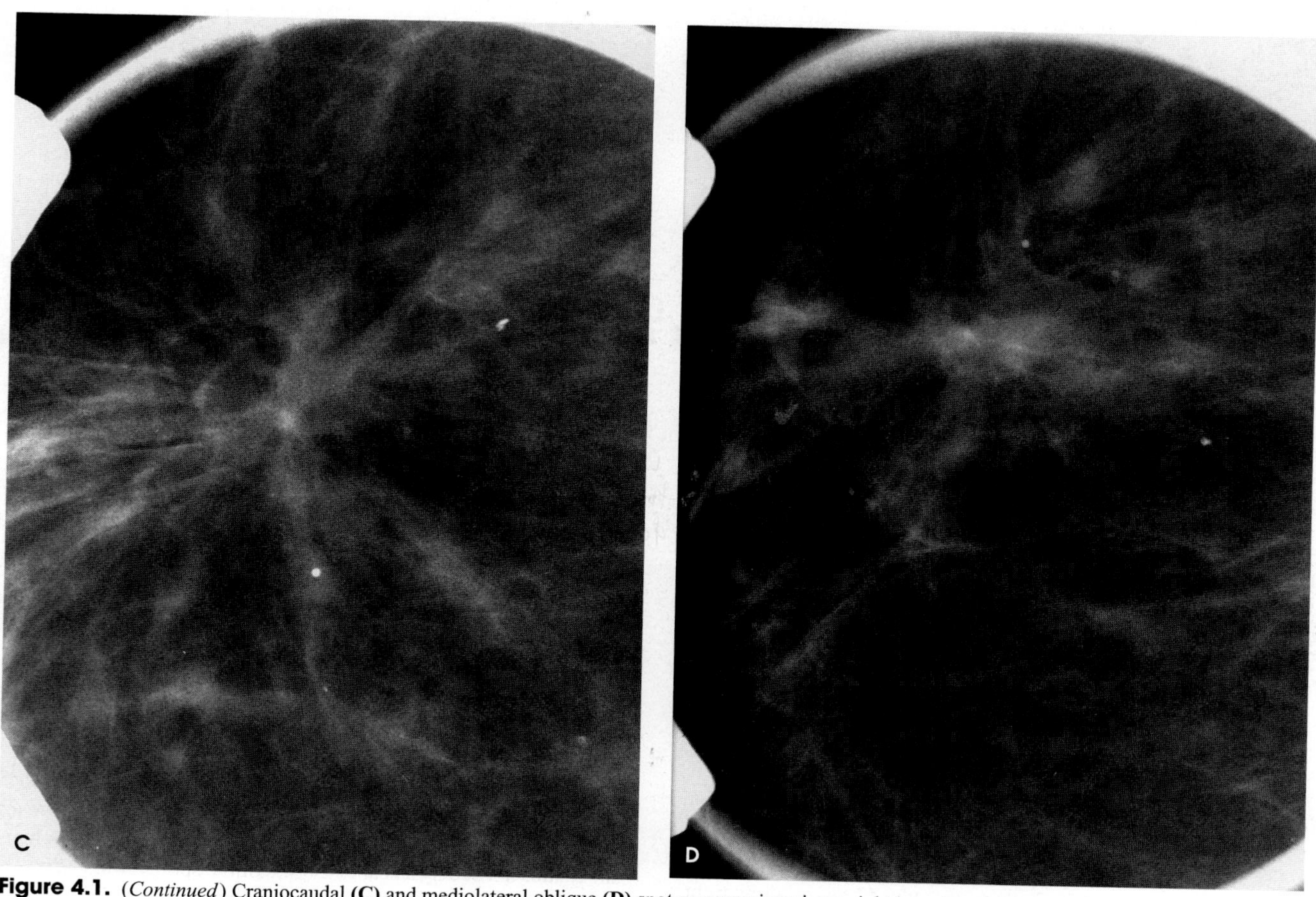

Figure 4.1. (*Continued*) Craniocaudal **(C)** and mediolateral oblique **(D)** spot compression views, right breast.

PATIENT 2

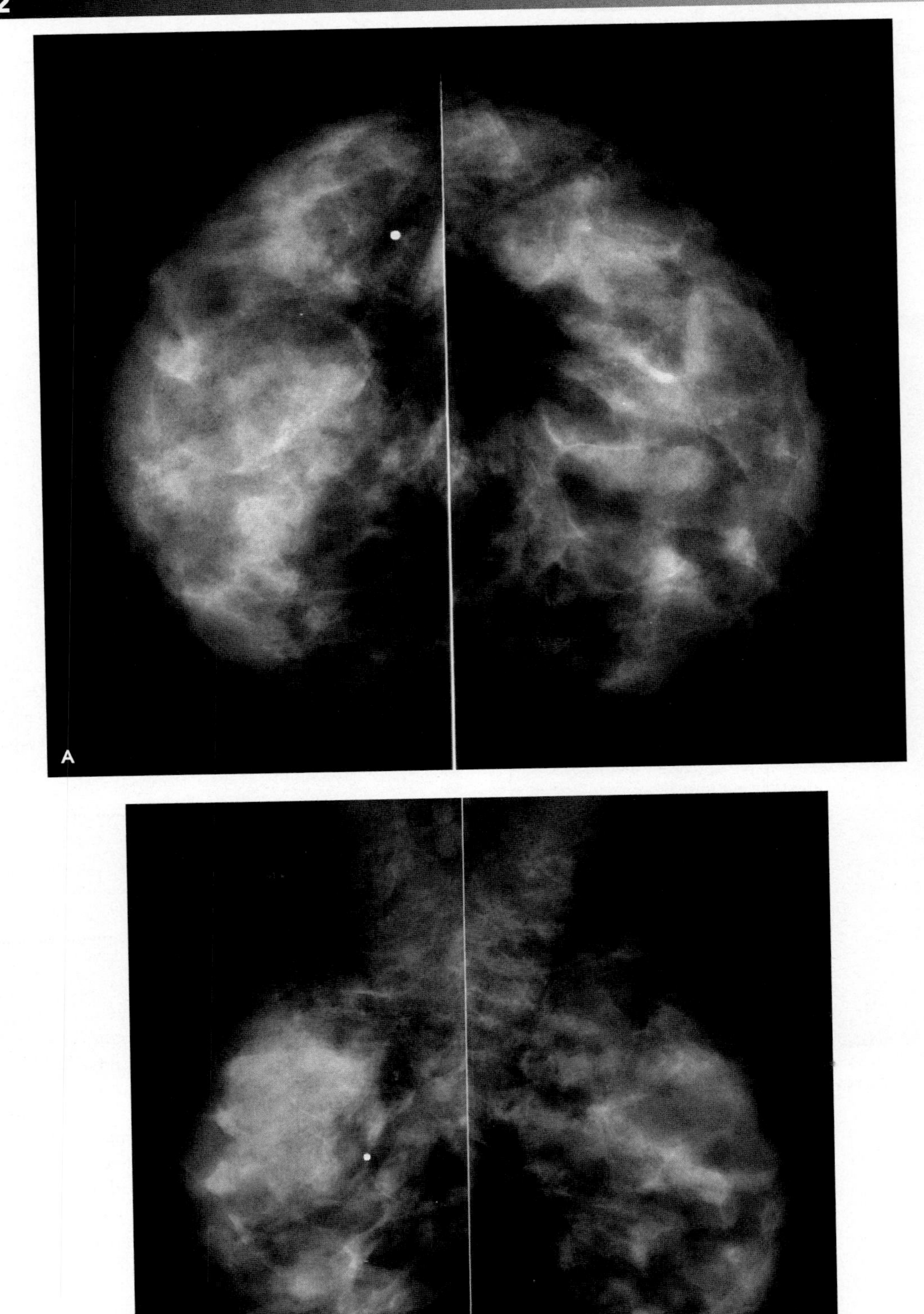

Figure 4.2. Diagnostic evaluation, 33-year-old patient presenting with a "lump" in the right breast. Craniocaudal **(A)** and mediolateral oblique **(B)** views, metallic BB used to mark location of "lump" described by the patient.

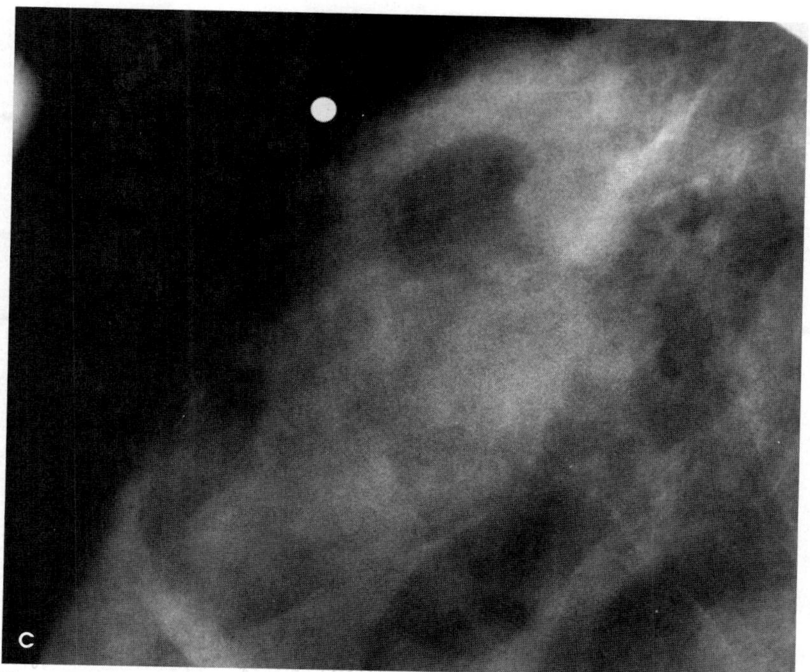

Figure 4.2. (*Continued*) Spot tangential (**C**) view of the palpable finding, right breast.

What do you think? What would you do next?

There is dense fibroglandular tissue, and no focal abnormality is apparent on the spot tangential view. Correlative physical examination and an ultrasound are indicated for further evaluation.

On physical examination, a hard, fixed mass is palpated at the 9 o'clock position, 5 cm from the right nipple. On ultrasound, (Fig. 4.2D, E), an irregular mass with a heterogeneous echotexture, indistinct margins, and areas of shadowing and enhancement is imaged corresponding to the palpable finding. This mass measures at least 5 cm. The clinical and sonographic findings are consistent with a malignant process, most likely an invasive ductal carcinoma. A biopsy is indicated.

What else should you do to evaluate this patient further?

For patients in whom we suspect a malignancy, we examine the ipsilateral axilla for potentially abnormal lymph nodes. If any potential abnormality is identified in the axilla, a fine-needle aspiration or a needle biopsy is also done. Patients with metastatic disease to the axilla will undergo a full axillary dissection at the time of the lumpectomy, bypassing the need for a sentinel lymph node biopsy.

In this patient, an oval hypoechoic mass is imaged in the right axilla (Fig. 4.2F). Given the thickening of the cortex and the lack of a hyperechogenic hilar region, this is a potentially abnormal lymph node. Biopsies of the right breast and axillary masses confirm the suspected diagnoses. At the time of her definitive surgery, a grade III invasive ductal carcinoma with extensive lymphovascular space involvement measuring at least 5.7 cm in size is reported histologically. Tumor is also reported in the dermal lymphatics surrounding the right nipple [pT3, pN2, pMX; Stage IIIA].

In patients with palpable findings and normal-appearing dense glandular tissue mammographically, correlative physical examination and an ultrasound are indicated for further evaluation. In this group of patients, ultrasound is an excellent adjunctive tool in evaluating the clinical findings. If our focus is optimal, efficient, and expeditious patient care, then clinical, mammographic, and sonographic evaluations and, when needed, imaging-guided biopsies of the breast and axilla, are done in one visit. With a 24-hour turnaround time on core biopsy results, histology findings are available the following day and the patient is scheduled to see the surgeon for definitive treatment. As clinical breast imagers, we are in a unique position to affect the care our patients receive. Evaluations, which in many communities take weeks, with significant associated anxiety for the patient and her family, can be accomplished accurately in 24 hours. By providing this type of service, we also effectively eliminate the fragmentation of care (and with that the potential for miscommunication) among providers that can result when evaluations are carried out over several weeks (e.g., one radiologist doing the initial mammogram, another doing the ultrasound, and possibly a third doing the biopsies).

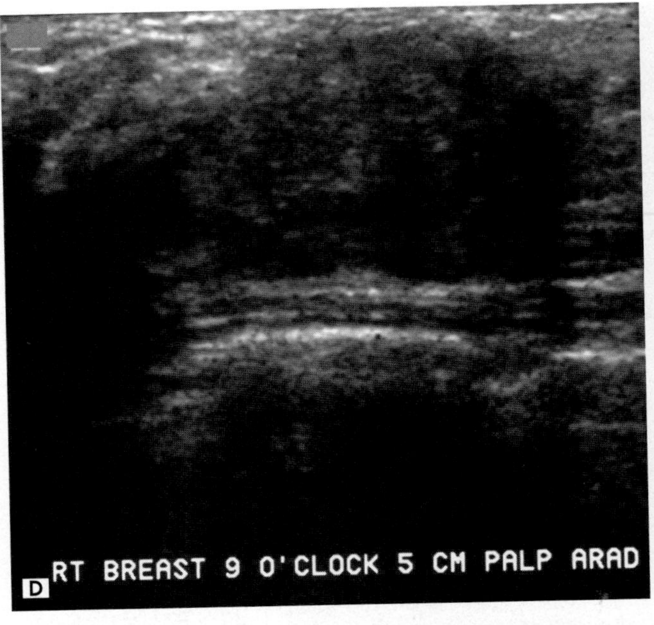

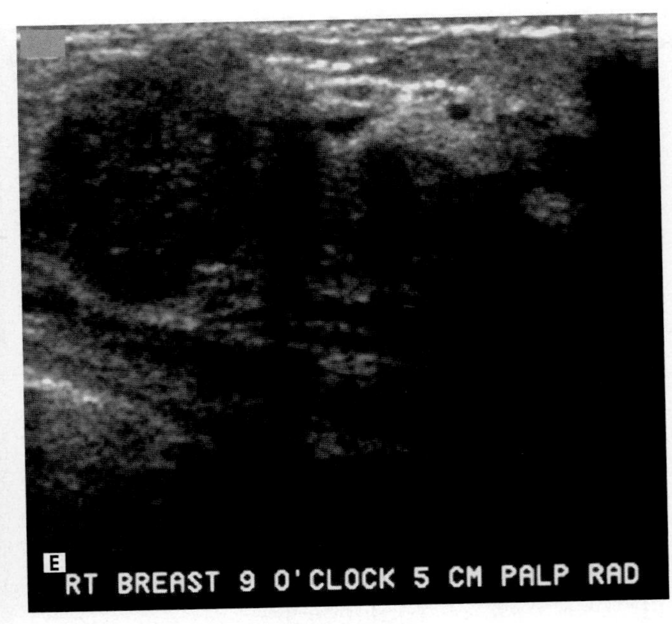

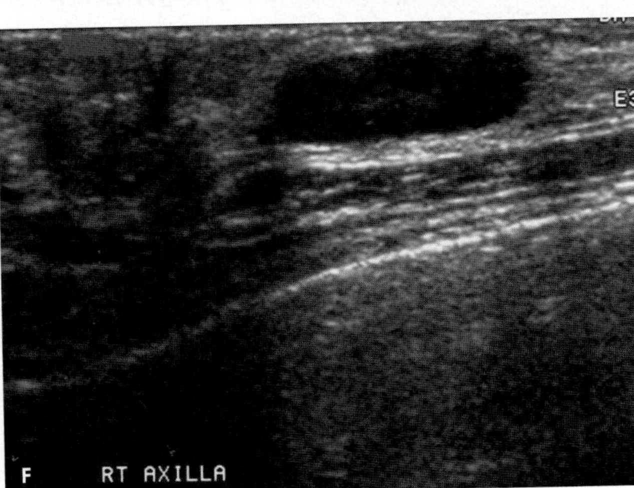

Figure 4.2. Ultrasound images, radial (RAD) **(D)** and antiradial (ARAD) **(E)** projections, corresponding to the area of concern to the patient in the right breast. Ultrasound image **(F),** right axilla.

PATIENT 3

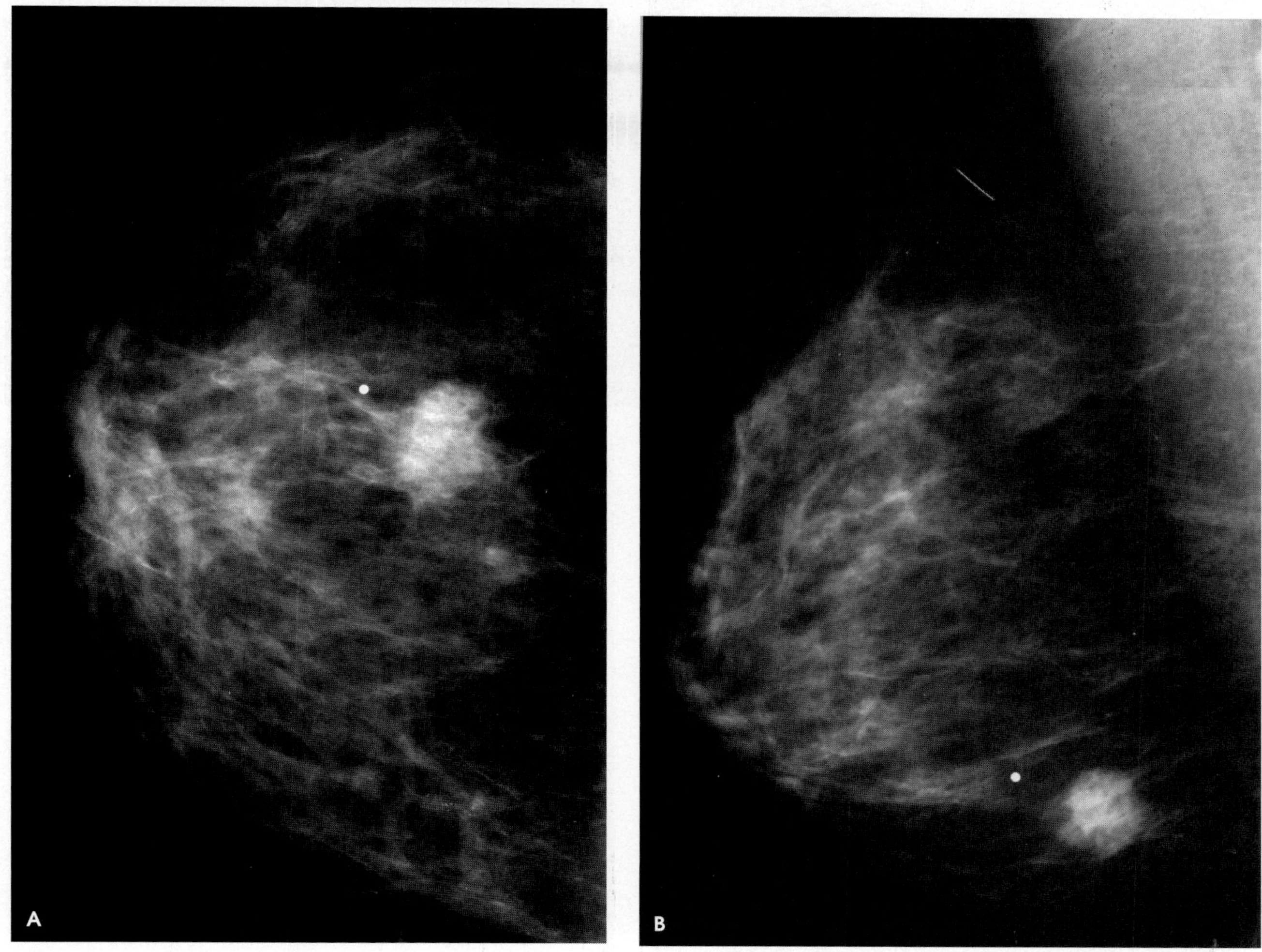

Figure 4.3. Diagnostic evaluation, 38-year-old patient presenting with a palpable mass in the right breast. Craniocaudal **(A)** and mediolateral oblique **(B)** views of the right breast. Metallic BB used to mark "lump" described by the patient.

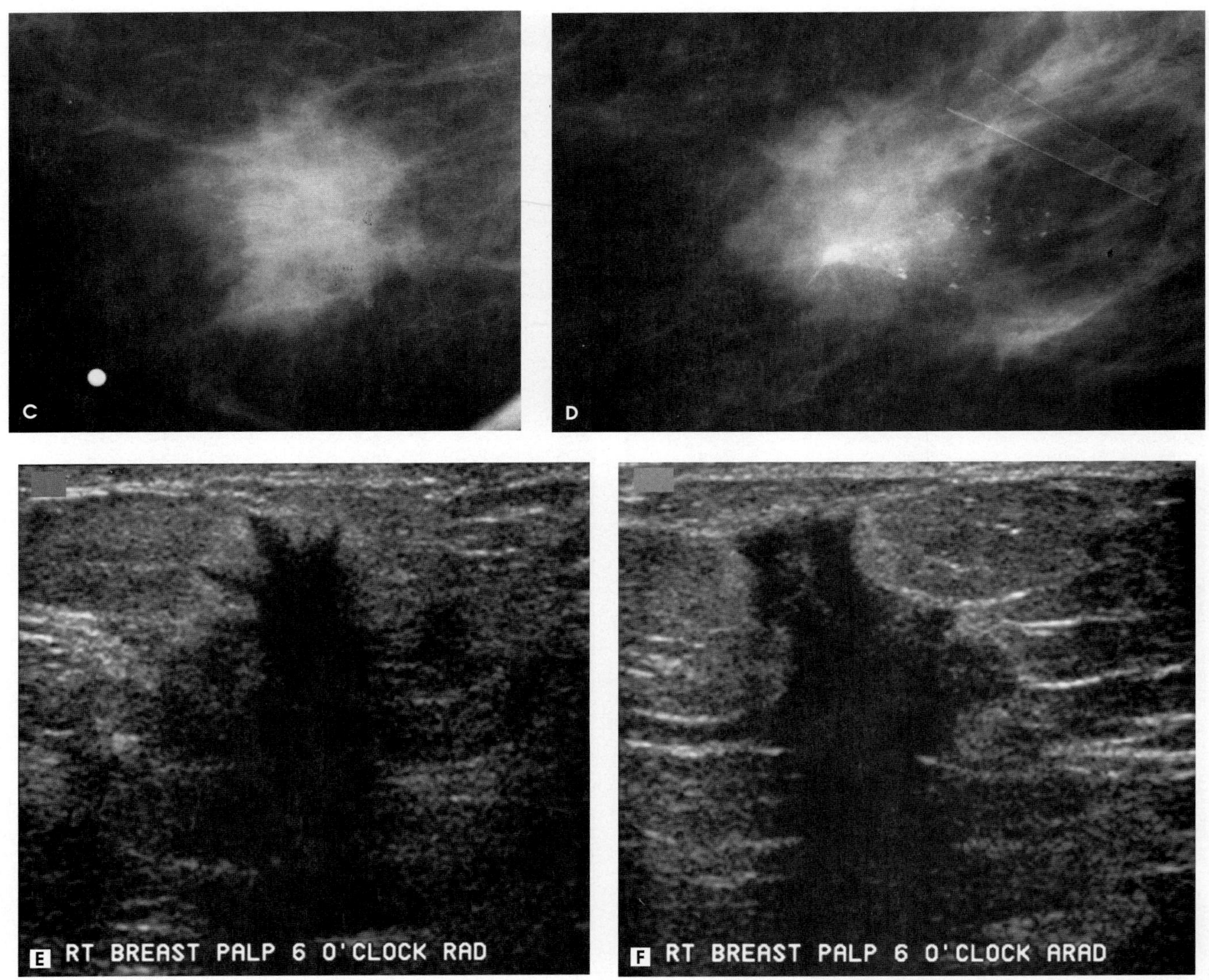

Figure 4.3. (*Continued*) Spot compression views of mass in craniocaudal **(C)** and mediolateral oblique **(D)** views. Ultrasound images in radial (RAD) **(E)** and antiradial (ARAD) **(F)** projections of palpable finding at the 6 o'clock position, approximately 12 cm from the right nipple.

What do you think?

A round, solid, 2-cm mass with spiculated, indistinct, and angular margins and associated shadowing is imaged in the right breast, corresponding to the area of concern to the patient. Although no calcifications are identified associated with the mass on the craniocaudal spot compression view, or on the ultrasound, a cluster of pleomorphic calcifications is evident on the mediolateral oblique spot compression view. Why are these not seen on the spot craniocaudal view? Did you see them on the routine craniocaudal view, or was your eye drawn to the clinical finding? Remember, do not let yourself be distracted by obvious benign or malignant mammographic/clinical findings. Even when you are presented with an obvious finding, make sure to evaluate the remainder of the mammogram and the contralateral side thoroughly.

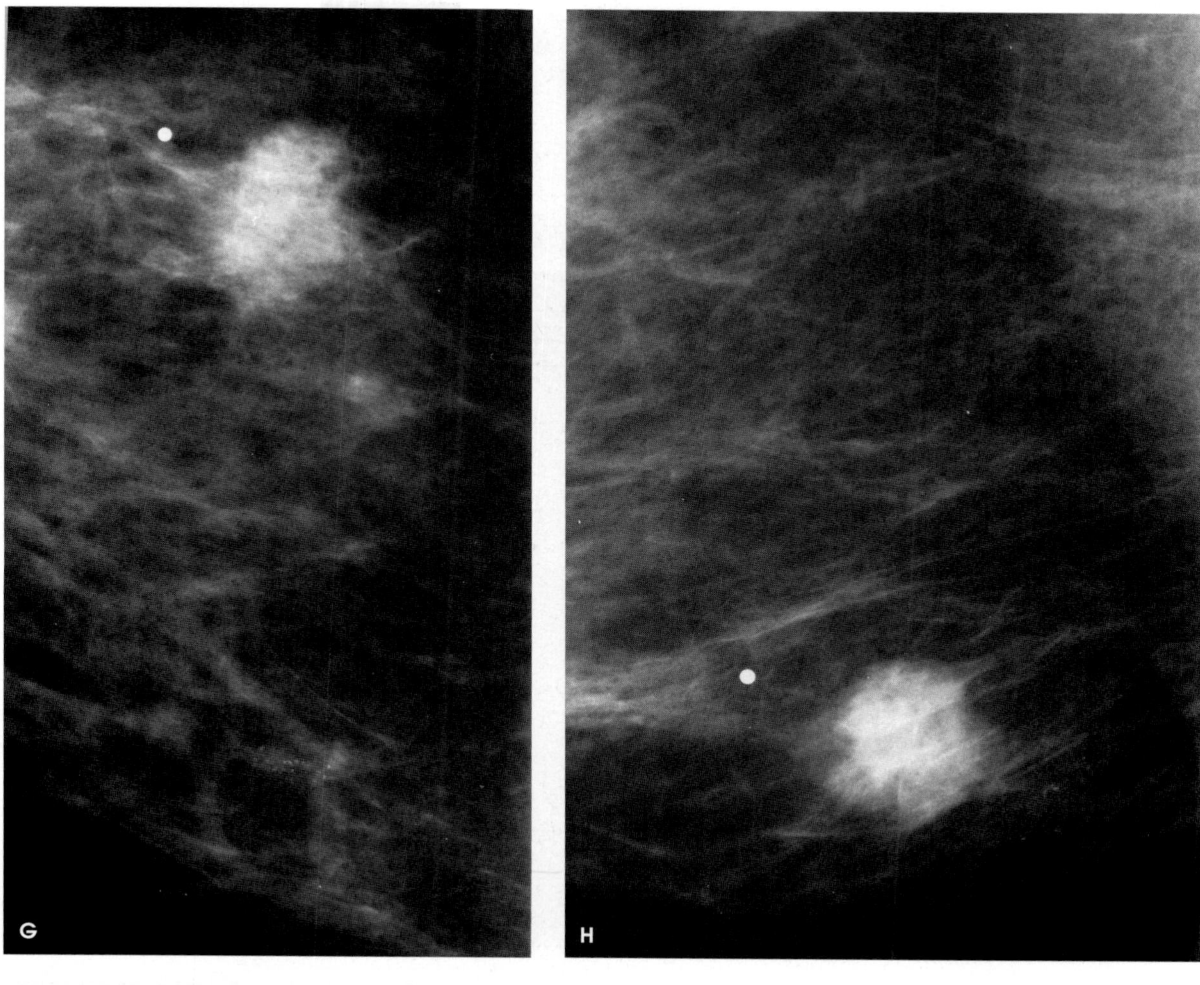

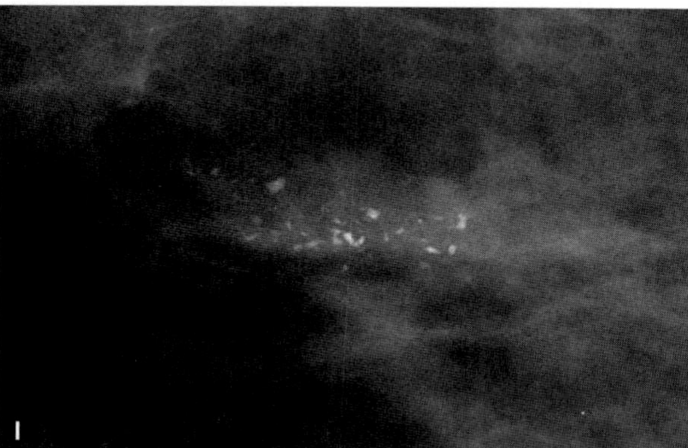

Figure 4.3. (*Continued*) Craniocaudal **(G)** and mediolateral oblique **(H)** views, right breast, photographically coned. Double spot compression magnification **(I)** view, right breast.

What do you think now? What is your recommendation?

The calcifications project on the mass in the mediolateral oblique view, but they are medial in location on the craniocaudal view and at a distance from the mass. On the magnification views, the calcifications are pleomorphic and there are associated linear forms consistent with ductal carcinoma in situ with central necrosis, likely high-nuclear-grade. Biopsies of the mass and calcifications are indicated because if these confirm the suspected diagnoses, this represents multicentric disease and a mastectomy is probably indicated for this patient.

Histologically, a complex ductal carcinoma in situ is diagnosed, corresponding to the cluster of calcifications seen mammographically, and a 2.5-cm, grade III, invasive ductal carcinoma with associated lymphovascular space involvement is described for the mass. Micrometastatic disease is reported in the sentinel lymph node [pT2, pN1mi(sn) (i), pMX, Stage IIB].

Given the incidence of multifocal, multicentric, and bilateral lesions, thorough evaluation of patients who are likely to have a malignancy is critical preoperatively. The mammogram needs to be reviewed carefully. Complete ultrasound evaluations of the breasts and ipsilateral axilla, as well as magnetic resonance imaging, are also helpful in evaluating patients diagnosed with breast cancer. With appropriate imaging protocols, magnetic resonance imaging also makes the evaluation of internal mammary, axillary, supraclavicular, and neck lymph nodes possible for our patients.

PATIENT 4

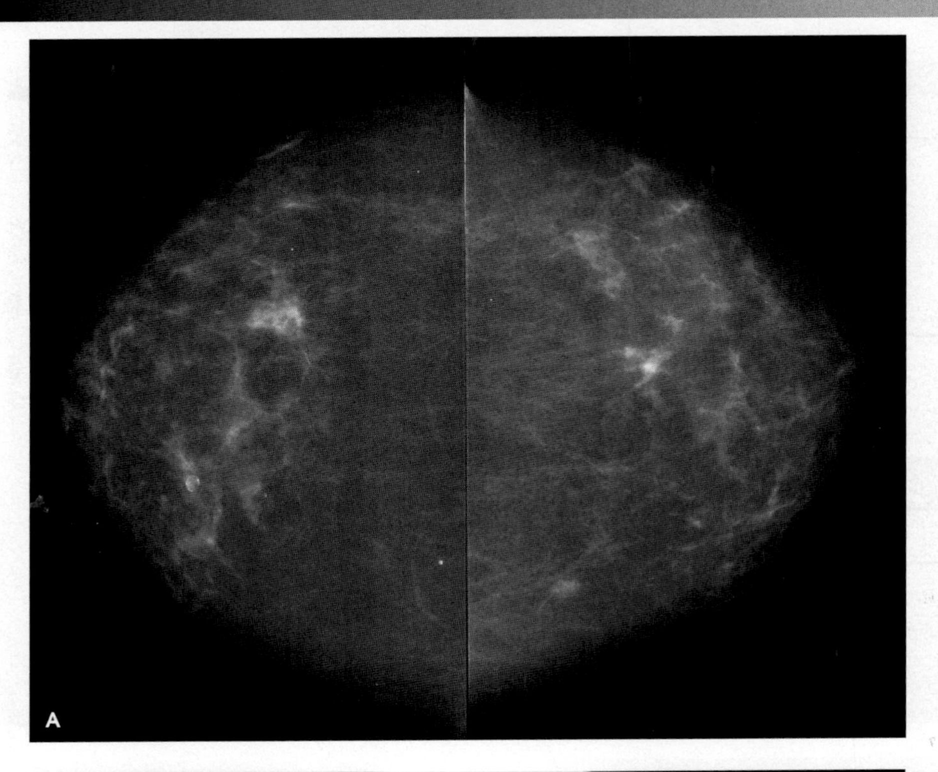

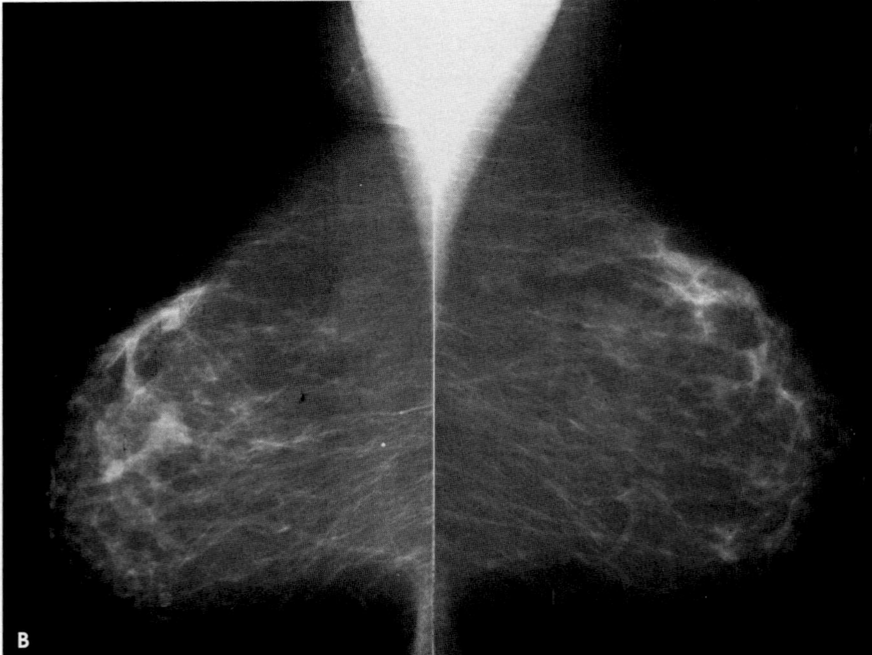

Figure 4.4. Screening study, 57-year-old woman. Craniocaudal **(A)** and mediolateral oblique **(B)** views.

What do you think? Is this a normal study, or is there a potential abnormality?

A lucent-centered, benign-type calcification is present in the right breast medially. In reviewing these images systematically, a potential abnormality is noted medially in the left craniocaudal (CC) view. Based on the expected location of this abnormality on the CC view, a low-density nodule is suspected inferiorly on the left mediolateral oblique view. If they are available, prior films would be helpful in assessing whether this finding is new, stable, or decreasing in size. If prior films are not available or this represents a new or enlarging mass, additional evaluation is indicated.

BI-RADS® category 0: need additional imaging evaluation.

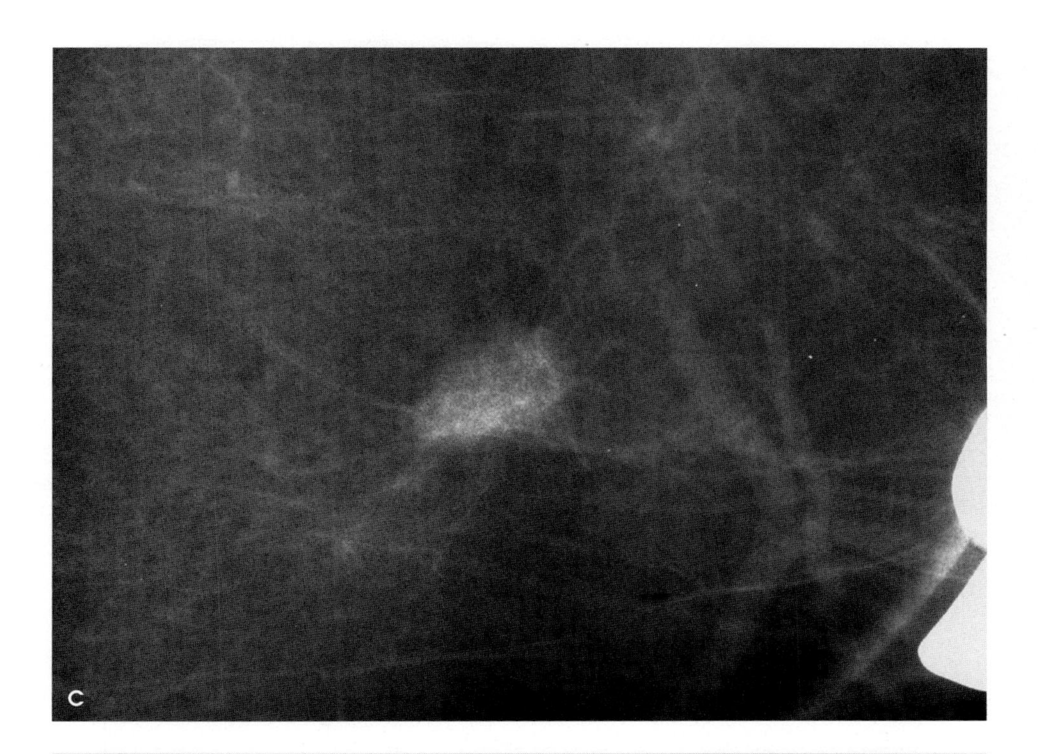

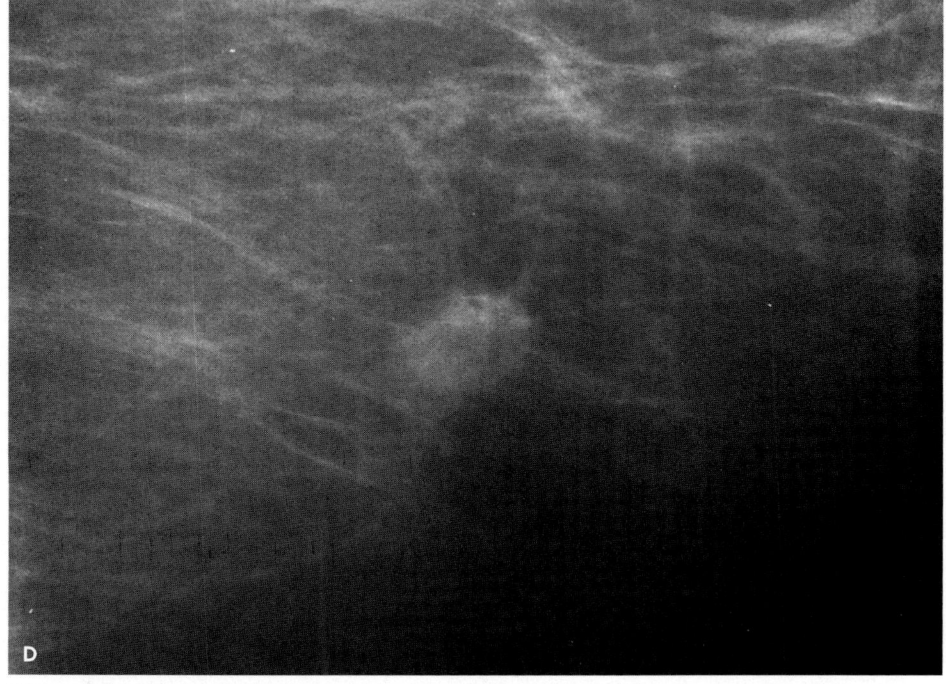

Figure 4.4. (*Continued*) Craniocaudal **(C)** and mediolateral oblique **(D),** spot compression views.

What do you think now, and with what level of certainty can you make a recommendation?

Did you notice the fingerprint superimposed on the mass in the craniocaudal spot compression view? This is a plus-density artifact that reflects improper film handling after the film was exposed but before processing. An oval mass with indistinct and spiculated margins is confirmed on the spot compression views. Based on the mammographic findings, this mass requires biopsy. In planning the biopsy, an ultrasound is done because, if the lesion is identified on ultrasound, ultrasound guidance can be used to do the biopsy. If the mass is not identified sonographically, a stereotactically guided biopsy can be done.

BI-RADS® category 4: suspicious abnormality, biopsy should be considered.

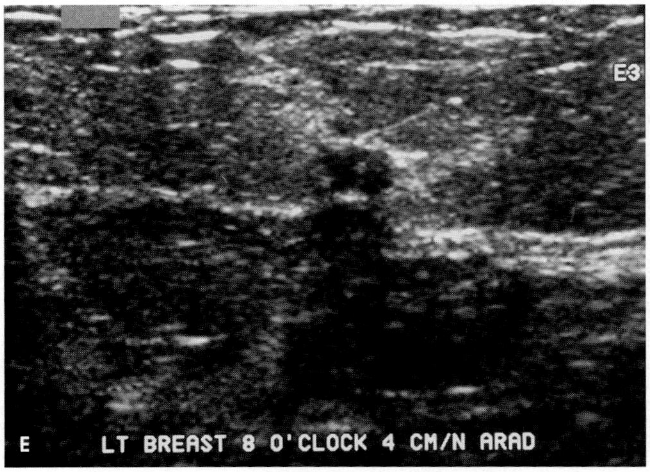

E LT BREAST 8 O'CLOCK 4 CM/N ARAD

E3

Figure 4.4. (*Continued*) Ultrasound image, antiradial (ARAD) projection **(E),** at the eight o'clock position, 4 cm from the left nipple.

Based on the mammographic and sonographic findings, what will you accept as a diagnosis for this mass?

A hypoechoic mass is imaged at the eight o'clock position, 4 cm from the left nipple. Using ultrasound guidance, a biopsy of this mass is done. Fibrocystic changes are reported histologically. What do you think? What would you recommend for this patient? The imaging and pathology findings are not congruent. Given the mammographic features of this mass, the likelihood of malignancy is high and a benign diagnosis on the cores is not acceptable.

In assessing this situation and problem solving in general, it is helpful to go back to basics. The pathologist should be asked if additional sectioning of the cores can be done, because sometimes the lesion is deep in the cores and it is possible that the lesion has not yet been examined histologically. If all available tissue has been sectioned and examined, the mammographic and ultrasound images should be reviewed. Do the images obtained during the biopsy confirm adequate positioning of the needle through the mass? Ideally, orthogonal images of the needle are obtained during the biopsy to document final needle positioning. With small lesions it is particularly important to document that the needle is associated with the mass longitudinally as well as in cross section (Fig. 4.4F [I and III] and Fig. 4.4G, I). There are times when the needle appears to be through the mass longitudinally, but the needle is actually just at the edge of the mass (and not in it) when the needle is imaged in cross section (Fig. 4.4F [II] and Fig. 4.4H). Lastly, you have to ask yourself: Does what is seen sonographically correlate with the mammographic finding?

In this patient, the pathologist has reviewed all available material and the images during the biopsy document adequate needle positioning. What do you think relative to the correlation of the lesion seen mammographically with what is imaged on ultrasound? At what clock position would you expect to find the mammographic finding, and at what distance should this lesion be from the nipple? The lesion is expected at the 8 o'clock position; however, in measuring back from the nipple, this lesion is closer to 8 cm and not 4 cm (Fig. 4.4J–L) from the nipple. When the patient is scanned at the 8 o'clock position, 8 cm from the nipple, a 9-mm spiculated mass with angular margins and associated shadowing is imaged at this site (Fig. 4.4M, N). This corresponds with the mass seen mammographically and its ultrasound features suggesting a malignant process correlate closely with those seen mammographically. Ultrasound guidance is used preoperatively to localize the mass at the 8 o'clock position, 8 cm from the left nipple (Fig. 4.4O). A 0.8-cm, well-differentiated invasive ductal carcinoma not otherwise specified is reported following the lumpectomy. No metastatic disease is identified in two excised sentinel lymph nodes [pT1b, pN0, pMX; Stage I].

Correlation is critically important. For clinical findings, does what is seen mammographically correlate with what the patient or the clinician is describing? In this situation, talking directly to the patient while doing a physical examination and the ultrasound study can provide the needed correlation. Specifically, ask the patient to show you the location of what she is feeling. For mammographic findings, is what is seen on the ultrasound the same thing as what is on the mammogram? If I am doing an ultrasound for a mammographic finding, I walk into the ultrasound room with an expected clock position in mind and an estimated distance from the nipple. This is my starting point for the physical examination and where I place the transducer. After I have evaluated this area fully, I scan the remainder of the quadrant or the breast as needed. For findings on magnetic resonance imaging (MRI), is what is seen on the ultrasound the same thing as what is on the MRI? Knowing slice thickness, the distance of the lesion with respect to the nipple can be estimated and used as the starting point for the ultrasound study. If an imaging-guided biopsy is done, are the imaging and histologic findings congruent? If they are not congruent, is the problem with the imaging or is there a possibility the lesion has not been evaluated histologically (i.e., has all tissue been sectioned?)?

Lastly, following excisional biopsies, is there correlation between clinical and imaging findings and the reported histology? Specimen radiography is used to confirm that a clinically occult, preoperatively (wire) localized lesion is excised and the location of the lesion in the specimen is marked for the pathologist, thereby assuring that the lesion is examined. However, for patients in whom preoperative localization and specimen radiography are not done, we have had situations in which a solid, water-density mass is reportedly excised based on palpable findings and a lipoma or other noncongruent lesion is reported histologically. In this situation either the lesion was not excised or the pathologist did not evaluate the lesion of interest in the specimen. In these patients, repeating the mammogram is helpful in determining whether the lesion of interest has been excised.

If we are methodical in our approach and provide the needed correlation at every step of the process, the clinical breast imager is a critical factor in optimizing patient care. We are in a unique position to provide the needed correlation among clinical, imaging, and histologic findings.

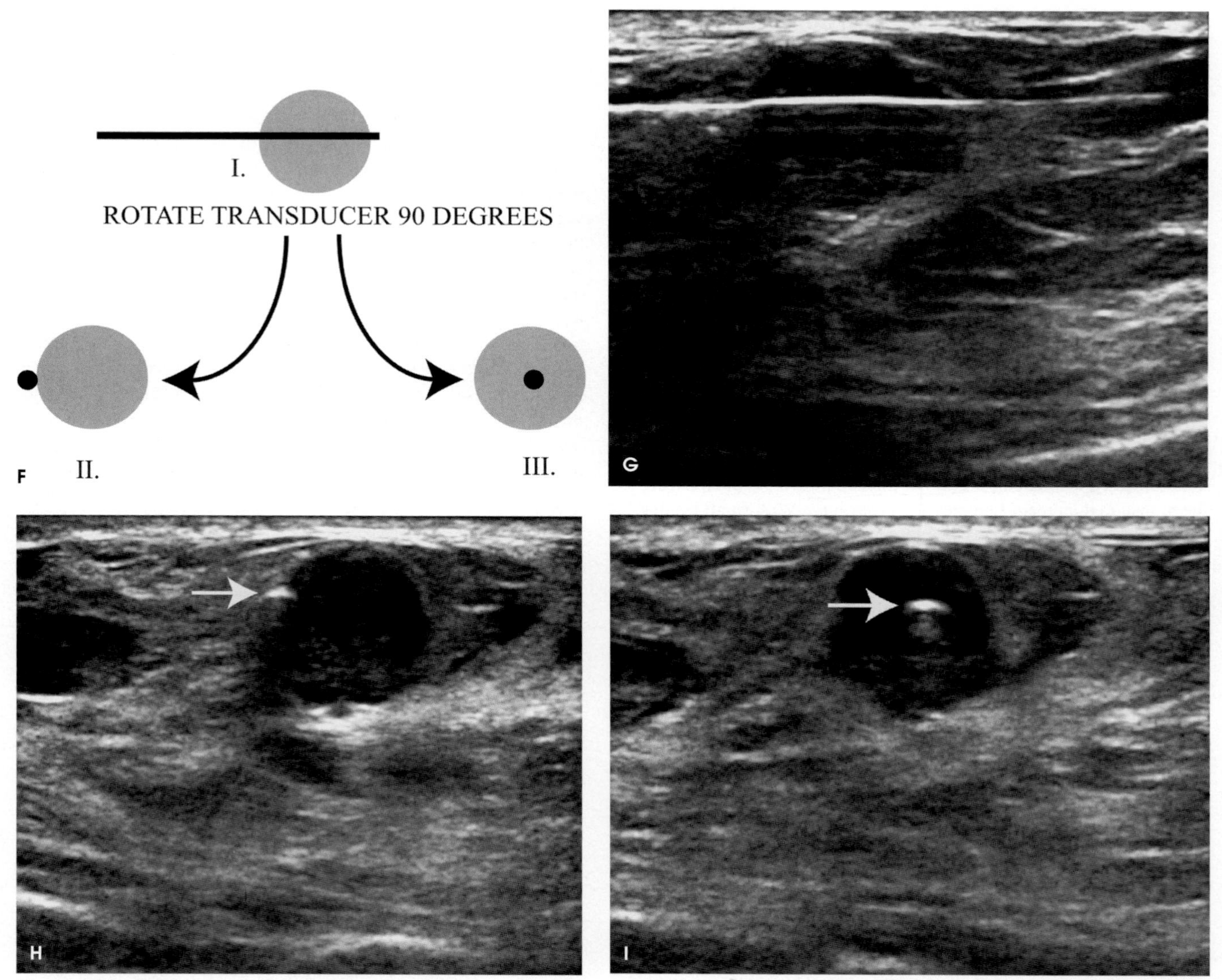

Figure 4.4. (*Continued*) Diagram **(F)** illustrating orthogonal images of needle positioning. Obtaining orthogonal images to document final needle positioning is particularly critical when sampling small lesions. The needle may appear to be through the lesion (I); however, on the orthogonal image, the needle is along the edge of the mass (II). Ideally, the needle is surrounded by the lesion on the orthogonal (III) image. Ultrasound images in a different patient demonstrating the needle through the lesion **(G)** longitudinally. When the transducer is rotated for the orthogonal image **(H),** the needle is seen at the edge of the mass (*arrow*) and not through it. Ideally, when the transducer is rotated for the orthogonal image **(I),** the needle is seen within the mass (*arrow*).

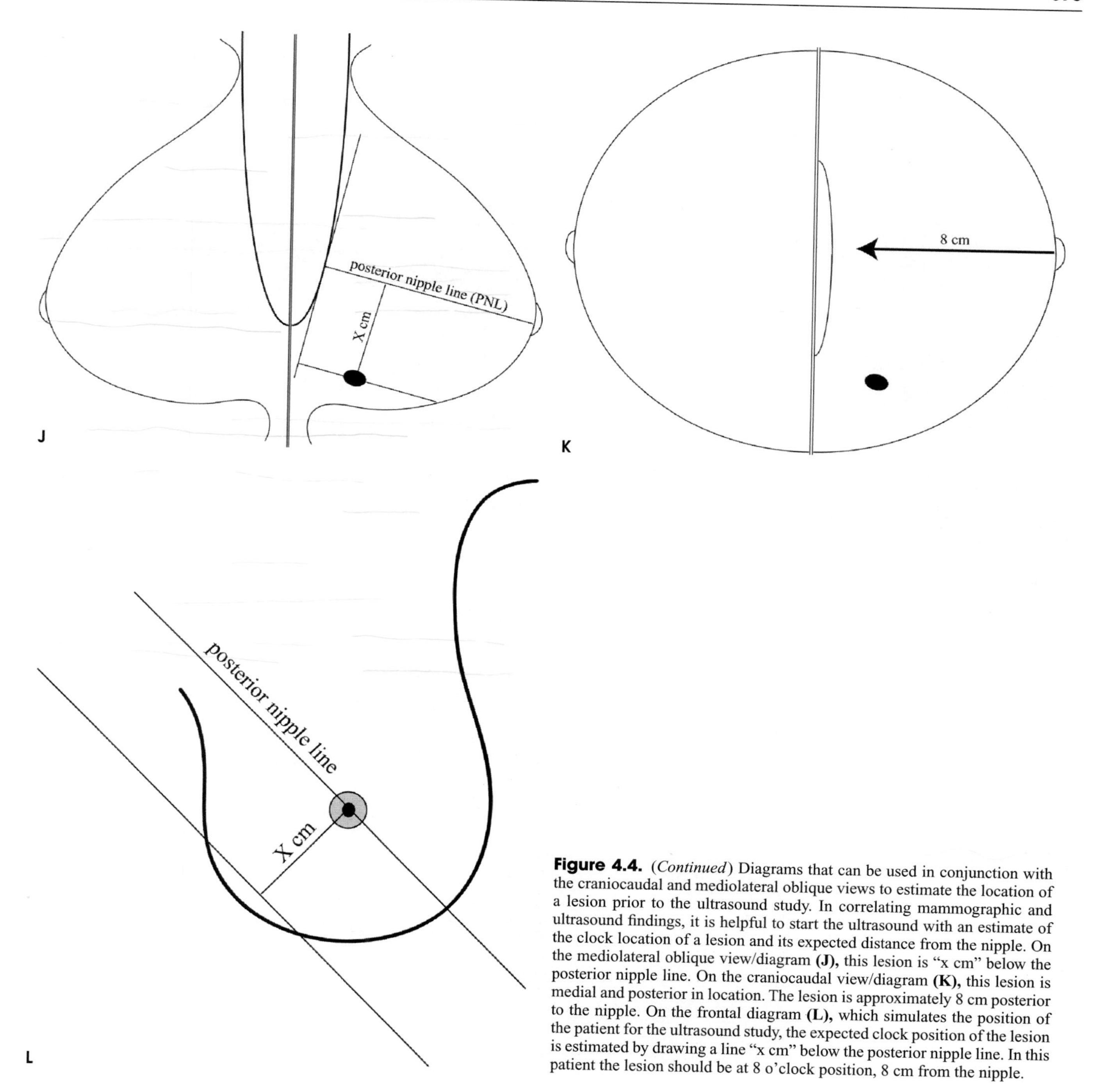

Figure 4.4. (*Continued*) Diagrams that can be used in conjunction with the craniocaudal and mediolateral oblique views to estimate the location of a lesion prior to the ultrasound study. In correlating mammographic and ultrasound findings, it is helpful to start the ultrasound with an estimate of the clock location of a lesion and its expected distance from the nipple. On the mediolateral oblique view/diagram **(J),** this lesion is "x cm" below the posterior nipple line. On the craniocaudal view/diagram **(K),** this lesion is medial and posterior in location. The lesion is approximately 8 cm posterior to the nipple. On the frontal diagram **(L),** which simulates the position of the patient for the ultrasound study, the expected clock position of the lesion is estimated by drawing a line "x cm" below the posterior nipple line. In this patient the lesion should be at 8 o'clock position, 8 cm from the nipple.

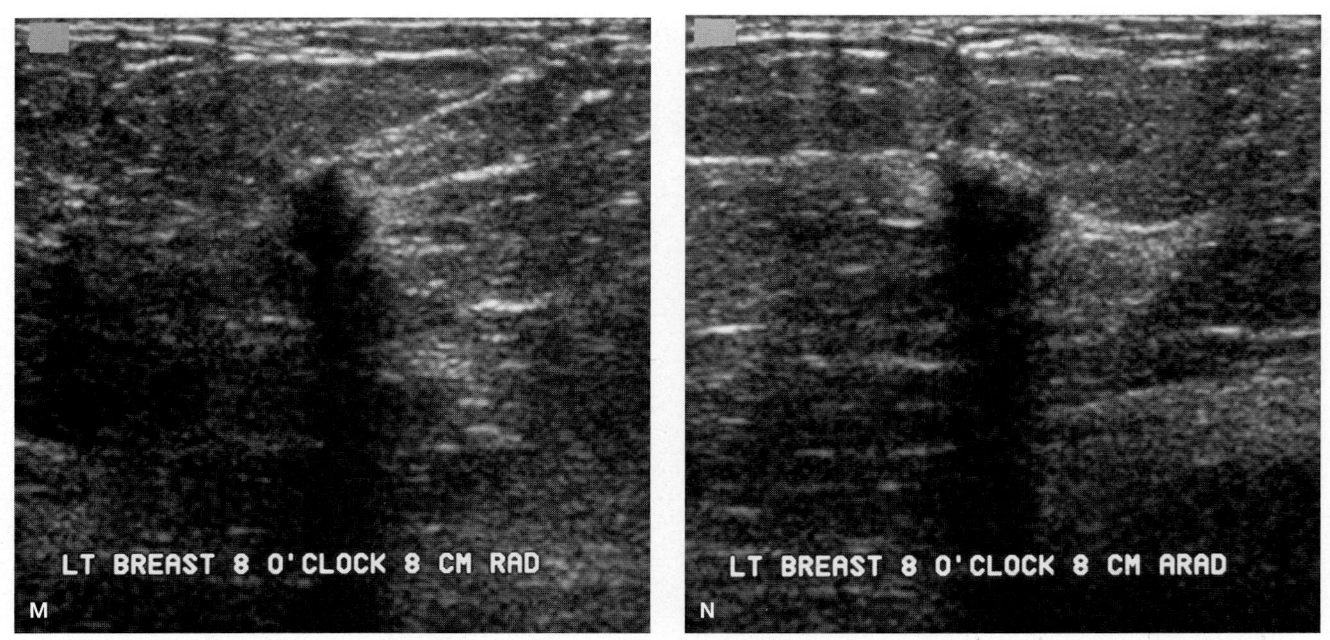

Figure 4.4. (*Continued*) Ultrasound images, radial (RAD) **(M)** and antiradial (ARAD) **(N)** projections obtained at the 8 o'clock position, 8 cm from the left nipple, confirm the location of a mass that corresponds with the mammographic finding. Its sonographic features more closely resemble those of the mass seen mammographically.

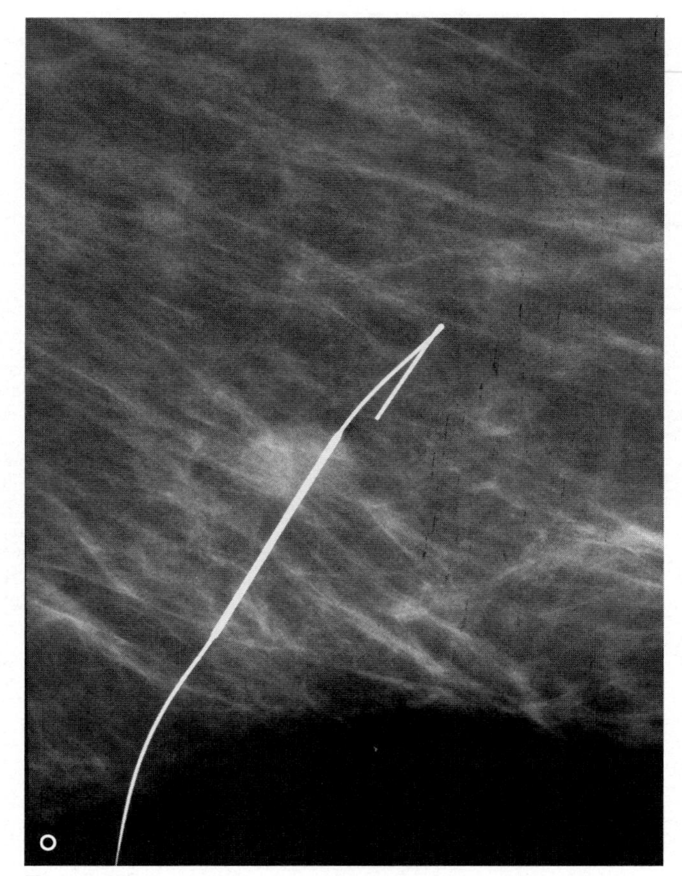

Figure 4.4. (*Continued*) Single mammographic view **(O)** obtained following an ultrasound-guided wire localization of the lesion at the 8 o'clock position, 8 cm from the left nipple. The localization wire is through the mass.

PATIENT 5

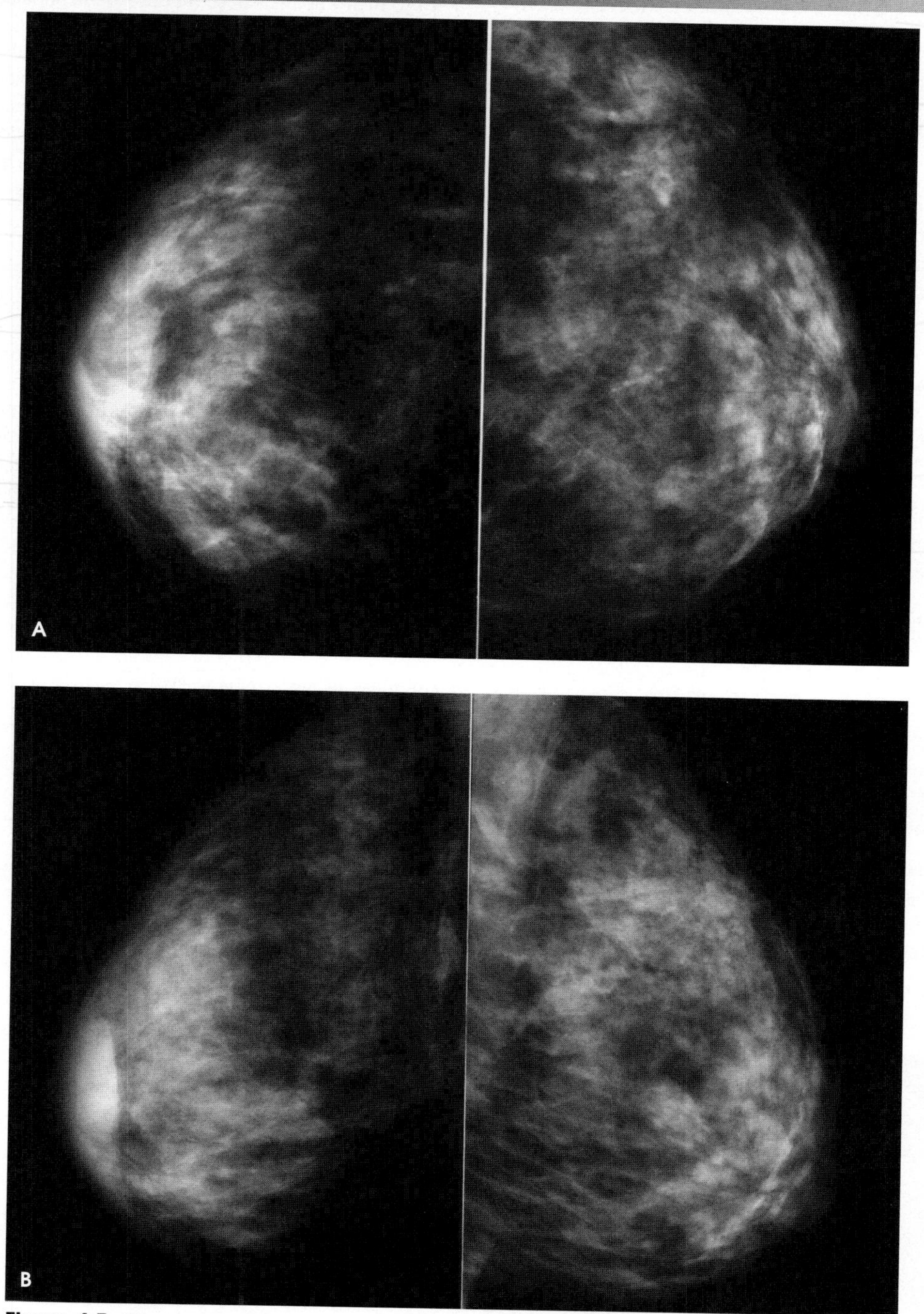

Figure 4.5. Diagnostic evaluation in 43-year-old patient presenting with a tender "lump" in the right subareolar area. Craniocaudal **(A)** and mediolateral oblique **(B)** views.

What are your observations?

There is increased density in the right subareolar area corresponding to the site of concern to the patient. In looking at the technical factors, the right breast is less compressible and a higher kilovoltage and milliamperage were needed for exposure when compared with the left breast. Physical examination and an ultrasound are indicated for further evaluation.

On physical examination, erythema and *peau d'orange* changes are noted in the periareolar area. Significant tenderness is elicited with gentle compression. A mass is palpated in the right subareolar area. Sonographically, a mass with posterior acoustic enhancement is imaged in the subareolar area, corresponding to the palpable finding (Fig. 4.5C). Based on the clinical presentation and the imaging findings, an ongoing inflammatory process is suspected. The patient is started on antibiotics.

The patient returns within 72 hours, describing progressive symptoms and purulent fluid draining from the periareolar area. On physical examination, erythema and *peau d'orange* changes are again noted, but these are now much more extensive and there is now a protuberant mass extending into the upper inner quadrant of the right breast. The overlying skin is thinned and there is a fistula draining purulent fluid at the areolar margin at the 1 o'clock position (Fig. 4.5D). On ultrasound, the abscess has increased in size (Fig. 4.5E). Given the rapid progression of symptoms, the formation of a fistula, and the subareolar location of this abscess, the patient is transferred to the hospital for consultation and surgical drainage.

When considering mastitis and abscess formation, what groups of patients should you consider?

Three different patient populations can be considered relative to mastitis and breast abscess formation. Most commonly, we associate these inflammatory conditions with women who are breastfeeding: This is *puerperal mastitis.* Reportedly, mastitis occurs in approximately 2.5% of women who breastfeed, and abscess formation affects <1 in 15 of all women who breastfeed. In this patient population, *Staphylococcus aureus* is the most common causative agent. Patients with mastitis alone are usually treated effectively with antibiotics. If an abscess develops, percutaneous drainage can be helpful, and surgical drainage may be required for some patients. These patients are usually treated by their obstetricians and are not usually referred for imaging.

The second group of patients to consider in terms of breast infections is those with recurring *subareolar abscess formation* unrelated to nipple piercing or nipple rings. These patients are nonlactating, premenopausal women, most with a history of heavy smoking. As seen in this patient, many of these patients develop periareolar fistulas spontaneously *(Zuska's disease)*. Squamous metaplasia involving the subareolar ducts is seen histologically in these patients, and it is postulated that this process leads to obstruction of the ducts, with inspissation of secretions, duct wall erosion, and the development of periductal mastitis and abscess formation. Antibiotic therapy alone is not usually effective in these patients. Although some have advocated percutaneous drainage, this also is not always effective, and wide surgical excision is required. Even in the patients who undergo surgical drainage, however, there is a high incidence of recurrence. With recurrent episodes, the nipple begins to flatten and some patients develop horizontal inversion centrally in the nipple (Fig. 4.5F, G). Bilateral abscess formation is seen in as many as a quarter of these patients, either simultaneously or at different times. A mixture of aerobic and anaerobic organisms is often cultured in these patients. It has been reported that these patients have a higher incidence of acne, hidradenitis suppurativa, and perineal inclusion cysts.

Lastly, *peripheral mastitis or abscess formation can be seen unrelated to pregnancy and lactation.* Rarely, some of these patients are diabetic; most of the women in this group, however, are otherwise healthy, with no identifiable source of infection. These patients respond well to antibiotic therapy and infection usually does not recur. They are also unlikely to present with bilateral findings.

Figure 4.5. *(Continued)* Ultrasound image **(C)** of the right subareolar area at the site of the palpable finding.

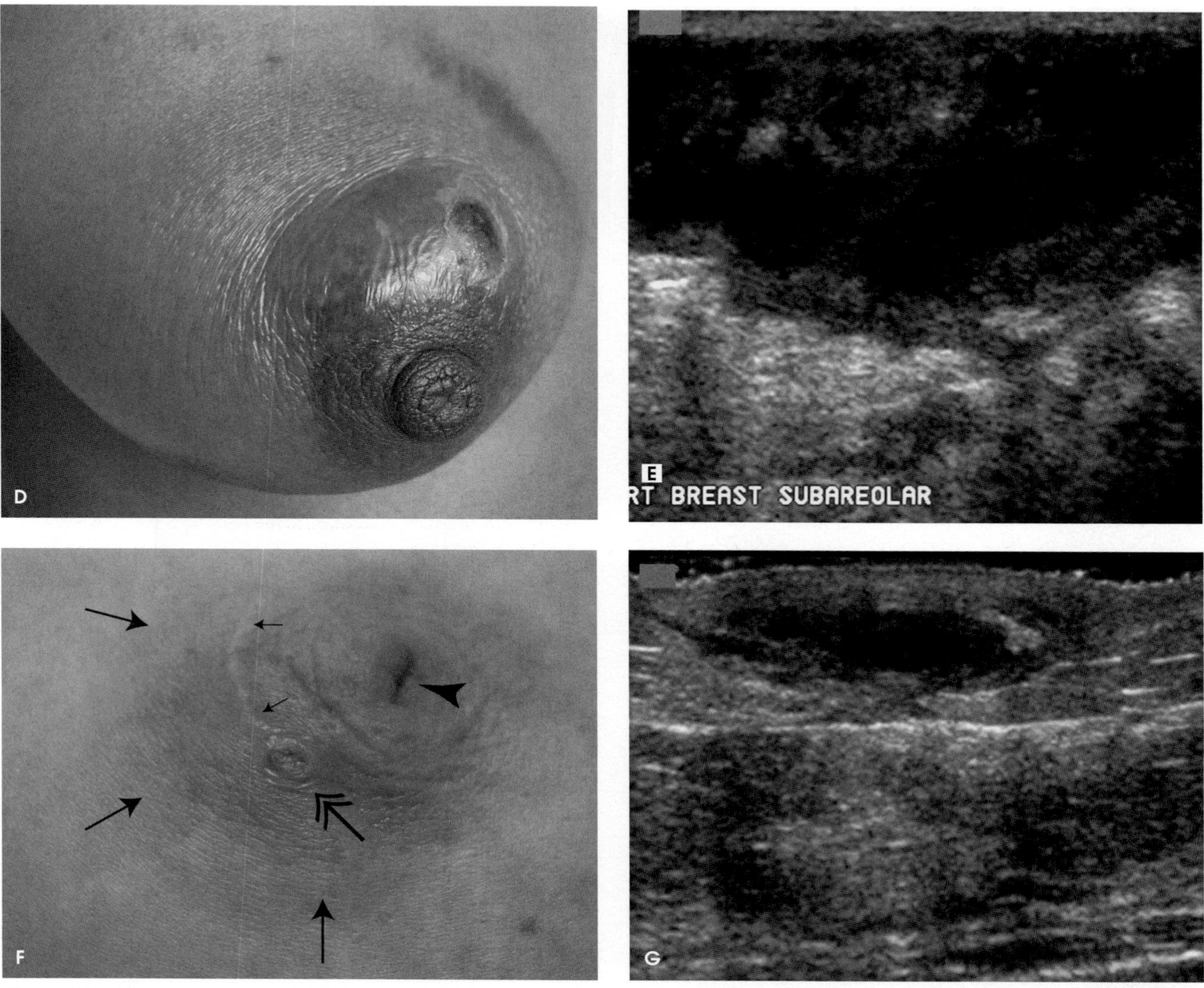

Figure 4.5. (*Continued*) Photograph of the breast **(D)** and ultrasound image **(E)** of the right subareolar area, 72 hours following **(C).** Second patient presenting with a tender mass in the right subareolar area. On physical examination **(F),** there is erythema (*long arrows*) in the periareolar region laterally. Other pertinent observations include a periareolar scar (*small arrows*) and a healed fistula (*double-headed arrow*). This patient has had multiple recurrent episodes of subareolar abscess formation with prior surgery and fistula formation. Also note the horizontal inversion (*arrowhead*) of the nipple. It is postulated that this type of nipple inversion is a reflection of periductal fibrosis resulting from recurrent episodes of inflammation. In this patient, the ultrasound examination **(G)** demonstrates a lenticular-shaped complex cystic mass in the subcutaneous tissues of the subareolar area (as though dissecting through the subcutaneous tissues), a common ultrasound appearance of early subareolar abscess formation.

PATIENT 6

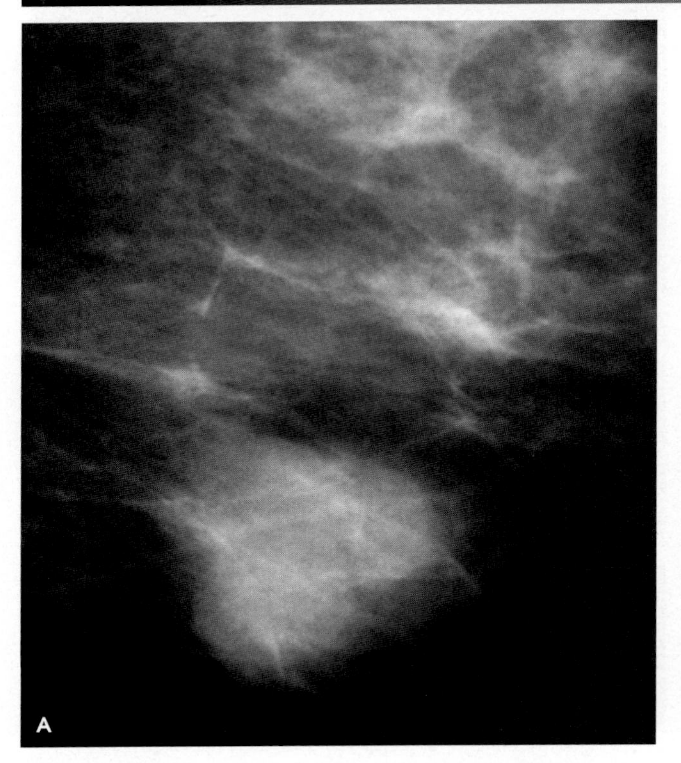

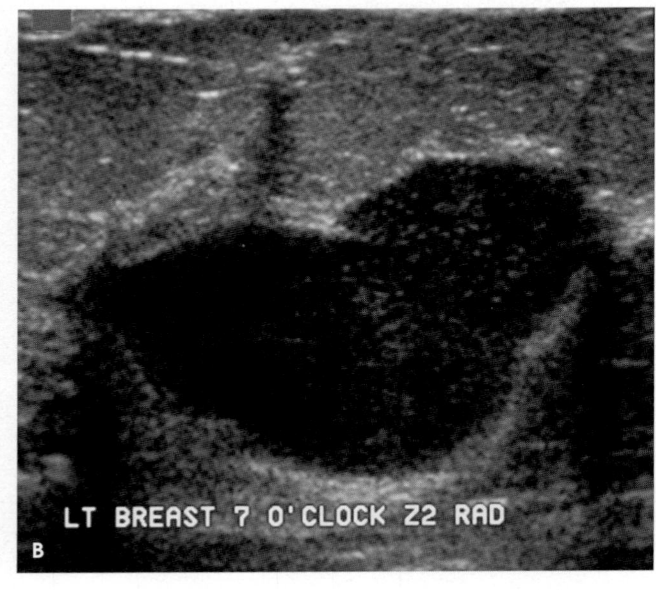

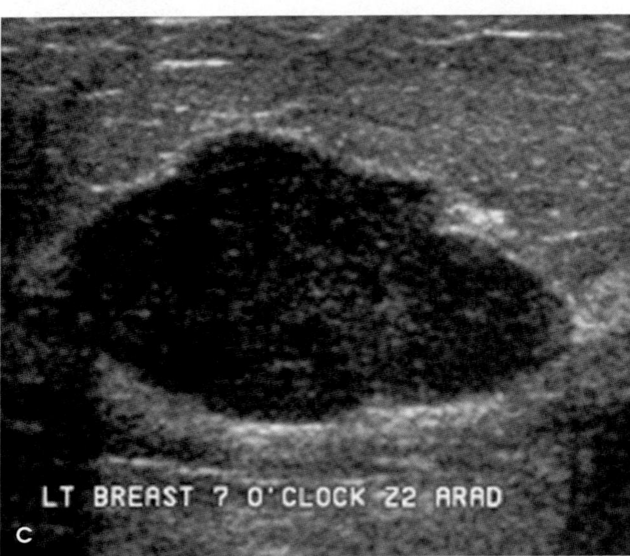

Figure 4.6. Diagnostic evaluation, 54-year-old woman called back for a mass in the left breast detected on her screening study. Left mediolateral oblique **(A),** photographically coned view. Ultrasound images, radial (RAD) **(B)** and antiradial (ARAD) **(C)** projections corresponding to the area of the mammographic abnormality at the 7 o'clock position, zone 2 (Z2).

How would you describe the imaging findings?

A 2-cm, macrolobulated mass, with partially well circumscribed and indistinct margins, is seen mammographically. On ultrasound, a well-circumscribed, irregular mass with posterior acoustic enhancement is imaged at the 7 o'clock position, zone 2 (Z2), corresponding to the mammographic finding. Although a cyst is suspected, the presence of internal echoes and the irregular shape of this mass are such that this cannot be called a simple cyst. A cyst aspiration is undertaken. In discussing this with the patient, I tell her that if I do not obtain fluid, or if there is a residual abnormality postaspiration, I will do a needle biopsy and obtain tissue for histologic evaluation.

After establishing an approach that allows me to advance the needle parallel to the transducer, I clean the skin and use lidocaine to anesthetize the skin. Then, using ultrasound guidance, I inject lidocaine into the tissue leading up to, but taking care to not go into, the lesion. I use ultrasound guidance for administering the anesthesia and for doing the aspiration, even in those patients in whom the mass is palpable. Commonly, the advancing needle displaces the mass, or indents the wall, but does not penetrate into the mass

(I think this explains many of the patients who present for evaluation of a palpable mass following attempted aspirations that yielded no fluid and yet we find a cyst corresponding to the palpable finding). By visualizing the trajectory of the advancing needle, I can gauge the amount of compression I need to apply to effectively immobilize the mass and the amount of controlled pressure I need to exert with the needle so that the cyst wall is punctured. Once the needle is in the mass, I pull the stylet out of the 20G spinal needle, attach a 10-mL syringe, and aspirate. I watch on real-time ultrasound as I aspirate to be sure there is no residual abnormality postaspiration. Also, in some patients, the needle may need to be redirected (i.e., the tip of the needle put against the cyst wall) during the aspiration to be sure that all of the fluid is aspirated. If I do not obtain fluid, I may try using an 18G spinal needle, and if I still do not obtain fluid, or if there is a residual abnormality postaspiration, I proceed with core biopsies using the 14G needle.

In this patient, 8 mL of greenish fluid is aspirated and no residual abnormality is seen following the aspiration. At this point, I inject 4 mL of air (50% of the aspirated fluid volume) into the cyst cavity, because it has been suggested that by doing this we can lower the incidence of cyst recurrence. The air does not hurt the patient, and if it is helpful in minimizing the likelihood of a recurrence, it can be beneficial to the patient. If I am concerned about the presence of a mural or intracystic abnormality, spot compression magnification views of the mass are done following the injection of air in the cyst (i.e., a pneumocystogram) to further evaluate the wall of the cyst.

As a routine, I discard aspirated fluid. Intracystic carcinomas are rare (0.5% of all carcinomas and <0.1% of cysts), and even when an intracystic carcinoma is present, negative cytology is obtained in more than half of patients. I submit fluid for cytology if I obtain bloody fluid following an atraumatic tap, if there is a residual abnormality postaspiration, or if requested by the patient. It has also been recommended that fluid be submitted for cytology when a repeat aspiration is done in a patient who presents with rapid reaccumulation of fluid. As mentioned previously, in addition to submitting aspirated fluid for cytology, when a residual abnormality is seen postaspiration, I do core biopsies through the residual lesion.

Cysts have a variable mammographic appearance. They are usually round or oval masses with marginal characteristics that range from well circumscribed to obscured, to indistinct (particularly when inflamed). Mural and intracystic calcifications (milk of calcium) may be present. On ultrasound, simple cysts are well-circumscribed, anechoic masses with posterior acoustic enhancement and thin edge shadows. Less common appearances include the presence of intracystic echoes that during real time are characterized by movement (e.g., "gurgling"), and persistent, nonmovable echoes that sometimes have an S-shaped (yin-yang sign) interface with the more anechoic portion of the cyst. If the cyst is small and deep in the breast, posterior acoustic enhancement may not be apparent.

PATIENT 7

What would you do to evaluate this patient? When would you obtain a mammogram for a 20-year-old woman?

Correlative physical examination and an ultrasound are our starting point in evaluating focal signs and symptoms in women under the age of 30 years or those who present during pregnancy or lactation regardless of age. A full mammogram is done only if breast cancer is suspected based on the clinical and ultrasound findings.

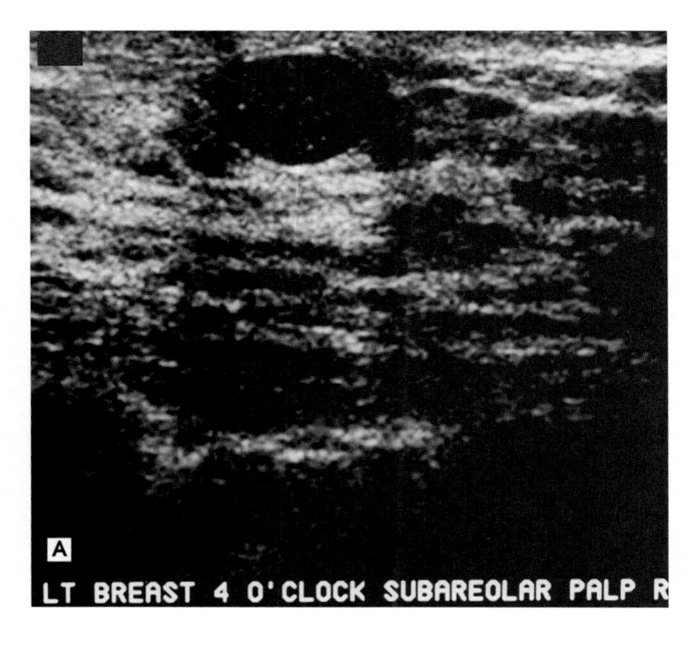

Figure 4.7. Diagnostic evaluation, 20-year-old patient presenting with a "lump" in the left breast. Ultrasound image **(A)** in the radial projection of the palpable finding at the 4 o'clock position, left subareolar area.

How would you describe the finding, and what is your differential? What would you recommend next?

An oval, well-circumscribed complex cystic mass with posterior acoustic enhancement is imaged corresponding to the palpable finding. Although the appearance is somewhat atypical for a cyst, this is the main diagnostic consideration. Alternative possibilities include a fibroadenoma, papilloma, and pseudoangiomatous stromal hyperplasia. A galactocele, abscess, or posttraumatic or postsurgical fluid collection would be considerations in the appropriate clinical context. Although a cyst with atypical features is suspected, aspiration is undertaken.

The preaspiration image documents needle placement in the mass (Fig. 4.7B). A little less than 1 mL of serous fluid is aspirated. No residual abnormality is seen postaspiration (Fig. 4.7C). On ultrasound, simple cysts are described as anechoic, well-circumscribed masses with posterior acoustic enhancement and thin edge shadows. In some patients, however, cysts can be seen with internal echoes that shift in position as you image them in real time (i.e., gurgling cysts), persistent echoes that form an abrupt linear or S-shaped (yin-yang sign) interface with the cystic component of the mass, or high spicular echoes that do not shift in position. Gurgling cysts do not require aspiration unless the patient is symptomatic. Depending on your level of concern, relative to the latter two types of cysts, aspirations are not absolutely indicated.

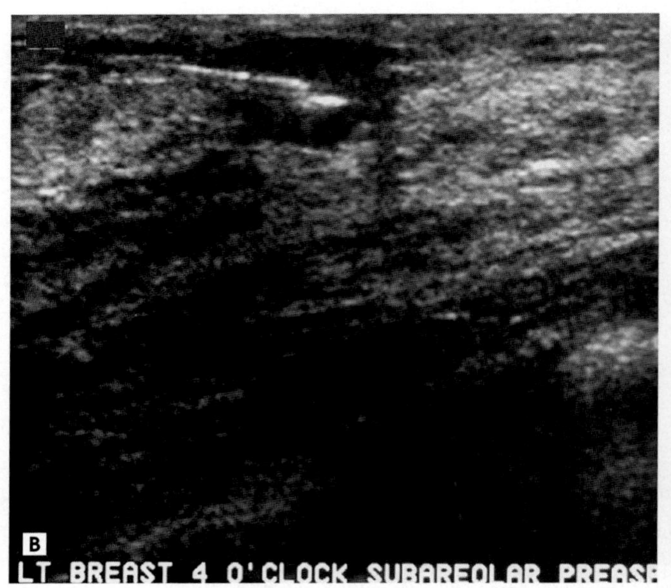

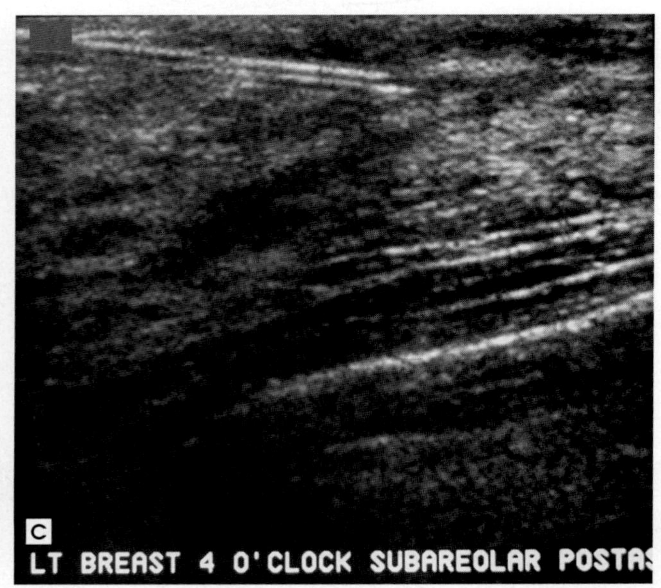

Figure 4.7. (*Continued*) Ultrasound images obtained during the ultrasound-guided aspiration. Preaspiration **(B)** image, documenting preaspiration needle positioning in the cyst, and postaspiration **(C)** image, demonstrating that there is no residual abnormality.

PATIENT 8

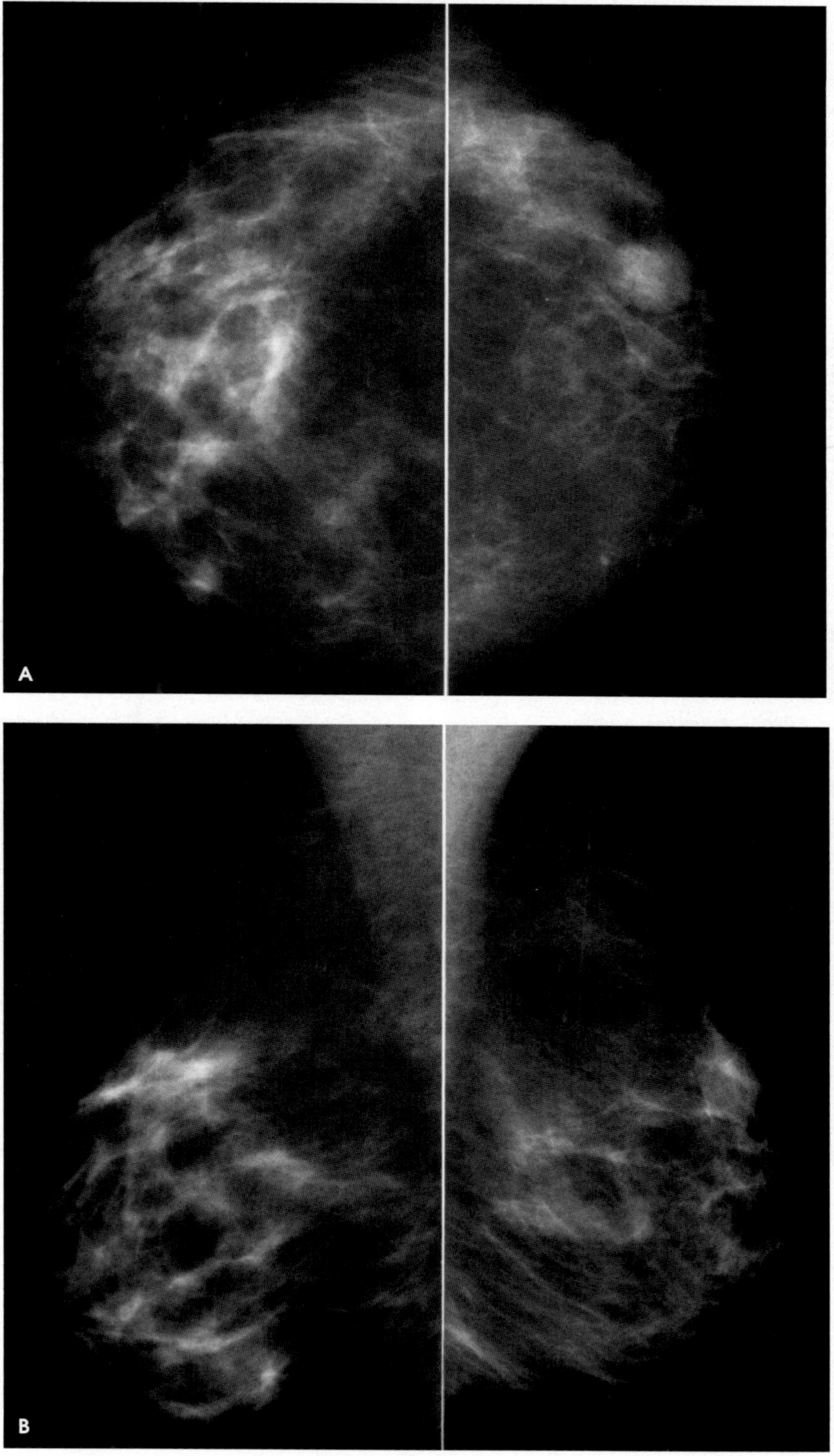

Figure 4.8. Screening study, 47-year-old woman. Craniocaudal **(A)** and mediolateral oblique **(B)** views. No prior films are available.

What do you think?

A round mass is present in the upper outer quadrant of the left breast. The patient is called back for additional evaluation, which includes spot compression views and an ultrasound. Differential considerations at this point include cyst, fibroadenoma (complex fibroadenoma, tubular adenoma), phyllodes, papilloma, pseudoangiomatous stromal hyperplasia, adenosis tumor, and focal fibrosis. Depending on the clinical context, sebaceous cyst, galactocele, postoperative or traumatic fluid collection, and an abscess are also in the differential. Given the seemingly circumscribed margins, malignancy is less likely; however, invasive ductal carcinoma not otherwise specified, medullary, mucinous, or papillary carcinoma, or metastatic disease, particularly if the patient has a known malignancy, are additional considerations.

Spot compression views (not shown) demonstrate a well-circumscribed mass with no associated calcifications. On ultrasound, a well-circumscribed, anechoic mass with posterior acoustic enhancement is imaged, consistent with a simple cyst. In an asymptomatic patient, this requires no additional intervention or short-interval follow-up. The patient is reassured that what we are seeing is not cancer, that cysts do not turn into cancer, and that they are common, with many women developing them at various times.

BI-RADS® category 2: benign finding. Annual screening mammography is recommended.

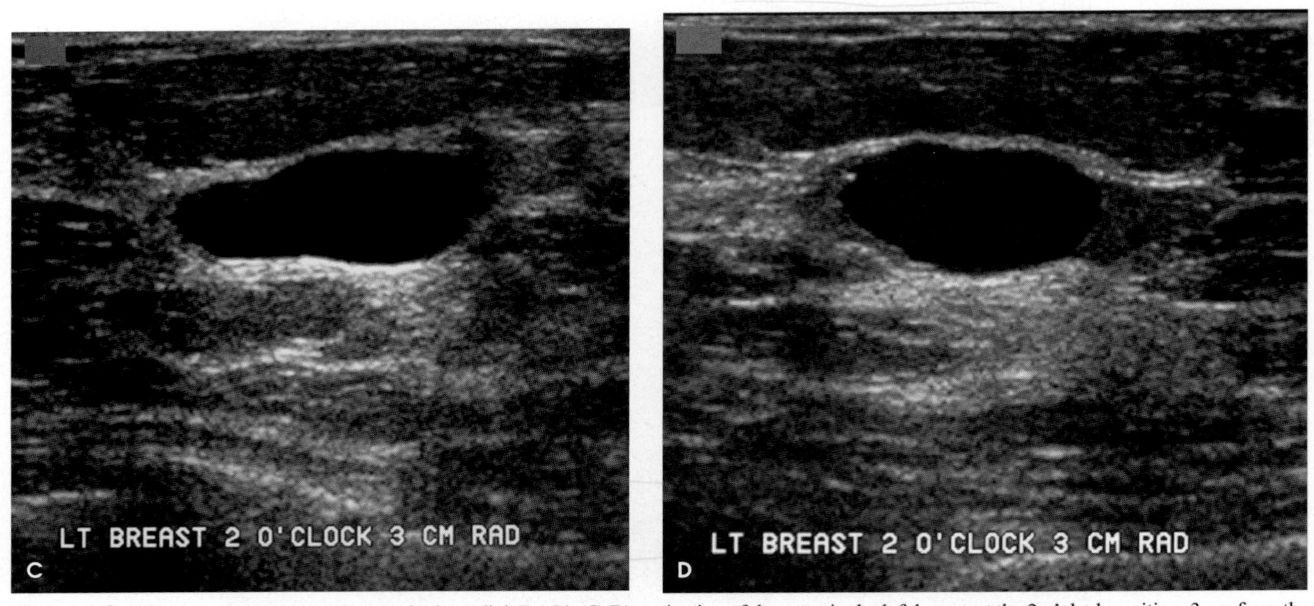

Figure 4.8. (*Continued*) Ultrasound images in the radial (RAD) **(C, D)** projection of the mass in the left breast, at the 2 o'clock position, 3 cm from the left nipple.

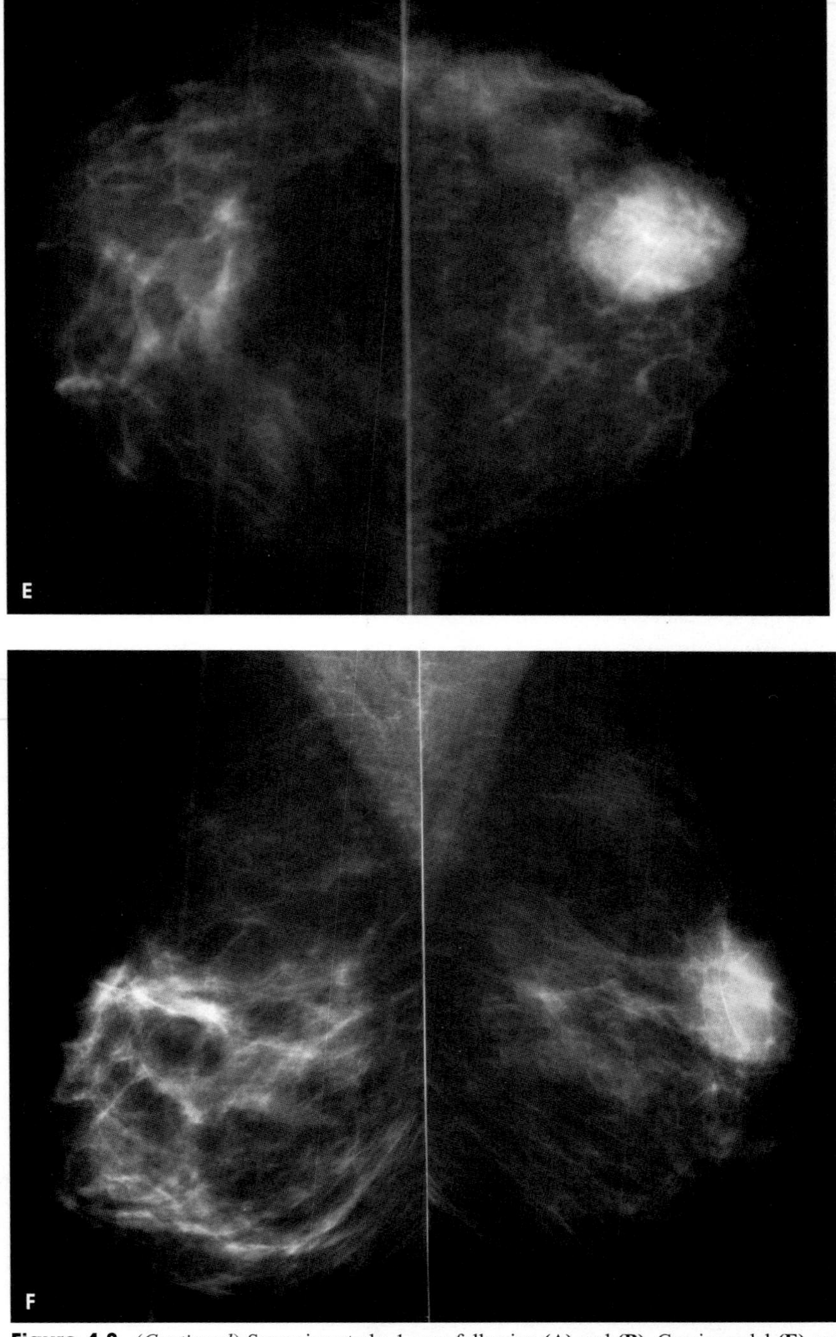

Figure 4.8. (*Continued*) Screening study, 1 year following **(A)** and **(B).** Craniocaudal **(E)** and mediolateral oblique **(F)** views.

What would you do next?

The mass in the left breast has enlarged. In determining the next appropriate step, I review the evaluation done the previous year. I focus on the ultrasound study. If, as in this patient, the ultrasound demonstrates a "classic" simple cyst, I do not call the patient back for a repeat evaluation. Cysts fluctuate in size, and as long the patient remains asymptomatic, I do not call the patient back. If, in reviewing the prior ultrasound there is any question about the diagnosis of a cyst (e.g., internal echoes, shadowing, or irregular margins), I will call the patient back for a repeat ultrasound.

BI-RADS® category 2: benign finding. Annual screening mammography is recommended.

PATIENT 9

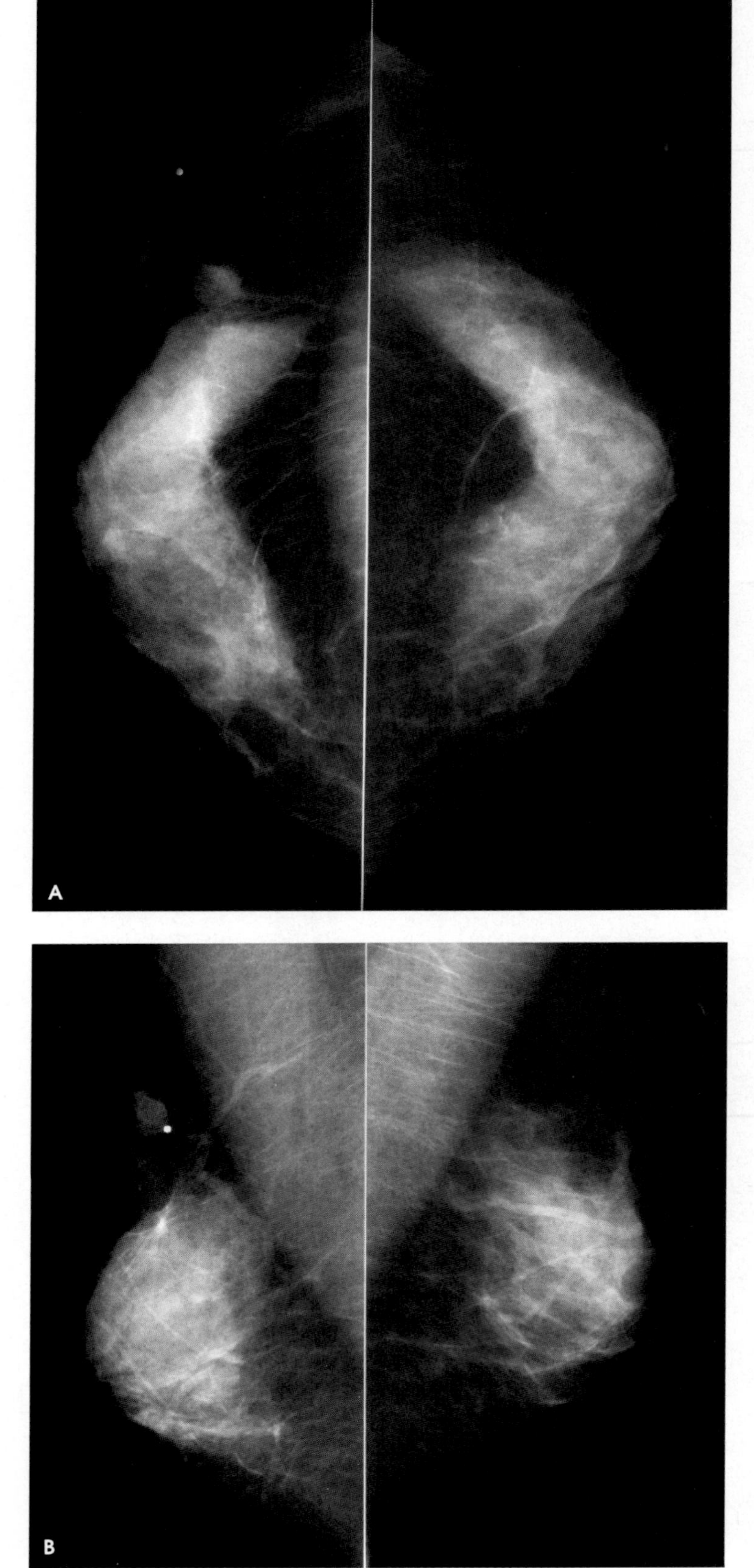

Figure 4.9. Diagnostic evaluation, 47-year-old patient presenting with a "lump" in the right breast. Craniocaudal **(A)** and mediolateral oblique **(B)** views, metallic BB used to mark location of palpable finding.

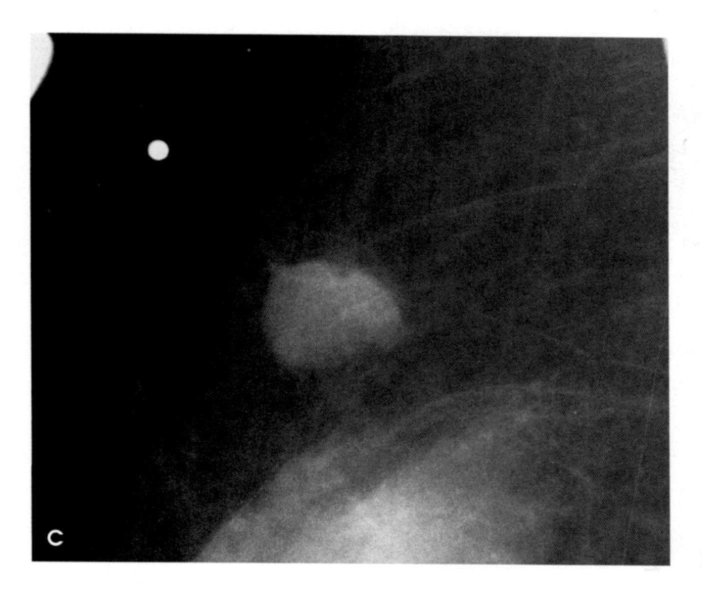

Figure 4.9. (*Continued*) Spot tangential **(C)** view of palpable finding.

How would you describe the findings, and what would you recommend next?

A well-circumscribed mass is imaged corresponding to the palpable finding. On the tangential view, this appears to be a mixed-density lesion such that differential considerations include a lymph node, fat necrosis, hematoma, galactocele, or a fibroadenolipoma. The patient does not recall any recent trauma, and there is no history of a recent pregnancy.

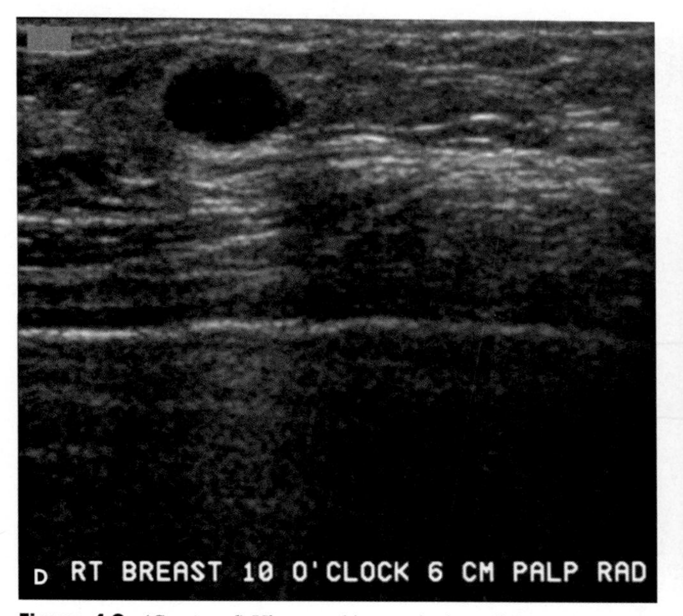

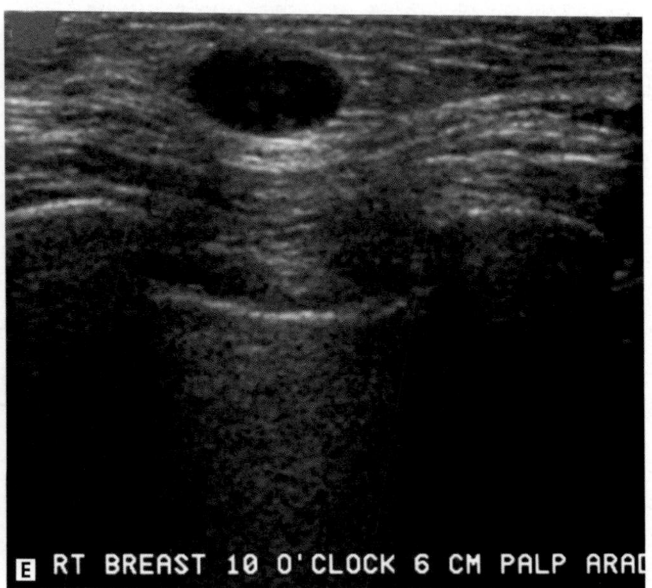

Figure 4.9. (*Continued*) Ultrasound images in the radial (RAD) **(D)** and antiradial (ARAD) **(E)** of the palpable finding.

How would you describe the findings, and what is your recommendation?

On physical examination a discrete, mobile, hard mass is palpated at the 10 o'clock position, 6 cm from the right nipple. A well-circumscribed, oval 1-cm mass that is nearly anechoic with posterior acoustic enhancement is imaged corresponding to the palpable finding. Although a cyst is suspected given the presence of internal echoes and following a discussion with the patient, an aspiration is undertaken.

The mass is atraumatically punctured using a 20G spinal needle and grossly bloody fluid is aspirated. Although several attempts are made to reposition the needle, no additional fluid is obtained and a residual abnormality persists. Core biopsies are done through the persistent abnormality. On inspection of the cores, a central area of hemorrhagic tissue (i.e., a lesion) is noted, on either side of which fatty tissue is seen. This correlates with what is seen mammographically: The lesion is surrounded by fat. The appearance of the cores, in conjunction with that of the aspirate, suggests either a hematoma or fat necrosis. The aspirated fluid is submitted for cytology and the cores are submitted for histologic evaluation. Predominantly blood and hemosiderin-laden macrophages are reported on the cytology. Fibroadipose tissue with granulation tissue, necrosis, hemosiderin-laden macrophages, chronic inflammation, fat necrosis, and foreign-body giant cells are reported on the cores. These findings are congruent with the clinical and imaging findings and the gross appearance of the cores. Annual mammography is recommended for this patient.

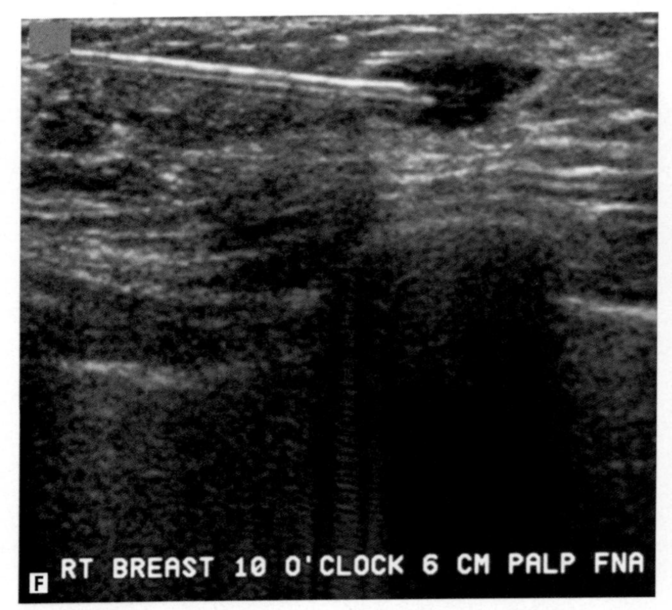

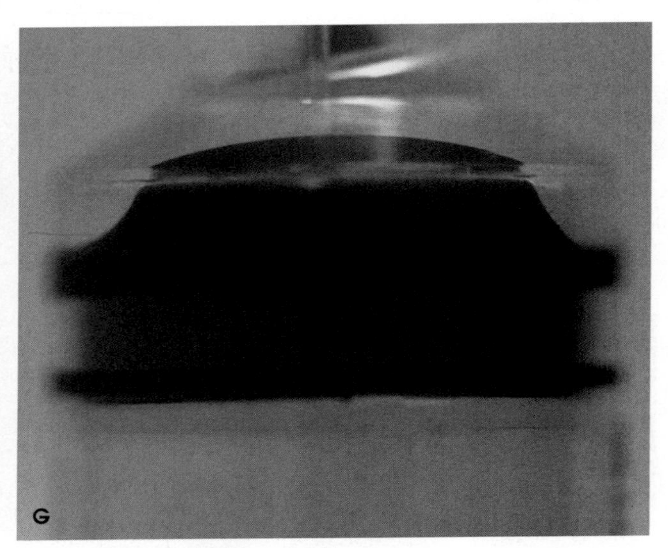

Figure 4.9. (*Continued*) Ultrasound image **(F)** after approximately 0.5 mL of grossly bloody fluid **(G)** is aspirated.

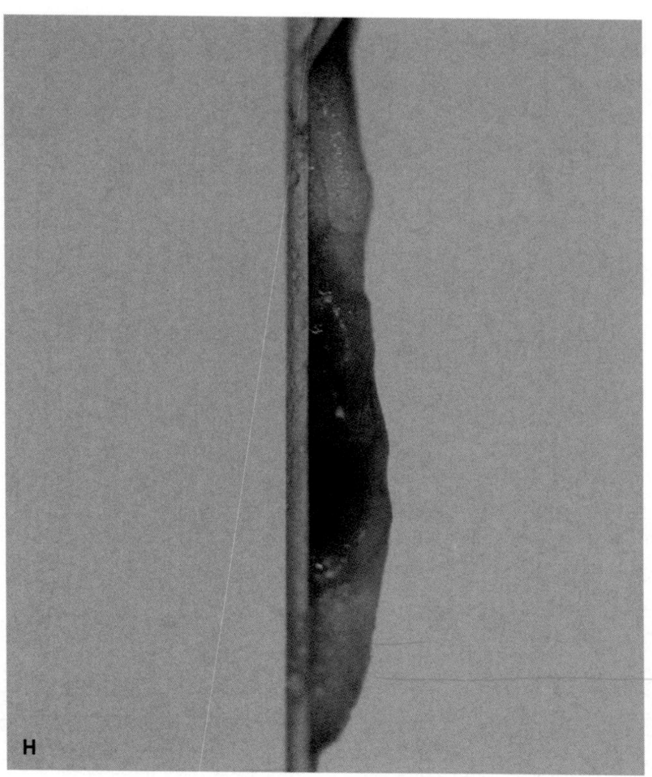

Figure 4.9. (*Continued*) Image of one of the core samples **(H)** demonstrating hemorrhagic tissue flanked by fatty tissue.

PATIENT 10

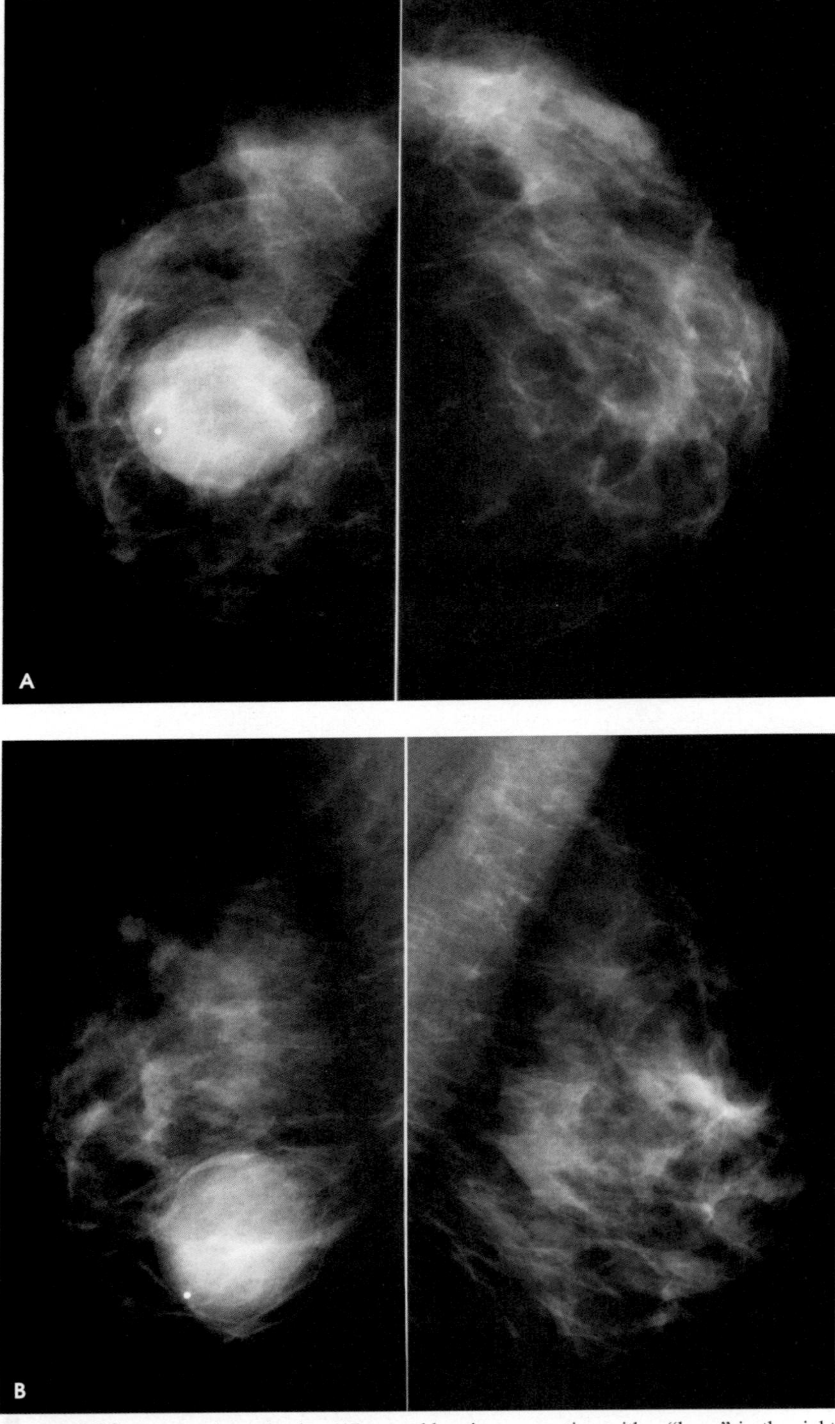

Figure 4.10. Diagnostic evaluation, 47-year-old patient presenting with a "lump" in the right breast. Craniocaudal **(A)** and mediolateral oblique **(B)** views with a metallic BB placed at site of the palpable finding, right breast.

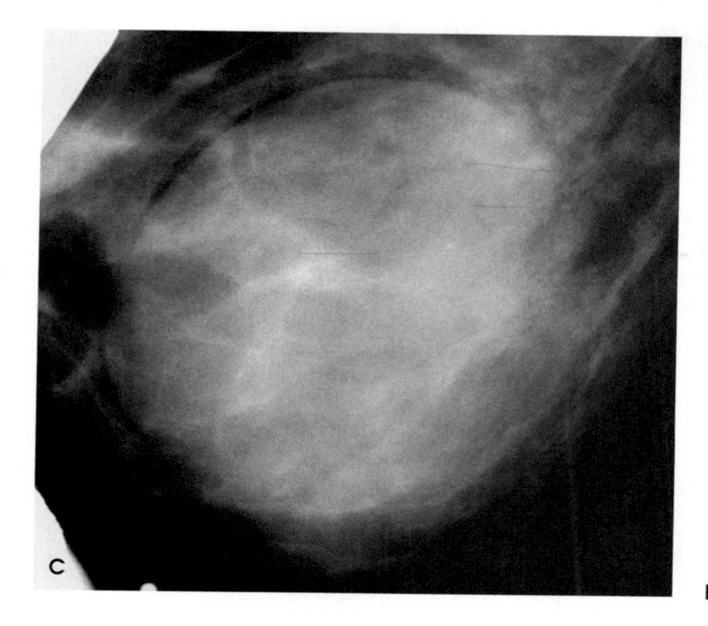

Figure 4.10. (*Continued*) Spot compression view **(C)** of the palpable finding.

A round mass with partially well-circumscribed margins is present in the right breast, corresponding to the site of clinical concern. The differential considerations for the mammographic findings in this patient include cyst, fibroadenoma (tubular adenoma, complex fibroadenoma), papillary lesion, focal fibrosis, pseudoangiomatous stromal hyperplasia (PASH), adenosis tumor, and phyllodes tumor. Depending on the clinical context, galactocele, postoperative or traumatic fluid collection, and an abscess are also in the differential. Given the seemingly circumscribed margins, malignancy is less likely; however, invasive ductal carcinoma not otherwise specified, medullary, mucinous, or papillary carcinoma, or metastatic disease, particularly if the patient has a known malignancy, are additional considerations. An ultrasound is indicated for further evaluation.

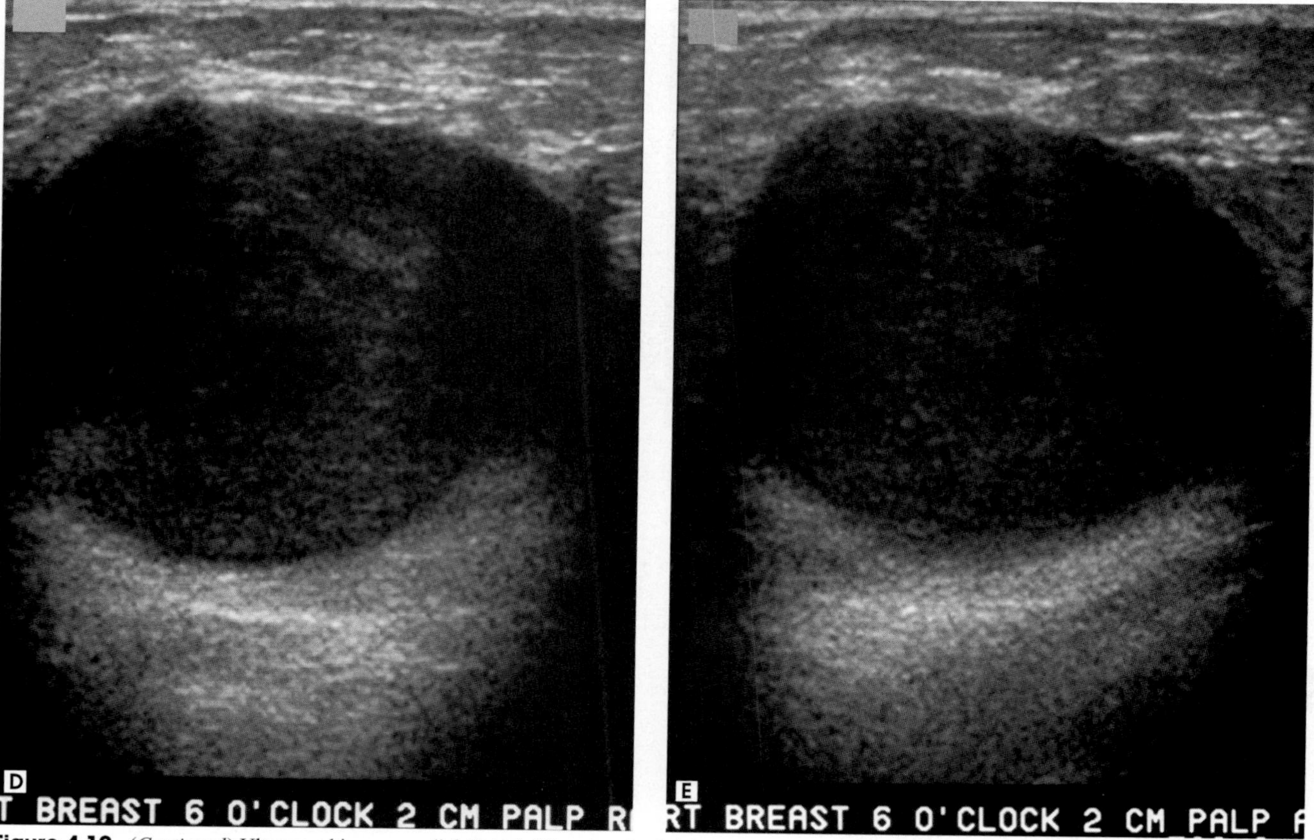

Figure 4.10. (*Continued*) Ultrasound images, radial (RAD) **(D)** and antiradial (ARAD) **(E)** projections of the palpable finding at the 6 o'clock position of the right breast, 2 cm from the nipple.

How would you describe the findings, and what is your recommendation?

There is no history of a recent pregnancy, trauma, surgery, or significant tenderness. On physical examination, a hard but mobile mass is palpated at the 6 o'clock position, 2 cm from the right nipple. A well-circumscribed mass with internal echoes and posterior acoustic enhancement is imaged corresponding to the palpable finding. Although a cyst is suspected, the echoes did not change in position during the ultrasound study and so an aspiration is undertaken. The mass is easily and atraumatically punctured, and approximately 8 mL of grossly bloody fluid is aspirated. No residual abnormality is seen postaspiration. The fluid is submitted for cytologic evaluation. Abundant red blood cells in a background of acellular debris are reported on the thin prep, and the cell block material is submitted for cytology. No malignant cells are identified.

The fluid reaccumulated in a matter of days. This, in combination with the bloody fluid obtained during the initial aspiration, suggests that further action is indicated. An excisional biopsy is performed, and an intermediate-grade, intracystic papillary carcinoma confined within a fibrous capsule (i.e., ductal carcinoma in situ) is reported on the excisional biopsy [pTis, pN0(sn), pMX; Stage 0]. There is no evidence of invasion. Atypical ductal hyperplasia is reported in the surrounding tissue.

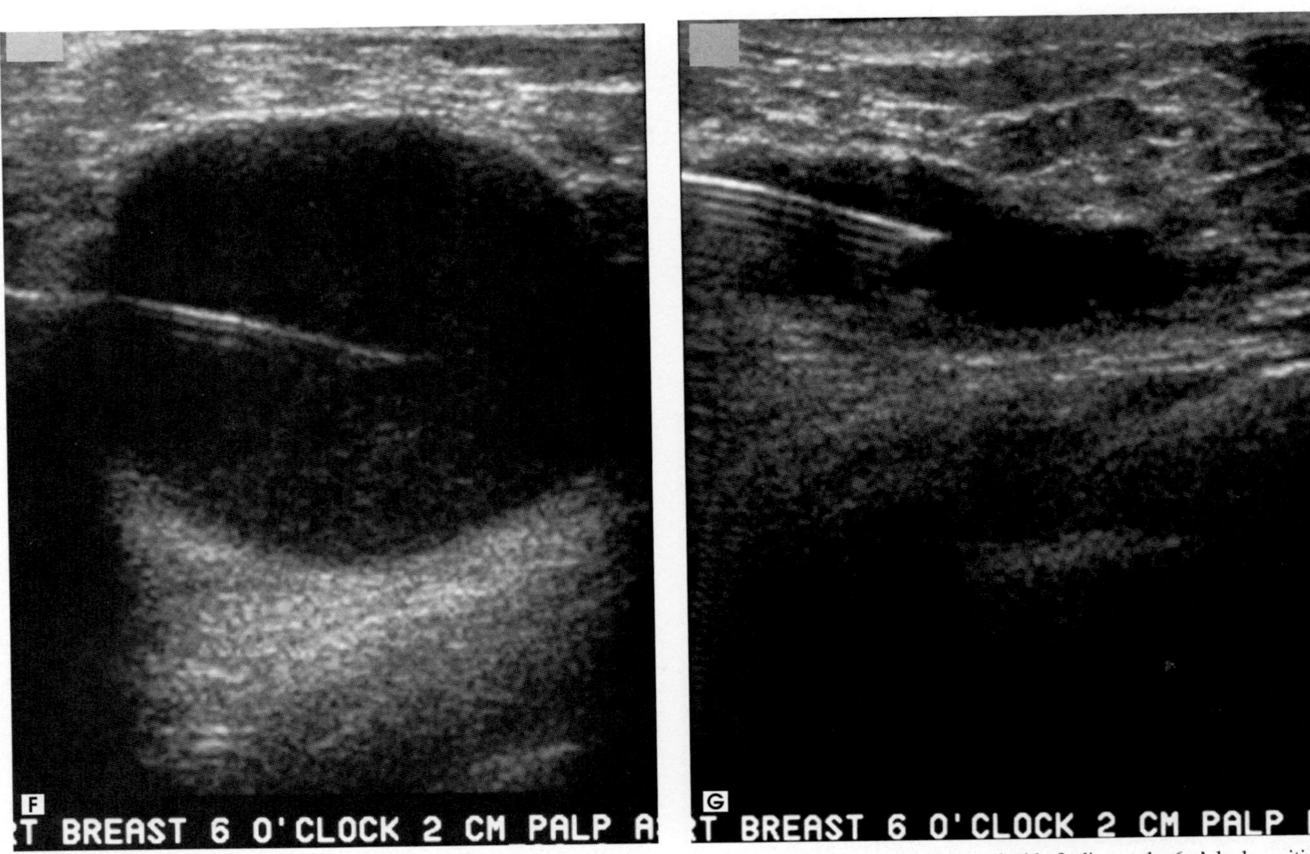

Figure 4.10. *(Continued)* Ultrasound images, radial (RAD) **(D)** and antiradial (ARAD) **(E)** projections of the palpable finding at the 6 o'clock position of the right breast, 2 cm from the nipple. Ultrasound images **(F, G)** obtained during aspiration.

Intracystic papillary carcinomas are rare, but they should be suspected if bloody fluid is aspirated following an atraumatic tap, if there is a residual abnormality following the aspiration, or if fluid reaccumulates rapidly. It is also important to emphasize that cytology is negative in a significant number (>50%) of patients with intracystic carcinomas, so if there is a mural or intracystic component, core biopsies through these areas may be useful in establishing the correct diagnosis.

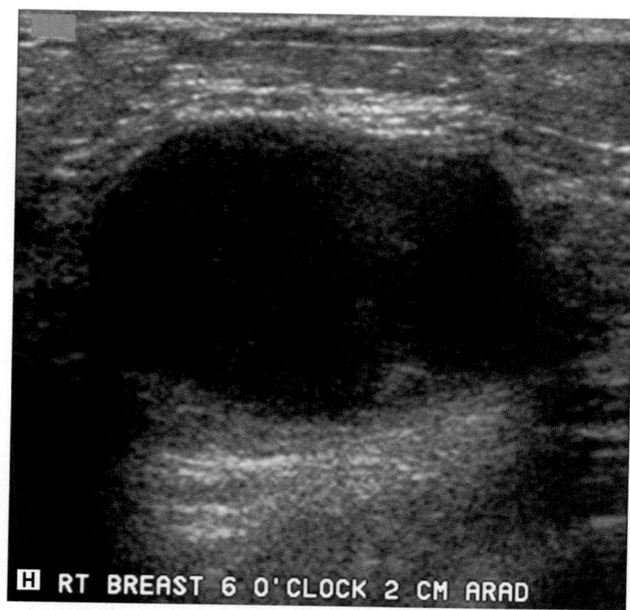

Figure 4.10. Ultrasound image **(H)**, approximately 72 hours following the aspiration.

PATIENT 11

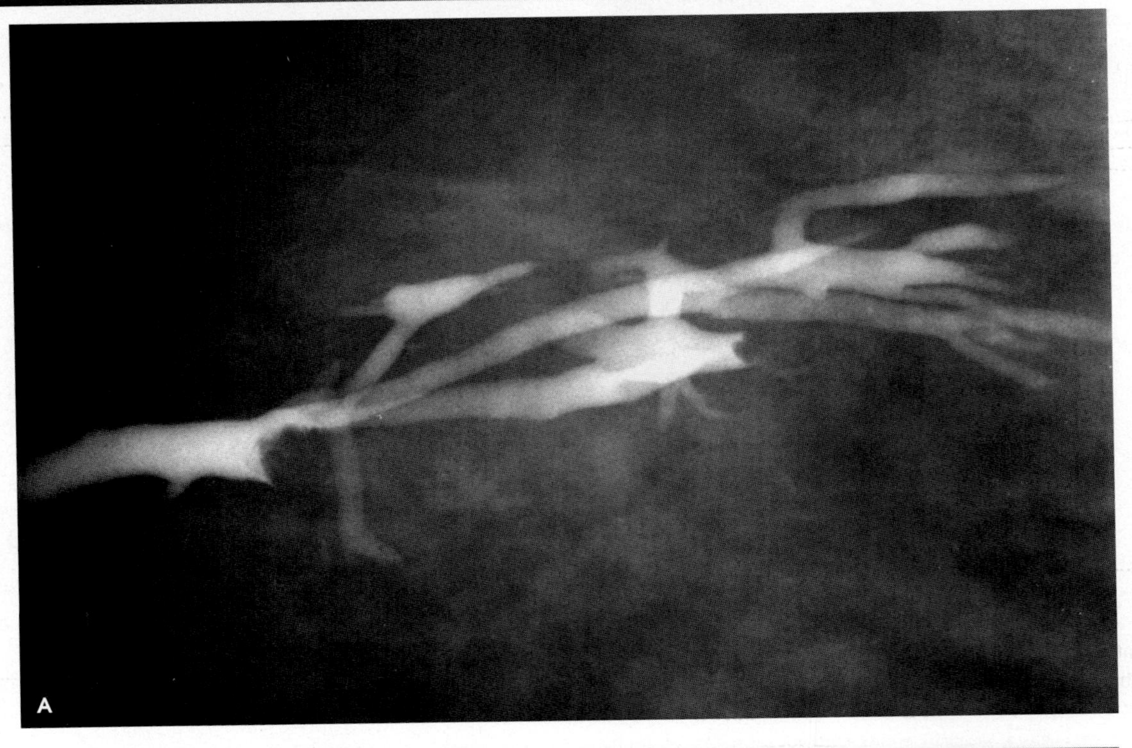

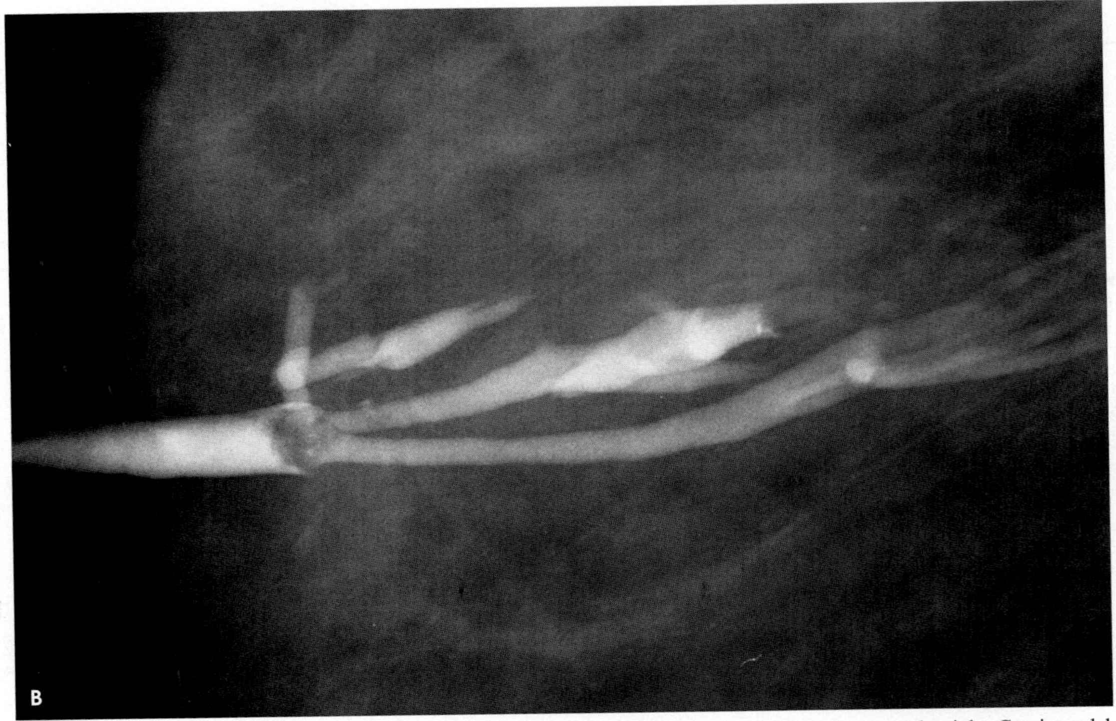

Figure 4.11. Diagnostic evaluation, 58-year-old patient who presents describing nipple discharge on the right. Craniocaudal **(A)** and 90-degree lateral **(B)** magnification views of the right breast following a ductogram. Magnification view, craniocaudal projection, right breast.

How should patients presenting with nipple discharge be evaluated? What do you think of this ductogram?

For patients presenting with nipple discharge, a full mammogram is done (images not shown for this patient), history is obtained, and a physical examination is done. If it is determined that the nipple discharge is spontaneous, a ductogram is done. In this patient, the cannulated duct is dilated (arbitrarily, we use the cannula as an internal reference for duct size; normal ducts are one to three cannulas in diameter) and there are two lesions in the duct. The anterior-most lesion is a filling defect; the second lesion is obstructing a side branch of the involved duct (Fig. 4.11C, arrows). These are likely to be papillomas, but excisional biopsy is recommended. Excisional biopsy in this patient confirms the presence of intraductal papillomas with no atypia or other associated proliferative changes.

Ultrasound is sometimes used to evaluate women with nipple discharge. It is important to recognize that this is useful when the lesion or lesions are close to the nipple and in a dilated duct. However, this is not always the situation. Intraductal lesions can be found several centimeters away from the nipple in nondilated ducts and therefore are not always identified by ultrasound.

Ductography can provide information relative to the course of the abnormal duct, the number and location of lesions, and the likely etiology of the lesions. It is not appropriate to assume, as many surgeons do, that lesions causing nipple discharge are in the subareolar area or that the ducts containing the lesions are dilated and therefore identifiable intraoperatively. Even if the abnormal duct is identifiable at the time of surgery, the number and location of potential lesions cannot be established reliably through visual inspection intraoperatively. When patients are taken to the operating room because of discharge but in the absence of preoperative evaluation, blind excisions are done, with no assurance that the cause of the discharge has been excised and evaluated histologically. Following duct excision, the discharge is usually eliminated. The patient may be relieved, but what have we accomplished if the underlying lesion, possibly a ductal carcinoma in situ, has not been excised?

What information is useful in evaluating women who present with nipple discharge?

Obtaining a good history is a helpful starting point in evaluating patients who present describing nipple discharge. We ask the patient: "How did you notice the discharge?" Invariably, patients with significant nipple discharge provide one, or all, of three descriptions: They notice dark brown spots in the cup of their bra, dark spots on their night clothes, or they have just gotten out of a hot bath or shower, dried their breasts, and notice fluid coming from their nipple. This is spontaneous nipple discharge, and regardless of its appearance (e.g., clear, serous hem-occult-negative or bloody), requires further evaluation. It should be contrasted with expressed nipple discharge that is physiologic in etiology and does not usually require additional evaluation. A variable amount of fluid is found in normal ducts, so nipple discharge can be obtained from multiple duct openings, bilaterally, in most women following vigorous breast and nipple manipulation.

The next step in evaluating women with nipple discharge is physical examination. A bright source of light (e.g., a halogen lamp) focused on the nipple and magnification of the nipple are helpful. I start by examining the surface of the nipple for any crusting or a duct opening that appears erythematous or more patulous than the others. These may be indicators of a duct opening that needs to be cannulated for ductography. I next use an alcohol wipe to clean the surface of the nipple (this clears any keratin plugs that may be partially or completely occluding the duct opening) and I examine the breast for any palpable mass. In doing the exam, I check to see if I am able to elicit discharge. In many patients with an intraductal lesion, it is possible to identify the trigger point described by Haagensen. When you apply pressure over the trigger point, discharge is elicited. As you move away from the trigger point, the discharge stops. In many patients with an intraductal lesion, the discharge is projectile (shoots out at you and can hit you in the eyes if you are not careful) and copious.

If the patient provides a history of spontaneous nipple discharge, and single-duct discharge is elicited on physical examination, a ductogram is undertaken even in women with hem-occult-negative discharge. If fluid is difficult to obtain, and it originates from multiple duct openings bilaterally, ductography is not indicated. We do not routinely submit nipple discharge for cytology, and we do not routinely do hem-occult testing. A negative cytology report does not exclude significant pathology, however, and if atypical cells are described, the issue of establishing the presence and location of a lesion in the duct remains.

There is a misconception that only bloody nipple discharge is significant. On the contrary, clear or serous hem–occult-negative discharge may reflect the presence of underlying ductal carcinoma in situ, so if nipple discharge is spontaneous, it warrants additional evaluation. Although ductography is not a perfect test and it is associated with a 15% false negative rate, ductography can be helpful in identifying the presence of one or multiple intraductal lesions, the location and course of the duct containing the lesions, and the extent of the lesion. It seems to be a more helpful study than doing cytology and blind surgical excisions that can potentially cut through tumor or leave a lesion in the breast while eliminating the presenting symptom. Duct openings are closely apposed on the surface of the nipple, so a 15% false negative rate for ductography is not surprising. If a normal ductogram is obtained in a patient with a history and physical examination that is highly suggestive of an intraductal lesion, I assume the normal ductogram is a false negative study and ask the patient to return in 1 week for a repeat study.

How is a ductogram done?

The secreting duct opening is cannulated using a blunt-tipped 30G straight sialography needle. As a starting point, 0.2 mL of contrast is injected into the duct. The cannula is left in the duct and taped onto the breast. Craniocaudal and 90-degree lateral magnification views of the breast are obtained. The initial amount of contrast injected is small, so that the subareolar portion of the duct can be evaluated. If more contrast is injected at the onset, the density of the contrast may mask small lesions close to the nipple, resulting in a false negative study. By leaving the cannula in the duct, additional contrast material can be injected as needed.

What are the common causes of spontaneous nipple discharge, and what are the more common findings on ductography?

Papillomas, fibrocystic changes, duct ectasia, and breast cancer (usually ductal carcinoma in situ) are the more common causes of spontaneous nipple discharge. Findings on ductography include one or multiple filling defects, duct obstruction, wall irregularity, displacement of the duct, extravasation, and duct dilatation.

What can be done preoperatively to assure excision of the abnormal duct, and how can we facilitate the histologic evaluation of intraductal lesions?

In addition to doing diagnostic ductograms to establish the presence, location, and extent of intraductal lesion, we also do preoperative ductograms. A methylene blue contrast (1:1) combination is injected into the duct on the day of surgery. The contrast allows us to verify that we have cannulated the previously evaluated duct (i.e., the duct with the intraductal lesions), and the methylene blue stains the duct for the surgeon and pathologist. Having the ability to identify the duct stained in blue intraoperatively can effectively limit the excision to the abnormal duct. Of equal importance is facilitating identification of the abnormal duct for the pathologist, because even if the duct is dilated intraoperatively, it collapses as the fluid drains out after excision. The methylene blue is used to identify the duct grossly and direct the dissection for identification of the lesion. Rarely, if the intraductal lesion(s) is peripheral in location (i.e., not in the subareolar area) or if it is in a small branch of the main duct, the ductogram is done the day of surgery and used to guide a mammographically guided preoperative wire localization.

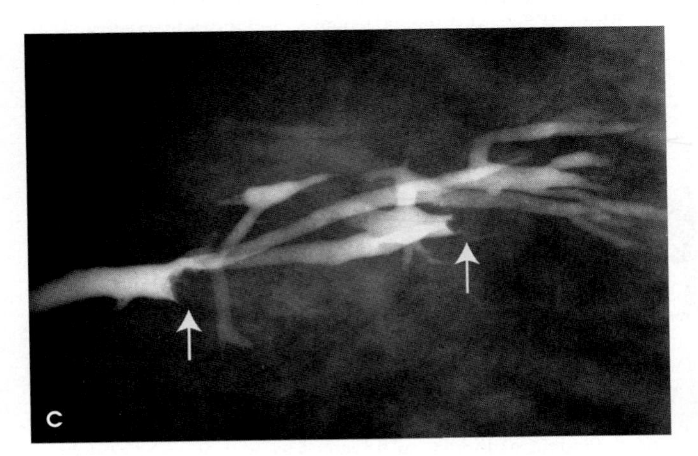

Figure 4.11. (*Continued*) Two intraductal lesions (*arrows*) are present **(C)** in a dilated duct. Excisional biopsy confirms the preoperative diagnosis of papillomas.

PATIENT 12

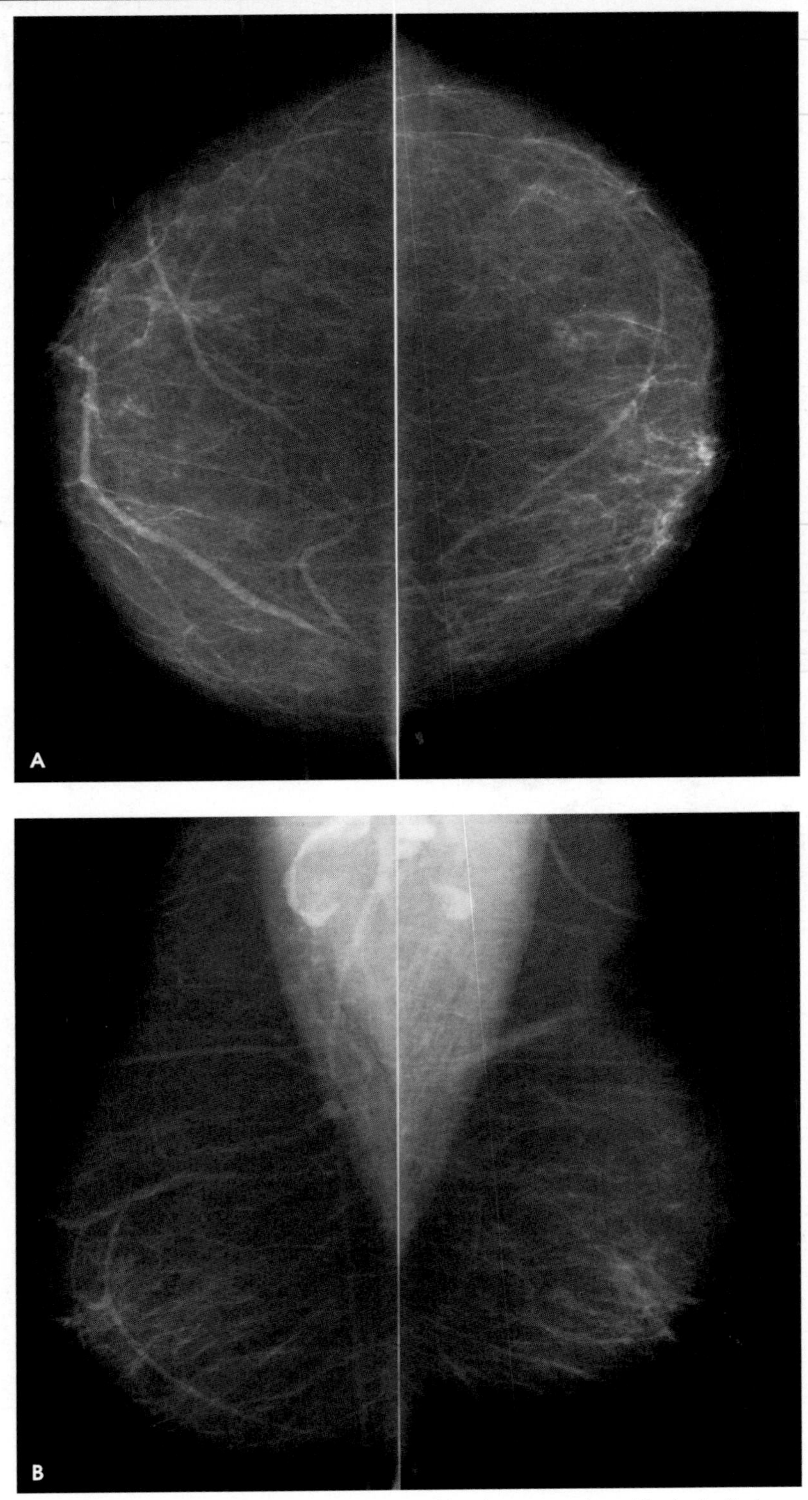

Figure 4.12. Diagnostic evaluation, 61-year-old patient presenting with nipple discharge on the left. Craniocaudal **(A)** and mediolateral oblique **(B)** views.

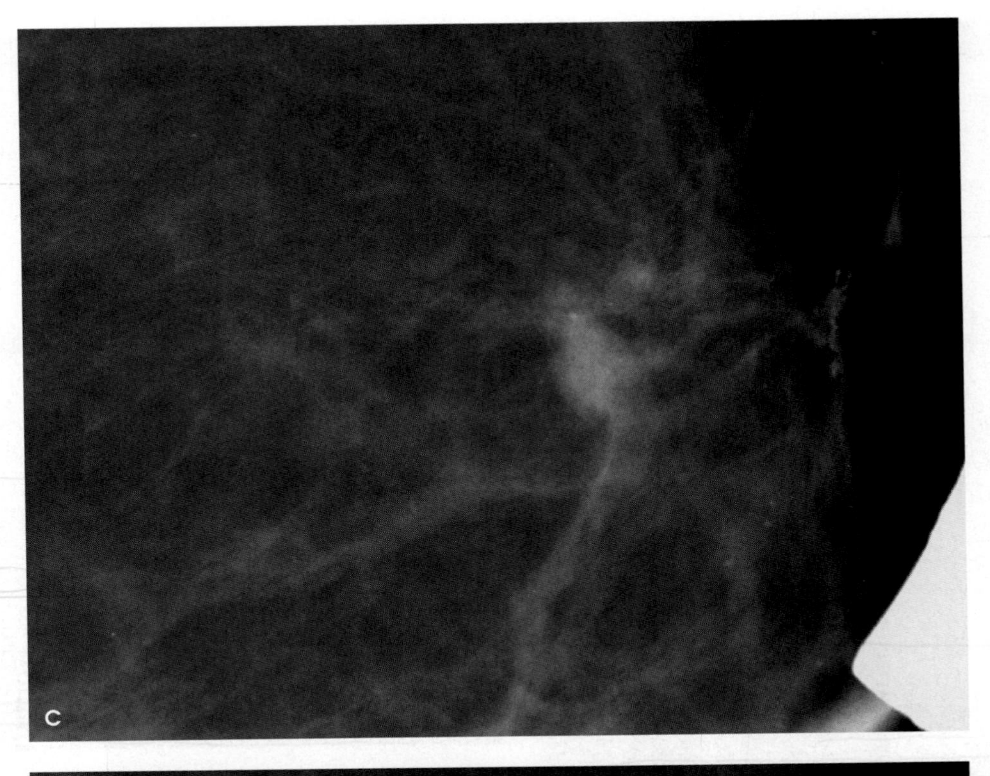

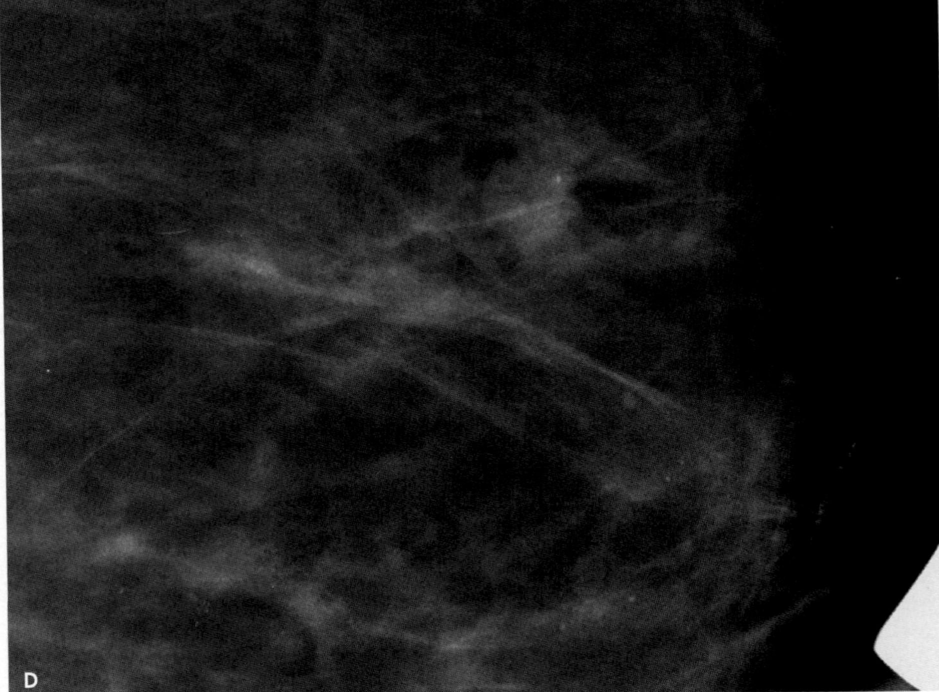

Figure 4.12. (*Continued*) Spot compression views of the left subareolar area, craniocaudal **(C)** and mediolateral oblique **(D)** views.

What do you think? What would you do next?

A predominantly fatty pattern is present, with axillary lymph nodes noted bilaterally. Scattered round calcifications, arterial calcifications, and a 1-cm mass with relatively well circumscribed margins and a round calcification are noted on the subareolar spot compression views. Given the described nipple discharge, a more detailed history of the discharge and a physical examination are indicated.

The patient describes a several-month history of dark brown spots on her bra cup and dripping from her left nipple after hot showers. On physical examination, there is some crusting involving one of the duct openings on the left nipple. An alcohol wipe is used to clear the crusting. With gentle compression of the left subareolar area, discharge is elicited easily from the opening that originally had the crusting. This duct is cannulated and 0.2 mL of contrast is injected.

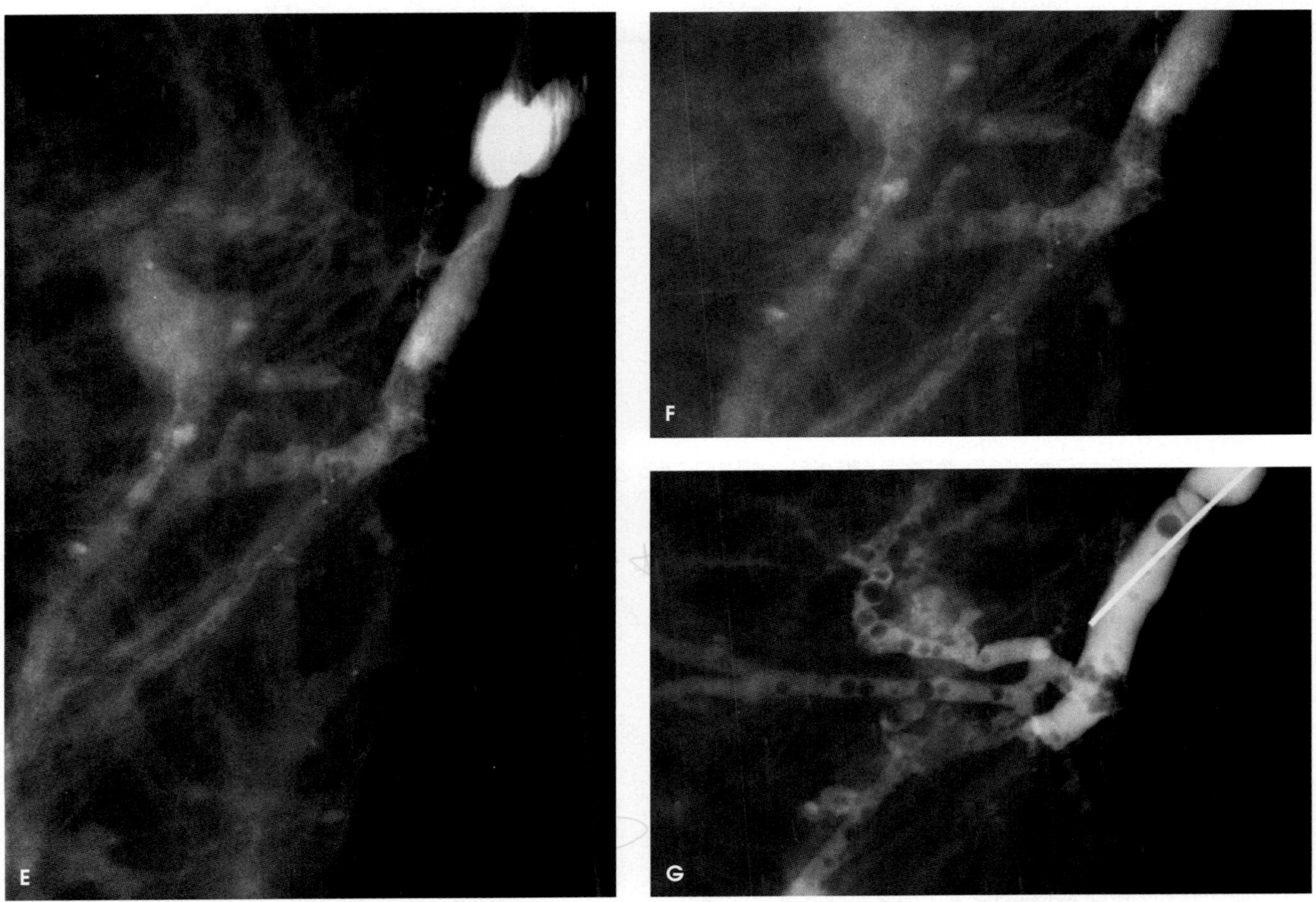

Figure 4.12. Ductogram, magnification views of the subareolar area: 90-degree lateral **(E),** 90-degree lateral photographically coned **(F),** and craniocaudal **(G)** views, left breast.

What do you think? What is your differential, and what would you recommend?

The opacified duct is minimally distended. Multiple filling defects and areas of duct wall irregularity are present (arrows, Fig. 4.12H, I). The duct leads up to the mass noted in the spot compression views. On the craniocaudal view, round, well-defined lucencies consistent with air bubbles are seen in addition to the filling defects and wall irregularity. Differential considerations for the findings include papilloma(s), ductal carcinoma in situ (DCIS), or fibrocystic changes (e.g., hyperplasia, atypical ductal hyperplasia). Given the multiplicity of findings in conjunction with the wall irregularity, DCIS is a significant consideration in this patient. Excisional biopsy is recommended. A high-nuclear-grade ductal carcinoma in situ is diagnosed at the time of the excisional biopsy [pTis, pN0(sn) (i−), pMX; Stage 0].

What are the likely causes of spontaneous nipple discharge, and what can be seen on ductography?

Papillomas are the most common cause of spontaneous discharge, diagnosed in slightly more than 50% of patients who present with spontaneous nipple discharge. One or multiple filling defects, duct obstruction, and wall irregularity are the most common findings on ductography in patients with papillomas. Most ducts that contain papillomas are dilated.

Fibrocystic changes represent the second most common cause of nipple discharge, reported in approximately 35% of patients. Filling of cysts with contrast, multiple filling defects, duct obstruction, and a more diffuse wall irregularity than that seen with a papilloma are the findings related to fibrocystic changes on a ductogram.

Distended ducts in close proximity to the nipple characterize duct ectasia; the opacified ducts assume a more normal caliber peripherally in the tissue. No focal intraductal abnormality is identified in patients with duct ectasia.

Breast cancer, commonly ductal carcinoma in situ, is diagnosed in 5% to 15% of patients who present with spontaneous nipple discharge. In some of these patients, a mass or pleomorphic calcifications may be seen on the mammogram; for many patients, however, the mammogram is normal. The findings on ductography overlap with those described for papillomas and include one or multiple filling defects, duct obstruction, wall irregularity, displacement of the duct, and contrast extravasation. In general, ducts involved with ductal carcinoma in situ are normal in caliber or only minimally distended. In contrast, ducts with associated papillomas are often moderately to significantly distended. Given the inability to distinguish between papillomas and ductal carcinoma in situ on ductography, excision is recommended for all patients identified with an intraductal lesion.

Potential pitfalls on ductography include false negative studies, air bubbles, masking of lesions, duct perforation, and contrast extravasation. The duct openings are closely apposed on the surface of the nipple. If too much discharge is elicited when trying to identify the duct opening, an adjacent opening may be flooded with fluid and inadvertently cannulated. If the history and physical examination are suggestive of an intraductal lesion, a normal ductogram is considered a false negative study and the patient is asked to return for a repeat ductogram. Because we do diagnostic and preoperative ductograms (repeat ductogram on the day of surgery using a methylene blue:contrast combination), we know that our false negative rate for ductography is approximately 15%.

In preparing for the ductogram, contrast is drawn into a 3-cc luer lock syringe and the contrast is run through the tubing of the sialography needle. Every effort should be made to eliminate air bubbles from the system prior to cannulation. If air bubbles inadvertently enter the duct system they are usually easy to distinguish from a lesion. Air bubbles are well defined, lucent, and shift in position between films. Intraductal lesions are characterized by irregular contours, and they do not shift in position between films.

A small amount (0.2 mL) of contrast is injected initially because otherwise, small lesions, particularly when close to the nipple, can be masked. Because we leave the cannula in the duct, we are able to inject additional contrast as needed to distend the more peripheral portions of the duct.

Perforation of a normal duct is rare; it takes significant pressure, and the patient describes a sharp pain when the duct is perforated and burning as soon as you inject contrast. Adhering to some simple guidelines during cannulation can prevent this possible complication. After identifying the secreting duct opening, I angle the cannula approximately 45 degrees, place the tip at the secreting duct opening, and straighten the cannula. It usually "falls" into the duct. If it does not, I gently twirl the cannula between my thumb and index fingers but do not apply any pressure or try to advance the cannula forcefully. If I have identified a trigger point, I try to angle the cannula in the direction of the trigger point. Sometimes, lifting the nipple up so as to "straighten" the duct in the subareolar portion can also be helpful. As I am manipulating the cannula, I repeatedly ask the patient if she is feeling anything sharp. If the patient describes any discomfort, I stop and reposition the cannula. Ductography is a painless procedure, so if the patient describes discomfort it is commonly an indication that the cannula is not in a duct opening.

Contrast extravasation can be seen in the context of duct perforation. In this situation, the patient describes a burning sensation as soon as you attempt to inject contrast, and an amorphous collection of contrast is seen in the subareolar area. Alternatively, peripheral extravasation can be seen as an amorphous collection of contrast surrounding the side branches of normal or hypoplastic ducts. In this situation, the patient experiences no discomfort as you start injecting the contrast, but she will describe a burning sensation after some volume of contrast has been introduced into the duct system. Opacification of lymphatic channels is sometimes also seen in patients with peripheral contrast extravasation.

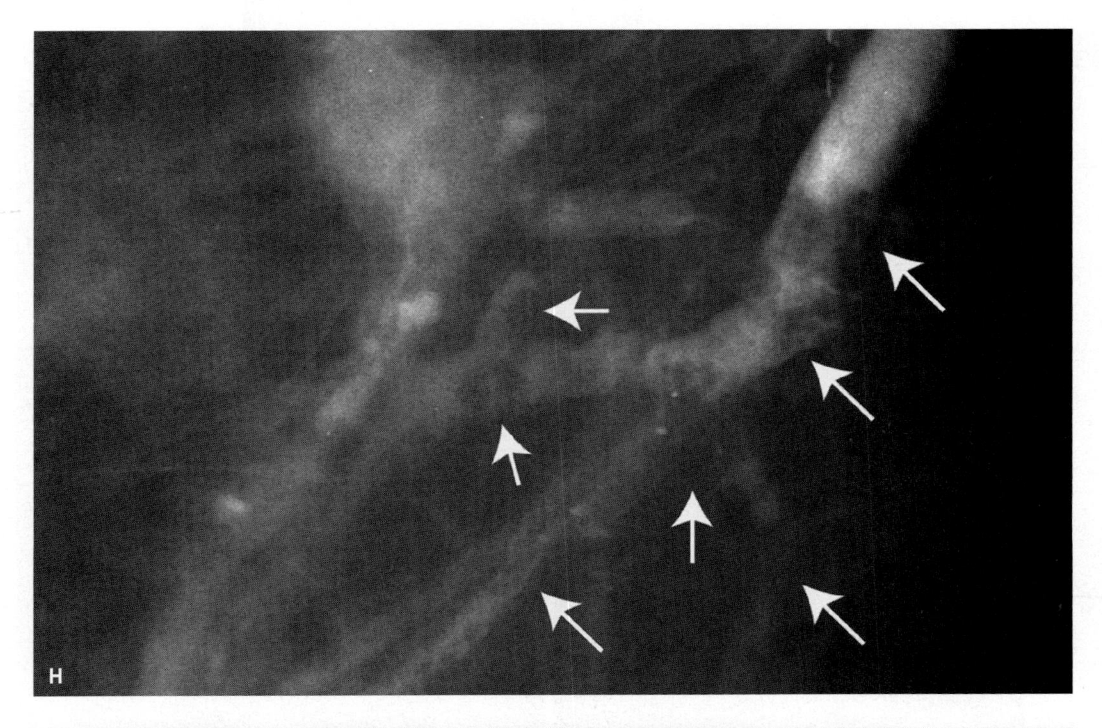

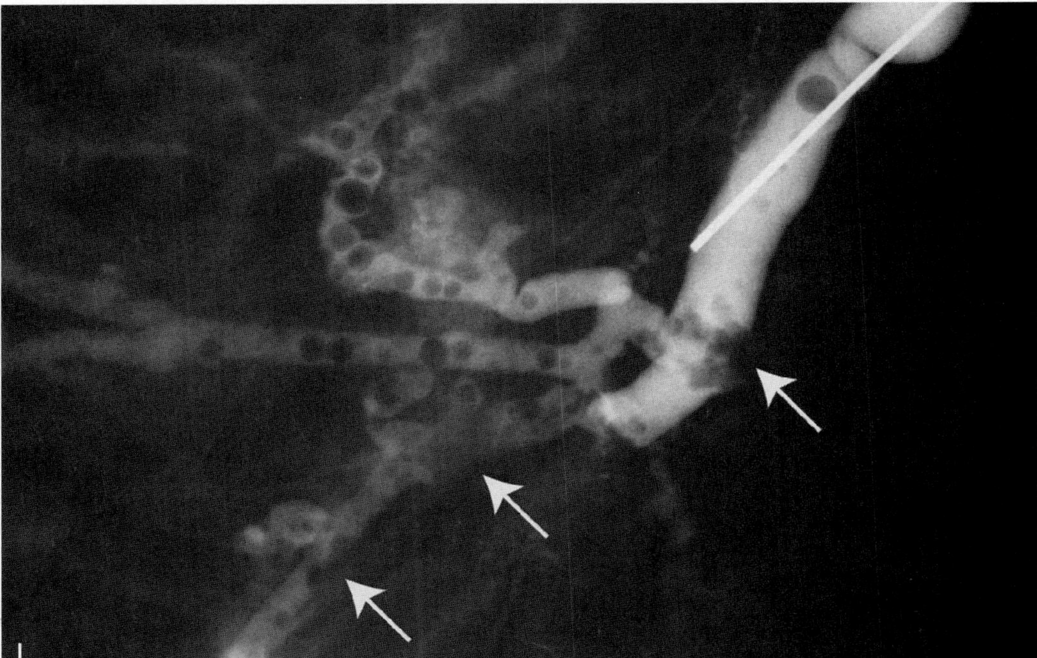

Figure 4.12. (*Continued*) Magnification views of the subareolar area: 90-degree lateral photographically coned **(H)** and craniocaudal **(I)** views, left breast. Multiple filling defects are present in the opacified duct and there are several areas of wall irregularity (*arrows*). A portion of the cannula and multiple air bubbles are also evident on the craniocaudal view.

PATIENT 13

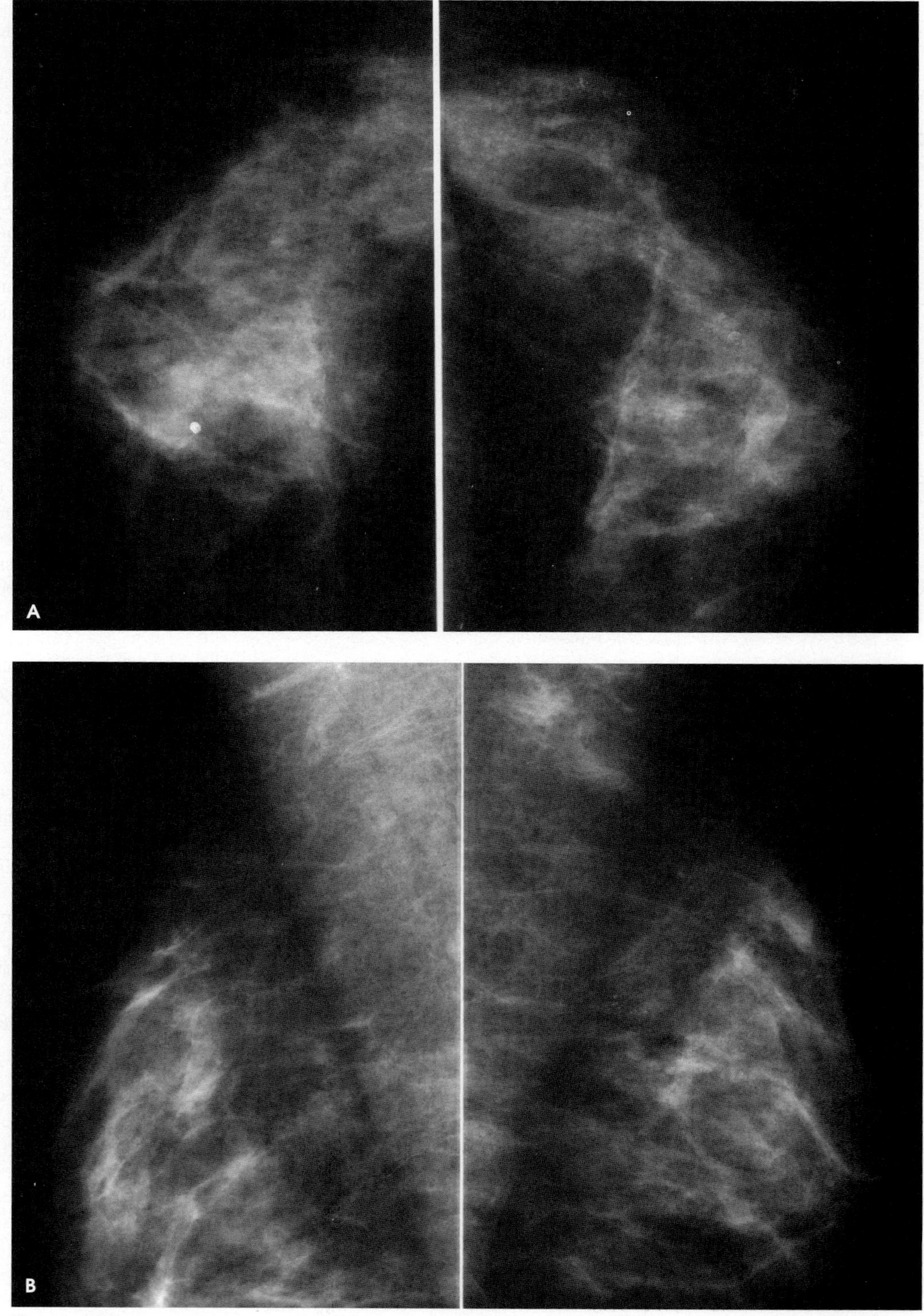

Figure 4.13. Screening mammogram, 54-year-old woman. Craniocaudal **(A)** and mediolateral oblique **(B)** views.

What do you think? What is indicated next?

There is dense tissue. A cluster of calcifications is present posterolaterally in the left breast. Magnification views are indicated for further characterization.

BI-RADS® category 0: need additional imaging evaluation.

What is your differential and recommendation?

A cluster of pleomorphic calcifications is confirmed on the magnification views (Fig. 4.13C, D). Fibrocystic changes including hyperplasia, atypical ductal hyperplasia, columnar alteration with prominent apical snouts and secretions (CAPSS), and sclerosing adenosis as well as fibroadenoma, papilloma, and ductal carcinoma in situ (usually low- or intermediate-nuclear-grade) are in the differential for this cluster of calcifications. An imaging-guided biopsy is indicated.

BI-RADS category 4: suspicious abnormality, biopsy should be considered. A stereotactically guided biopsy is done, and ductal carcinoma in situ is reported on the cores.

What would you recommend next?

Surgical consultation is indicated. Additionally, we recommend magnetic resonance imaging (MRI) for all of our patients with a diagnosis of breast cancer. This is particularly helpful in women with dense tissue mammographically. The purpose of the MRI is to better evaluate the extent of disease, including the presence of multifocal or multicentric disease in the ipsilateral breast, and to further evaluate the contralateral breast for synchronous lesions.

Irregular and clumped linear enhancement is noted, corresponding to the area of the patient's known DCIS in the upper outer quadrant of the left breast (Fig. 4.13E). Additionally, two masses with kinetic curves demonstrating rapid wash-in and wash-out of contrast are present in the lower outer quadrant of the left breast (Fig. 4.13F). The patient is asked to return for ultrasound evaluation of the MRI findings.

A mass with associated shadowing is imaged at the 4:30 o'clock position of the left breast, 5 cm from the left nipple. An ultrasound-guided biopsy is done and an invasive ductal carcinoma is reported histologically. Given the presence of multicentric disease (synchronous lesions in different quadrants), a mastectomy is recommended. On the mastectomy specimen, two foci (1.5 cm and 1.2 cm) of intermediate-grade invasive ductal carcinoma and associated DCIS (cribriform and micropapillary) are identified, and metastatic disease is reported in one of two excised sentinel lymph nodes; an additional positive lymph node is reported following the axillary dissection [pT1c, pN1a, pMX; Stage IIA].

What are some of the current indications for magnetic resonance imaging (MRI) of the breasts?

The role of MRI in breast imaging is evolving, and appropriate indications vary, depending on availability and experience. Described indications include the evaluation of women with an identified malignancy, particularly if they have dense tissue mammographically. In these patients, unsuspected multifocal or multicentric disease, or a breast cancer in the contralateral breast, may be identified, potentially altering the management of the patient. Other described uses include the evaluation of patients with metastatic disease to the axilla with an unknown (but presumed) breast primary, to potentially identify the primary; in monitoring the response of a tumor in patients undergoing neoadjuvant therapy; for assessing the presence of residual tumor in patients with positive margins postlumpectomy; and in distinguishing tumor recurrence from scar tissue at a prior lumpectomy site. The use of MRI to screen women for breast cancer is indicated in patients with dense tissue mammographically and a high risk of breast cancer, particularly BRCA1 or -2–positive patients, or those at least 10 years after chest wall radiation for lymphoma.

Scanning protocols for magnetic resonance imaging of the breast are still evolving. Bilateral, simultaneous imaging of the breasts is critical in assessing areas of asymmetry, hormonal influence, or diffuse change. A dedicated breast coil, at least a 1.5-T magnet, 1-mm spatial resolution in all planes, high temporal resolution, a 2-mm slice thickness, subtraction or fat suppression, and biopsy capability are minimal requirements for doing magnetic resonance imaging of the breast. As with mammography and ultrasound, meticulous technique is critical. This includes positioning of the breasts in the coil with no significant compression as well as arm positioning, and which vein is used to administer the contrast bolus for the dynamic portion of the scan. Lesions are assessed for signal characteristics and morphology, using T1- and T2-weighted images and for contrast enhancement patterns and kinetic analysis on the dynamic T1 scans obtained following the administration of contrast.

Lesions with high T2 signal intensity are usually benign and include cysts, lymph nodes, and some myxomatous fibroadenomas. Except for some mucinous carcinomas and necrotic tumors, most malignant lesions are characterized by low T2 signals. The shape of masses detected on MRI can be described as round, oval, lobulated, or irregular, and their margins as smooth, irregular, or spiculated. Margin analysis is best done on the first post-contrast image and is dependent on the size of the lesion and spatial resolution. In considering contrast enhancement, lesions may demonstrate homogenous or heterogeneous enhancement, central or rim enhancement, or enhancing internal septations. Alternatively, dark internal septations may be seen in a mass, reflecting the lack of enhancement. Homogeneous enhancement is more common in benign lesions. Inflammatory cysts and fat necrosis may exhibit rim enhancement. Inflammatory cysts, however, are bright on T2-weighted images, and the use of fat-suppression images, in conjunction with mammographic findings and clinical history, are helpful in the diagnosis of fat necrosis.

Enhancement can also be seen without the presence of a mass. In these situations, descriptive terms in the ACR lexicon for lesions detected on MRI include: focal area, linear, ductal (i.e., pointing toward the nipple and possibly branching), regional (not conforming to expected distribution of a duct), segmental (triangular enhancement with the apex toward the nipple), multiple regions, or diffuse. Non-mass-like enhancement can be further qualified as homogeneous, heterogeneous, stippled/punctate, clumped, reticular/dendritic, symmetric, or asymmetric. Linear enhancement, particularly when clumped or irregular, is suggestive of DCIS.

With contrast administration and dynamic imaging, kinetic data can be evaluated. Breast cancers typically enhance rapidly (i.e., "wash in"), with the enhancement stabilizing (plateau) or gradually decreasing in signal intensity (i.e., "wash out"). This is thought to reflect tumor neovascularity and shunting. Normal tissue, and most benign lesions, demonstrate gradual and continuous contrast enhancement. In describing the signal intensity–time curve, *slow, medium,* and *rapid* are used to describe the enhancement pattern of a mass within the first 2 minutes or when the curve starts to change. The delayed phase of the curve (after the first 2 minutes or after the curve starts to change) should be described as *persistent* if the enhancement continues to increase over time, *plateau* if the signal intensity does not change over time after the initial increase, or *wash-out* if the signal intensity decreases after the initial rise.

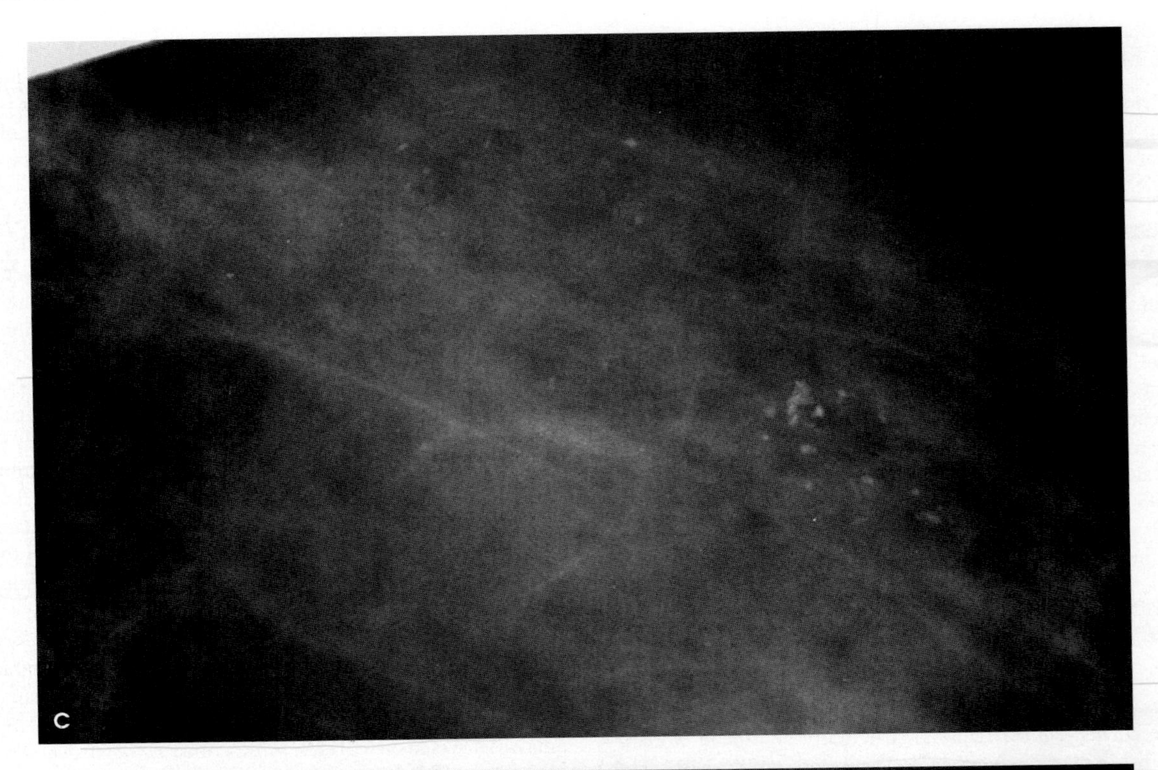

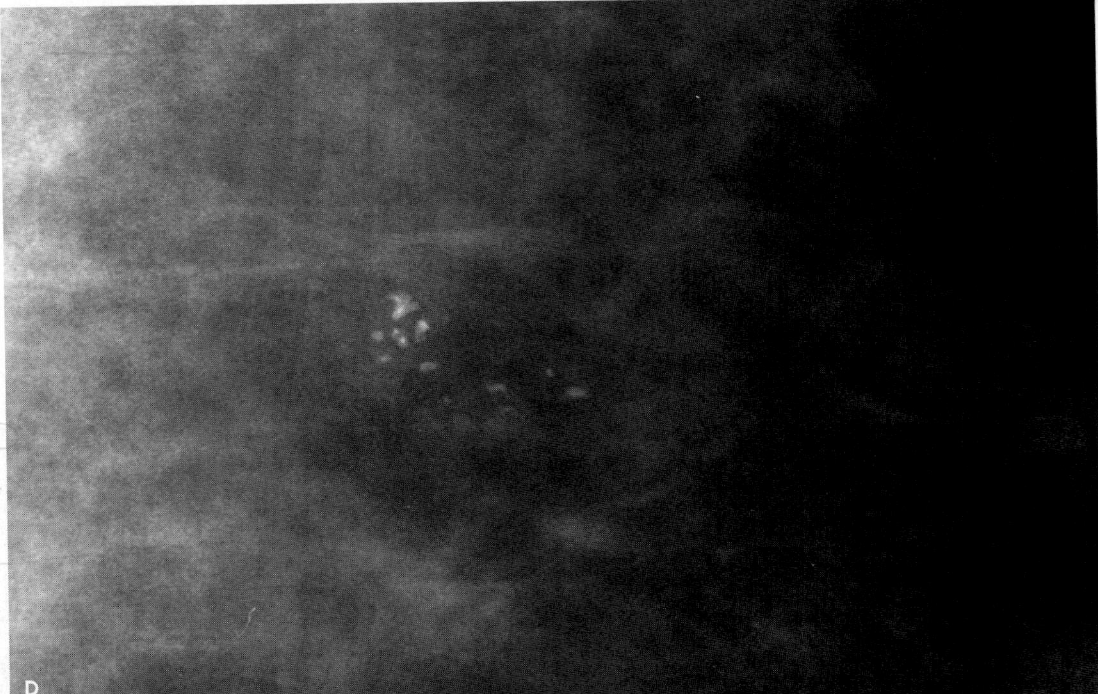

Figure 4.13. (*Continued*) Craniocaudal **(C)** and mediolateral oblique **(D)** double spot compression magnification views of the left breast.

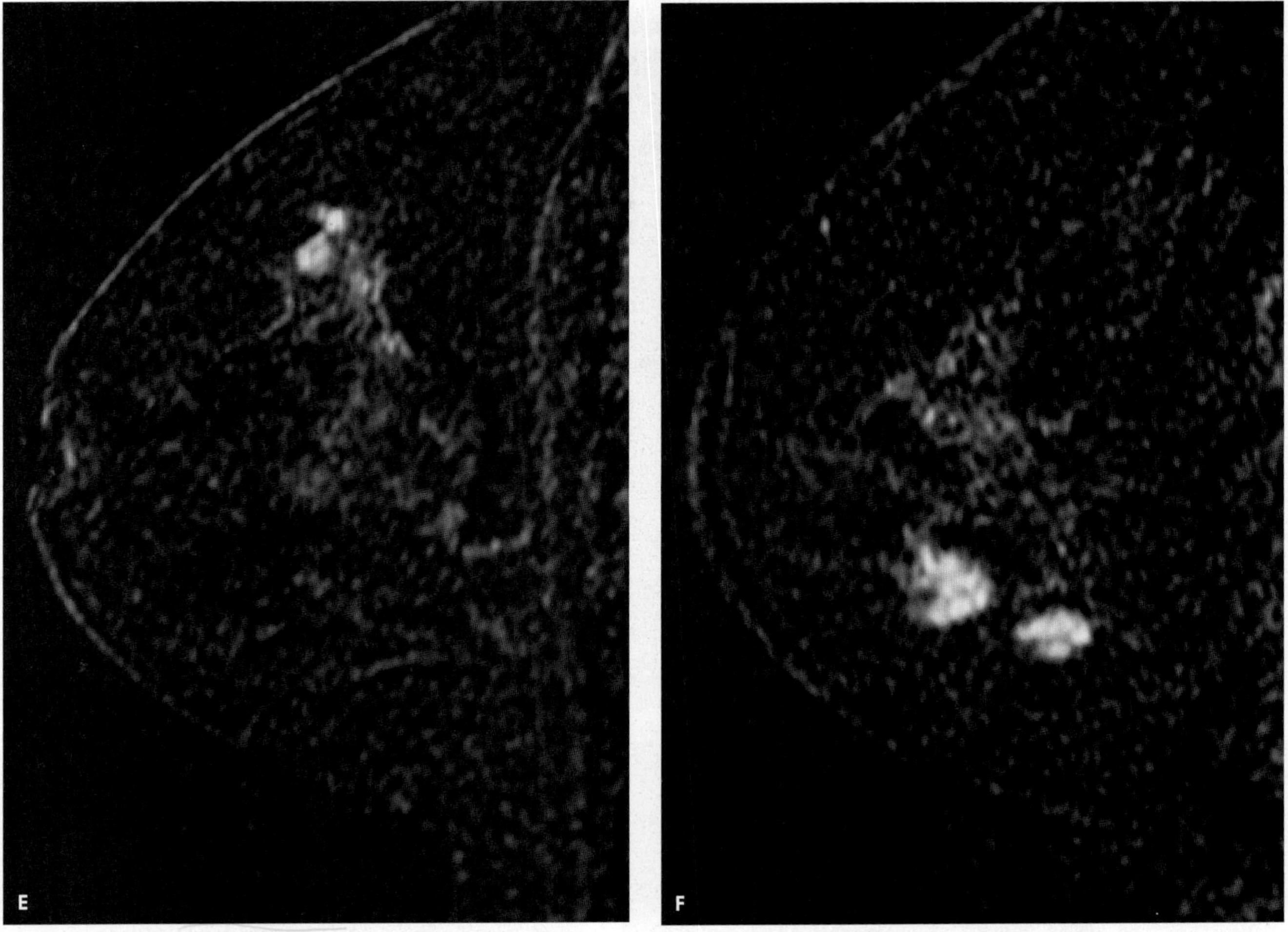

Figure 4.13. (*Continued*) Subtraction images **(E, F)** obtained from precontrast and sequential sagittal T1-weighted images done after the intravenous bolus administration of gadolinium.

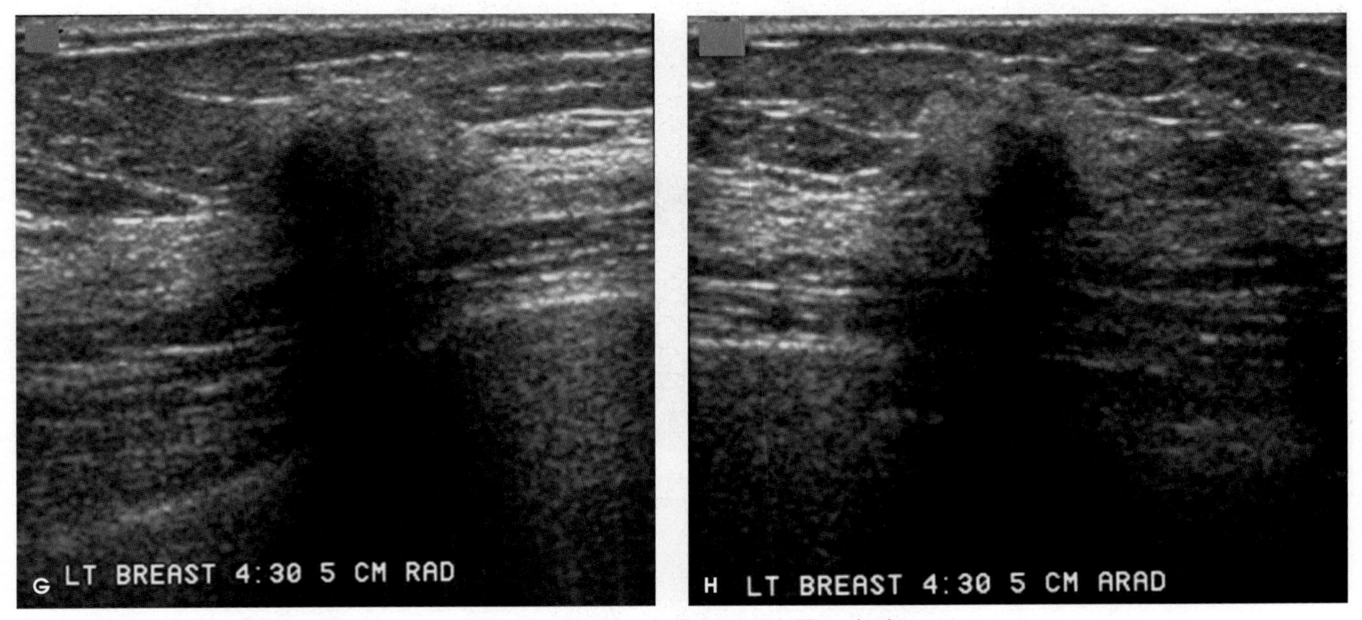

Figure 4.13. (*Continued*) Ultrasound images, radial (RAD) **(G)** and antiradial (ARAD) **(H)** projections.

PATIENT 14

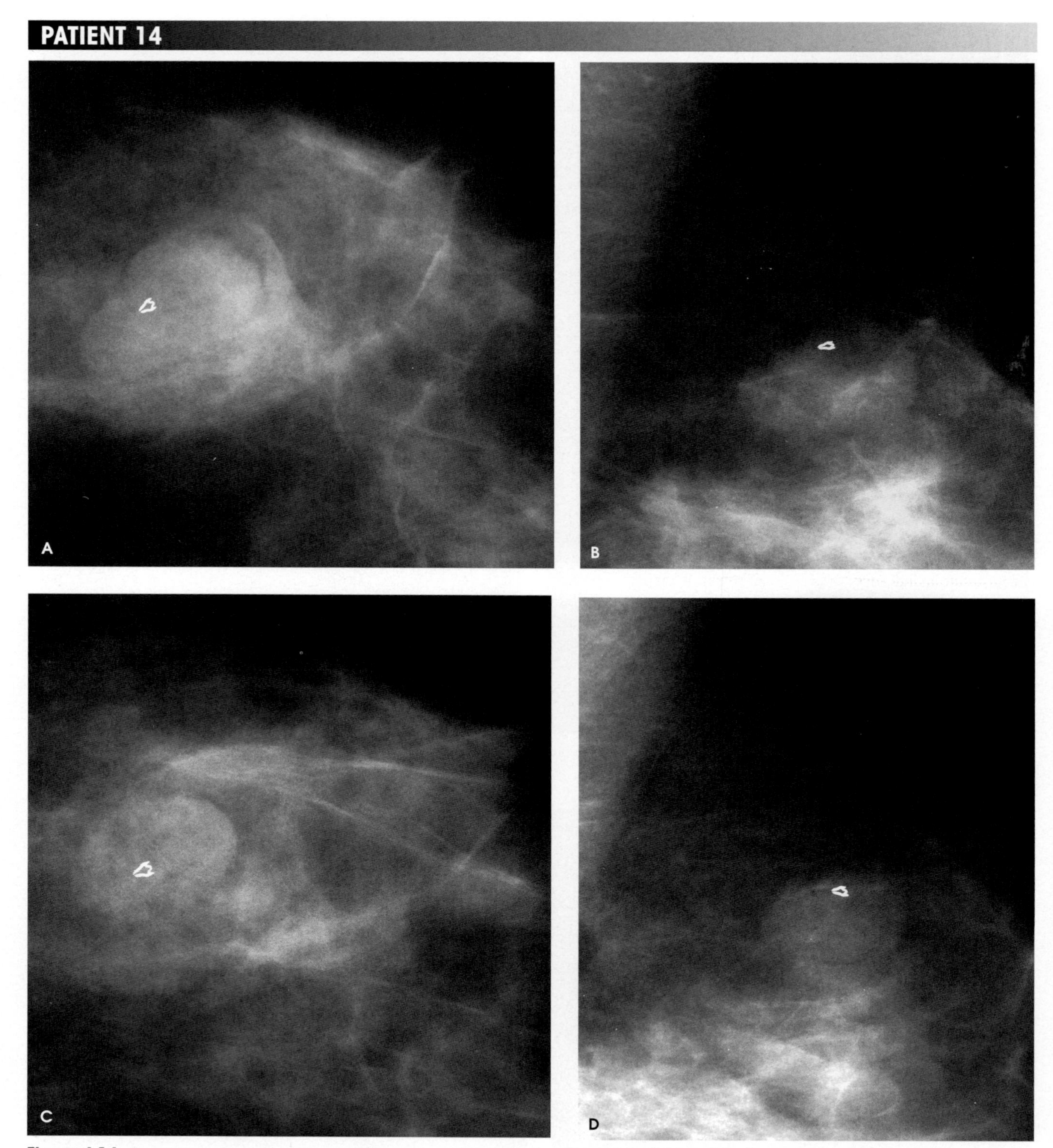

Figure 4.14. Screening mammograms, 50-year-old woman, craniocaudal **(A)** and mediolateral oblique **(B)** views, left breast, photographically coned to a mass in the upper outer quadrant of the left breast. Craniocaudal **(C)** and mediolateral oblique **(D)** views, 1 year before **(A)** and **(B),** left breast, photographically coned to the mass in the upper outer quadrant of the left breast.

How would you describe the findings, and why is there a metallic clip in the breast?

An oval, well-circumscribed mass is present in the upper outer quadrant of the left breast. A metallic clip is present in the mass, consistent with a prior imaging-guided core biopsy. Metallic clips are deployed at the time of imaging-guided biopsy procedures when complete removal of the lesion may occur as a result of the biopsy (e.g., biopsy of a cluster of calcifications or small mass using an 11G vacuum-assisted device). If the lesion is diagnosed as a malignancy or high-risk lesion, and it is removed in its entirety, the clip marks the location of the original lesion so that the tissue around the lesion can be localized and evaluated histologically for residual tumor at the time of the lumpectomy. In reviewing the prior biopsy report in this patient, a fibroadenoma is reported. The mass is now larger.

What is your recommendation at this point? Because the mass is enlarging, is an excisional biopsy indicated?

The original diagnosis of a fibroadenoma is congruent for a well-circumscribed oval mass seen mammographically. In premenopausal women, fibroadenomas can enlarge, and a change in size alone does not constitute an indication for excisional biopsy. It has been reported that volume growth rates of $<16\%$ per month in women under the age of 50 years, and 13% per month in those over the age of 50 years, or up to a 20% mean change in dimension in a 6-month interval, regardless of age, are acceptable, and the patient can be followed.

In this patient, the mass has enlarged, but the change in size falls within the acceptable limit. Nevertheless, the next step I take is to call pathology and request a review of the previous biopsy material in the context of a mass that has increased slightly in size. The pathologist confirms the diagnosis of a fibroadenoma; specifically, that the histologic findings do not suggest the possibility of a phyllodes tumor. Annual mammography is recommended for this patient.

BI-RADS® category 2: benign finding.

In most patients, the diagnosis of a fibroadenoma on core biopsy is reliable. In some women, the distinction between fibroadenoma and phyllodes tumor is an issue. In these patients, appropriate management decisions require placing the imaging findings in the proper clinical and pathologic context. Fibroadenomas are common lesions in younger, premenopausal women. Phyllodes tumors are uncommon lesions that occur predominantly in perimenopausal or postmenopausal women.

Fibroadenomas and phyllodes tumors are biphasic (fibroepithelial) lesions, arising in the lobules and characterized by proliferating epithelial and stromal elements. It is the cellularity of the stroma, not the appearance of the epithelial elements, that is used to distinguish between these lesions. In young women, fibroadenomas may be characterized as having a cellular stroma. As estrogen levels decrease with advancing age, epithelial elements and stromal cellularity in fibroadenomas normally decrease and hyalinization (i.e., fibrosis) increases. When fibroadenomas are described as "cellular," or when the descriptive term "hypercellular stroma" is used relative to a fibroadenoma, particularly if it is an older, perimenopausal or postmenopausal patient, a direct discussion with the pathologist regarding the possibility of phyllodes tumor is helpful. If the distinction cannot be made reliably based on the core samples, excisional biopsy is recommended.

PATIENT 15

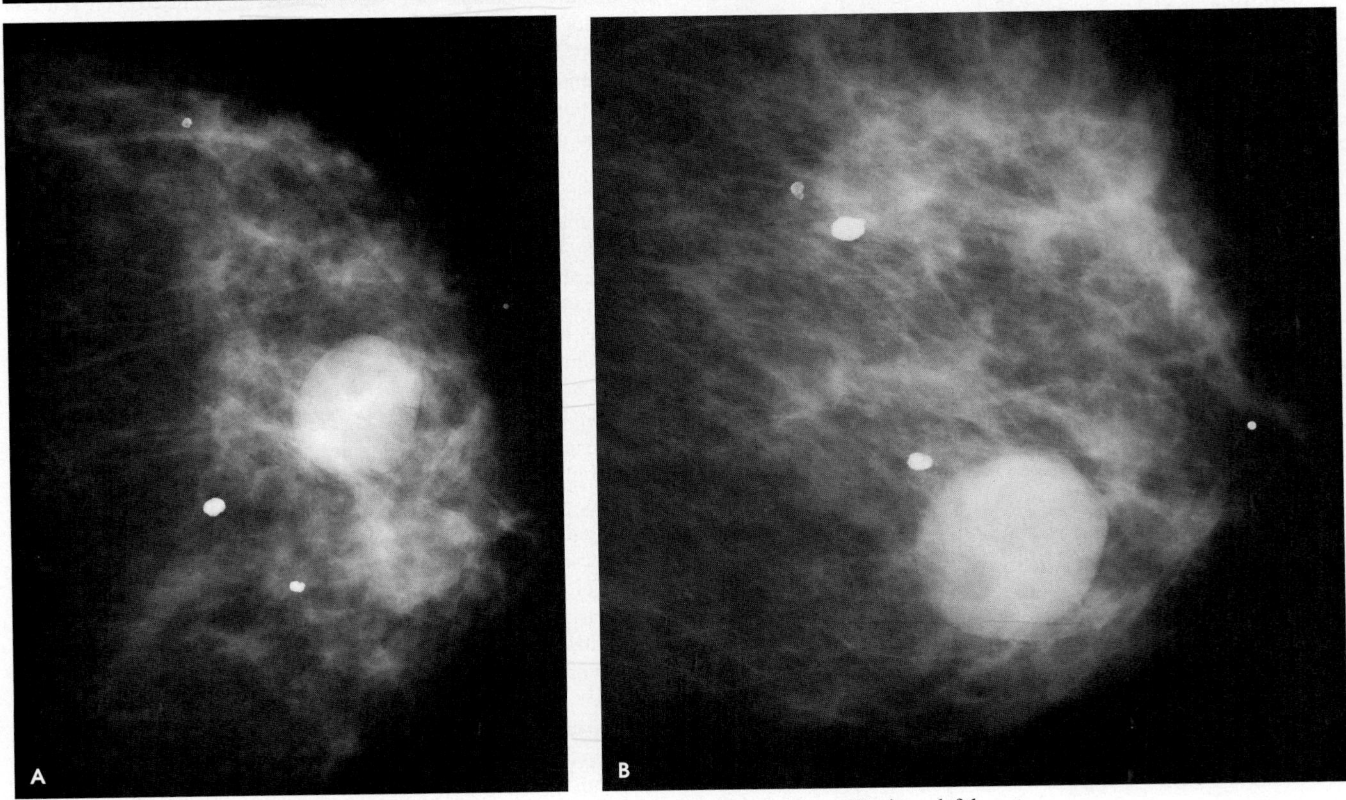

Figure 4.15. Screening study, 62-year-old woman. Craniocaudal **(A)** and mediolateral oblique **(B)** views, left breast.

What do you think? What would you do next?

Dense glandular tissue with several coarse calcifications, possibly reflecting fibroadenomas undergoing hyalinization and calcification, is noted. Additionally, there is a round, well-circumscribed mass in the lower outer quadrant of the left breast. Prior films would be helpful in determining the next appropriate step.

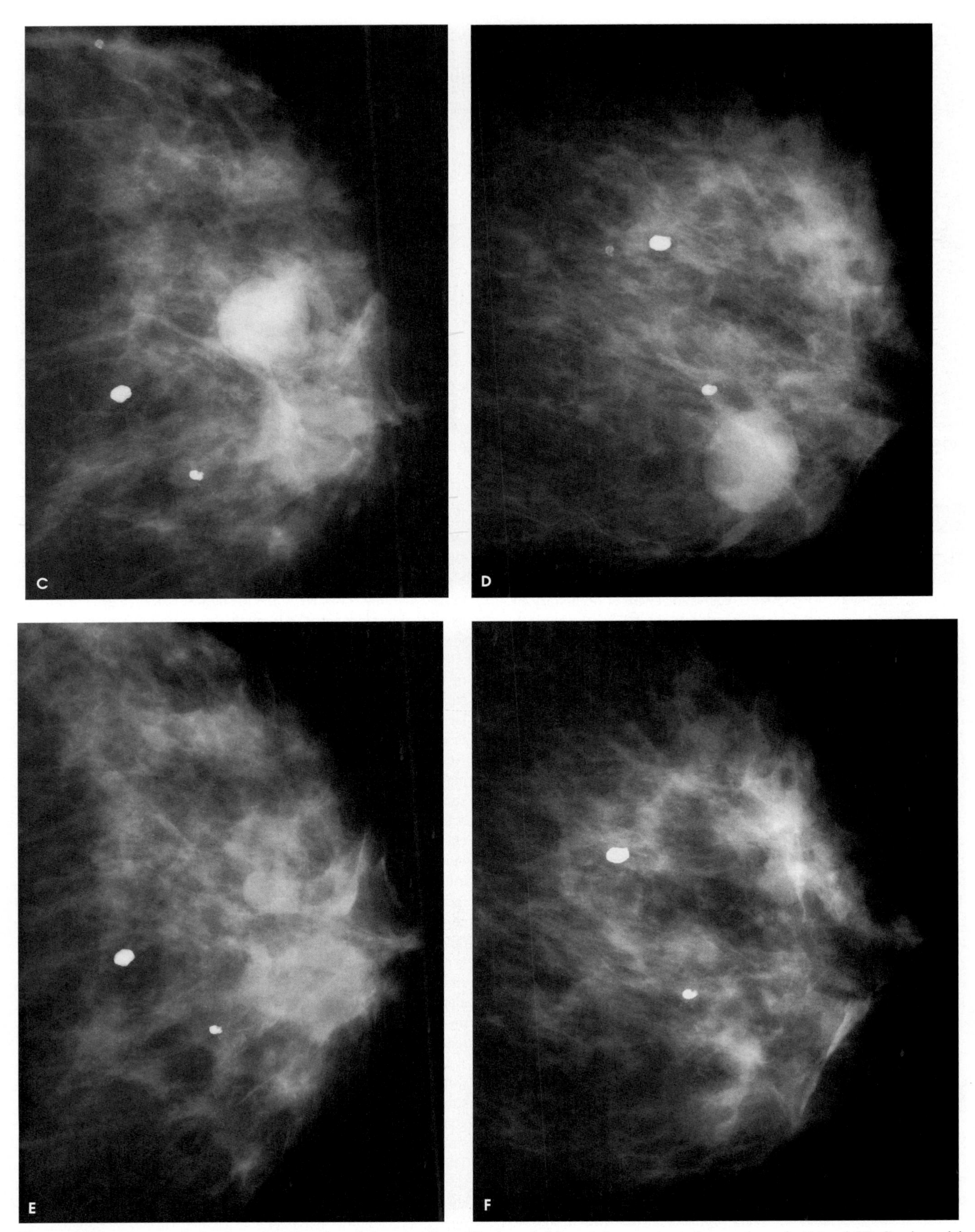

Figure 4.15. (*Continued*) Craniocaudal **(C)** and mediolateral oblique **(D)** views, left breast, 1 year prior to images shown in **(A)** and **(B).** Craniocaudal **(E)** and mediolateral **(F)** views, left breast, 2 years prior to images shown in **(A)** and **(B).**

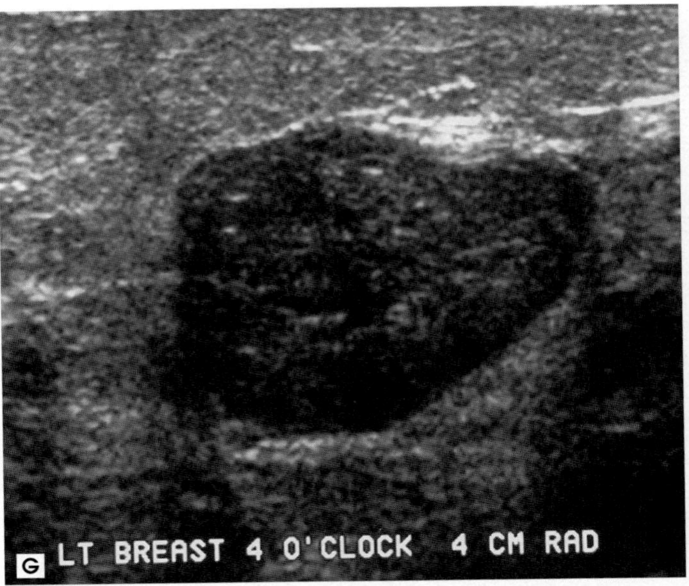

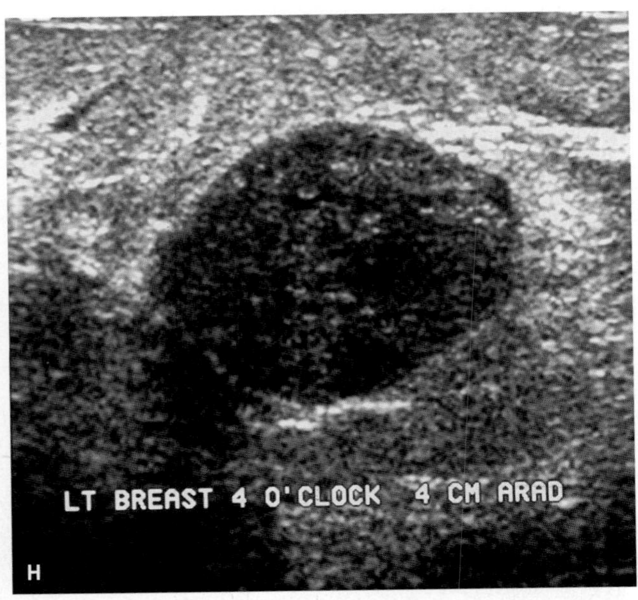

Figure 4.15. (*Continued*) Ultrasound images, radial (RAD) **(G)** and antiradial (ARAD) **(H)**, 1 year ago, at the time of **(C)** and **(D)**.

What do you think?

The solid, well-circumscribed mass in the left breast is enlarging. A fibroadenoma was reported on core samples obtained following an ultrasound-guided biopsy done 1 year ago. There is no history of hormone replacement therapy. What do you think? Are the clinical, imaging, and histologic findings congruent? Given the most recent mammogram (Fig. 4.15A, B), what is your main concern, and what would you recommend at this time?

The diagnosis of a fibroadenoma is a congruent diagnosis for a round, well-circumscribed solid mass, particularly in younger, premenopausal patients. In such a patient, an increase in the size of a fibroadenoma diagnosed with a needle biopsy is not an absolute indication for excision unless the change in size is significant. In a 61-year-old woman, however, particularly if she is not on hormone replacement therapy, the diagnosis of a fibroadenoma should be considered carefully and discussed with the pathologist directly. Fibroadenomas may develop in the early postmenopausal period, particularly if a patient is started on hormone replacement therapy. They are not expected to develop and enlarge years following menopause in a patient with no history of hormone replacement therapy. The pathologist should be asked specifically about the possibility of a phyllodes tumor. In this postmenopausal patient, the original diagnosis should have been challenged and now, a year later, as you review all available studies and note the progressive change in the size of this mass, an excisional biopsy is indicated.

A benign phyllodes tumor is diagnosed on the excised tissue.

What are phyllodes tumors, and how do they present?

Phyllodes tumors are rare, representing between 0.3% and 1% of all breast tumors. They are biphasic (fibroepithelial) tumors, diagnosed more commonly in perimenopausal and postmenopausal patients. The median age (45 years) of patients with phyllodes tumors is approximately 15 years higher than the median age of women who present with fibroadenomas. Phyllodes tumors commonly present as a single, well-circumscribed, hard mass; rarely, patients may present with multiple phyllodes tumors in one or both breasts. These tumors develop from lobules, and their resemblance to fibroadenomas has led some to suggest that they arise from preexisting fibroadenomas. Alternatively, some have postulated that they arise de novo.

Histologically, phyllodes tumors are characterized by the presence of clefts or cystic spaces lined by epithelial cells and a cellular stroma. The epithelial elements in these lesions are normal and similar to those seen in fibroadenomas. It is the appearance of the stroma that is used to distinguish phyllodes tumors from fibroadenomas. Attempts have been made to subclassify phyllodes tumors into malignant, benign, and borderline lesions based on their margins, stromal cellularity and overgrowth, stromal cell atypia, and mitotic activity. Features that are suggestive of malignancy include the presence of infiltrative margins, marked stromal cellular overgrowth, moderate to marked atypia of the stromal cells, and 10 or more mitotic figures per 10 high-power fields. Features of benign tumors include expansile margins, moderate stromal cellularity, minimal atypia of the stromal cells, and 0 to 4 mitoses per 10 high-power fields. A borderline tumor is described when a lesion demonstrates expansile or infiltrative margins, moderate atypia of the stromal cells, and 5 to 9 mitoses per 10 high-power fields. Rarely, sarcomatous elements including angiosarcoma, liposarcoma, chondrosarcoma, myosarcoma, or osteosarcoma are described in the stroma of phyllodes tumors.

It is important to emphasize that fibroadenomas in younger women are characterized by the presence of epithelial elements and a stroma that may be described as cellular. As patients age, and estrogen levels decrease, the epithelial elements and cellularity of the stroma decrease, and fibrosis and hyalinization of the lesion occurs. The diagnosis of a "cellular" fibroadenoma is acceptable in young women (teens and 20s, early 30s), but care should be exercised in accepting the diagnosis of a "cellular" fibroadenoma, or one characterized as having a "hypercellular stroma," in perimenopausal and postmenopausal women. In this latter group of patients, the pathologist needs to be asked specifically about the possibility of a phyllodes tumor, and if this is a concern, excisional biopsy is appropriate.

Local recurrence is the main concern in patients diagnosed with a phyllodes tumor, but distant metastases and death can occur. Wide surgical excision is critical in minimizing the likelihood of local recurrence. A hematogenous route of spread is described in patients with metastatic disease. Consequently, axillary dissections are not indicated for patients with phyllodes tumors. Benign phyllodes tumors do not usually metastasize, have a lower incidence of local recurrence, and the interval to recurrence is longer.

PATIENT 16

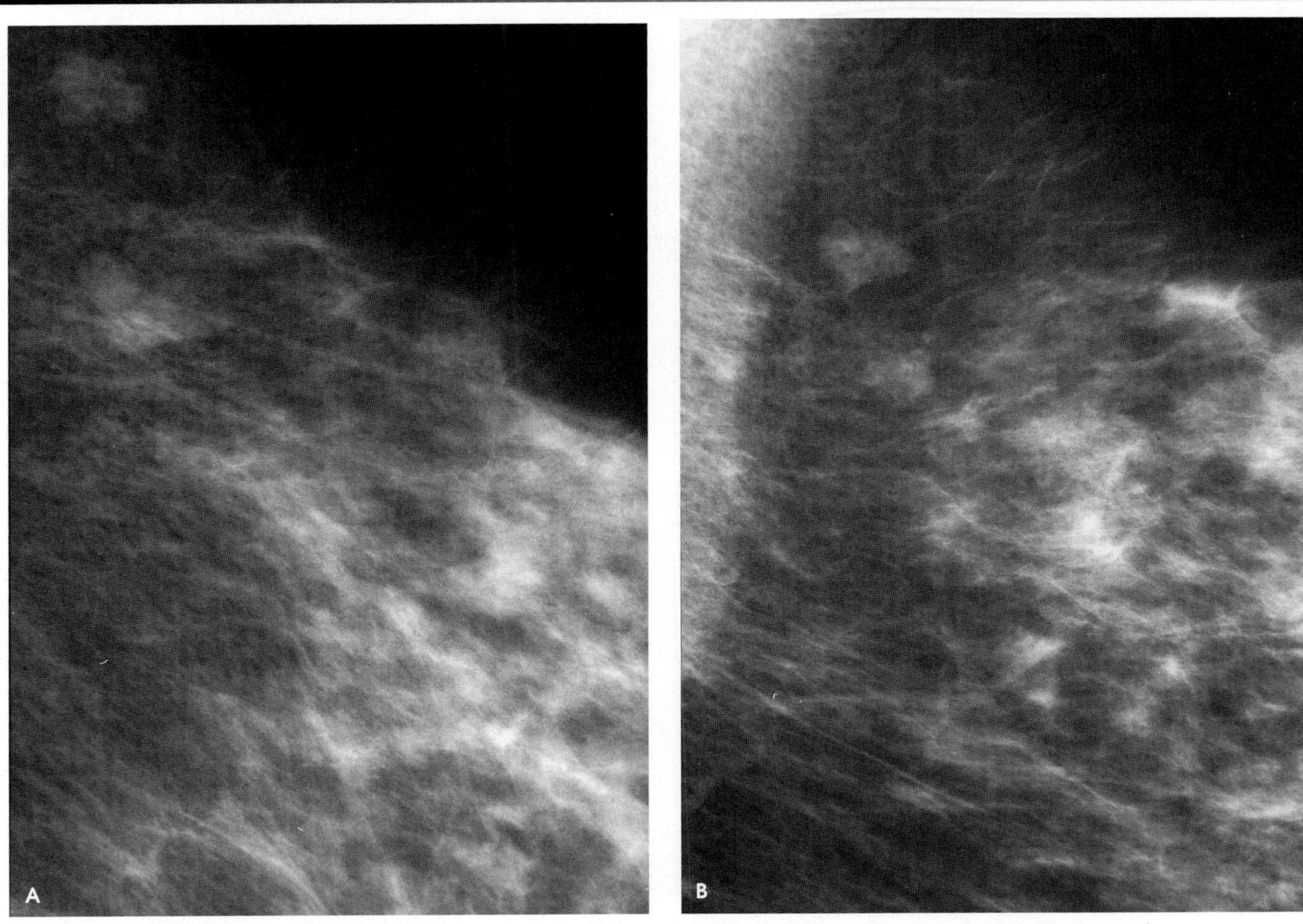

Figure 4.16. Screening study, 64-year-old woman. Left craniocaudal **(A)** and mediolateral oblique **(B)** views, photographically coned.

How would you describe the findings?

Two masses are present in the upper outer quadrant of the left breast. The more superior and lateral of the lesions is characterized by microlobulated and irregular margins. The second mass has partially well circumscribed margins. Compared with prior studies (not shown), these findings represent a change. Imaging-guided biopsy is done of the more superior and lateral of the lesions. A sclerosing lesion with associated atypical ductal hyperplasia and mucin dissecting in the sclerosing lesion and adjacent stroma is reported on the cores.

Is this congruent with the imaging findings? At this point, what is your recommendation for this patient and why?

The mammographic and histologic findings are congruent. However, with a sclerosing lesion, atypical ductal hyperplasia, and dissecting mucin reported in the lesion and stroma, an excisional biopsy is recommended. Both masses, seen mammographically, are excised following wire localization (Fig. 4.16C, D). An intraductal papilloma with apocrine atypical ductal hyperplasia and adjacent mucocele-like tumor were reported for the lesion biopsied previously. An intraductal papilloma with no atypia is reported for the second excised mass.

What are mucocele-like lesions of the breast, and how should they be managed following diagnosis on core biopsy?

Mucocele-like lesions of the breast are made up of multiple cysts or dilated ducts containing mucinous material that is extruded into the surrounding stroma. The epithelial cells lining these cysts or ducts are uniformly flat or cuboidal to columnar in appearance. Although they were initially described as benign lesions, there are now reports in the literature of associated atypical ductal hyperplasia, ductal carcinoma in situ (DCIS), or invasive carcinoma with some of these lesions. The associated DCIS is usually micropapillary or cribriform type, and the invasive lesion is usually mucinous carcinoma. Consequently, the diagnosis of a mucocele-like lesion, or the presence of mucinous material dissecting in the stroma on core biopsy samples, should prompt consideration of an excisional biopsy of the lesion.

What imaging findings have been reported for mucocele-like lesions of the breast?

In screening programs, these lesions are usually diagnosed on core biopsies done for indeterminate or suspicious microcalcifications; some of the described calcifications are coarse and eggshell-shaped. Masses with margins ranging from well circumscribed to indistinct, with or without associated calcifications, have also been reported. On ultrasound, cysts with noncalcified or calcified mural nodules, hypoechoic masses characterized by low-level internal echoes, or tubular structures with low-level internal echoes may be seen in these patients.

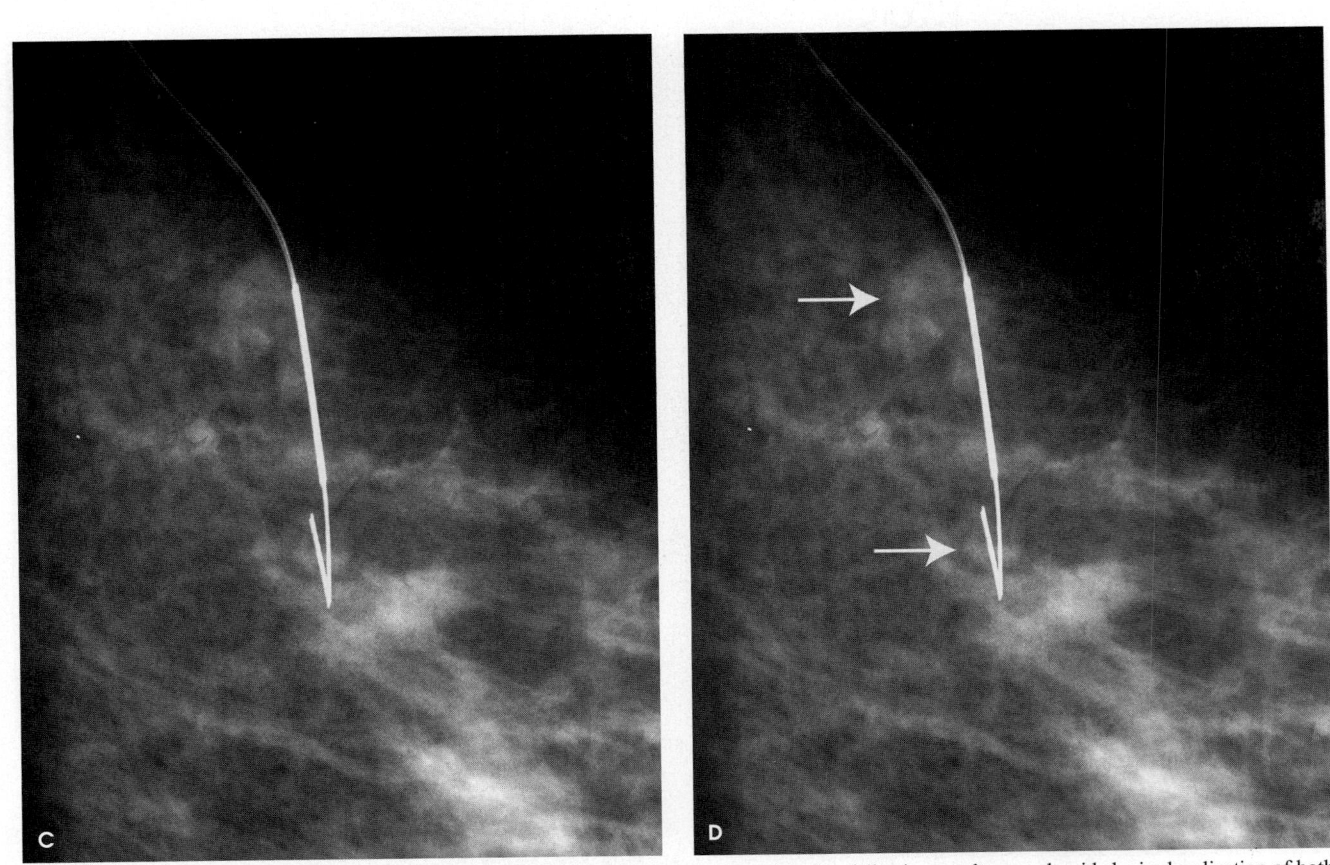

Figure 4.16. (*Continued*) Ninety-degree lateral **(C)** view documenting final wire positioning following an ultrasound-guided wire localization of both lesions [*arrows* in **(D)**] in the upper outer quadrant of the left breast.

PATIENT 17

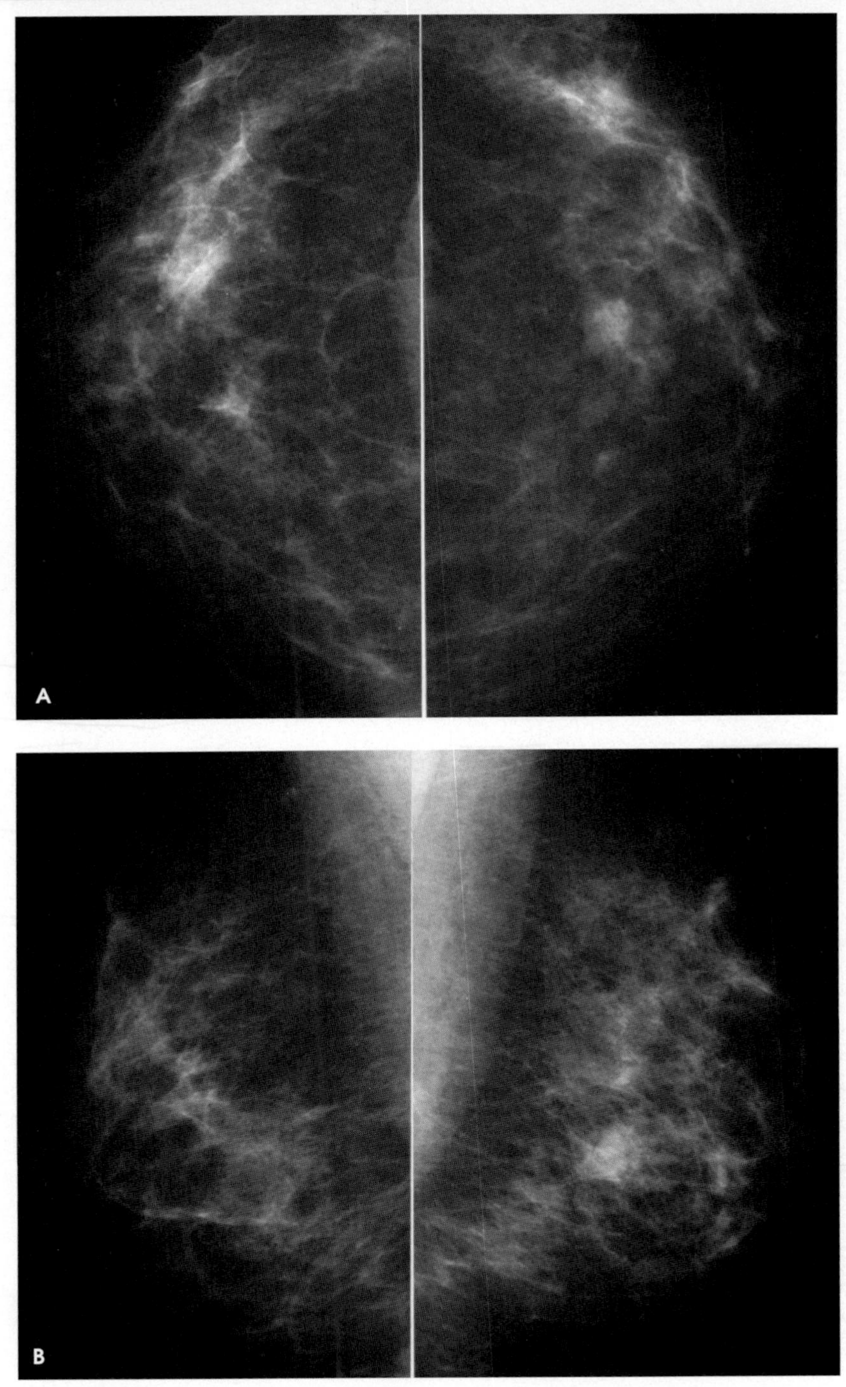

Figure 4.17. Screening study, 42-year-old woman. Craniocaudal **(A)** and mediolateral oblique **(B)** views.

What do you think?

A potential mass is described in the left breast. If no prior films are available, or if this finding represents an interval change, the patient should be called back for spot compression views and possibly an ultrasound.

BI-RADS® category 0: need additional imaging evaluation.

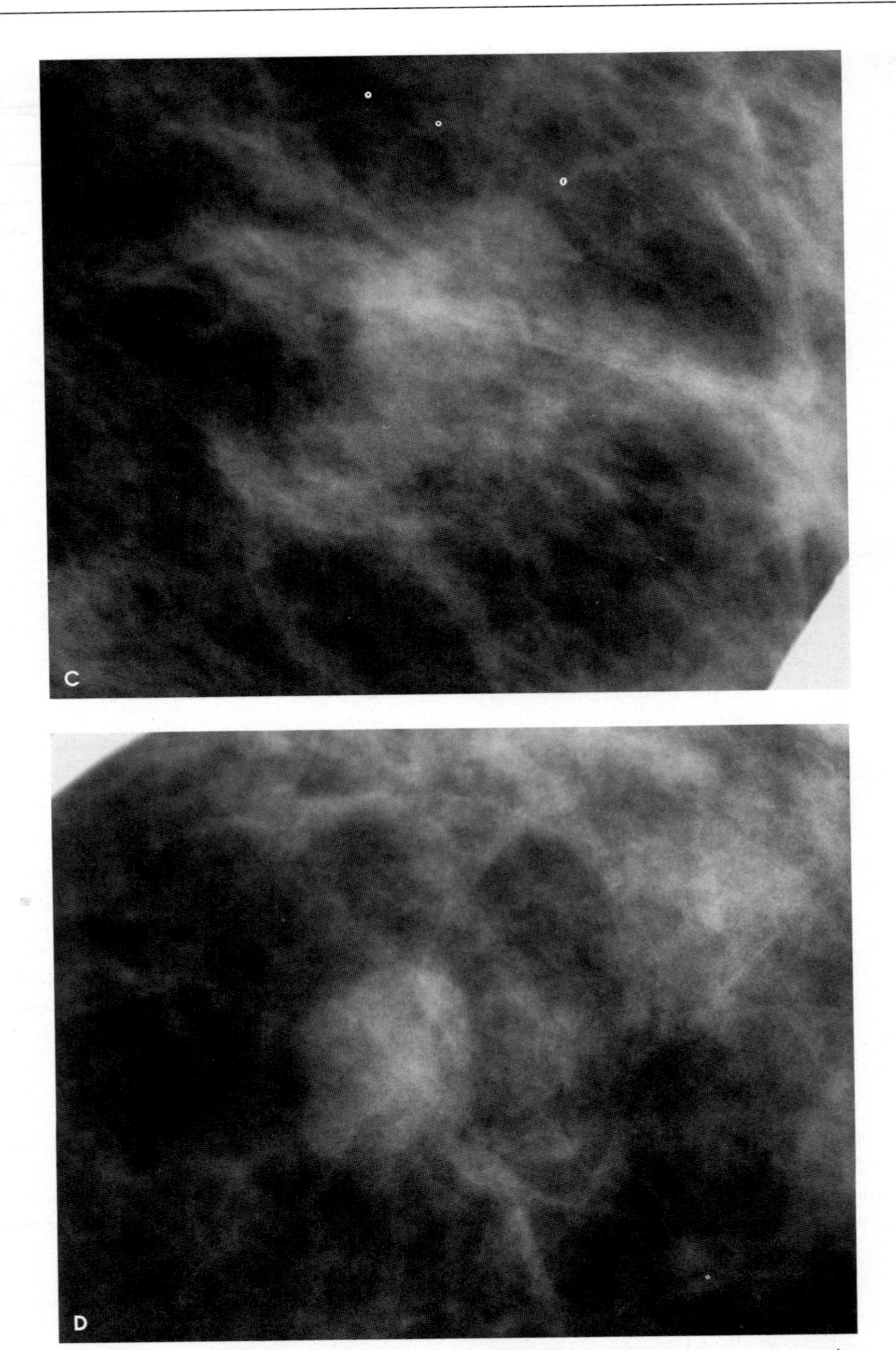

Figure 4.17. (*Continued*) Craniocaudal **(C)** and mediolateral oblique **(D)** spot compression views, left breast.

What do you think now, and what would you recommend next?
At what clock position would you place the ultrasound transducer to find this mass?

A mass is confirmed on the spot compression views. Although the margins are obscured on the craniocaudal projection, they are better seen and appear partially well circumscribed on the oblique projection. Benign considerations in a 42-year-old woman include cyst, fibroadenoma (complex fibroadenoma, tubular adenoma), papilloma, focal fibrosis, pseudoangiomatous stromal hyperplasia, papilloma, adenosis tumor, phyllodes tumor, and granular cell tumor. Depending on history and clinical findings, an inflammatory process, posttraumatic/postsurgical fluid collection, and a galactocele might also be included in the differential. Malignant considerations include invasive ductal not otherwise specified, medullary carcinoma, or metastatic disease. Although they are less likely given the patient's age, mucinous and papillary carcinomas are also in the differential.

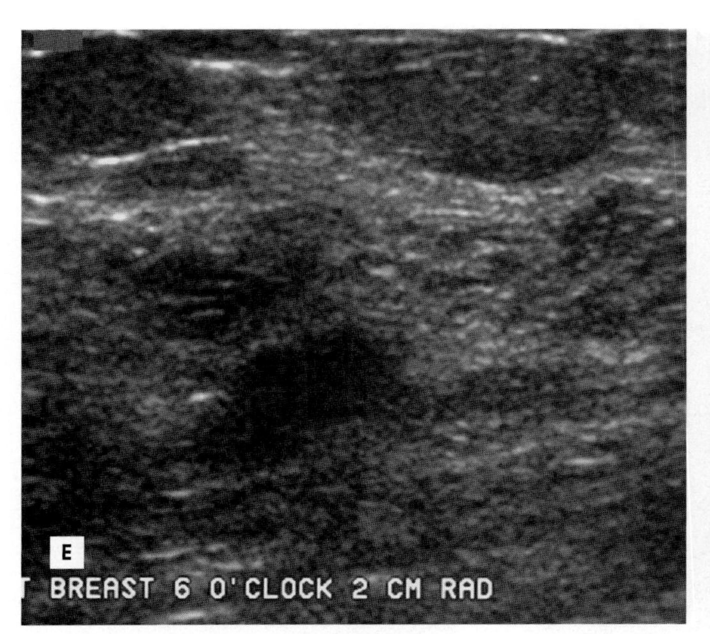

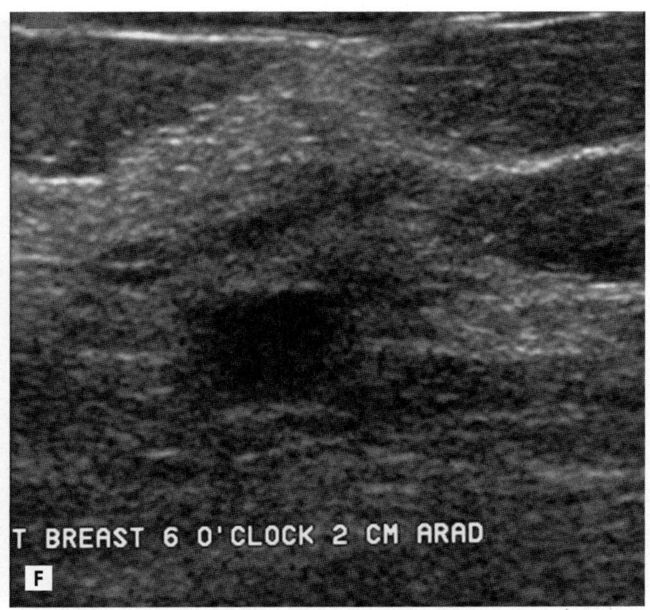

Figure 4.17. (*Continued*) Ultrasound images, radial (RAD) **(E)** and antiradial (ARAD) **(F)** projections corresponding to the area of mammographic concern, 6 'clock position, 2 cm from the left nipple.

What do you think based on the ultrasound images, and what is your recommendation?

On ultrasound, a hypoechoic oval mass is imaged at the 6 o'clock position, 2 cm from the left nipple, corresponding to the mammographic finding. The margins are not well defined and there is no posterior acoustic enhancement; although you may be tempted to call this a cyst, it does not fulfill the diagnostic criteria for a cyst and therefore further evaluation is indicated.

How would you approach this patient's evaluation?

For patients in whom a cyst is a possibility, I approach their interventional procedures in a stepwise manner. The first step, after injecting lidocaine in the skin and expected needle course, is to attempt an aspiration. If no fluid is obtained, or a residual abnormality is noted following aspiration, I do core biopsies through the mass. In this patient, no fluid is aspirated and atypical ductal hyperplasia (ADH), apocrine type, is reported on the core biopsies.

Is this histology concordant with the imaging findings? What would you recommend next, and why?

Pleomorphic calcifications with round, punctate, and amorphous forms are the most common mammographic finding reflecting the presence of atypical ductal hyperplasia (ADH) and ductal carcinoma in situ (DCIS). Rarely, ADH and DCIS can present as parenchymal asymmetry, distortion, or a mass with well-circumscribed, often macrolobulated margins that may be further characterized as indistinct and sometimes spiculated. So the diagnosis of ADH in this patient with a mass is concordant. However, depending on whether a 14G automated spring-loaded or an 11G vacuum-assisted device is used for sampling, ADH is upgraded to DCIS or invasive ductal carcinoma on excision in as many as 56% and 27% of patients, respectively. Consequently, excisional biopsy is the appropriate management of patients diagnosed with ADH on core biopsy, regardless of the finding (e.g., calcifications, mass, or distortion).

In this patient, an excisional biopsy is done following an ultrasound-guided preoperative wire localization of the mass in the left breast. A 1.1-cm ductal carcinoma in situ, apocrine type, is diagnosed in the excised tissue [pTis, pNX, PMX; Stage 0].

PATIENT 18

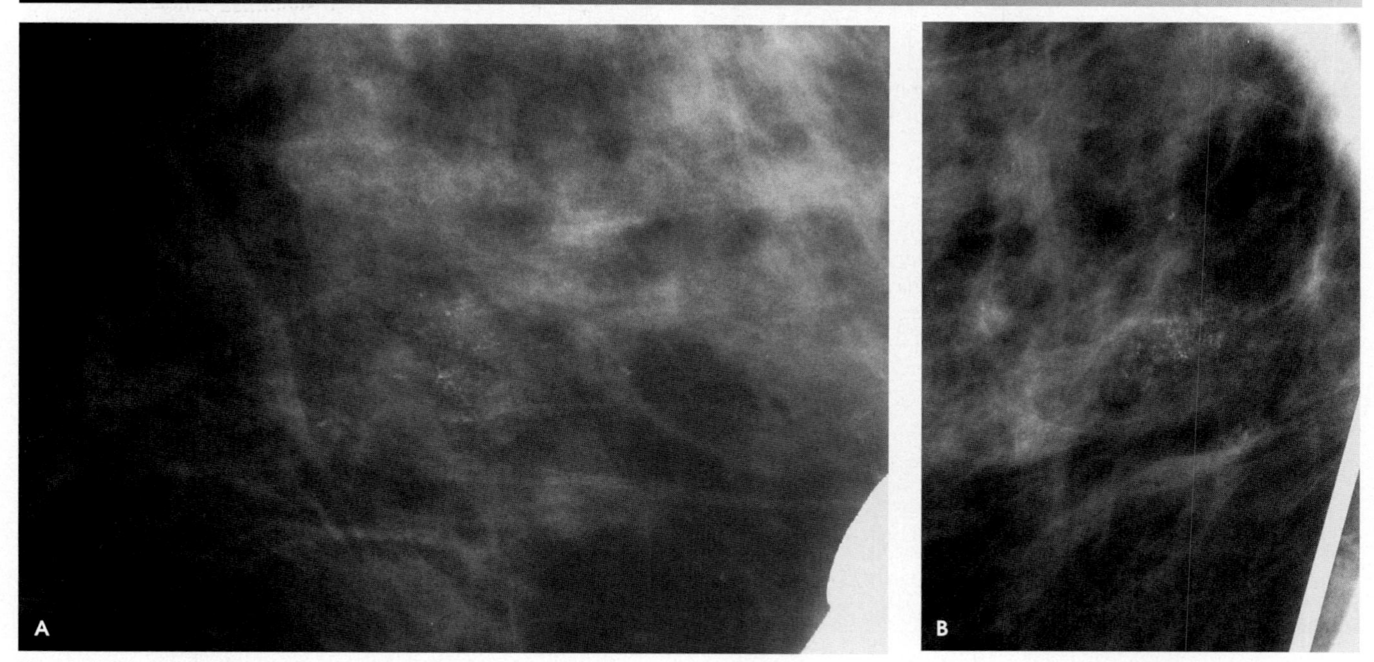

Figure 4.18. Diagnostic evaluation, 72-year-old patient called back for evaluation of calcifications detected in the left breast on her screening mammogram. Craniocaudal **(A)** and mediolateral oblique **(B)** double spot compression magnification views, left breast.

How would you describe the findings?

A cluster of round, punctate, and amorphous calcifications is confirmed on the double spot compression magnification views. No linear forms, linear orientation, or change in configuration of the calcifications (i.e., no milk of calcium) is noted on the magnification views. Fibrocystic changes including hyperplasia, atypical ductal hyperplasia, columnar alteration with prominent apical snouts and secretions (CAPSS), and sclerosing adenosis, as well as fibroadenoma, papilloma, and ductal carcinoma in situ (usually low- or intermediate-nuclear-grade) are in the differential for this cluster of calcifications. Biopsy is indicated.

BI-RADS® 4: suspicious abnormality, biopsy should be considered.

Stereotactically guided core biopsies are done on this patient. Depending on the size of the lesion, the needle used (e.g., 14G, 11G, 8G), the number of cores taken, and the device used for the biopsy (e.g., vacuum-assisted or wire basket), the lesion may actually be completely "excised" during the biopsy. If this is a possibility, a metallic clip needs to be deployed at the time of the biopsy so that the location of the original lesion is marked. If a malignancy or a high-risk lesion is diagnosed, the clip deployed at the time of the imaging-guided biopsy can be used to localize the area for excision and further histological evaluation. Craniocaudal and 90-degree lateral views are obtained after a clip is deployed to document the location of the clip immediately following the biopsy. In this patient, a 14G needle in a spring-loaded device is used for the biopsy. Complete removal of the lesion is not expected, so no clip is deployed. Atypical ductal hyperplasia with associated microcalcifications arising in a background of columnar alteration with prominent apical snouts and secretions (CAPSS) is reported on the core biopsy.

What is indicated next?

A diagnosis of atypical ductal hyperplasia on core biopsy requires excisional biopsy. This is done following preoperative wire localization of the calcifications in the left breast.

The calcifications are confirmed to be in the specimen (Fig. 4.18C). Based on this radiograph, the location of the calcifications is marked for the pathologist. Residual atypical ductal hyperplasia arising in a background of columnar alteration with prominent apical snouts and secretions (CAPSS) with associated microcalcifications is reported on the excised tissue. The pathologist comments that "The area of CAPSS is partially involved with a monotonous low-grade cell population which is insufficient in extent for a diagnosis of low-grade ductal carcinoma in situ." Atypical ductal hyperplasia (ADH) is considered a high-risk marker lesion. Patients with ADH have four to five times increased risk for developing breast cancer compared to the reference population. This risk is increased further in women with ADH and a family history of breast cancer.

A contiguous layer of epithelial cells and an intermittent basilar layer of myoepithelial cells line the basement membrane of normal ducts and lobules in the breast. *Hyperplasia* refers to an increase in the number of cells (usually epithelial, though in some processes it is the myoepithelial cells that are hyperplastic) lining the ducts. In *usual hyperplasia,* the number of epithelial cells lining the ducts is increased and secondary spaces in the ducts are irregular in size and shape and commonly elongated or slitlike. In *atypical ductal hyperplasia,* the number of cells lining the ducts is increased, and secondary spaces of varying sizes and shapes, though somewhat more rigid and fixed than those seen in usual hyperplasia, are present in the duct. These proliferative changes in the duct can progress to *ductal carcinoma in situ* (usually low- or intermediate-nuclear-grade), characterized by a monomorphic cell population and rigid secondary spaces in the duct. Descriptive terms used for these types of DCIS include *cribriform, micropapillary,* and *solid*. This spectrum of cellular changes in the duct is not typically associated with rapid cell proliferation or central necrosis. The calcifications that develop in association with these proliferative processes develop in secretions (not in necrotic debris). The resulting calcifications are typically variable in density (possibly reflecting the variably sized spaces in which they develop) and pleomorphic, including round, punctate, and in some patients amorphous (tiny calcifications below the resolution obtainable with magnification views in a patient).

These processes involve the duct in a multifocal manner so that in some patients you can have hyperplasia next to DCIS, next to another area of hyperplasia, next to ADH, etc. Several studies have reported the presence of ADH in a peripheral location to areas of DCIS. In some patients, the proliferative changes have no associated calcifications. In other patients, the proliferative changes have associated calcifications but these are not necessarily closely associated with the malignant cells. Consequently, when you target these calcifications you may or may not be targeting the malignant cells. Additionally, the distinction between ADH and DCIS can be problematic, particularly given the small amounts of tissue submitted following imaging-guided needle biopsies. There is a need to increase the number and size (e.g., 14G vs. 11G) of the cores and a need to recommend excision if ADH is reported following core biopsies.

The complexity of the situation in managing some patients with these processes is further compounded because, although efforts have been made to define and standardize classification schemes for these processes, the diagnosis of hyperplasia, atypical ductal hyperplasia, and low-nuclear-grade DCIS remains subjective. Also, as described in this patient, some of the criteria for DCIS may be present, but the changes are insufficient to qualify for the diagnosis. A study by Rosai in 1991 reported that there was no agreement on a diagnosis in 17 borderline cases submitted for review to five leading breast pathologists, and the diagnoses rendered in some of the cases ranged from hyperplasia to DCIS.

This spectrum of disease should be contrasted with DCIS that is characterized by rapid cell proliferation (high thymidine labeling) and central necrosis. These lesions are thought to arise de novo in the duct, without antecedent hyperplasia or atypical hyperplasia. Although these are usually high-nuclear-grade cells, some may be intermediate- or low-nuclear-grade. The cells lining these ducts are pleomorphic, do not demonstrate polarization relative to the duct lumen, and have multiple nucleoli. Mitotic figures, cell necrosis, and autophagocytosis may be seen involving the cells lining the ducts. In these patients, the malignant cells circumferentially narrow the duct lumen and there is necrotic debris in the center of the duct. The calcifications seen mammographically develop in necrotic debris and consequently are closely apposed to the malignant cells (i.e., the calcifications are molded by the proliferating cells). In targeting this type of proliferative process, when you target the calcifications you target the malignant cells. The number and size of the cores is not as critical in these patients. If you remove calcifications in your cores, you are likely to have made the diagnosis of DCIS.

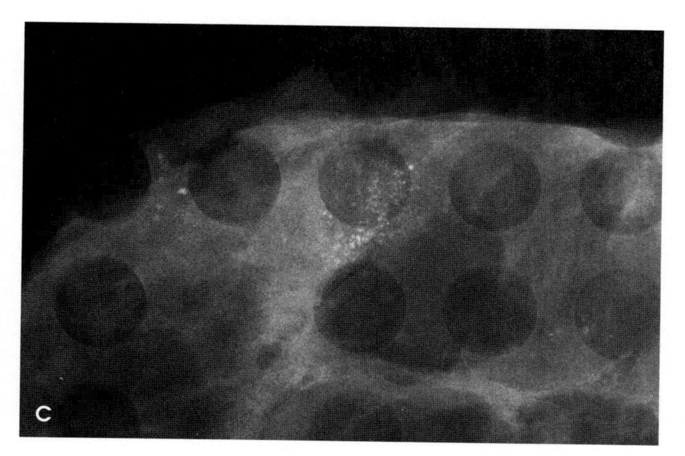

Figure 4.18. (*Continued*) Specimen radiograph **(C)** of excised tissue.

PATIENT 19

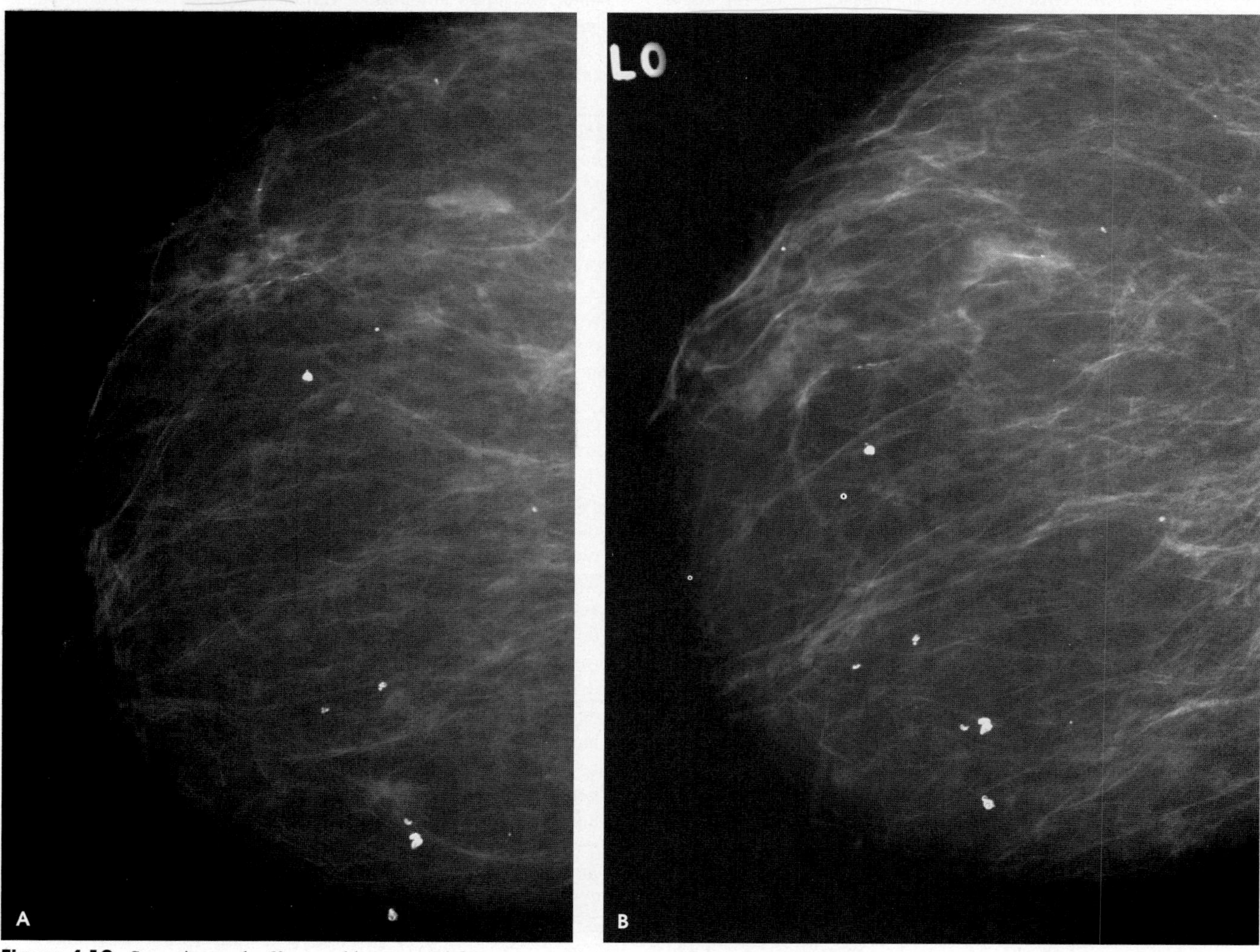

Figure 4.19. Screening study, 69-year-old woman. Right craniocaudal **(A)** and mediolateral oblique **(B)** views.

How would you describe the findings?

Several coarse, dystrophic-type calcifications are present in the right breast. Additionally, a cluster of calcifications, some of which may be linear with possible linear orientation, is noted in the upper outer quadrant of the breast anteriorly. Magnification views are indicated for further characterization.

BI-RADS® category 0: need additional imaging evaluation.

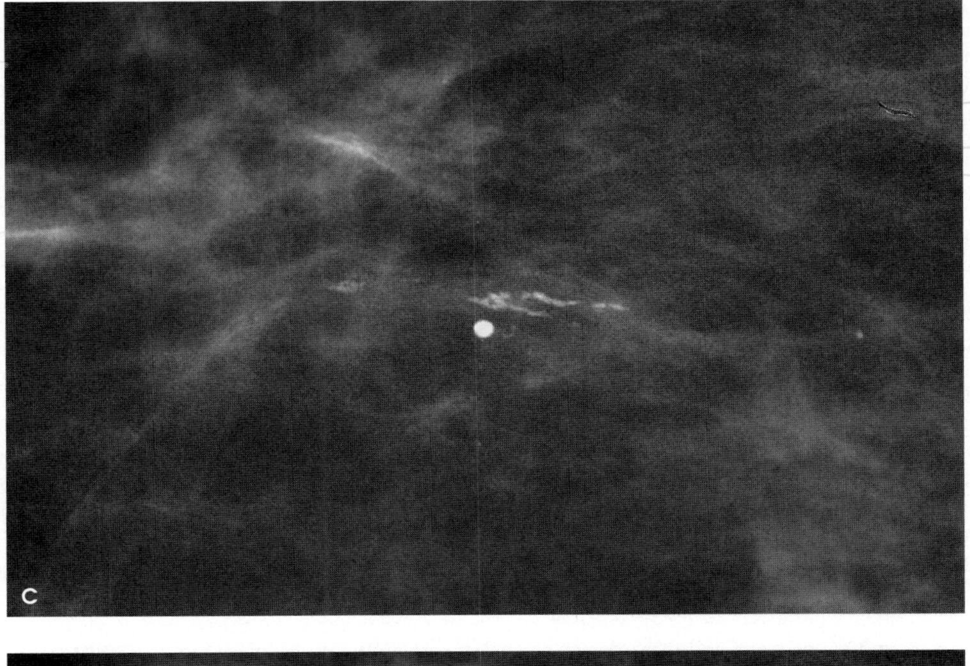

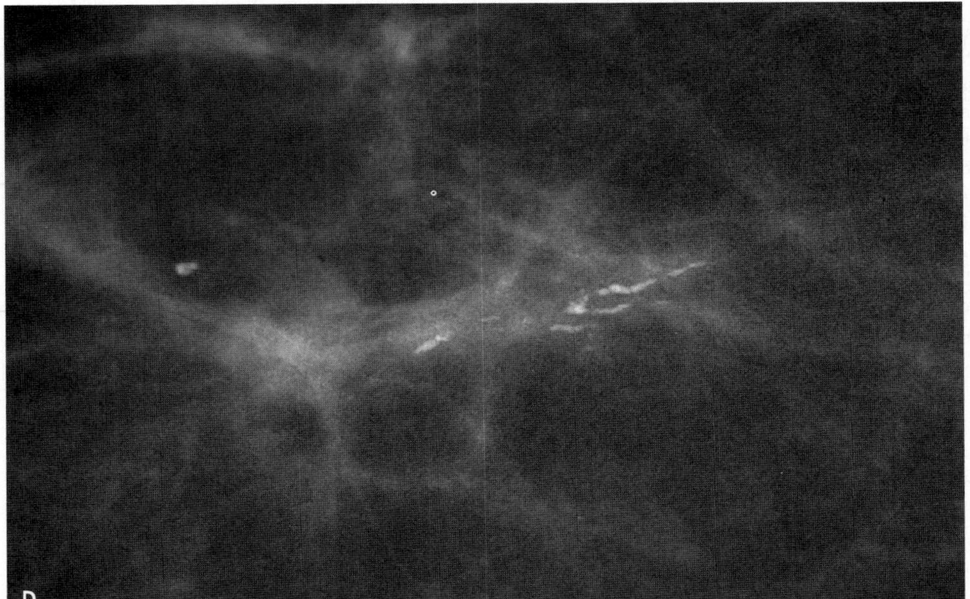

Figure 4.19. (*Continued*) Craniocaudal **(C)** and mediolateral oblique **(D),** double spot compression magnification views, right breast.

The double spot compression magnification views confirm the presence of linear calcifications demonstrating a linear orientation. The margins of these calcifications are irregular and there are associated clefts in the calcifications. Ductal carcinoma in situ (DCIS) with associated central necrosis (usually high-nuclear-grade) is the primary consideration with calcifications having these features. Biopsy is indicated.

What is your recommendation?

BI-RADS® category 4: suspicious abnormality, biopsy should be considered.

An invasive mammary carcinoma with predominantly lobular features and ductal carcinoma in situ, high-nuclear-grade, with central necrosis is diagnosed on the core samples. A 1.2-cm, grade III, invasive ductal carcinoma with associated high-nuclear-grade ductal carcinoma in situ with central necrosis is diagnosed on the lumpectomy specimen. The sentinel lymph node is negative for metastatic disease [pT1c, pN0, pMX; Stage I].

Ductal carcinoma in situ used to be considered a "rare" disease, with only scattered descriptions in the literature regarding its histologic appearance and biologic significance. With the widespread use of screening mammography, and our ability to detect and biopsy microcalcifications, DCIS now constitutes a significant proportion of the breast cancer that is diagnosed and treated. Driven by mammographic findings, our knowledge and understanding of this disease process has been significantly advanced in the last two decades. It is now recognized that DCIS is not one disease but several diseases characterized by clinical, mammographic, and biologic heterogeneity. Based on histology, biologic markers, and associated invasive lesions, we can consider at least two main paths of origins. One group of DCIS arises or evolves through proliferative changes in the duct that include hyperplasia, atypical ductal hyperplasia, and ductal carcinoma in situ. These proliferative lesions coexist and are multifocal in the involved duct. They are characterized by low rates of proliferation, long intraductal phases, and not all of the DCIS arising through this pathway is thought to progress to invasion. In some patients, these are thought to be precursors for low- or intermediate-grade invasive ductal carcinomas.

In contrast, a second group of DCIS develops in the duct without progressing through hyperplasia and atypical hyperplasia. This type of DCIS is characterized by rapid cell proliferation with high thymidine labeling rates, central necrosis in the duct, and a short intraductal phase. These types of lesions are all thought to progress to invasive disease (i.e., obligate invaders), giving rise to poorly differentiated invasive ductal carcinomas. Low-nuclear-grade DCIS is not thought to evolve (i.e., is not a precursor) to high-nuclear-grade DCIS.

Pleomorphic calcifications are the most common mammographic finding associated with DCIS. Depending on the underlying process in the duct, the calcifications have a variable appearance. In the first group of proliferative processes, the calcifications have been described as developing in secretions. Although they are pleomorphic and demonstrate variation in density, they are usually round, punctate, or amorphous. Multiple clusters may be seen. These calcifications may be associated with hyperplasia, atypical ductal hyperplasia, and DCIS (usually a low- or intermediate-grade DCIS). It is also important to recognize that these processes may be present in the breast without any associated calcifications. With this type of proliferative process, we underestimate the extent of disease in nearly 50% of patients. When doing biopsies of this type of calcification, it is important to assure adequate sampling by either increasing the number and size of the cores or even considering excisional biopsy in some patients. Removing some of the calcifications in these patients does not assure a correct diagnosis, as reflected by the high percentage of ADH that is upgraded to DCIS or invasive cancer when ADH is excised following diagnosis on core biopsy.

When there is central necrosis in the duct reflecting rapidly proliferating cells, the calcifications are often linear and may demonstrate a linear orientation. In this type of proliferative process, the calcifications are intimately associated with the malignant cells; the calcifications are being molded by the proliferating cells and develop in the necrotic debris. Targeting the calcification in essence targets the malignant cells. If calcifications are removed in one or two cores, you are likely to have made the diagnosis. Complete workups with optimal magnification views are helpful in these patients, because mammography is good at estimating the extent of the disease. Disease is found where we see the calcifications. In patients with lesions occupying several centimeters, the use of multiple wires for the preoperative localization facilitates complete removal of the lesion. Aggressive pursuit of these types of calcifications is critical because of the short intraductal phase of the disease and the almost certain, and in some patients rapid, development of invasive disease (often poorly differentiated).

PATIENT 20

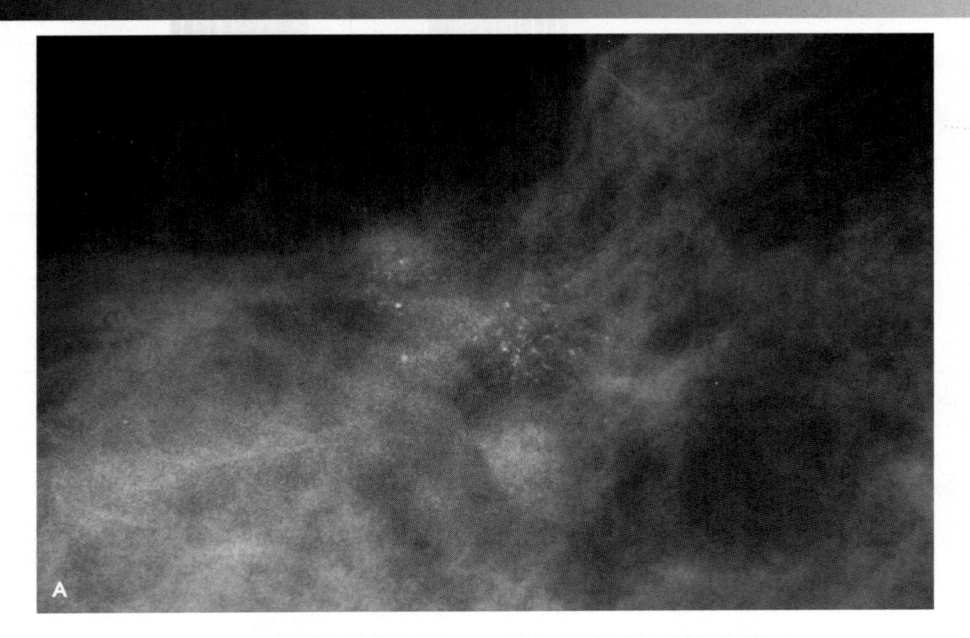

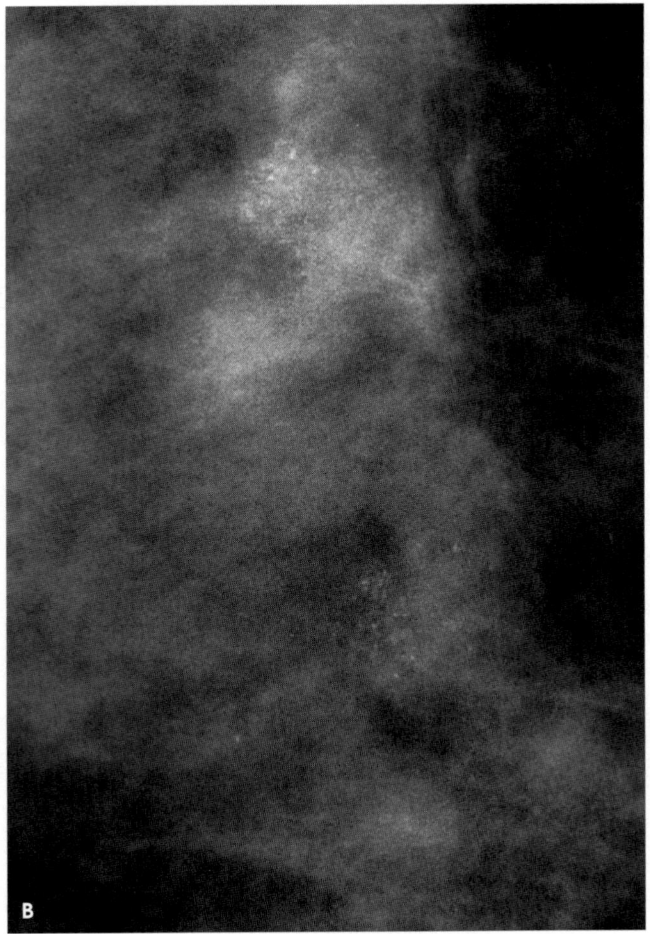

Figure 4.20. Diagnostic evaluation, 51-year-old patient called back for calcifications detected in her right breast on the screening study. Double spot compression magnification views, craniocaudal **(A)** and mediolateral oblique **(B)** projections.

How would you describe the findings?

The magnification views confirm the presence of two adjacent clusters of calcifications. The calcifications composing the clusters demonstrate pleomorphism and variable density; however, there are no linear forms and there is no linear orientation. The calcifications do not change significantly in configuration between the craniocaudal and oblique projections (i.e., these do not reflect milk of calcium). Although there are well-defined round and oval calcifications, some of these would fall under the "amorphous" terminology currently provided by the ACR lexicon. It is important to recognize that these are not really amorphous but rather tight clustering of punctate calcifications that fall below the resolution of the magnification we can obtain when imaging a patient. If these are magnified three or four times, as can be done with a specimen, some of the seemingly amorphous calcifications can be resolved into individual, tightly clustered punctate calcifications. Fibrocystic changes including hyperplasia, atypical ductal hyperplasia, columnar alteration with prominent apical snouts and secretions (CAPSS), and sclerosing adenosis, as well as fibroadenoma, papilloma, and ductal carcinoma in situ (usually low- or intermediate-nuclear grade, with no central necrosis) are in the differential for these clusters of calcifications. A biopsy is indicated.

BI-RADS® category 4: suspicious abnormality, biopsy should be considered.

A stereotactically guided core biopsy is done, and fibrocystic changes including sclerosing adenosis, CAPSS with associated atypia, and atypical lobular hyperplasia are reported on the core samples. In discussing the findings directly with the pathologist, he confirms that the calcifications are found in sclerosing adenosis and CAPSS; the atypical lobular neoplasia is noted incidentally in surrounding breast tissue, with no associated calcifications.

At this point, what do you recommend for this patient?

Given the presence of CAPSS with associated atypia, and incidentally identified atypical lobular neoplasia, excisional biopsy is recommended for this patient. No malignancy is identified on the excisional biopsy, and the patient is returned to annual screening.

Lobular neoplasia is a term used to describe a spectrum of proliferative changes in the acini of lobules that ranges from atypical lobular hyperplasia (ALH) to lobular carcinoma in situ (LCIS). Continuous with that of the ducts, a two-cell layer above the basement membrane normally lines the acini in a lobule. A contiguous epithelial cell layer and a basilar, intermittent myoepithelial cell layer. Hyperplasia, defined as an increase in the number of cells, is present when there are three or more cells above the basement membrane. In both ALH and LCIS, a monomorphic cell population fills, distends, and distorts the acini in the lobular unit. In ALH, filling of the acini is incomplete, other cell types may be intermixed with the monomorphic cell population, and fewer than half of the acini in the lobular unit are expanded and distorted by the proliferating cells. In LCIS, the acini are filled with a monomorphic cell population and at least half of the acini are distended and distorted by the proliferating cells. In some patients the distinction between LCIS and ductal carcinoma in situ (DCIS) may be difficult for the pathologist. Immunohistochemical staining for E-cadherin, a cell adhesion molecule, is used in some patients to distinguish lobular lesions that do not stain from ductal lesions that do stain for E-cadherin.

Lobular neoplasia is an uncommon diagnosis, reported in 0.5% to 3.8% of benign breast biopsies. It is diagnosed predominantly in premenopausal women and is characterized as a multicentric and bilateral process. Although there are now reported cases of calcifications identified in foci of lobular neoplasia, this is the exception. In most patients, lobular neoplasia is an incidental finding in biopsies done for palpable or mammographic findings. Women with lobular neoplasia are at increased risk for developing invasive ductal or lobular carcinoma within the first 10 to 15 years following the diagnosis. The increased risk reportedly applies to both breasts, though more recently there has been a report suggesting that the risk is higher in the breast diagnosed with the lobular neoplasia.

It is postulated that lobular neoplasia regresses following menopause and that these processes are marker lesions for increased risk of subsequently developing breast cancer. However, unlike DCIS, which is thought to progress to invasive disease in some women, the traditional teaching has been that lobular neoplasia is not precancerous. It is interesting to note, however, that in close to 50% of postmenopausal women diagnosed with invasive lobular carcinoma, prominent lobular neoplasia is diagnosed in association with the invasive lesion. This seems to challenge the notion that this is not a precancerous lesion and that it regresses in all patients. Alternatively, it may be that this lesion recurs in some patients.

The management of patients with lobular neoplasia diagnosed incidentally on core biopsy is evolving and remains controversial. Unfortunately, available studies at this time are limited by the relatively low number of patients reported and the potential bias built into the retrospective nature of the studies. In the past, excisional biopsy was not usually recommended for most of these patients. More recently, some investigators have suggested that excision is required if there is an overlap in the histologic features between LCIS and DCIS, if the histologic and imaging findings are discordant (e.g., if lobular neoplasia is all that is reported histologically, this may be an inadequate explanation for the findings prompting the biopsy), or in those patients in whom the lobular neoplasia coexists with another high-risk lesion. Alternatively, a growing number of authors suggest that excision should be the recommendation for this small group of patients because available reports in the literature describe malignancy in 0% to 50% of patients in whom excision is recommended following a core biopsy with incidentally noted lobular neoplasia.

PATIENT 21

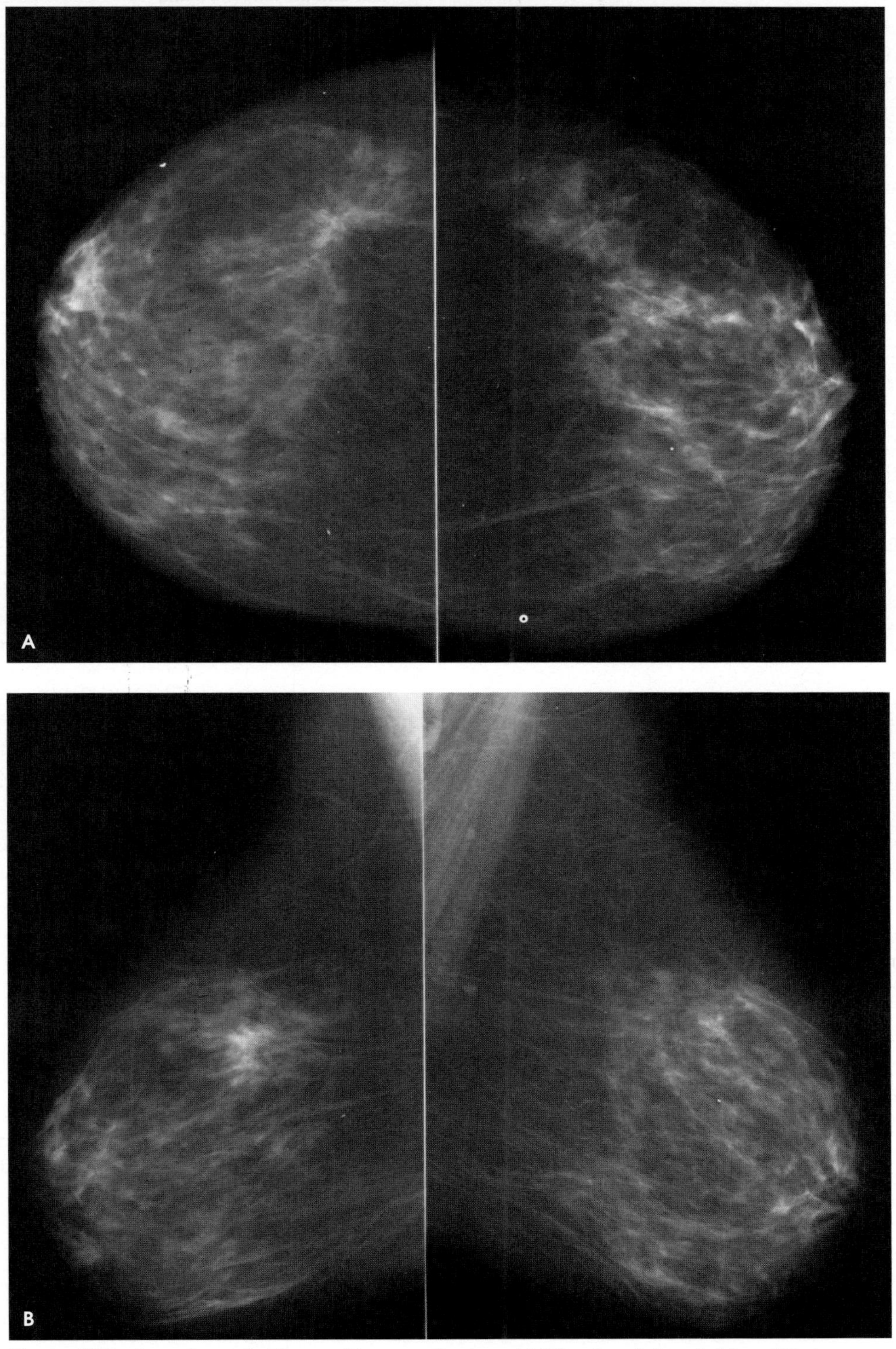

Figure 4.21. Screening study, 76-year-old woman. Craniocaudal **(A)** and mediolateral oblique **(B)** views.

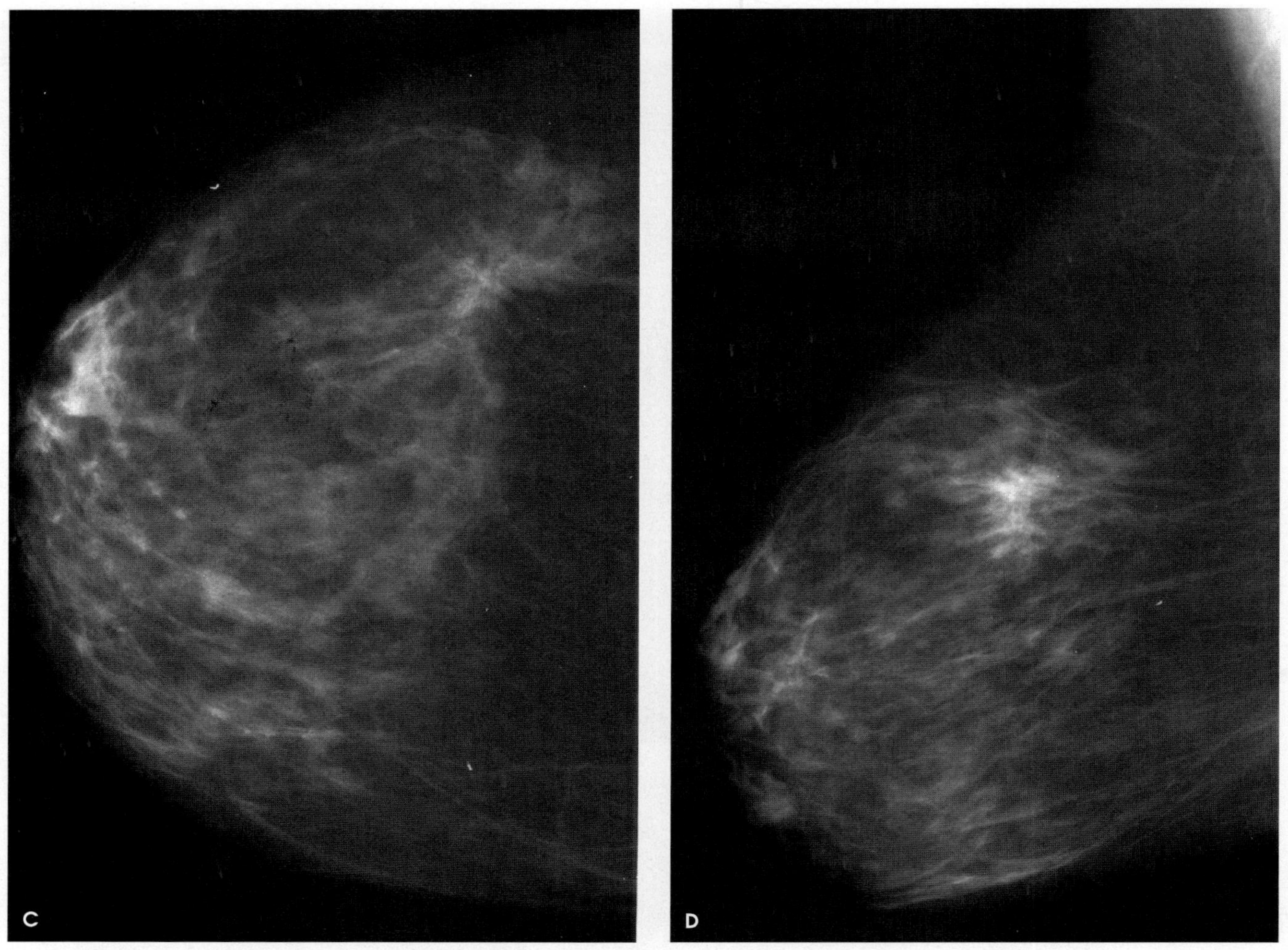

Figure 4.21. (*Continued*) Craniocaudal **(C)** and mediolateral oblique **(D)** views, right breast.

What do you think? Is this a normal study, or is additional evaluation indicated?

A possible area of distortion is imaged in the upper outer quadrant of the right breast. Additional evaluation is indicated.

BI-RADS® category 0: need additional imaging evaluation.

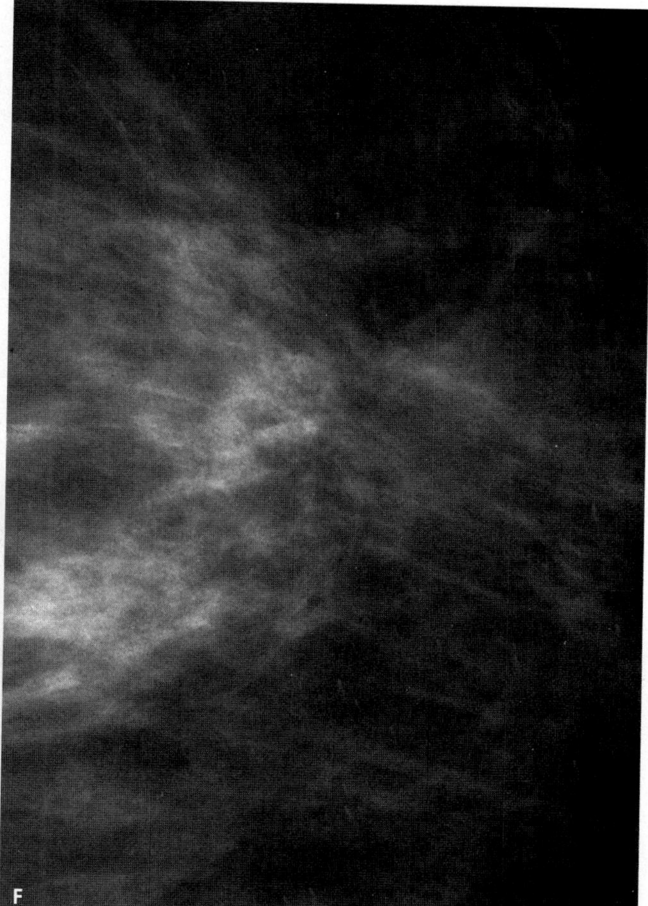

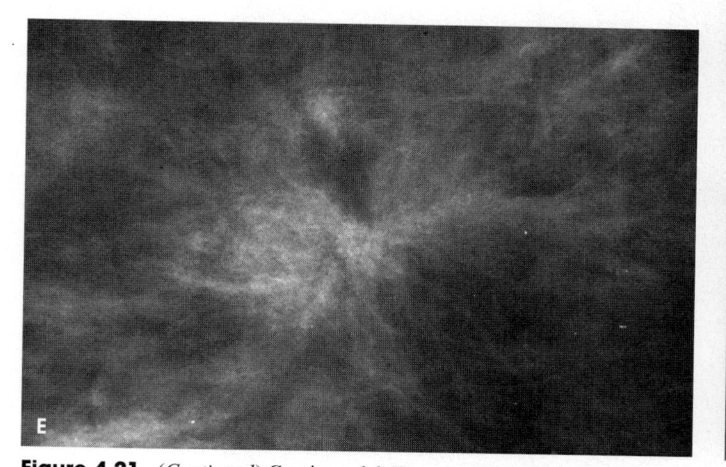

Figure 4.21. (*Continued*) Craniocaudal **(E)** and mediolateral oblique **(F)** spot compression views, right breast.

What do you think, and what is your differential?

The spot compression views confirm the presence of distortion. The finding is readily apparent on the craniocaudal view and although it is identifiable on the oblique spot compression view, it is less striking. Differential considerations include fat necrosis related to prior surgery or trauma, complex sclerosing lesion, sclerosing adenosis, papilloma, focal fibrosis, an inflammatory process, invasive ductal carcinoma not otherwise specified, tubular carcinoma, and invasive lobular carcinoma. Rarely, ductal carcinoma in situ can present with distortion in the absence of calcifications. On physical examination, no scar is identified at the expected location of the distortion and no tenderness is elicited with compression. Given the Leborgne sign, which is that on palpation invasive ductal carcinomas are larger than what is seen on the mammogram, one would expect this lesion to be palpable, but it is not. On ultrasound, no abnormality is seen at the expected location of the mammographic finding. This suggests either a complex sclerosing lesion or an invasive lobular carcinoma. Atypical ductal hyperplasia is reported on core biopsies. Excisional biopsy is recommended, and a complex sclerosing lesion with atypical ductal hyperplasia and sclerosing adenosis is reported on the excised tissue.

The management of patients with complex sclerosing lesions remains controversial. With respect to these lesions, we need to consider several related questions. On core samples, can the pathologist reliably distinguish a complex sclerosing lesion from tubular carcinomas and sclerosing adenosis? In a patient with distortion and spiculation, can we accept the diagnosis of a complex sclerosing lesion after core biopsy? Is the association of complex sclerosing lesions with other lesions, including atypical ductal hyperplasia (ADH), lobular neoplasia, low-nuclear-grade ductal carcinoma in situ, and tubular carcinomas, frequent enough to warrant excisional biopsy in all patients with complex sclerosing lesions? If a complex sclerosing lesion is suspected based on imaging and clinical findings, should an imaging-guided core biopsy be done?

In most patients, a complex sclerosing lesion can be diagnosed on core biopsy samples. Rarely, the distinction among this entity, sclerosing adenosis, and tubular carcinomas can be a challenge histologically. Because atypical ductal hyperplasia, lobular neoplasia, ductal carcinoma in situ (usually low- or intermediate-grade), or tubular carcinomas are reported in as many as 33% of patients with complex sclerosing lesions, I recommend excision of all complex sclerosing lesions. Alternatively, some have suggested that if the lesion is not associated with ADH, the biopsy included at least 12 specimens, and the mammographic findings are reconciled with the histologic findings, no excision is required.

Complex sclerosing lesions can demonstrate fairly distinctive mammographic, sonographic, and clinical findings. The mammographic findings for these lesions include distortion with central 1-to 2-mm locules of fat (i.e., no significant central density), long curvilinear spicules, and better visualization in one of the two projections, commonly the craniocaudal view. Round and punctate calcifications may be seen in as many as 30% to 40% of lesions. These lesions are not related to a prior biopsy and, although they are occasionally palpable, most have no associated clinical finding (unlike what would be expected for an invasive ductal carcinoma of comparable size). On ultrasound, normal tissue or a subtle area of distortion with some shadowing that is not necessarily confirmed on the orthogonal image may be noted.

Based on imaging and clinical features, the likelihood of a complex sclerosing lesion can be predicted in a high percentage of patients. In patients in whom I consider the likelihood of a complex sclerosing lesion to be high, I recommend an excisional biopsy and forgo the imaging-guided biopsy. For those patients in whom a complex sclerosing lesion is in the differential but the imaging and clinical findings are not diagnostic, I do an imaging-guided biopsy; if a complex sclerosing is reported on the cores, I recommend excisional biopsy.

PATIENT 22

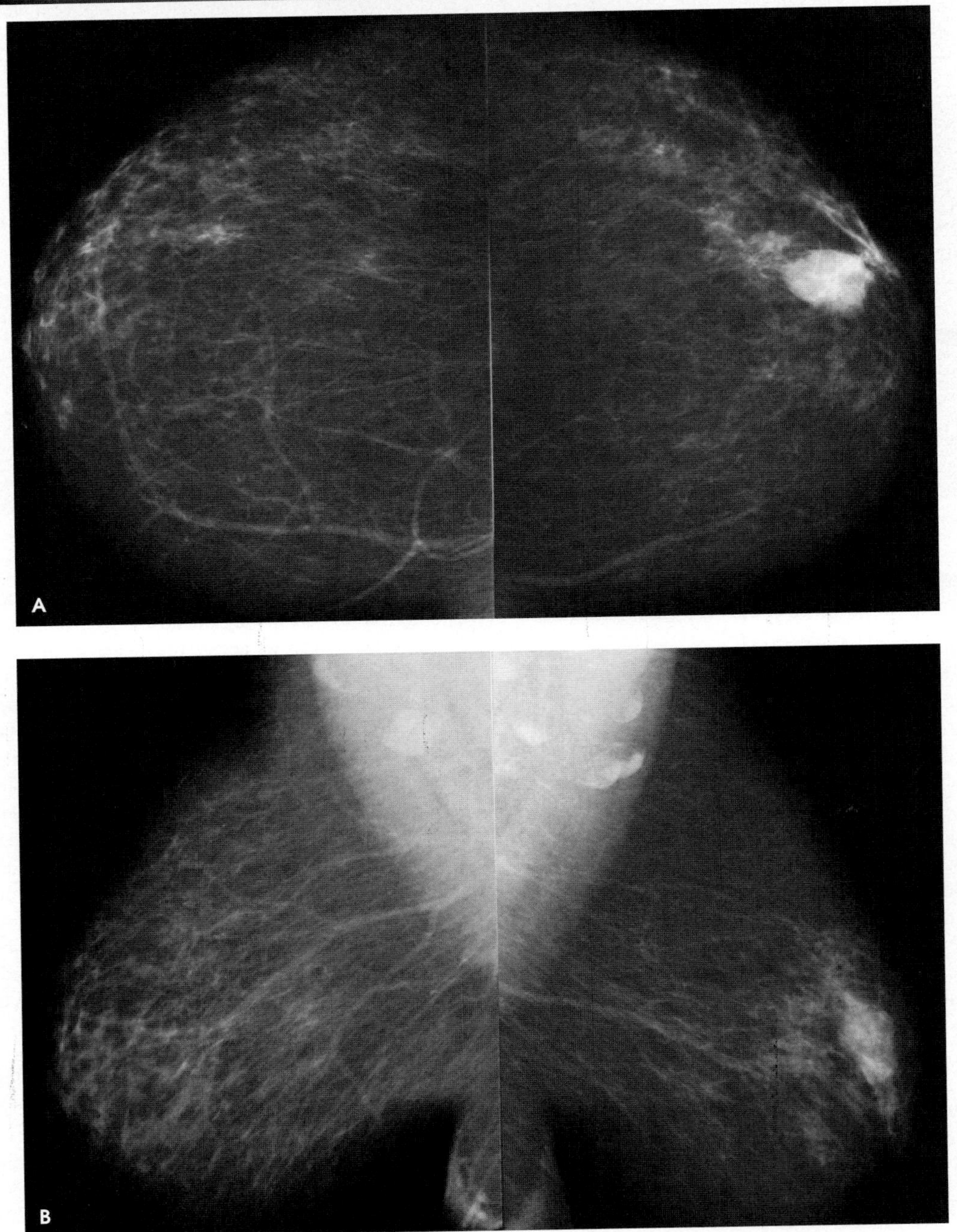

Figure 4.22. First screening study, 39-year-old woman. Craniocaudal (**A**) and mediolateral oblique (**B**) views.

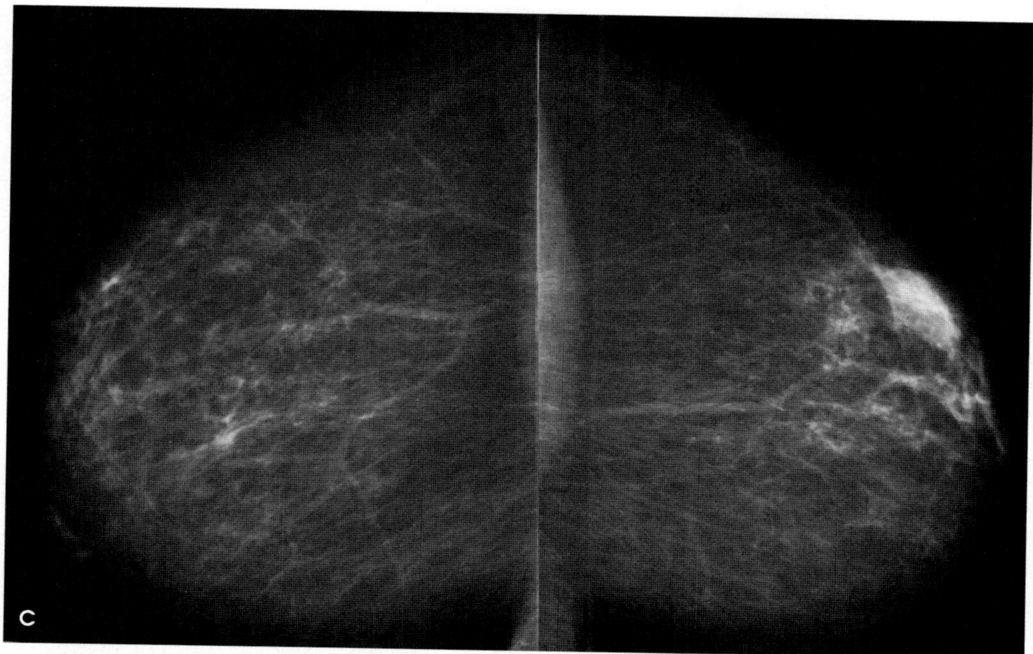

Figure 4.22. (*Continued*) Mediolateral oblique **(C),** anterior compression views obtained as part of her screening study.

Is this a normal or potentially abnormal mammogram? What are the pertinent observations?

An oval mass is imaged in the upper outer quadrant of the left breast. Are there any other observations? How about a possible area of distortion at the posterior edge of the obvious mass in the left breast?

BI-RADS® category 0: need additional imaging evaluation.

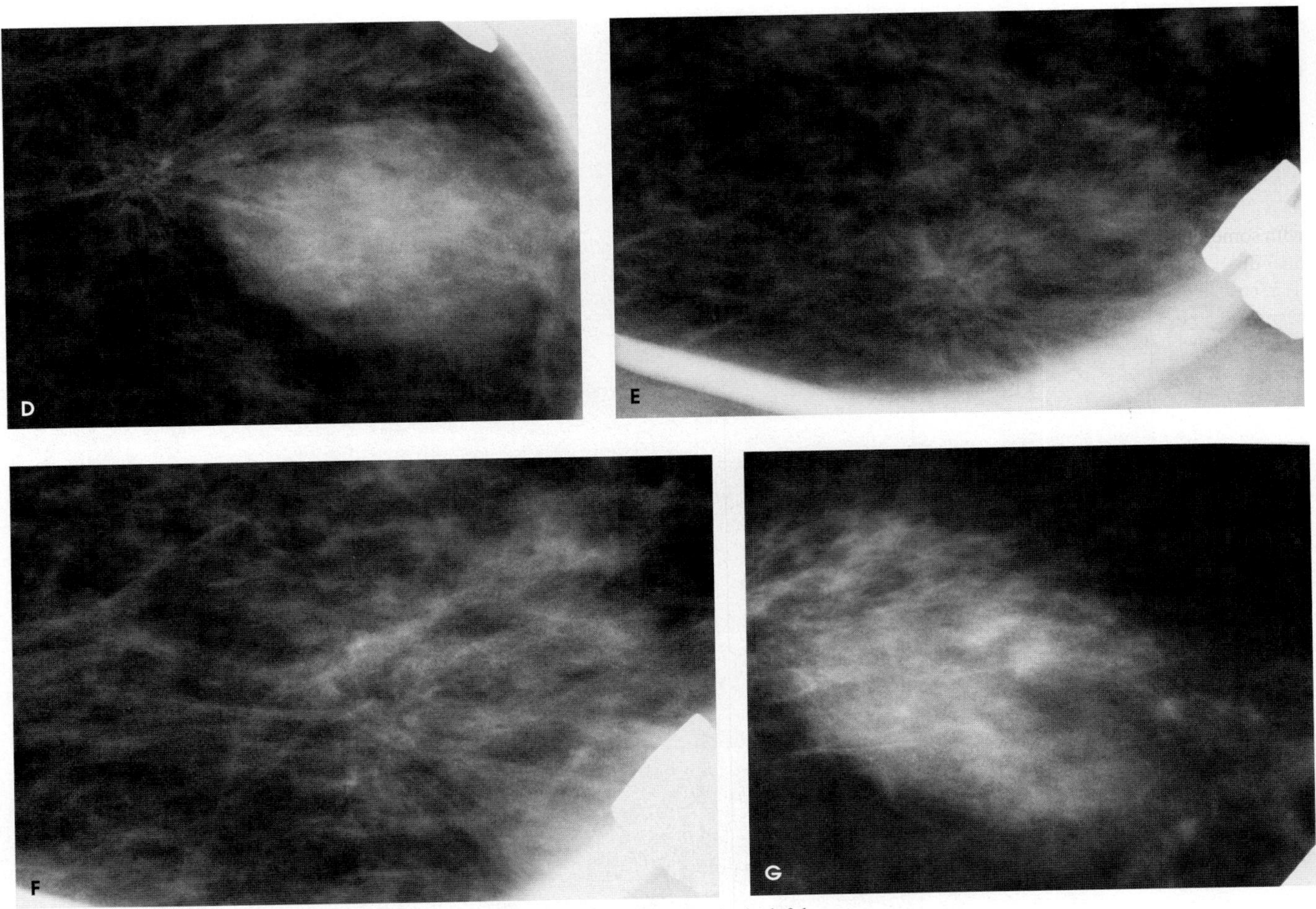

Figure 4.22. (*Continued*) Multiple spot compression **(D–G)** views of the findings in the left breast.

How would you describe the findings, and what is your differential?

An area of distortion is confirmed on the spot compression views (Fig. 4.22D–F). It is characterized by the presence of fatty tissue centrally and long radiating spicules. It is more apparent on the craniocaudal view (Fig. 4.22D). Differential considerations include postsurgical or traumatic change, complex sclerosing lesion, papilloma, inflammatory change, focal fibrosis, sclerosing adenosis, fibromatosis, invasive ductal carcinoma not otherwise specified, and tubular carcinoma. Rarely, ductal carcinoma in situ can present with distortion in the absence of calcifications. Invasive lobular carcinoma is also in the differential, however, given the patient's age this is less likely. The patient has no history of breast surgery or trauma, and she is otherwise asymptomatic. Her physical examination in the expected location of the area of distortion is normal. No abnormality is identified on ultrasound corresponding to the area of distortion seen mammographically. A complex sclerosing lesion is suspected and excisional biopsy is recommended.

BI-RADS® category 4: suspicious abnormality, biopsy should be considered.

An oval mass with partially obscured and indistinct margins is confirmed on the spot compression views (Fig. 4.22G). Differential considerations for this finding include cyst, fibroadenoma (complex fibroadenoma, tubular adenoma), phyllodes tumor, papilloma, pseudoangiomatous stromal hyperplasia, adenosis tumor, and focal fibrosis. Depending on the clinical context, galactocele, postoperative or traumatic fluid collection, and an abscess are also in the differential. Invasive ductal carcinoma not otherwise specified and medullary carcinoma are the main considerations in the malignant category. Mucinous and papillary carcinoma are less likely, given the patient's age.

On ultrasound, a well-circumscribed mass with a heterogeneous echotexture and associated cystic areas is imaged corresponding to the mass seen mammographically (Fig. 4.22H). Biopsy is indicated.

BI-RADS® category 4: suspicious abnormality, biopsy should be considered.

The specimen radiograph is used to confirm excision of the mass and adjacent area of distortion (Fig. 4.22I, J). The localizing wire is seen in the specimen between the two lesions. Based on this image, the location of the mass and distortion are marked for the pathologist. A complex sclerosing lesion with no associated proliferative lesions is diagnosed for the area of distortion, and an adenosis tumor with significant fibrosis is reported for the mass.

Complex sclerosing lesions can demonstrate fairly distinctive mammographic, sonographic, and clinical findings. The mammographic findings for these lesions include distortion with central 1- to

2-mm locules of fat (i.e., no significant central density), long curvilinear spicules, and better visualization in one of the two projections, commonly the craniocaudal view. Round and punctate calcifications may be seen in as many as 30% to 40% of lesions. These lesions are idiopathic and are not related to a prior biopsy or trauma. Unlike the palpable findings one would expect to find for a comparably sized invasive ductal carcinoma, complex sclerosing lesions are usually not palpable. On ultrasound, normal tissue or a subtle area of distortion with some shadowing that is not necessarily confirmed on the orthogonal image may be noted.

For patients in whom, based on imaging and clinical findings, I suspect a complex sclerosing lesion, I recommend excision so that the lesion can be evaluated in its entirety. In nearly 33% of patients with complex sclerosing lesions, atypical ductal hyperplasia, lobular neoplasia, ductal carcinoma in situ (usually low- or intermediate-grade), or tubular carcinoma is reported being associated with the lesion. For patients in whom a complex sclerosing lesion is in the differential, but the imaging and clinical findings are not diagnostic, I do an imaging-guided biopsy; if a complex sclerosing is reported, I recommend excisional biopsy.

Alternatively, some recommend doing imaging-guided core biopsies on all of these lesions. If the lesion is a breast cancer, the patient can then have definitive surgery. If a complex sclerosing lesion is diagnosed on the cores, some recommend excisional biopsy. Others have suggested that if the complex sclerosing lesion is not associated with ADH, the biopsy includes at least 12 specimens, and the mammographic findings are reconciled with the histologic findings, no excision is required.

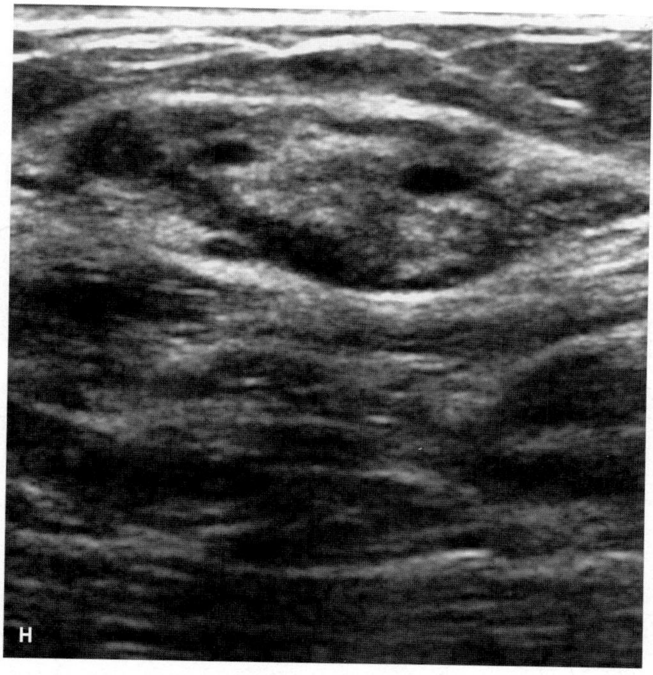

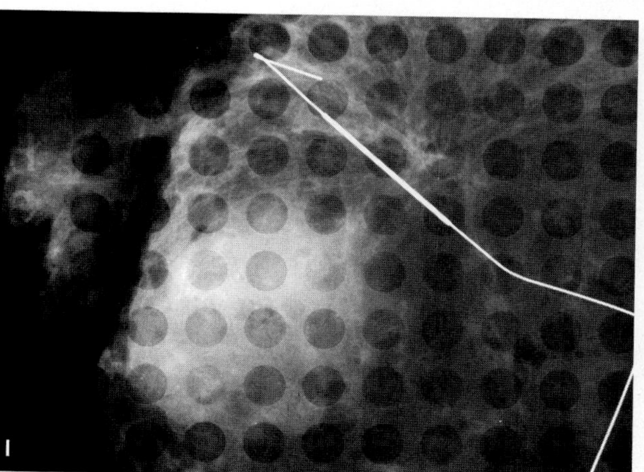

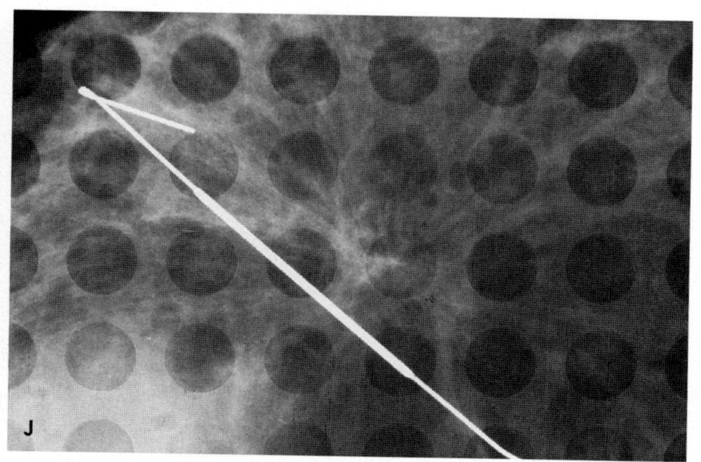

Figure 4.22. (*Continued*) Ultrasound image **(H)**, radial projection of the mass in the upper outer quadrant of the left breast. Specimen radiograph **(I)**, confirming excision of mass and adjacent area of distortion. Specimen radiograph **(J)**, photographically coned to area of distortion.

PATIENT 23

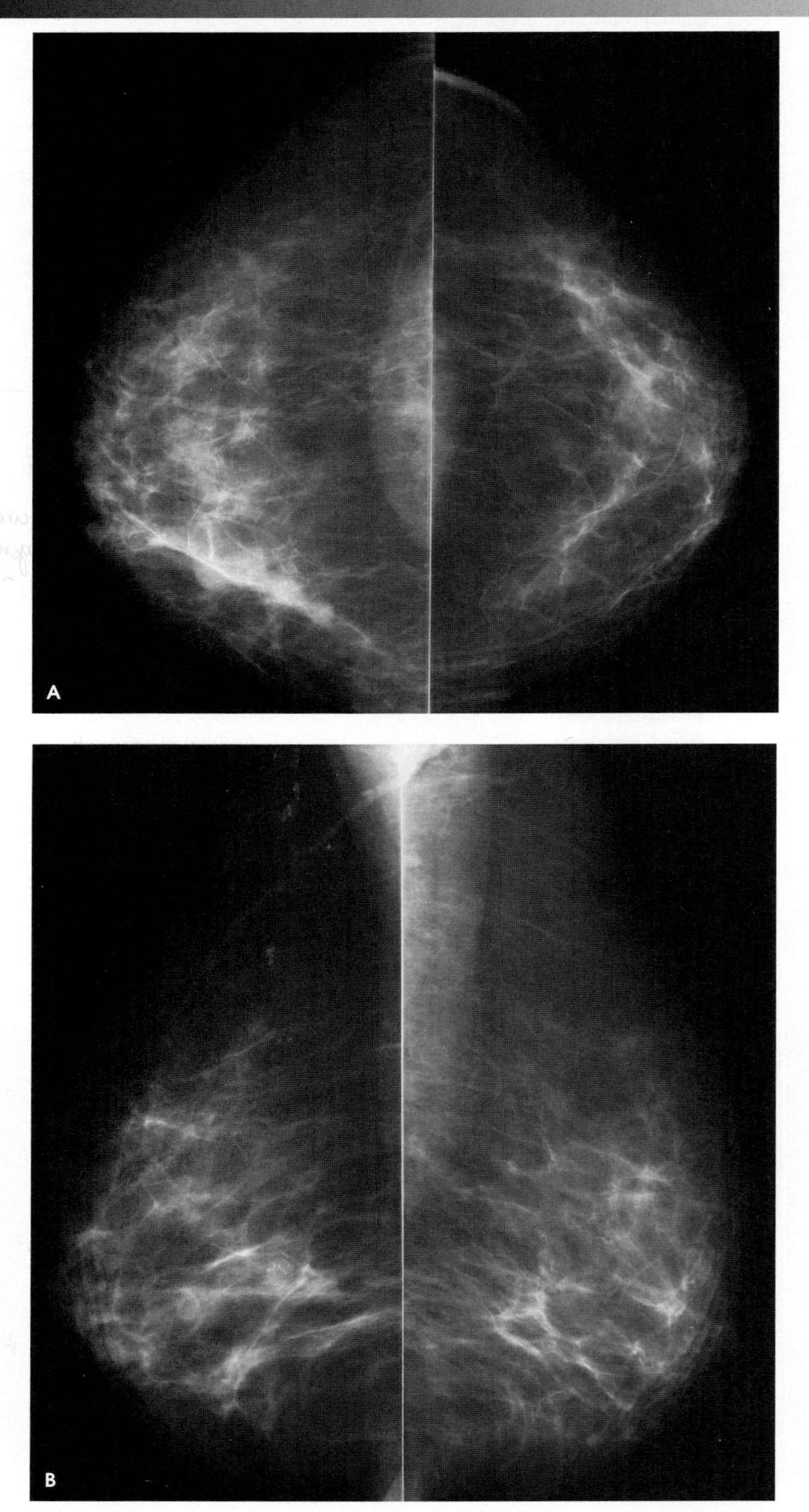

Figure 4.23. Screening study, 77-year-old woman. Craniocaudal **(A)** and mediolateral **(B)** oblique views.

Is this a normal study, or is additional evaluation indicated?

A mass with associated calcifications is present medially in the right breast. Additionally, at least on the craniocaudal view, nodularity is noted extending from the mass with calcifications towards the nipple.

BI-RADS® category 0: need additional imaging evaluation.

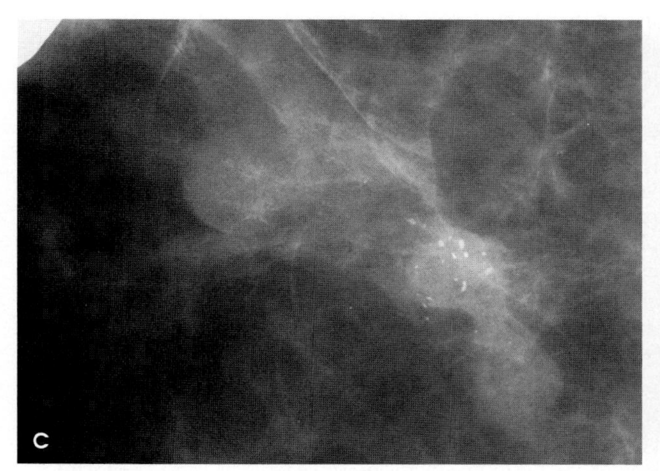

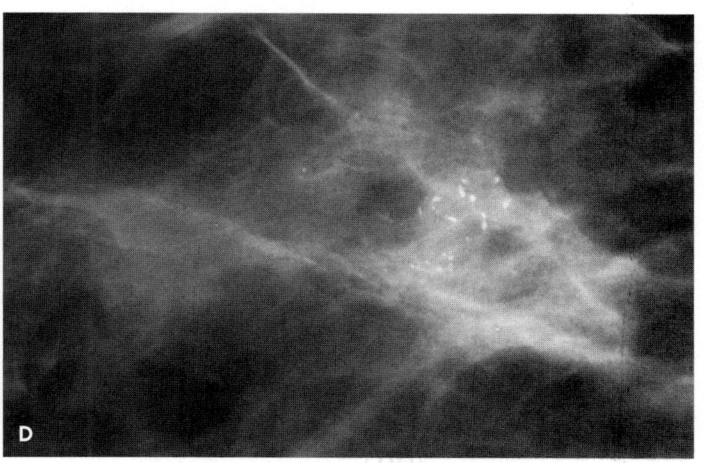

Figure 4.23. (*Continued*) Craniocaudal **(C)** and mediolateral oblique **(D)** spot compression magnification views, right breast. When positioning for the additional views, the technologist notes nipple discharge.

How would you describe the findings, and what would you do next?

A cluster of masses, one of which is associated with pleomorphic calcifications, is confirmed on the spot compression magnification views obtained of the right breast. A biopsy is indicated. An ultrasound is done to determine if the lesion can be identified for imaging-guided biopsy. Because of the nipple discharge noted by the technologist, additional history is obtained from the patient and, if indicated, physical examination and a ductogram are done.

On questioning, the patient relates having noticed her nipple dripping and dark brown spots on her bra and night clothes. On physical examination, nipple discharge is elicited easily from a single duct opening. A ductogram (not shown) and ultrasound are done for further evaluation.

Multiple intraductal masses are imaged in the subareolar area in moderately dilated ducts. These are confirmed on the ductogram (not shown). In addition, at least two solid masses, one of which has associated calcifications (Fig. 4.23I, thin arrow), are imaged at the 2 o'clock position, 4 cm from the right nipple. Given the clinical and imaging findings, multiple papillomas and associated invasive ductal carcinoma with ductal carcinoma in situ are the main considerations.

BI-RADS® category 4: suspicious abnormality, biopsy should be considered.

An ultrasound-guided biopsy of the mass with associated calcifications is done. An invasive ductal carcinoma with associated ductal carcinoma in situ, high nuclear grade with central necrosis, is reported on the core biopsy.

On the day of the lumpectomy, two wires are used to bracket the intraductal lesions seen on ultrasound, close to the nipple and the more peripheral cluster of masses. A 0.9-cm, grade III invasive ductal carcinoma with associated high-nuclear-grade ductal carcinoma with central necrosis is confirmed in the lumpectomy specimen. A 0.9-cm, high-nuclear-grade ductal carcinoma in situ with apocrine features is noted arising in an adjacent papilloma. Three excised sentinel lymph nodes are normal [pT1b, pN0, pMX, Stage I].

The management of patients diagnosed with papillomas on core needle biopsy remains controversial. Clearly, papillary lesions with atypia on core biopsy require excisional biopsy. The controversy centers on the diagnosis of a benign papillary lesion with no associated atypia on core biopsy. Many authors advocate that these can be followed with no excision required, while others recommend excision of all papillary lesions regardless of associated atypia. Among patients who have papillomas with associated atypia on core biopsy, 31% to 60% have been reported to have malignancy on excision. Among patients initially diagnosed with a papilloma (with no atypia), 0% to 18% have been reported to have malignancy on excision.

In considering the literature on papillary lesions, I think it is important to recognize the relatively low number of patients described, the retrospective nature of some of the studies, and the lack of adequate classification of lesions into central, usually solitary papillomas, and multiple peripheral papillomas. Additionally, the follow-up on many of these patients is limited; 2 or 3 years of follow-up is probably insufficient to truly assess the biologic significance of many of these lesions.

Patients with centrally occurring papillomas commonly present describing nipple discharge. The papillomas are often solitary, and on excision, no significant proliferative changes are typically reported in the surrounding breast parenchyma. In contrast, multiple peripheral papillomas are usually detected mammographically as one or multiple masses that may have associated calcifications or as multiple clusters of pleomorphic calcifications. Associated proliferative changes that include atypical ductal hyperplasia, lobular neoplasia, ductal carcinoma in situ (usually low-nuclear-grade), and invasive ductal carcinoma can be seen in nearly 50% of patients with multiple peripheral papillomas. Also, following excisional biopsy of these lesions, many patients present with recurrent lesions (new masses, or calcifications at the prior site). In the context of multiple peripheral papillomas, the term *papillomatosis* needs to be considered. This is a confusing term because some pathologists use it to describe multiple peripheral papillomas (i.e., lesions with a central fibrovascular core) and others use it for intraductal hyperplasia. I think it is best to avoid the term; however, when I am confronted with it, I specifically ask the pathologist how he or she is using the term.

As with so many other situations in breast imaging, the clinical context is important in determining the appropriate management of patients with papillary lesions. The larger the lesion, the greater the number of findings, and the older the patient, the more appropriate an excisional biopsy seems when a papilloma is diagnosed on core biopsy. It may be that patients with multiple peripheral papillomas should be treated more aggressively and that excisional biopsy may be appropriate in this patient population following an imaging-guided biopsy. In this context, it is also important to recognize that distinguishing benign papilloma from papillomas with atypia and papillary carcinoma may be difficult for the pathologist given core samples. As with the distinction between normal breast ductules and tubular carcinoma, it is the presence or absence of myoepithelial cells that distinguishes benign from malignant papillary lesions, and as much as 10% of a malignant papillary lesion has myoepithelial cells present, introducing the possibility of sampling bias.

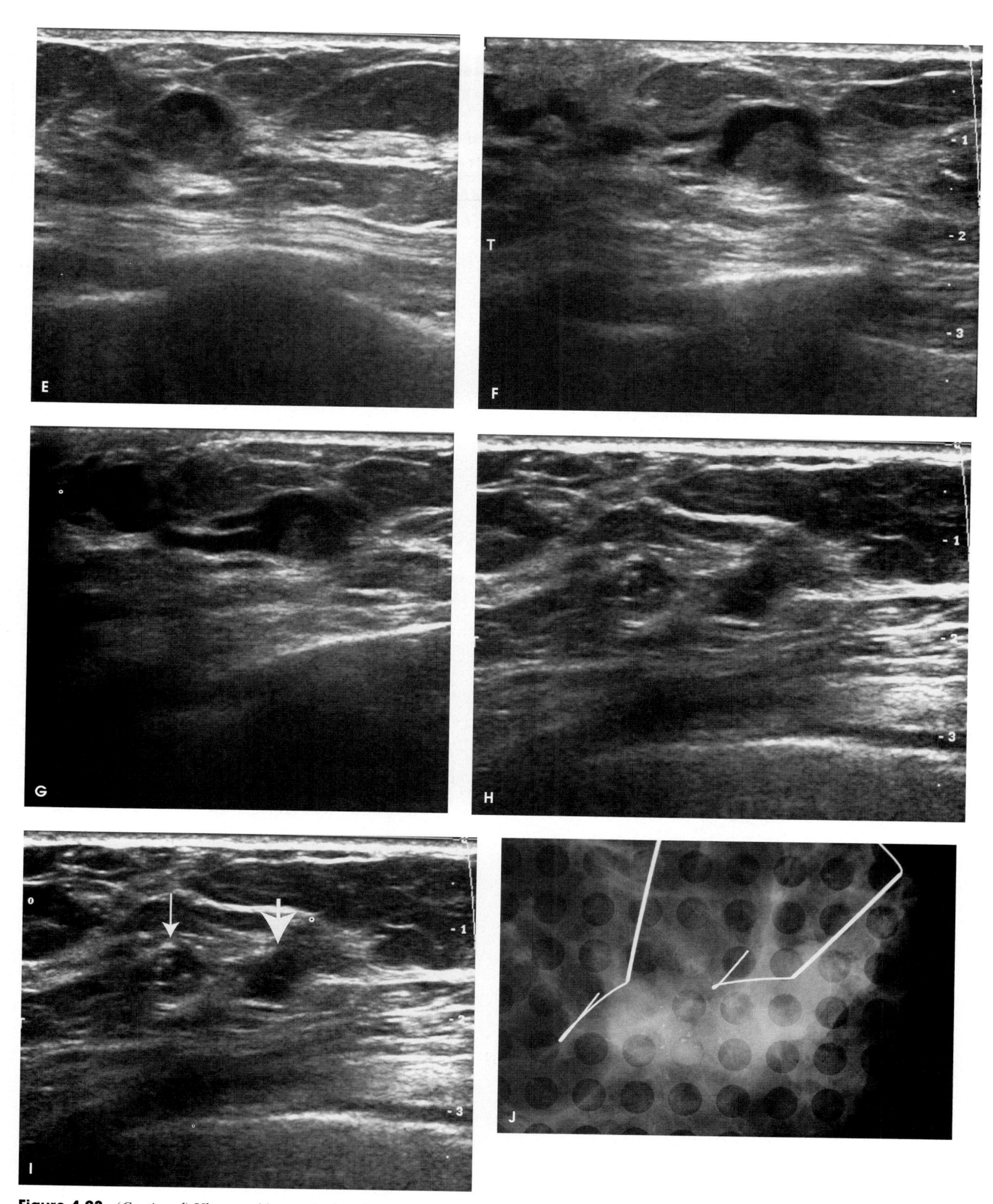

Figure 4.23. (*Continued*) Ultrasound images in the subareolar area **(E–G)** and at the 2 o'clock position, 4 cm from the right nipple **(H).** Ultrasound image **(I)** demonstrating the round solid mass with associated spicular echoes consistent with the calcifications seen mammographically (*thin arrow*) and a second adjacent, irregular solid mass (*thick arrow*) at the 2 o'clock position, 4 cm from the right nipple. Specimen radiograph **(J)** demonstrating multiple masses, one of which has associated calcifications in the specimen. The preoperative wire localization is done using ultrasound guidance. Two wires are used to bracket the location of the intraductal lesions (seen on ultrasound) and the more peripheral cluster of masses seen mammographically.

PATIENT 24

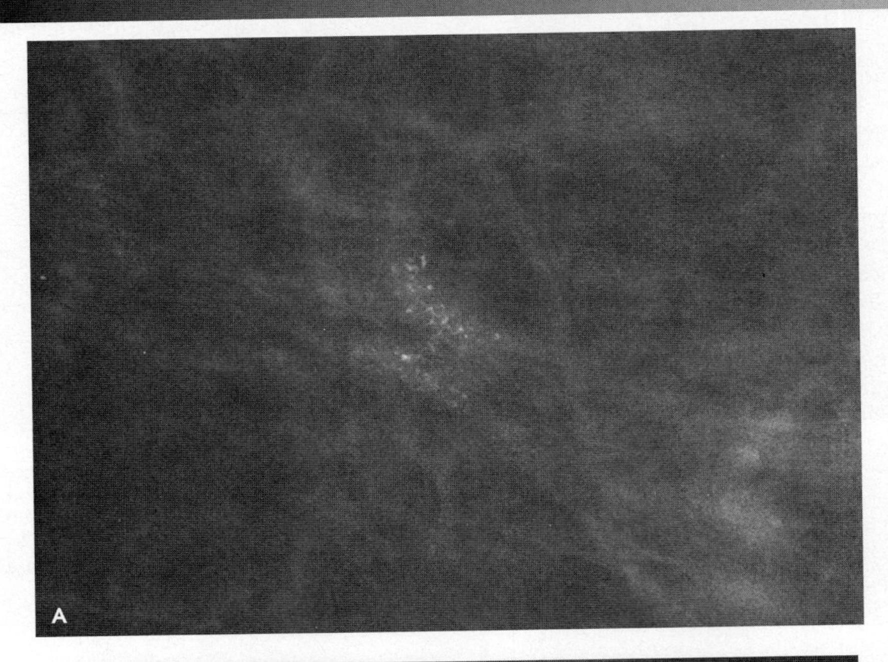

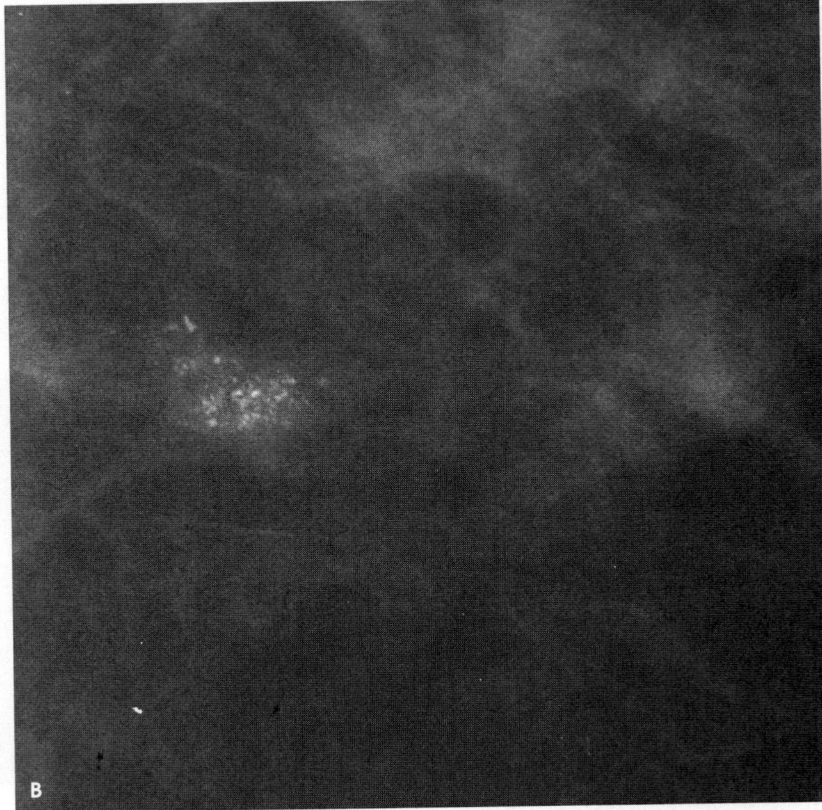

Figure 4.24. Diagnostic evaluation, 71-year-old woman called back for evaluation of calcifications in the left breast detected on her screening study. Craniocaudal **(A)** and mediolateral oblique **(B)** spot compression magnification views.

What would you recommend?

A cluster of pleomorphic calcifications with round, punctate, and amorphous forms is confirmed on the magnification views. No definite linear forms are present, and there is no linear orientation. Fibrocystic changes including hyperplasia, atypical ductal hyperplasia, columnar alteration with prominent apical snouts and secretions (CAPSS), and sclerosing adenosis, as well as fibroadenoma, papilloma, and ductal carcinoma in situ (usually low- or intermediate-nuclear-grade, with no central necrosis) are in the differential for this cluster of calcifications. A stereotactically guided needle biopsy is recommended; however, the patient is short of breath and unable to lie prone. Excisional biopsy is scheduled following wire localization of the cluster of calcifications.

The specimen radiograph is obtained for several reasons. Confirmation that the localized lesion is excised is the primary reason, and although the specimen is a two-dimensional representation of a three-dimensional structure, if the localized abnormality is in close proximity to the margins, it is equally important that this is communicated to the surgeon. In evaluating the specimen, you also want to make sure that the localization wire has been removed with the specimen. Rarely, additional unsuspected lesions may be detected on the specimen; and lastly, the location of the excised lesion in the specimen is marked for the pathologist to assure that the excised lesion is evaluated histologically.

For this patient, atypical ductal hyperplasia (ADH) is reported histologically on the excised tissue. No further intervention is recommended; however, a mammogram of this breast in 6 months is requested, to establish a new baseline for this patient. Our approach to patients diagnosed with a high-risk marker lesion (e.g., ADH, lobular carcinoma in situ, atypical lobular hyperplasia, papilloma with atypia, multiple peripheral papillomas, complex sclerosing lesions, CAPSS with atypia, and mucocele-like lesions) is to obtain a mammogram following the excisional biopsy so as to document post biopsy changes as they peak during the first 6 months following the biopsy. After the first 6 months, postbiopsy changes stabilize or slowly resolve. By evaluating the patient 6 months following the surgery, it is unlikely that a spiculated mass at the biopsy site represents interval development of an invasive lesion. Most important, we avoid finding ourselves with a spiculated mass at the biopsy site (of a high-risk lesion) 2 years or more after the surgery, and not knowing if this is postoperative change that is regressing or the development of a more significant lesion.

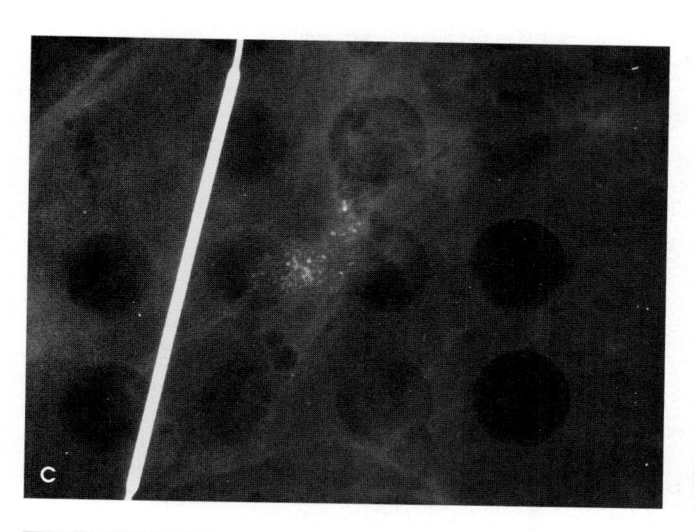

Figure 4.24. (*Continued*) Specimen radiography **(C)** obtained following wire localization of the breast lesion.

PATIENT 25

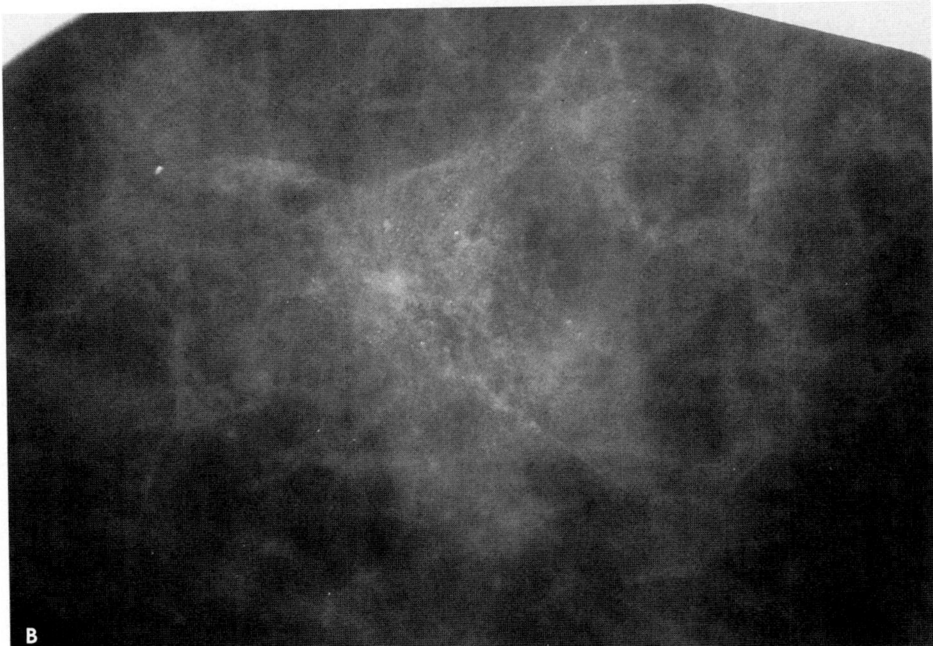

Figure 4.25. Diagnostic evaluation, 61-year-old woman called back for evaluation of calcifications detected in the right breast on her screening mammogram. Craniocaudal **(A)** and mediolateral oblique **(B)** double spot compression magnification views, right breast.

How would you define these findings?

An area of amorphous calcifications is demonstrated on the magnification views. Differential considerations include fibrocystic changes, hyperplasia, atypical ductal hyperplasia, sclerosing adenosis, columnar alteration with prominent apical snouts and secretions (CAPSS), fibroadenoma, papilloma, and ductal carcinoma in situ (usually low-nuclear-grade with no central necrosis).

BI-RADS® category 4: suspicious abnormality, biopsy should be considered.

Following preoperative wire localizations, the specimen is placed in a container that allows for compression of the specimen with an alphanumeric grid. Although we apply compression on the specimen, we try to minimize the amount of compression because recent reports in the literature suggest that vigorous specimen compression may result in "false positive" histologic interpretations of tumor extending to the margins. The specimen radiograph is done using magnification technique on a mammographic unit, or a dedicated specimen radiography unit. The use of an alphanumeric enables us to place a pin through the center of the lesion, or four pins can be used to delineate the margins of larger lesions for the pathologist. This assures that the area of mammographic concern is fully evaluated histologically. Extensive sclerosing adenosis with associated calcifications is reported histologically.

Are the imaging and histologic findings congruent? What do you recommend for this patient?

Yes, the imaging and histologic findings are congruent. The excised calcifications are identified as being associated with sclerosing adenosis, and no atypia or other high-risk lesion (e.g., complex sclerosing lesion or papilloma) is described by the pathologist. The patient is asked to return in 1 year.

Calcifications with this appearance typically occur in women with dense glandular tissue and may demonstrate a focal but loosely clustered distribution, as in this patient, or the calcifications may be diffusely scattered bilaterally. The differential to consider includes sclerosing adenosis, columnar alteration with prominent apical snouts and secretions (CAPSS), hyperplasia, atypical ductal hyperplasia, fibroadenoma, papilloma, and ductal carcinoma in situ (commonly low- or intermediate-grade with no associated central necrosis). The management of patients with this calcification type, particularly when diffusely involving the breast parenchyma bilaterally, can be a challenge. In women with focal findings, particularly if the calcifications represent a change compared with prior studies or they are in an unusual location (e.g., inner quadrants as opposed to the upper outer quadrant of the involved breast), I recommend a stereotactically guided biopsy. Patients with more diffuse and bilateral findings pose more of a management issue.

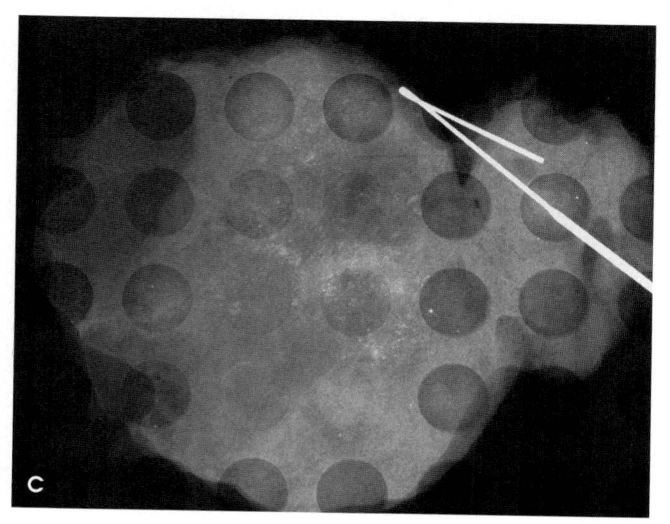

Figure 4.25. (*Continued*) Specimen radiograph **(C),** obtained to confirm excision of the localized lesion and the wire.

Do you sample or not? If you sample, how do you decide where? If you sample and the pathology is benign, can you be sure it is representative of all the calcifications?

My approach to patients with bilateral, diffusely scattered amorphous calcifications is annual follow-up with magnification views; I recommend biopsy when changes in the calcifications or the surrounding tissue are perceived on follow-up studies.

Sclerosing adenosis is a component of fibrocystic change most commonly seen in the perimenopausal period. It is a lobulocentric lesion characterized by disordered proliferation of epithelial, myoepithelial, and stromal elements. This process is characterized by an increased number of acini that are compressed and obliterated by the proliferating intralobular stroma predominantly in the center of lobules. More cystically dilated acini are seen at the periphery of the involved lobules. Sclerosing adenosis is also characterized by hyperplasia of the myoepithelial cells. It can occur as an isolated lesion or as a component of complex sclerosing lesions, papillomas, fibroadenomas (e.g., complex fibroadenomas), and invasive or in situ cancers.

The imaging features of sclerosing adenosis are variable. Sclerosing adenosis may present as a palpable or screen-detected mass, the margins of which may range from well circumscribed to indistinct to spiculated; it may also present as distortion or focal parenchymal asymmetry, and associated calcifications may be present. Alternatively, sclerosing adenosis may present with calcifications and no associated mass. One of three patterns may be seen relative to calcifications developing in areas of sclerosing adenosis: a tight cluster of round and punctate, well-defined calcifications; loosely clustered amorphous calcifications; or bilateral, diffusely distributed amorphous calcifications in the setting of dense glandular tissue.

PATIENT 26

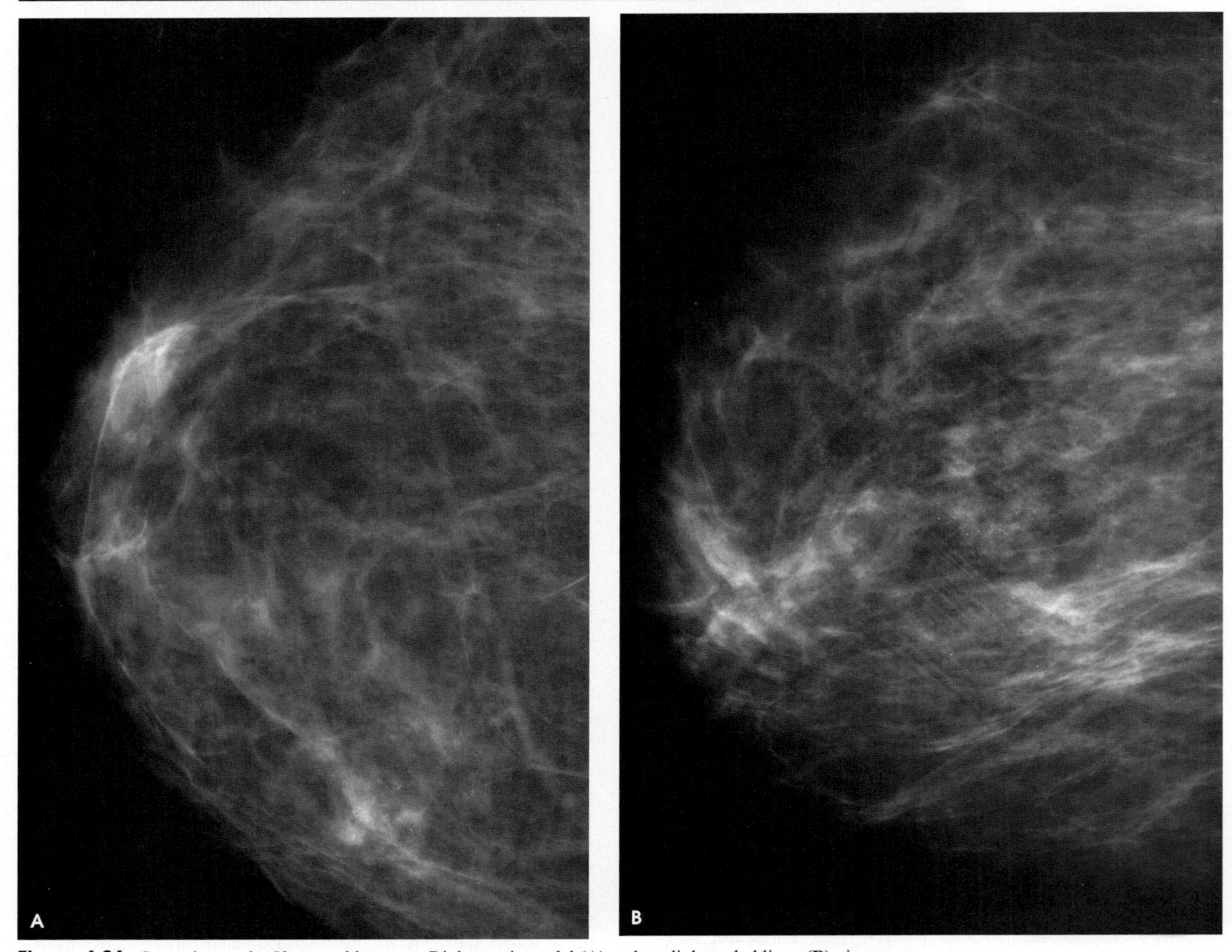

Figure 4.26. Screening study, 53-year-old woman. Right craniocaudal **(A)** and mediolateral oblique **(B)** views.

How would you describe these findings, and what would you recommend next?

A cluster of calcifications is detected medially in the right breast. Spot compression magnification views are indicated for further evaluation.

BI-RADS® category 0: need additional imaging evaluation.

The magnification views (the mediolateral oblique projection is not shown) confirm the presence of a cluster of pleomorphic calcifications in the right breast. Ductal carcinoma in situ (DCIS) is the main differential consideration for these calcifications, and therefore a biopsy is indicated. Because of the density associated with the calcifications, invasion may be present. DCIS is diagnosed following core biopsies, and is confirmed on the lumpectomy. In addition to the lumpectomy, the patient is treated with radiation therapy to the right breast.

Postlumpectomy changes and surgical clips are present in the right breast at the lumpectomy site. Immediately following the completion of the radiation therapy (Fig. 4.26D, E), there is increased density at the lumpectomy site. The density progressively resolves, and oil cyst formation is noted at the lumpectomy bed. What do you think about the findings in the last set of films (Fig 4.26J, K)? How would you report this study, and what is your recommendation?

At this time, there is an irregular 2-cm mass with indistinct margins, shadowing, and associated pleomorphic and linear calcifications, some of which demonstrate a linear orientation. The constellation of findings is consistent with recurrent disease. Ultrasound-guided biopsy is done and confirms the presence of invasive ductal carcinoma and associated high-nuclear-grade ductal carcinoma in situ (DCIS) with central necrosis. In retrospect, a density is seen developing at the lumpectomy bed on the last set of images (Fig. 4.26J, K), obtained 42 months following completion of treatment. A simple mastectomy with axillary dissection is done. A 3-cm invasive ductal carcinoma with associated high-nuclear-grade DCIS and lymphovascular space involvement is reported histologically. No metastatic disease is identified in two excised sentinel lymph nodes [pT2, pN0(sn) (i−), pMX; Stage II].

Local recurrence (i.e., ipsilateral breast tumor recurrence, IBTR) following breast-conserving therapy or mastectomy is defined as the development of cancer in remaining ipsilateral breast tissue or skin or on the ipsilateral chest wall or skin, respectively. Regional recurrence is defined as the development of cancer in remaining ipsilateral axillary lymph nodes, supraclavicular, infraclavicular, or internal mammary lymph nodes.

Follow-up protocols for patients after lumpectomy and radiation therapy are variable. Some facilities follow patients with a history of conservatively treated breast cancer at 6-month intervals for 3, 5, or 7 years, and the contralateral breast at yearly intervals. Other facilities obtain annual mammograms bilaterally on these patients. We recommend annual diagnostic mammography for these patients and obtain routine craniocaudal and mediolateral oblique views bilaterally as well as a spot magnification tangential view of the lumpectomy site for the first 7 years following the surgery, after which we return the patient to screening. The development of new pleomorphic calcifications, a mass, or increasing density and distortion at or close to the lumpectomy site are mammographic findings that may be associated with a recurrence. Less commonly, recurrences may be characterized by diffuse breast changes, including a change in the size of the breast, increased density of the parenchyma, prominence of the trabecular markings, and skin thickening.

Reported recurrence rates range from 5% to 19% in the first 5 to 12 years following lumpectomy with radiation therapy, and from 4% to 14% following mastectomy. Risk factors linked to recurrence following lumpectomy with radiation therapy include young age at the time of presentation, extensive intraductal component, multifocal disease, lymphovascular space involvement, large tumor size, high histologic grade, tumor necrosis, and positive margins at the time of the original resection. Most recurrences occur at or near the site of the original tumor within the first 5 years following treatment.

Postlumpectomy changes are variable but may include areas of increased density, distortion, and spiculation at the site of the lumpectomy, often associated with skin thickening and distortion. These changes are usually most prominent within the first year following the surgery and then stabilize or progressively resolve. In some patients, oil cyst formation and the development of dystrophic calcifications may be seen at the lumpectomy site as the area of density and distortion decreases. Some patients develop postoperative fluid collections; these may also stabilize or progressively decrease in size, sometimes resolving completely without the need for any intervention. Radiation therapy changes more commonly involve the entire breast and include increased density and prominence of the trabecular markings as well as diffuse skin thickening. Radiation therapy changes typically resolve within the first 2 years following completion of the therapy.

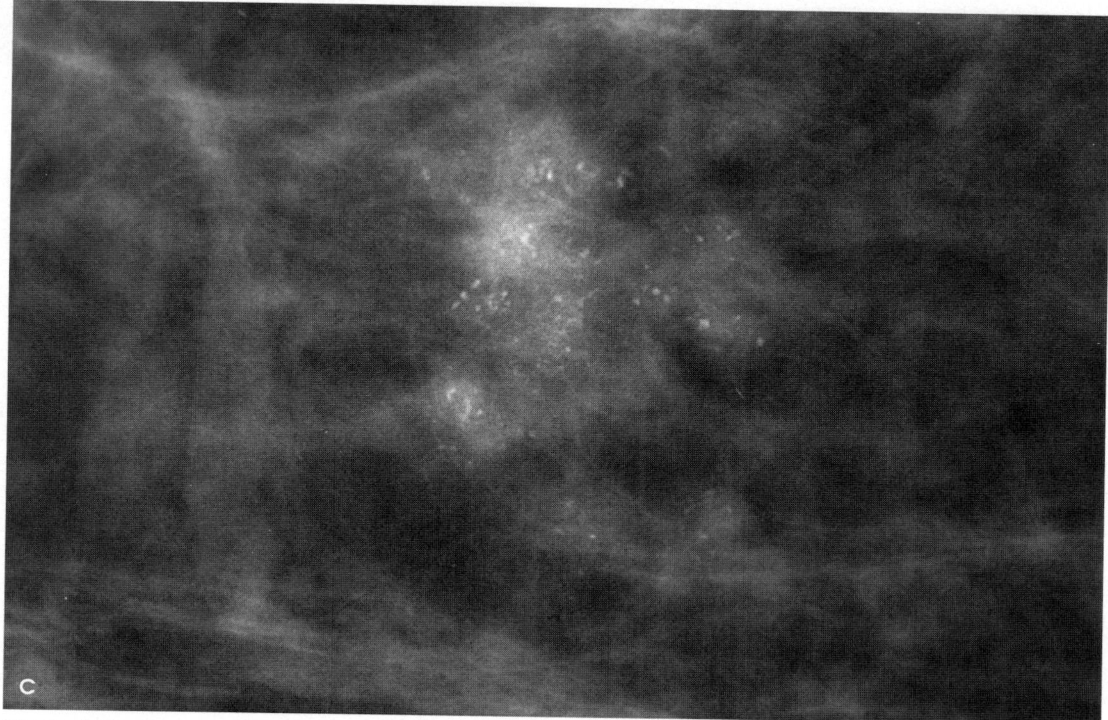

Figure 4.26. (*Continued*) Spot compression magnification craniocaudal view **(C)**, right breast.

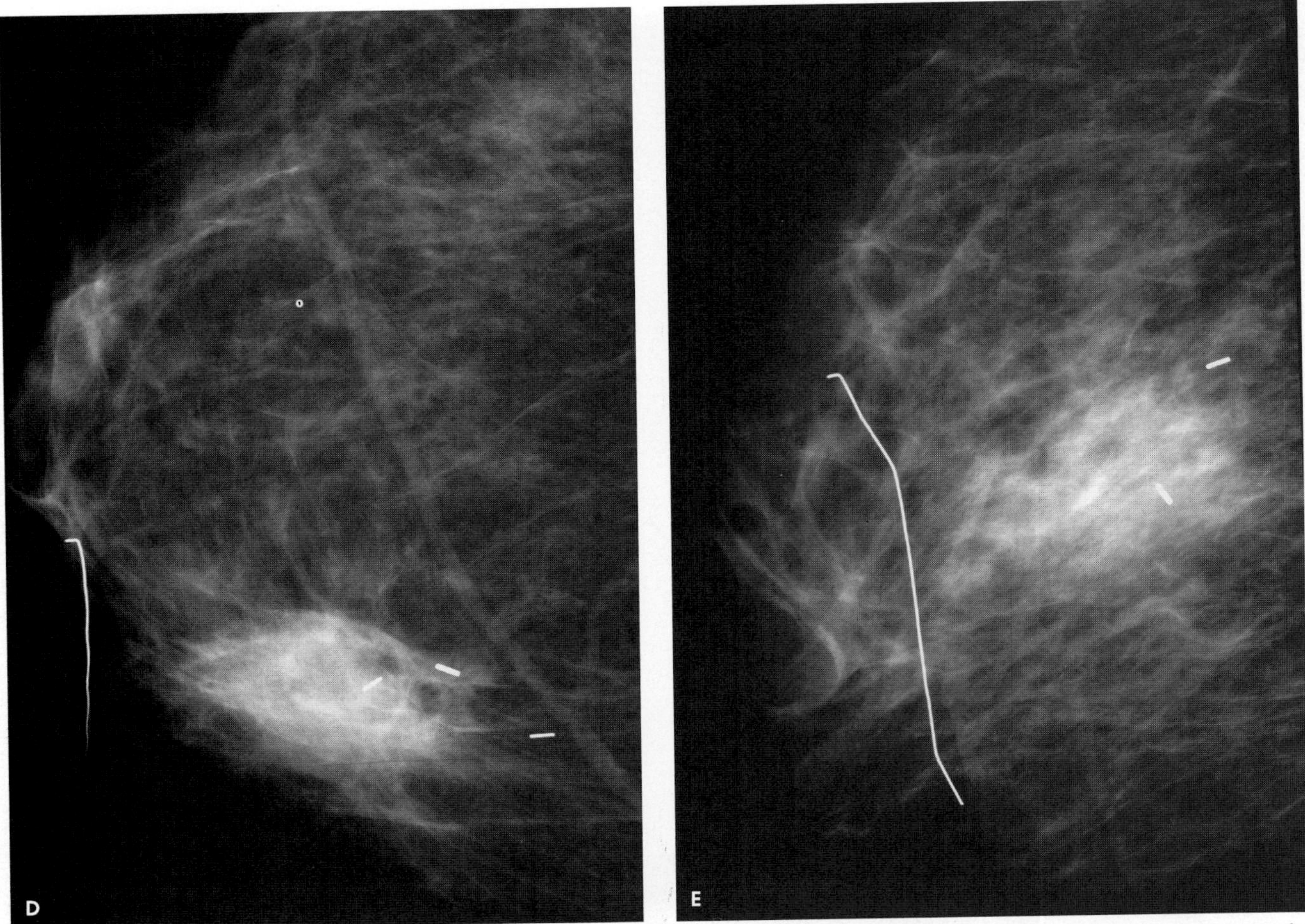

Figure 4.26. (*Continued*) Right craniocaudal **(D, F, H, J)** and mediolateral oblique **(E, G, I, K)** views, at 6, 18, 30, and 42 months following completion of the initial treatment. Linear metallic marker seen on some of the images is used to indicate the site of the lumpectomy scar.

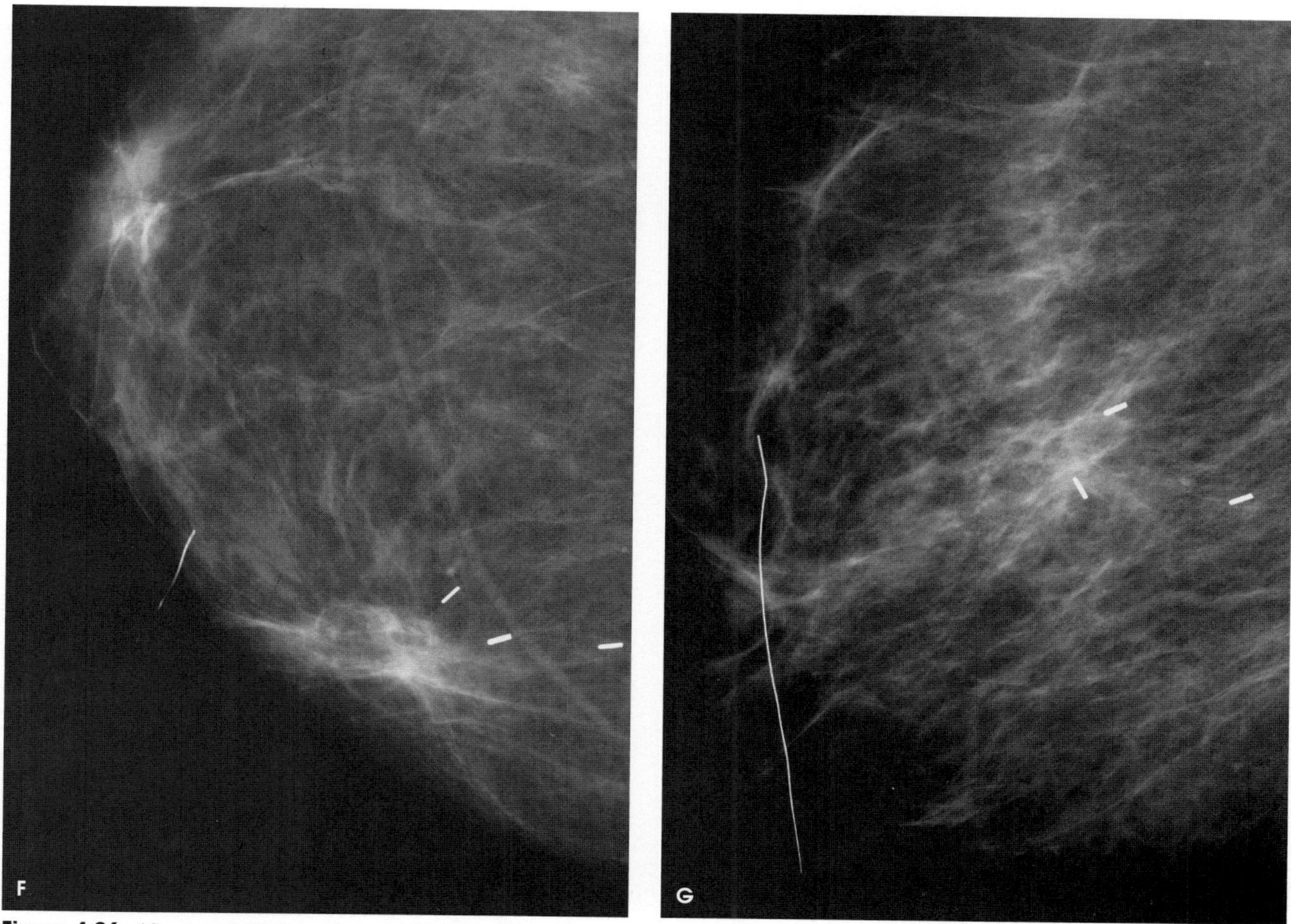

Figure 4.26. (*Continued*) Right craniocaudal **(D, F, H, J)** and mediolateral oblique **(E, G, I, K)** views, at 6, 18, 30, and 42 months following completion of the initial treatment. Linear metallic marker seen on some of the images is used to indicate the site of the lumpectomy scar.

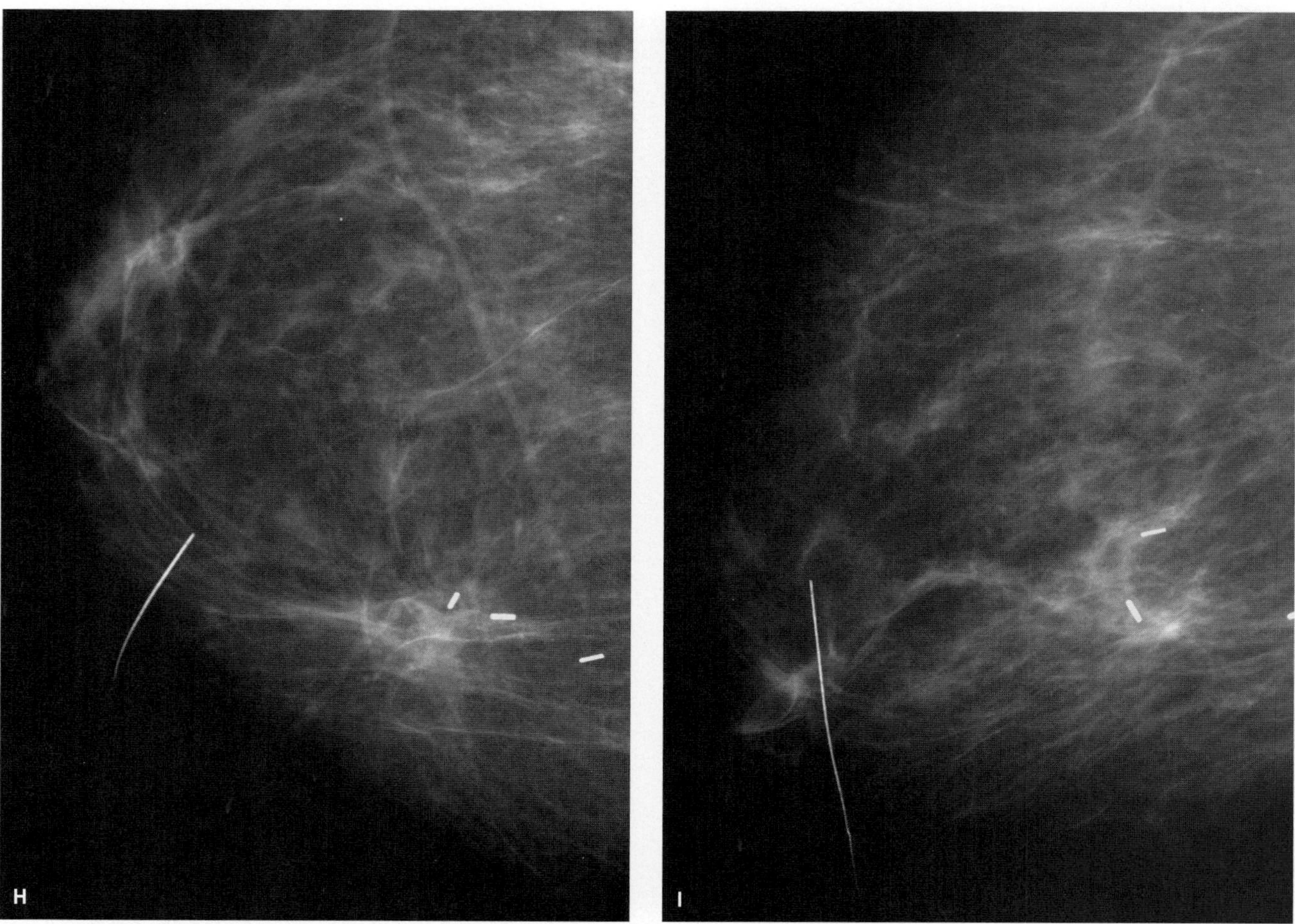

Figure 4.26. (*Continued*) Right craniocaudal **(D, F, H, J)** and mediolateral oblique **(E, G, I, K)** views, at 6, 18, 30, and 42 months following completion of the initial treatment. Linear metallic marker seen on some of the images is used to indicate the site of the lumpectomy scar.

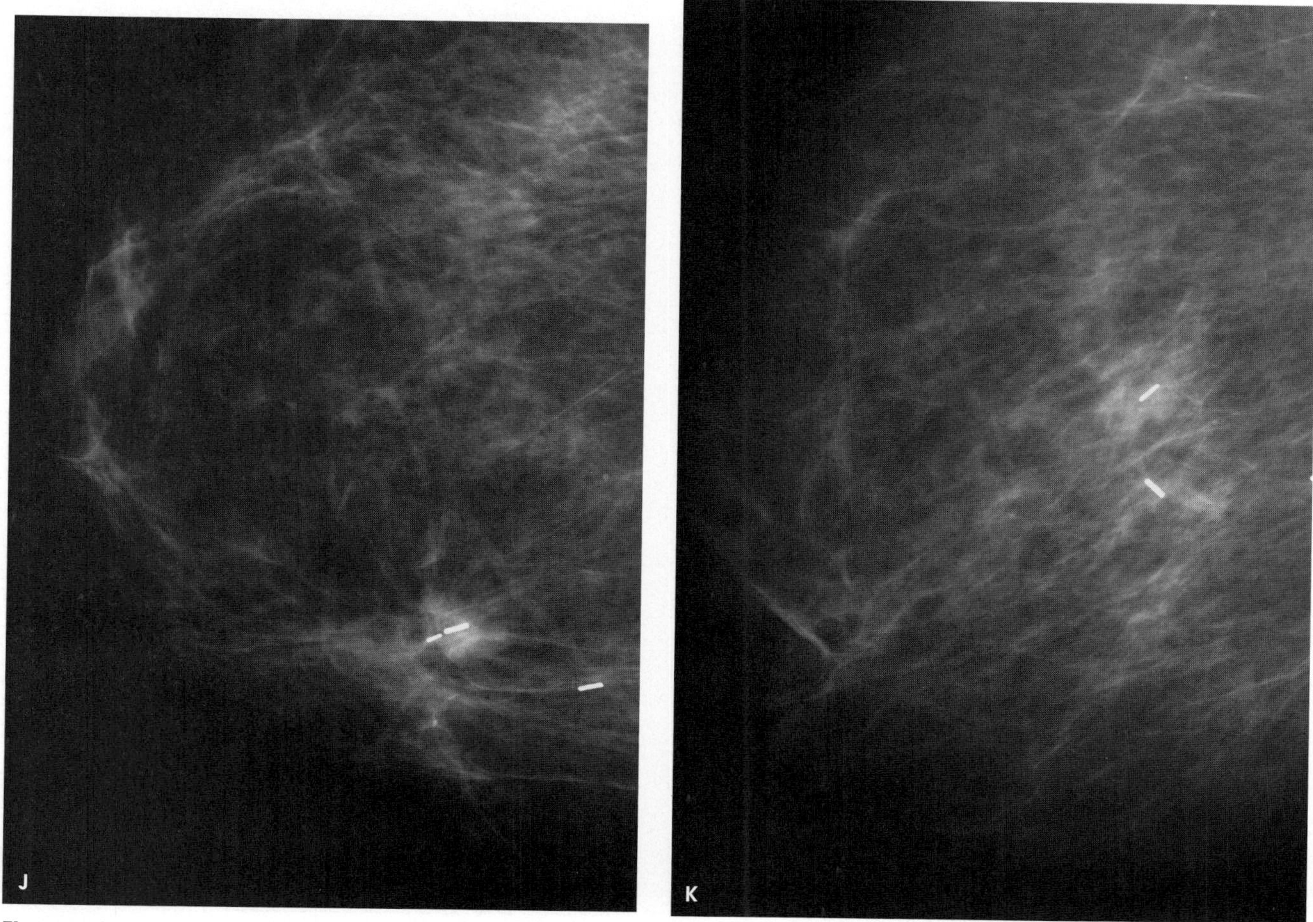

Figure 4.26. (*Continued*) Right craniocaudal **(D, F, H, J)** and mediolateral oblique **(E, G, I, K)** views, at 6, 18, 30, and 42 months following completion of the initial treatment. Linear metallic marker seen on some of the images is used to indicate the site of the lumpectomy scar.

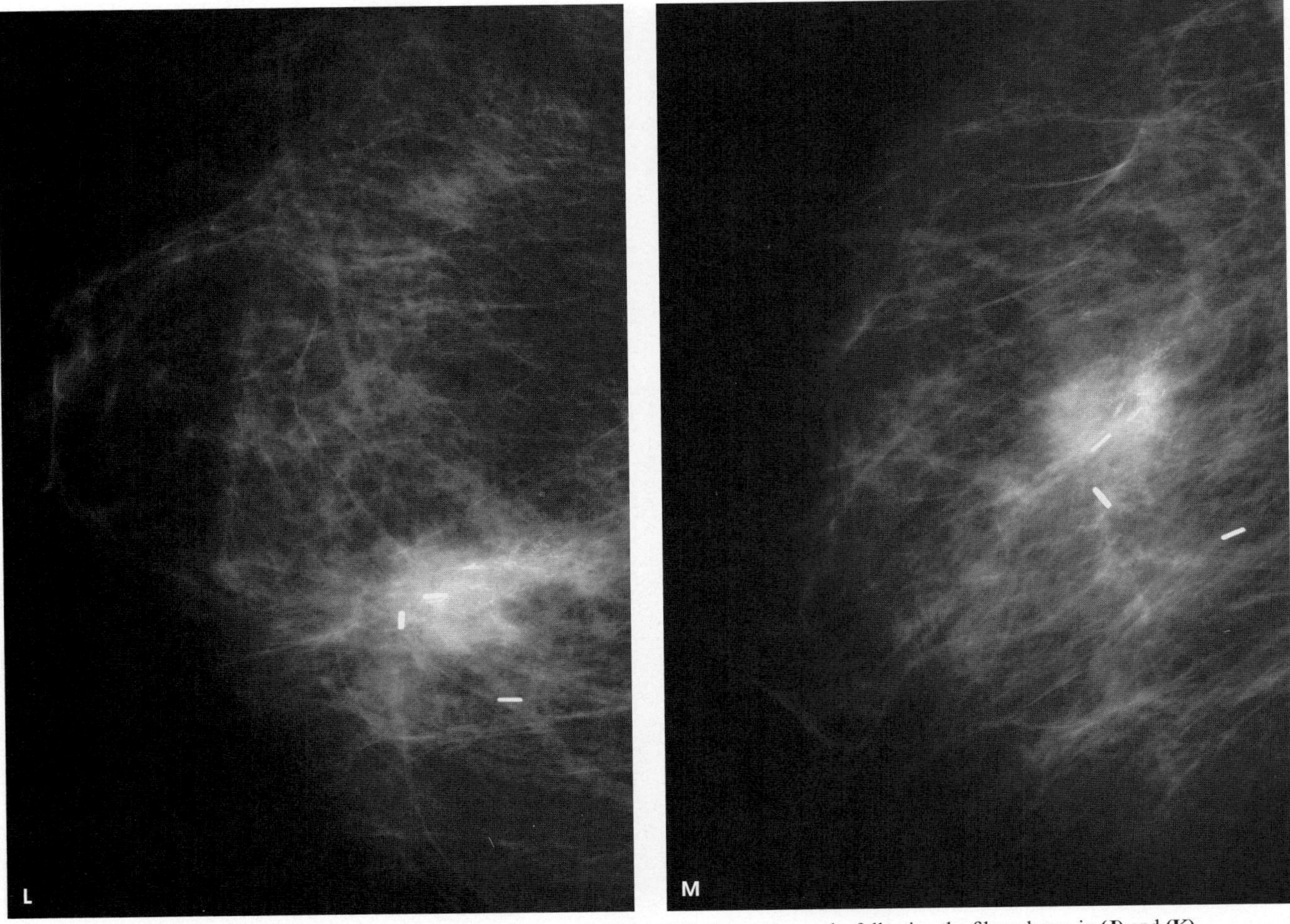

Figure 4.26. (*Continued*) Right craniocaudal **(L)** and mediolateral oblique **(M)** views, 11 months following the films shown in **(J)** and **(K)**.

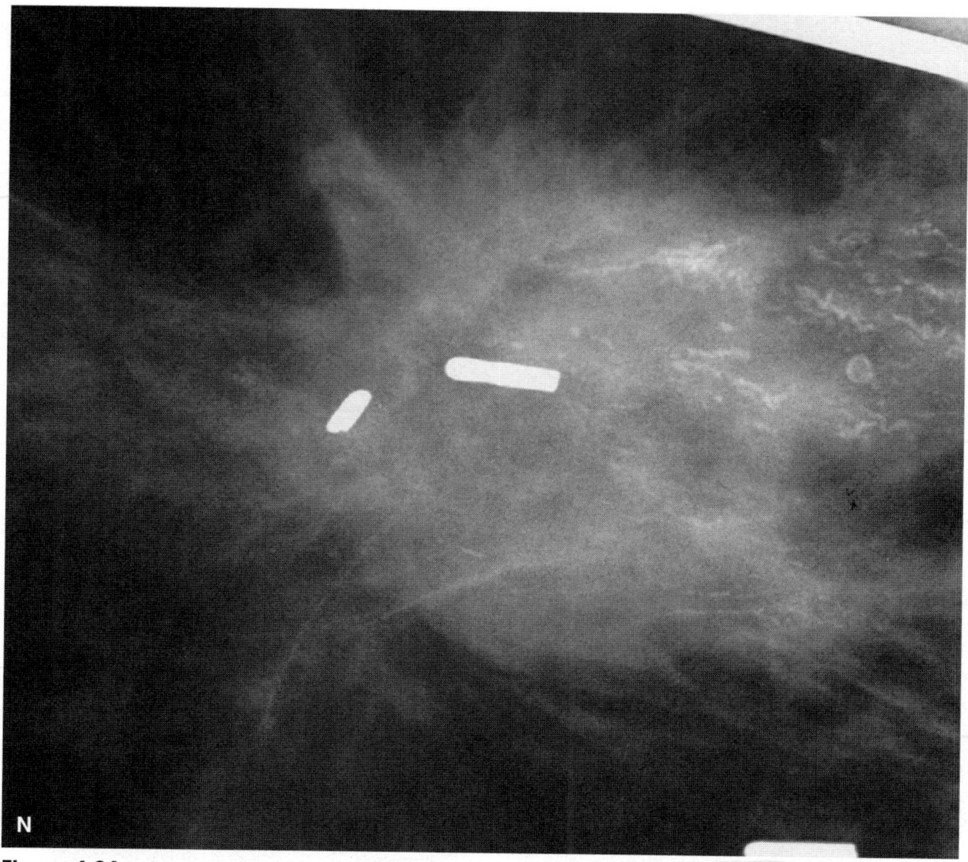

Figure 4.26. The patient now describes a "lump" at the lumpectomy site. Spot compression magnification craniocaudal view **(N),** right breast.

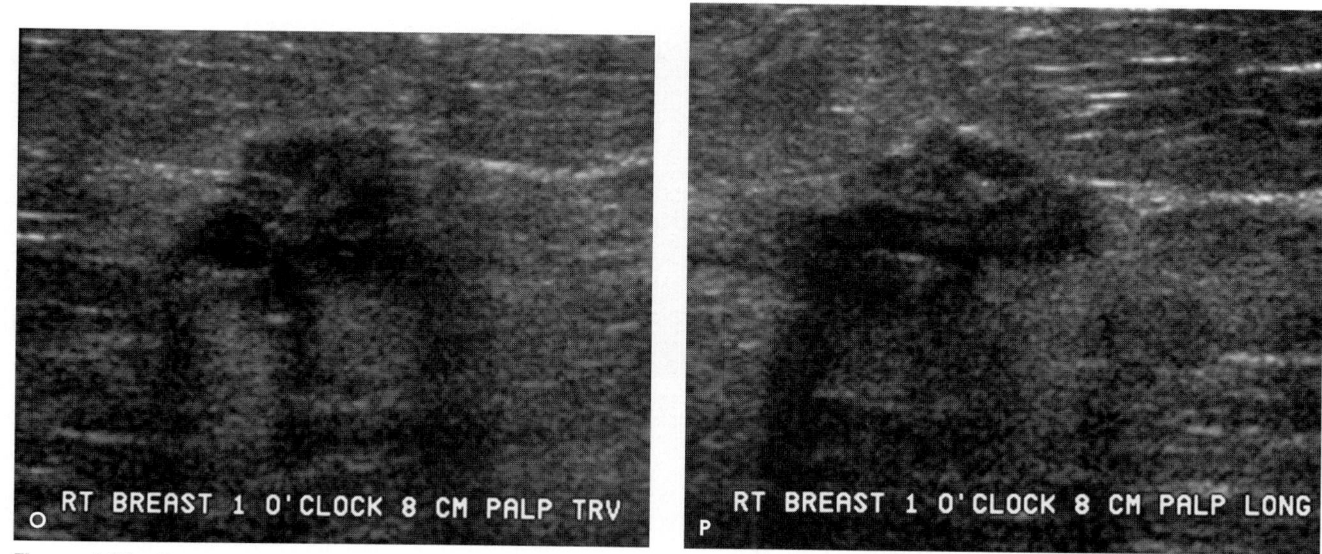

Figure 4.26. (*Continued*) The patient now describes a "lump" at the lumpectomy site. Spot compression magnification craniocaudal view **(N),** right breast. Ultrasound images, transverse (TRV) **(O)** and longitudinal (LON) **(P)** projections of the mass in the right breast at the 1 o'clock position, 8 cm from the nipple.

PATIENT 27

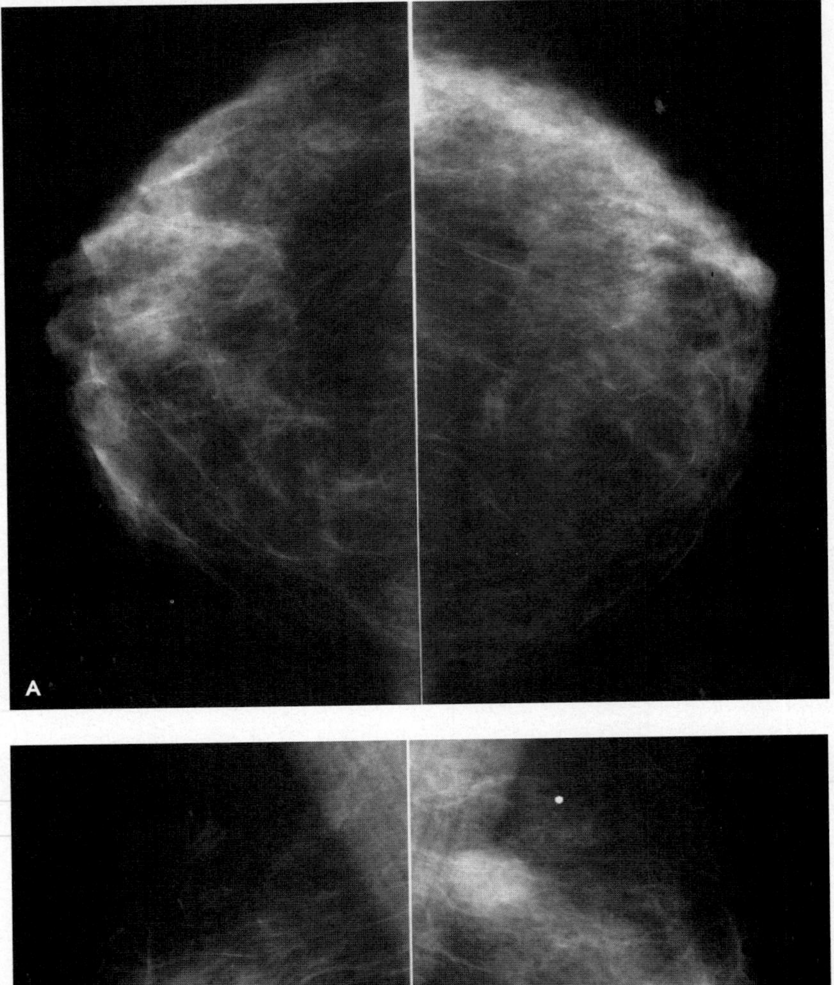

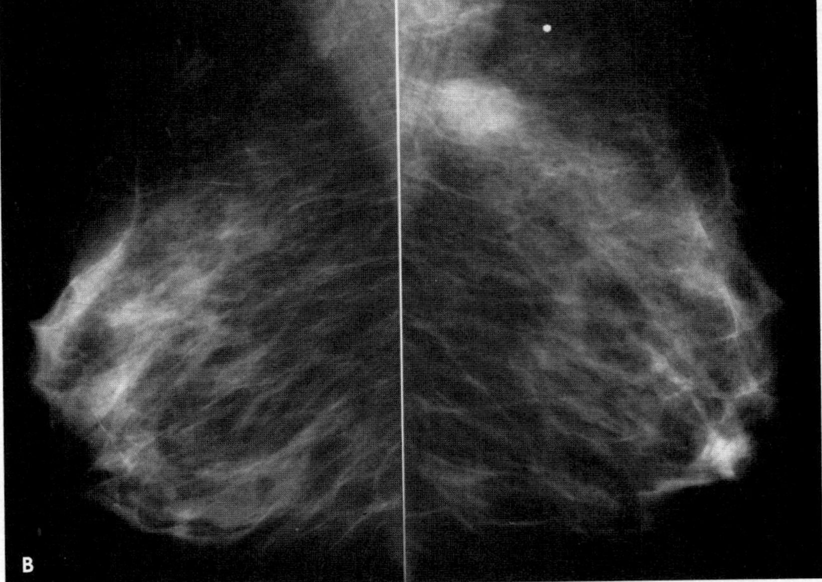

Figure 4.27. Diagnostic evaluation, 56-year-old patient presenting with a "lump" in the left breast. Craniocaudal **(A)** and mediolateral oblique **(B)** views.

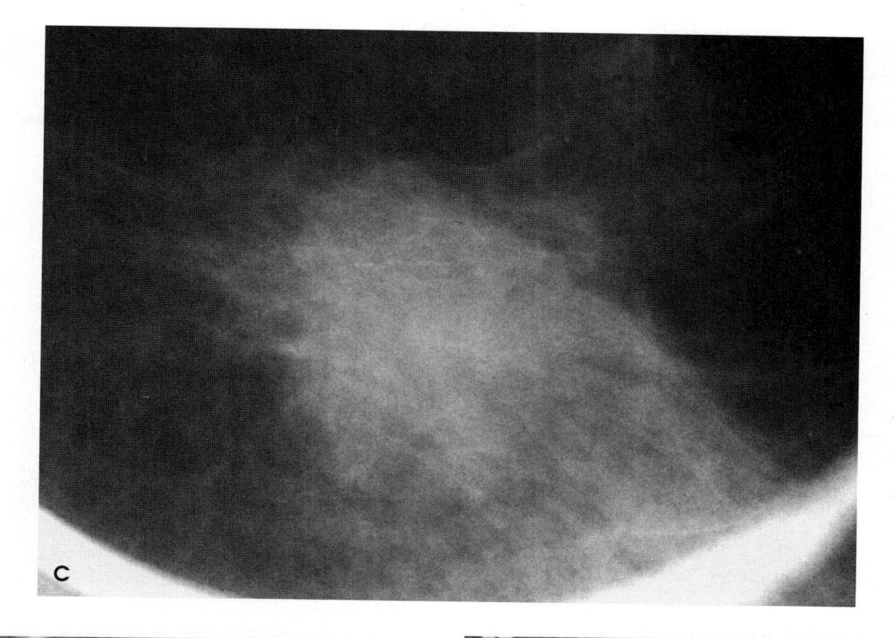

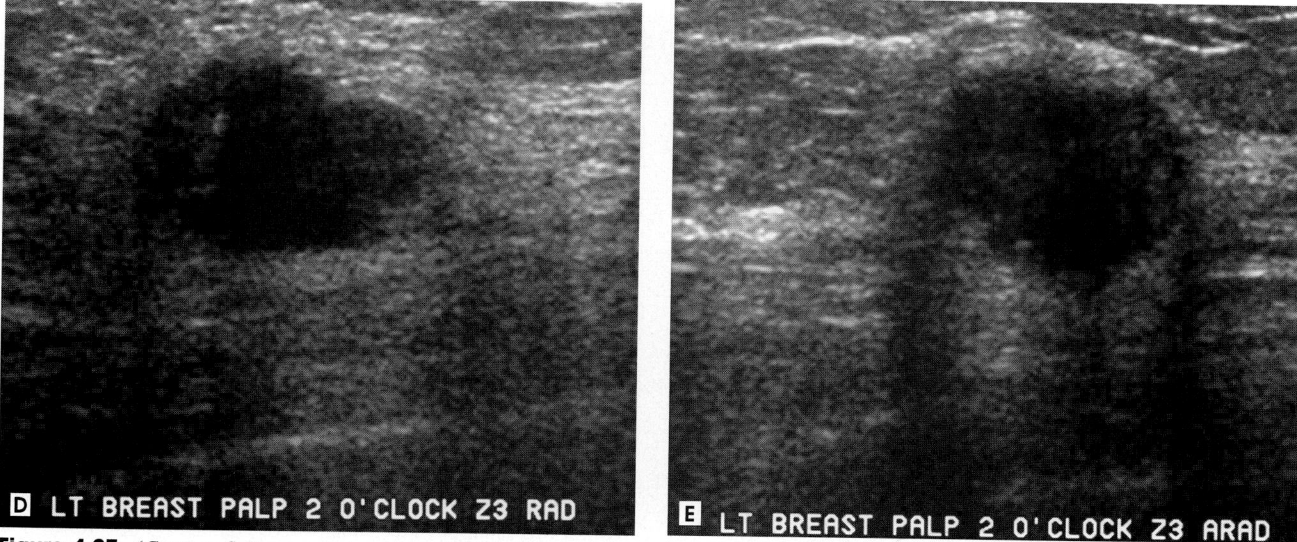

Figure 4.27. (*Continued*) Exaggerated craniocaudal **(C)** spot compression view of palpable finding, left breast. Ultrasound images, radial (RAD) **(D)** and antiradial (ARAD) **(E)** projections of palpable mass at the 2 o'clock position, posteriorly (Z3) in the left breast.

How would you describe the findings, and what is your recommendation?

On physical examination, a hard fixed mass is palpated at the site of concern to the patient. A solid, 2-cm mass with indistinct margins and spiculation, associated linear calcifications, and areas of shadowing and enhancement is imaged corresponding to the palpable finding. Given a round mass, with some enhancement and associated linear calcifications, the histologic diagnosis can be predicted fairly accurately. The clinical and imaging findings are consistent with a poorly differentiated invasive ductal carcinoma with associated ductal carcinoma in situ with central necrosis (probably high nuclear grade). In patients with a high likelihood of a malignancy, the remainder of the breast and the ipsilateral axilla are scanned to try and identify multifocal or centric disease and possibly abnormal axillary lymph nodes.

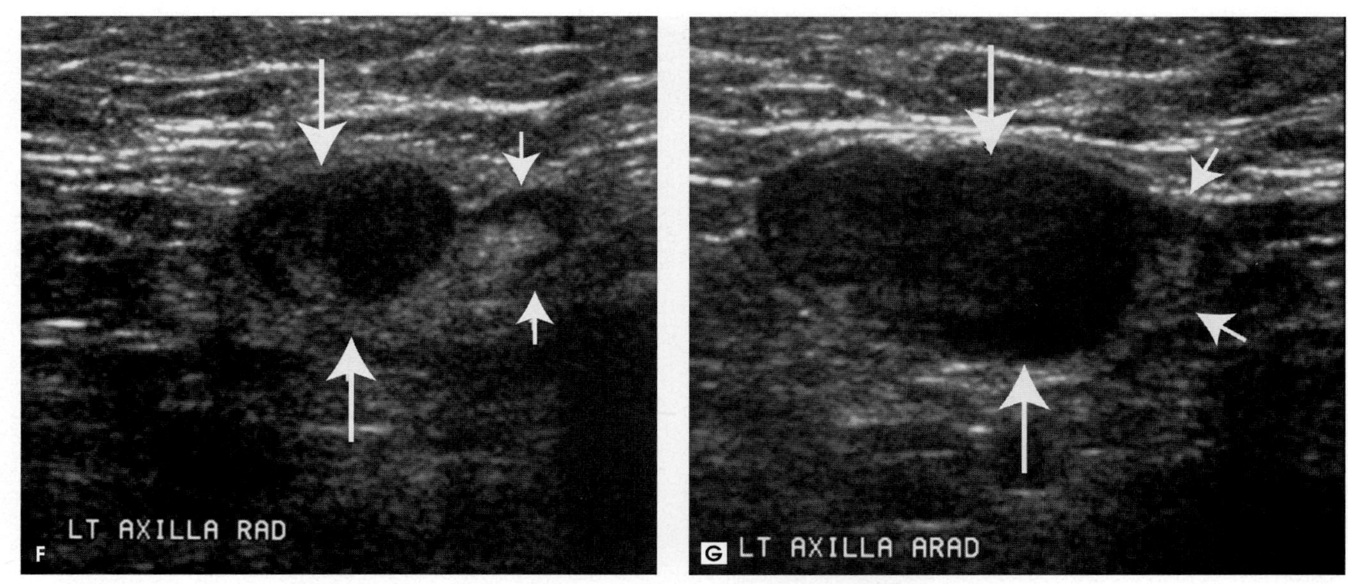

Figure 4.27. (*Continued*) Ultrasound images, radial (RAD) **(F)** and antiradial (ARAD) **(G)** projections, left axilla.

How would you describe the findings, and what is your recommendation?

A potentially abnormal lymph node is identified in the ipsilateral axilla. An adjacent normal-appearing lymph node is also noted. Potentially abnormal lymph nodes are characterized by absence or marked attenuation of the echogenic hilar region in conjunction with thickening and bulging of the hypoechoic cortex. In some patients, potentially abnormal lymph nodes are nearly anechoic and no hyperechoic hilar region is present. When a potentially abnormal lymph node is identified, we recommend fine-needle aspiration or, depending on the size and location of the lymph node, a core biopsy (if it can be done safely). In this patient, core biopsies are done on the mass in the breast and of the potentially abnormal axillary lymph node. An invasive ductal carcinoma with associated ductal carcinoma in situ and metastatic disease to the axillary lymph node are reported on the core biopsies. With the diagnosis of metastatic disease to an axillary lymph node, the patient will undergo a full axillary dissection (i.e., sentinel lymph node biopsy is not indicated).

Treatment options discussed with this patient include mastectomy and axillary dissection followed by chemotherapy; lumpectomy with axillary dissection followed by radiation therapy and chemotherapy; or, being used with increasing frequency, neoadjuvant therapy followed by either mastectomy or lumpectomy, an axillary dissection, and radiation therapy for those patients having a lumpectomy. If a mastectomy is done following neoadjuvant therapy, radiation therapy is not always recommended. Neoadjuvant therapy can decrease the size of, or eliminate, the tumor (i.e., downstage the lesion), enabling some patients, who might not otherwise be candidates for conservative therapy, to undergo lumpectomy. This patient elects to undergo neoadjuvant therapy.

After two courses of chemotherapy, the mass has decreased in size (Fig. 4.17H, I). In patients who undergo neoadjuvant therapy, the initial findings may resolve completely. Consequently, in patients who may elect to have a lumpectomy after neoadjuvant therapy, marking the location of the original lesion is important so that this area can be localized, excised, and evaluated for residual disease. Given the significant response in this patient after two courses of chemotherapy, and with a planned lumpectomy if the tumor continues to respond, a "marking" clip is placed in the mass using ultrasound guidance (Fig. 4.27J).

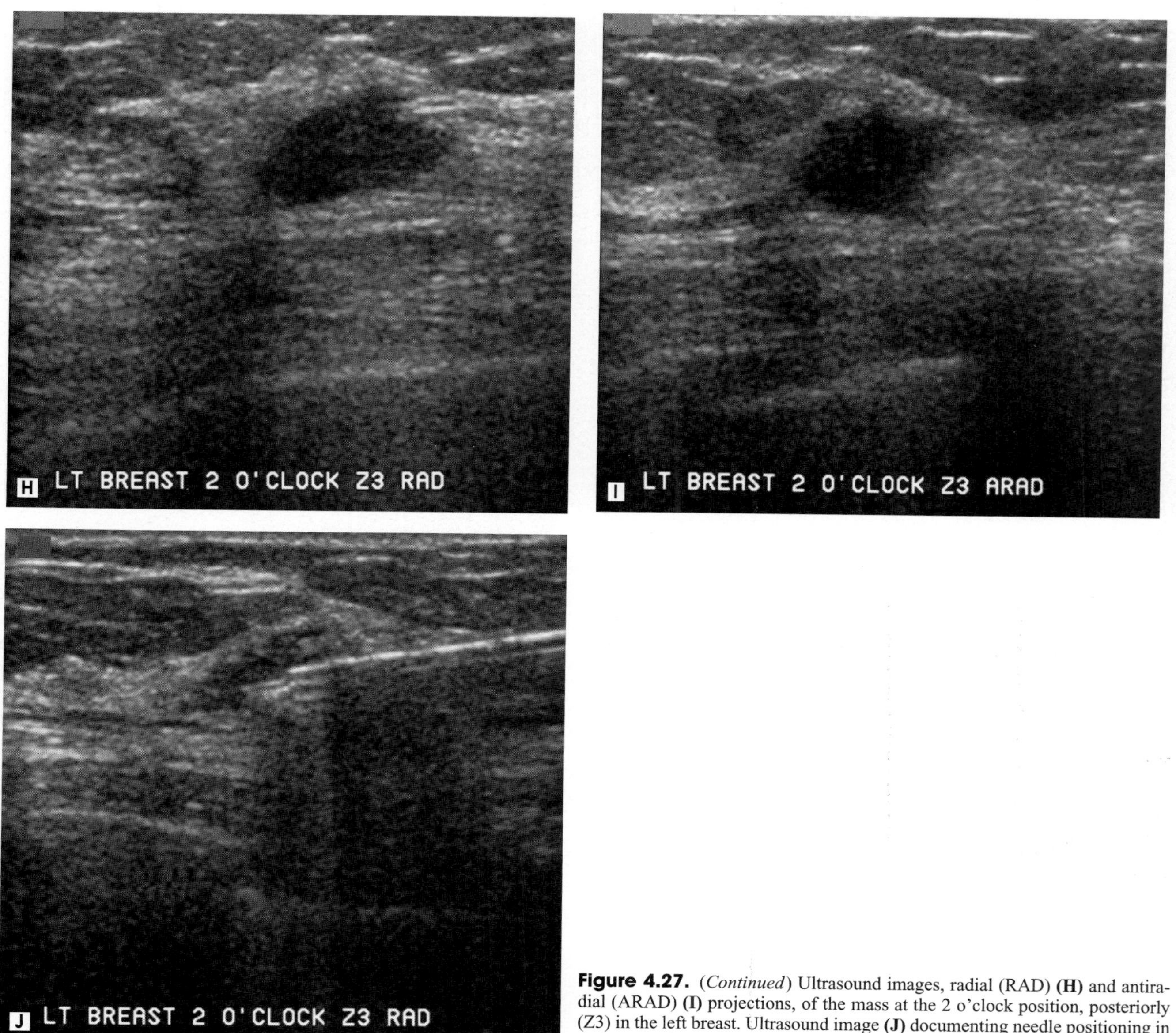

Figure 4.27. (*Continued*) Ultrasound images, radial (RAD) **(H)** and antiradial (ARAD) **(I)** projections, of the mass at the 2 o'clock position, posteriorly (Z3) in the left breast. Ultrasound image **(J)** documenting needle positioning in the center of the mass prior to deployment of the clip.

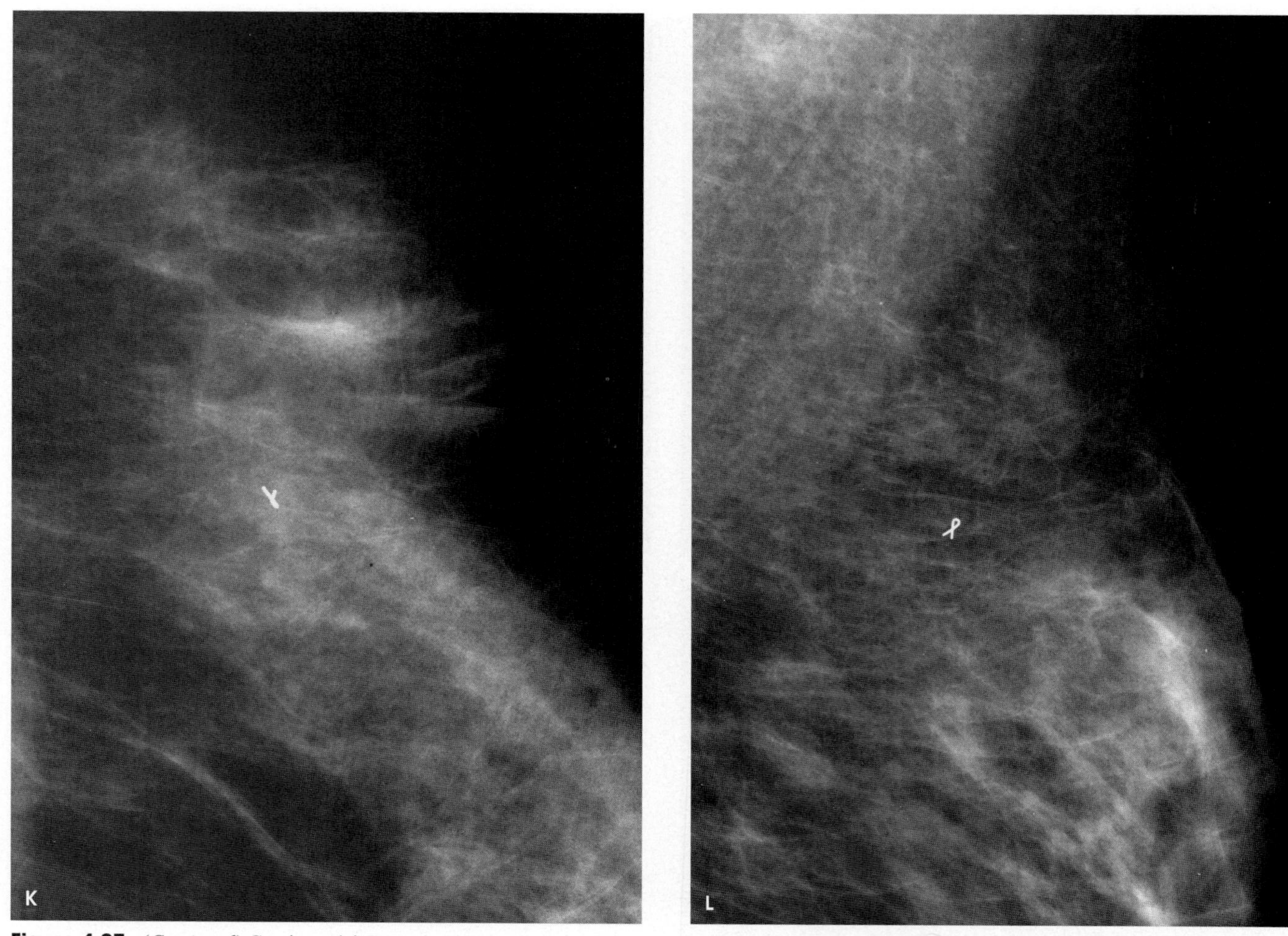

Figure 4.27. (*Continued*) Craniocaudal **(K)** and 90-degree lateral **(L)** views of the left breast, photographically coned, documenting clip location.

Clips to mark the location of a lesion are deployed at the time of imaging-guided biopsies when a lesion (e.g. a cluster of calcifications or a small mass being biopsied with an 11G vacuum-assisted device), which may be malignant, might be removed in its entirety as a result of the biopsy. In these patients, if a malignancy is diagnosed and the original lesion has been removed completely, the clip deployed at the time of imaging-guided biopsy marks the site of the lesion. At the time of the lumpectomy, the clip is localized so that the tissue surrounding the original lesion can be evaluated histologically for residual disease. Similarly, if it is known that a patient will undergo neoadjuvant therapy, and because the lesion may resolve as a result of the therapy, a clip can be deployed in the lesion at the time of the biopsy. If the lesion responds to therapy, the clip is localized preoperatively in those patients undergoing lumpectomy so that the tissue at the site of the treated lesion can be evaluated histologically for residual disease. Alternatively, as in this patient (because histology is not always predictable at the time of the biopsy and treatment choice is not always known), the clip can be deployed during the therapy in those patients in whom the original lesion is responding and may resolve completely prior to the surgery.

Following completion of her neoadjuvant therapy, the patient undergoes a lumpectomy and full axillary dissection. A 2-cm area of fibrosis, consistent with tumor regression, is described at the site of the clip. No residual tumor is identified. No metastatic disease is identified in 11 excised axillary lymph nodes. Several of the lymph nodes demonstrate areas of fibrosis consistent with tumor regression [ypTX, ypN0, ypMX]. As in this patient, approximately 15% to 20% of patients who undergo neoadjuvant therapy demonstrate complete response with no residual tumor identified histologically at the time of their surgical procedure. Reportedly, the subgroup of patients with a complete pathologic response has higher relapse-free survival and overall survival rates compared with patients with residual disease at the time.

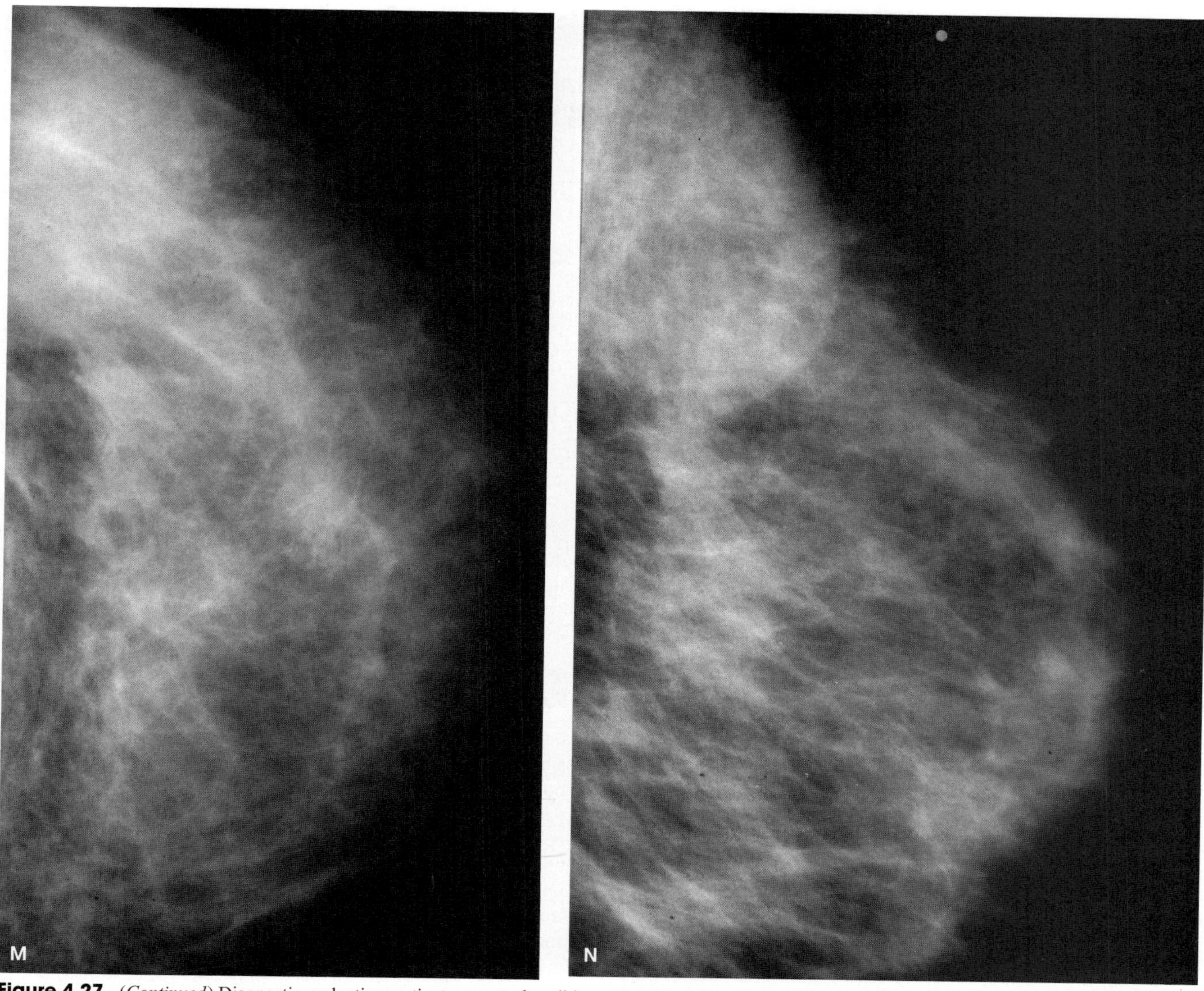

Figure 4.27. (*Continued*) Diagnostic evaluation, patient presents describing a "lump" at the lumpectomy site, 6 months following neoadjuvant therapy and, more recently, lumpectomy and radiation therapy. Craniocaudal **(M)** and mediolateral oblique **(N)** views, left breast.

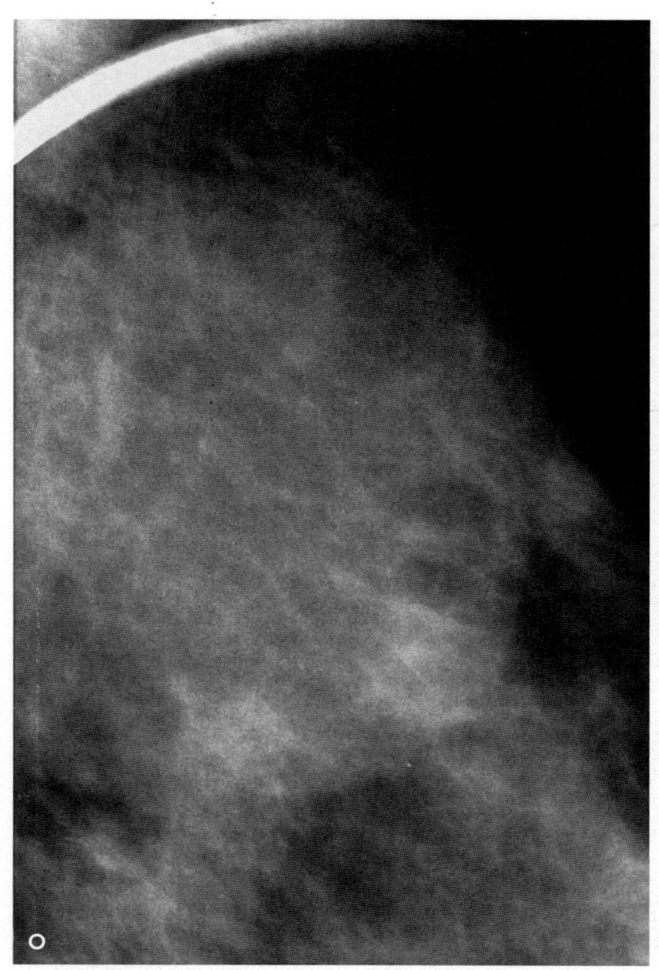

Figure 4.27. (*Continued*) Spot compression **(O)** view of palpable finding.

How would you describe the findings, and what is your main consideration at this point?

The overall density of the breast is increased, which is consistent with radiation therapy effect. A round mass with partially well circumscribed and obscured margins is imaged at the lumpectomy site and corresponds to the site of concern to the patient. Although this could represent a recurrence, given a complete pathologic response to neoadjuvant therapy and the short time interval between her lumpectomy and the development of this mass, a postoperative fluid collection is the primary consideration. An ultrasound is done for further evaluation.

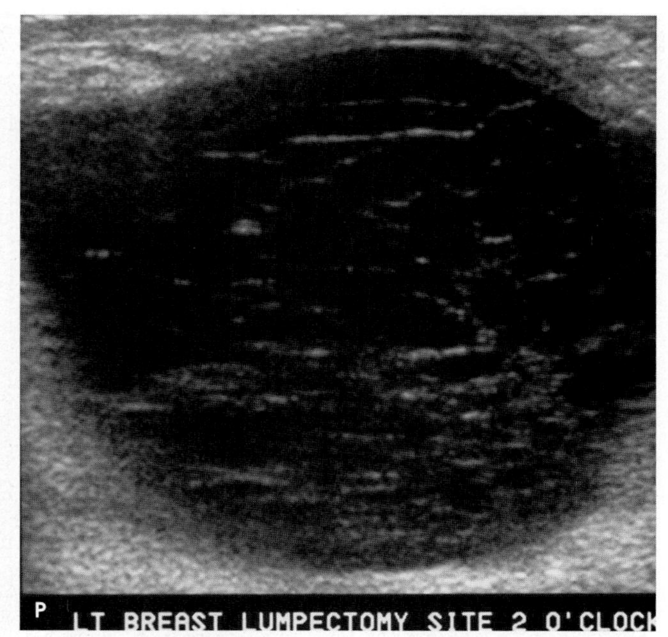

Figure 4.27. (*Continued*) Ultrasound image **(P)** of mass at the lumpectomy site, 2 o'clock position, left breast.

What is your diagnosis and recommendation?

On physical examination, a hard mass is palpated at the lumpectomy site. On ultrasound, a well-circumscribed, complex cystic mass with posterior acoustic enhancement is imaged corresponding to the palpable finding. During the real-time portion of the study, some of the spicular echoes and hyperechoic bands in the mass shift in position and appear to be "floating" in the mass, respectively. This is a postoperative fluid collection requiring no intervention unless a superimposed infection is suspected or it is causing significant discomfort. A high recurrence rate is associated with aspiration. It is critical, however, to reassure the patient that this is not a recurrence and that fluid collections are common following lumpectomy. We can expect that this will decrease in size and stabilize or resolve completely with time. Postoperative fluid collections typically have a complex cystic appearance on ultrasound. As in this patient, many can be characterized as predominantly cystic, with spicular echoes, septations, and mural nodules, whereas others have small cystic spaces in what otherwise appears to be a solid matrix.

PATIENT 28

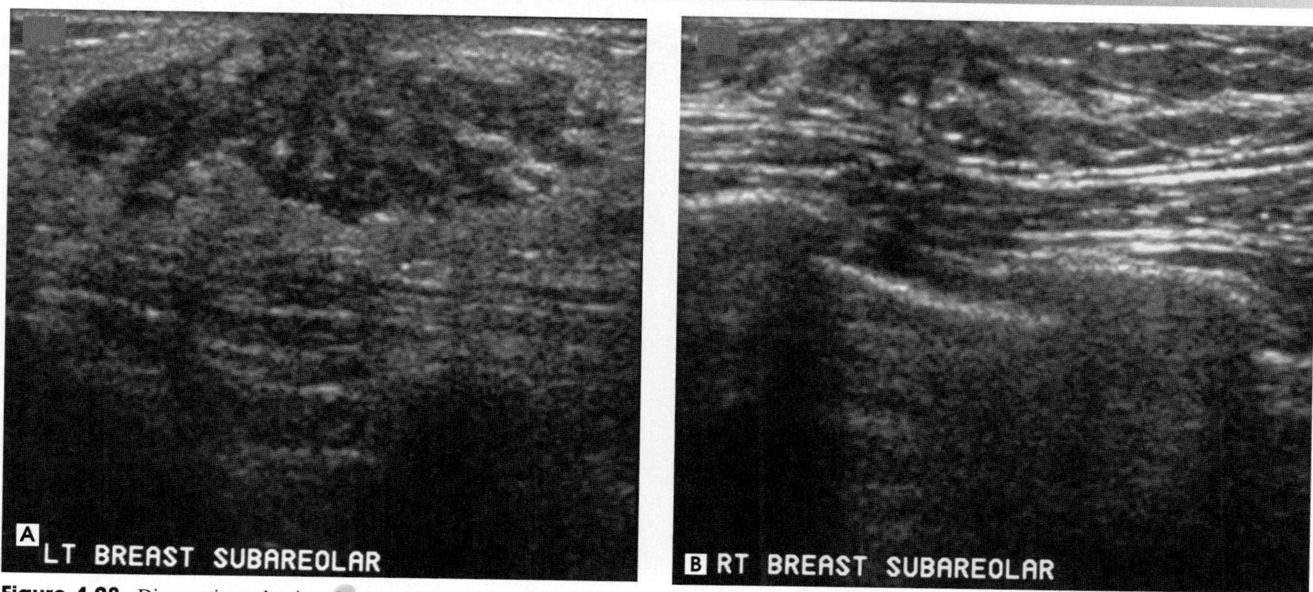

Figure 4.28. Diagnostic evaluation, 8-year-old girl with a mass in the left subareolar area. Ultrasound image **(A)** of left subareolar area. Ultrasound image **(B)** of the right subareolar area for comparison.

What is the diagnosis and recommendation?

On physical examination, the left breast is more prominent than the right, and a readily mobile mass is palpated in the left subareolar area. On ultrasound, an irregular area of hypoechogenicity with indistinct margins is imaged in the left subareolar area. A smaller but similar-appearing area is imaged in the right subareolar area. This is consistent with premature, asymmetric breast bud development (a very similar appearance is seen when an ultrasound study is done in men with gynecomastia). No further intervention is warranted.

Breast masses in children and adolescents are often benign and include inflammatory conditions, premature breast bud development, cysts, and fibroadenomas. Malignant causes are rare but include metastatic disease (rhabdomyosarcoma, neuroblastoma, lymphoma) and secretory carcinoma (a primary breast malignancy characterized by large amounts of intra- and extracellular secretion and neoplastic cells with granular eosinophilic cytoplasm). Although initially called juvenile carcinoma because it was associated with childhood and adolescence, it can occur in patients of all ages. Care is required in the management of these patients, because surgical removal of a developing breast bud results in significant deformity or failure of normal breast development. Consequently, fine-needle aspiration is the procedure of choice if a neoplastic process is a serious consideration in this patient population.

PATIENT 29

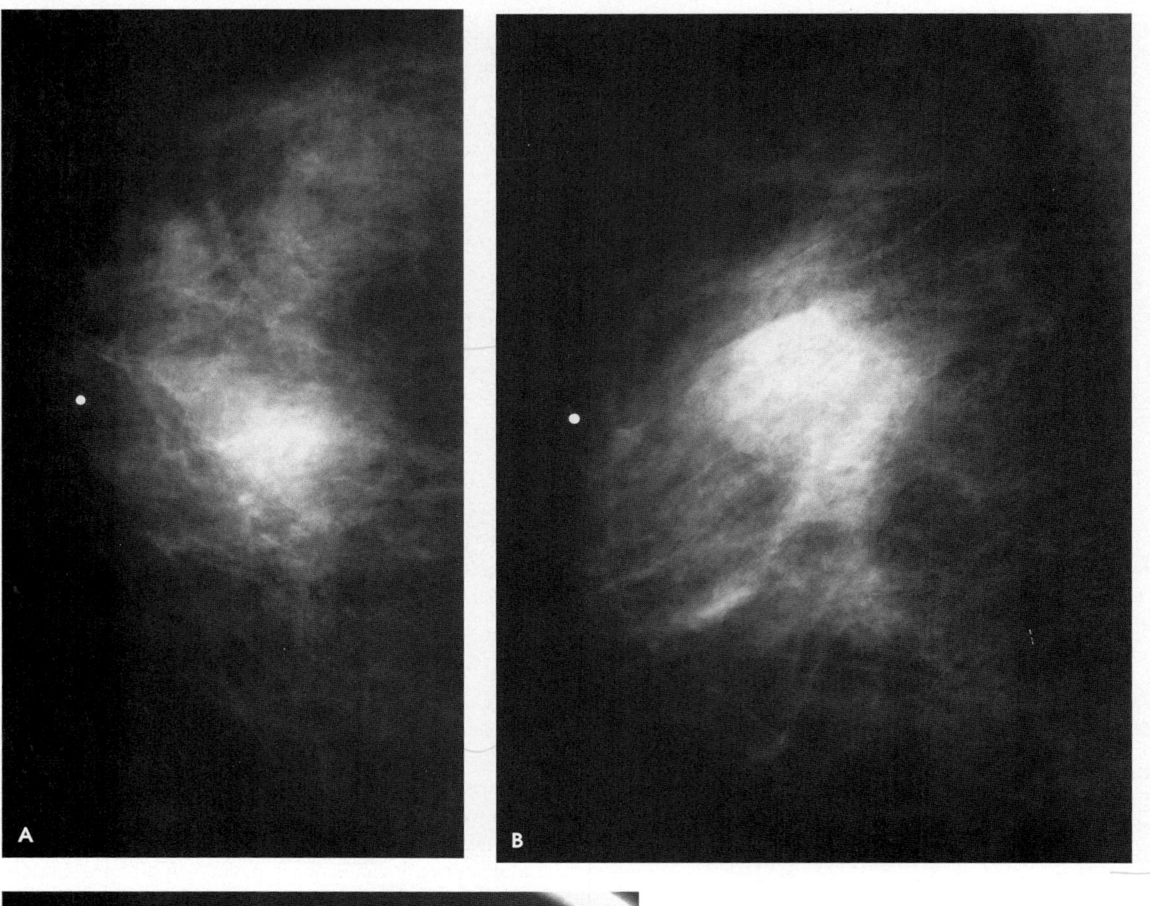

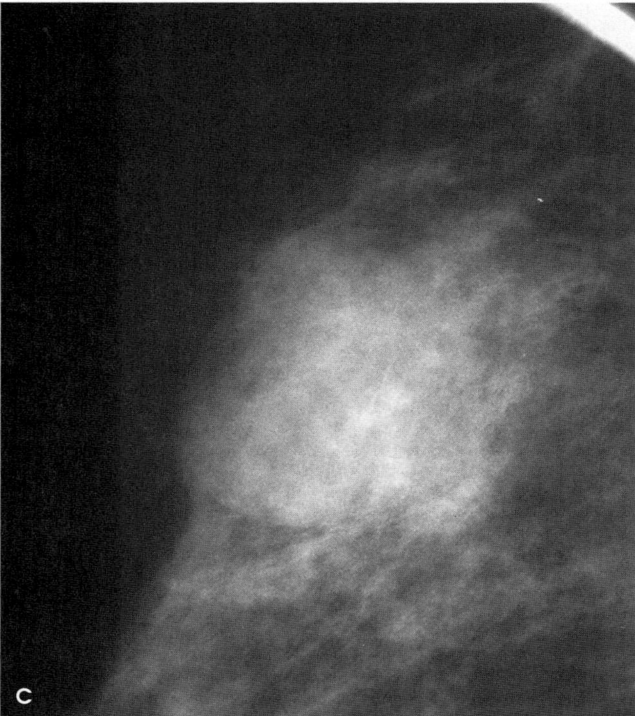

Figure 4.29. Diagnostic evaluation, 45-year-old patient presenting with a painful "lump" in the right breast. Craniocaudal **(A)** and mediolateral oblique **(B)** views, right breast, with a metallic BB at the site of concern to the patient. Spot tangential **(C)** view of the palpable finding.

How would you describe the findings, and what would you recommend next?

On the routine views, a mass with obscured margins is imaged corresponding to the palpable finding. On the spot tangential view, the margins of the mass are partially well circumscribed, indistinct and obscured. Differential considerations include cyst, fibroadenoma (complex fibroadenoma, tubular adenoma), phyllodes tumor, papilloma, pseudoangiomatous stromal hyperplasia, and focal fibrosis. Depending on history and clinical findings, an inflammatory process, posttraumatic/postsurgical fluid collection, and a galactocele might also be in the differential. Malignant considerations include invasive ductal carcinoma not otherwise specified, medullary carcinoma, or metastatic disease. Although they are less likely given the patient's age, mucinous and papillary carcinomas are also in the differential. Correlative physical examination and an ultrasound are indicated for further characterization.

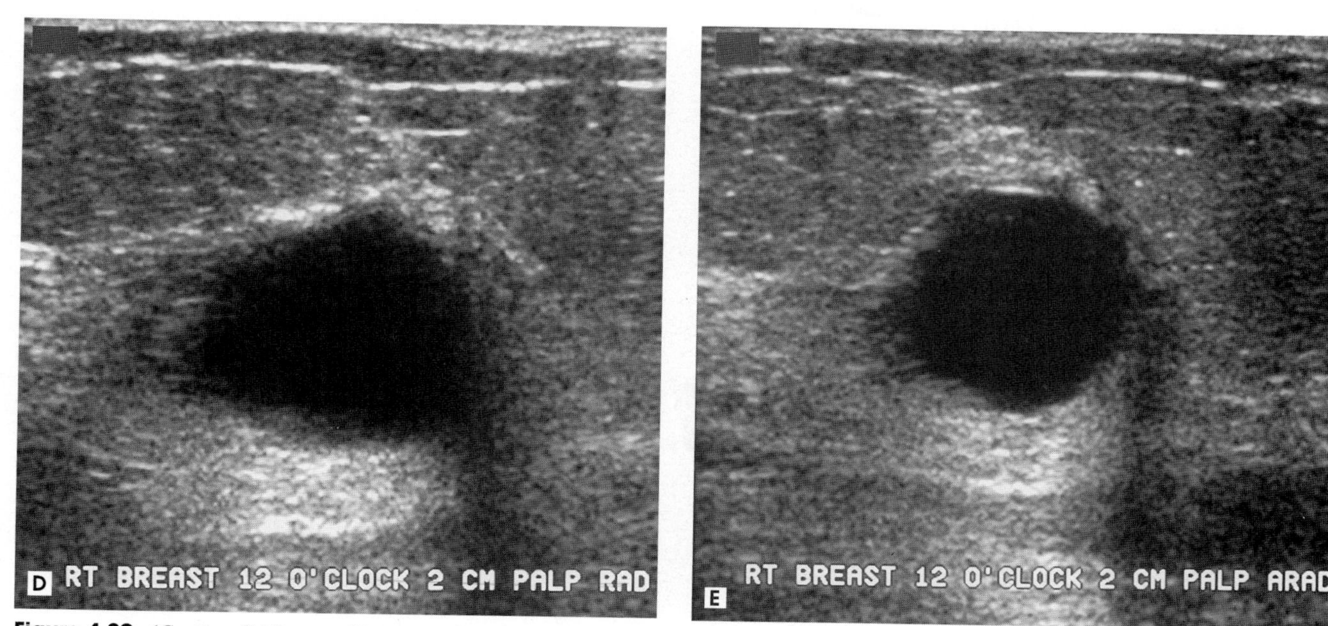

Figure 4.29. (*Continued*) Ultrasound images, radial (RAD) **(D)** and antiradial (ARAD) **(E)** projections of palpable finding, right breast.

What is the diagnosis, and what would you recommend?

On physical examination, there is a hard tender mass palpated at the 12 o'clock position, 2 cm from the right nipple. On ultrasound, this is an anechoic mass with posterior acoustic enhancement consistent with a cyst. There is some irregularity of a portion of the wall. Following discussion with the patient, an aspiration is undertaken, primarily for symptomatic relief. A pneumocystogram is also planned for further evaluation.

After establishing an approach that allows me to advance the needle parallel to the transducer, I clean the skin and use lidocaine to anesthetize the skin. Then, using ultrasound guidance, I inject lidocaine in the tissue leading up to, but taking care to not go into, the lesion. I use ultrasound guidance for administering the anesthesia and for doing the aspiration, even in patients in whom the mass is palpable. Commonly, the advancing needle displaces the mass, or indents the wall, but does not penetrate into the mass (I think this explains many of the patients who present for evaluation of a palpable mass following attempted aspirations that yielded no fluid and yet we find a cyst corresponding to the palpable finding). By visualizing the trajectory of the advancing needle, I can gauge the amount of compression I need to apply to effectively immobilize the mass and the amount of controlled pressure I need apply with the needle so that the cyst wall is punctured. With the needle in the cyst, I pull the stylet out of the 20G spinal needle, attach a 10-mL syringe, and aspirate. I watch on real time as I aspirate, to be sure there is no residual abnormality postaspiration. Also, in some patients, the needle may need to be redirected (i.e., the tip of the needle is against the cyst wall) during the aspiration, to be sure that all the fluid is aspirated. At this point, if I am doing a pneumocystogram, I stabilize the needle and replace the fluid-filled syringe with one holding air (half of the volume of the aspirated fluid), and I then inject the air into the cyst (Fig. 4.29H). The air is imaged as an echogenic line (Fig. 4.29I, arrows).

In this patient, 4 mL of serous fluid is aspirated and no residual abnormality is seen following the aspiration. For the pneumocystogram, half of the volume of fluid aspirated is replaced with air (Fig. 4.29H, I) and spot compression magnification views of the aspirated cyst are obtained (Fig. 4.29J, K). Possible wall irregularity and thickening or intracystic lesions can be further evaluated on the pneumocystogram. In this patient, the wall of the cyst is smooth and well defined. No intracystic lesion or wall abnormality is identified. Annual screening mammography is recommended.

BI-RADS® category 2: benign finding.

Following cyst aspiration, I routinely inject air into the cyst cavity. Some have suggested that air injection following aspiration can reduce the incidence of cyst recurrence. The air does not hurt the patient, and if it is helpful in minimizing the likelihood of a recurrence, it can be beneficial. For patients for whom I am concerned about the presence of a mural or intracystic abnormality, spot compression magnification views of the cyst are done following the injection of air (i.e., a pneumocystogram), to further evaluate the wall of the cyst.

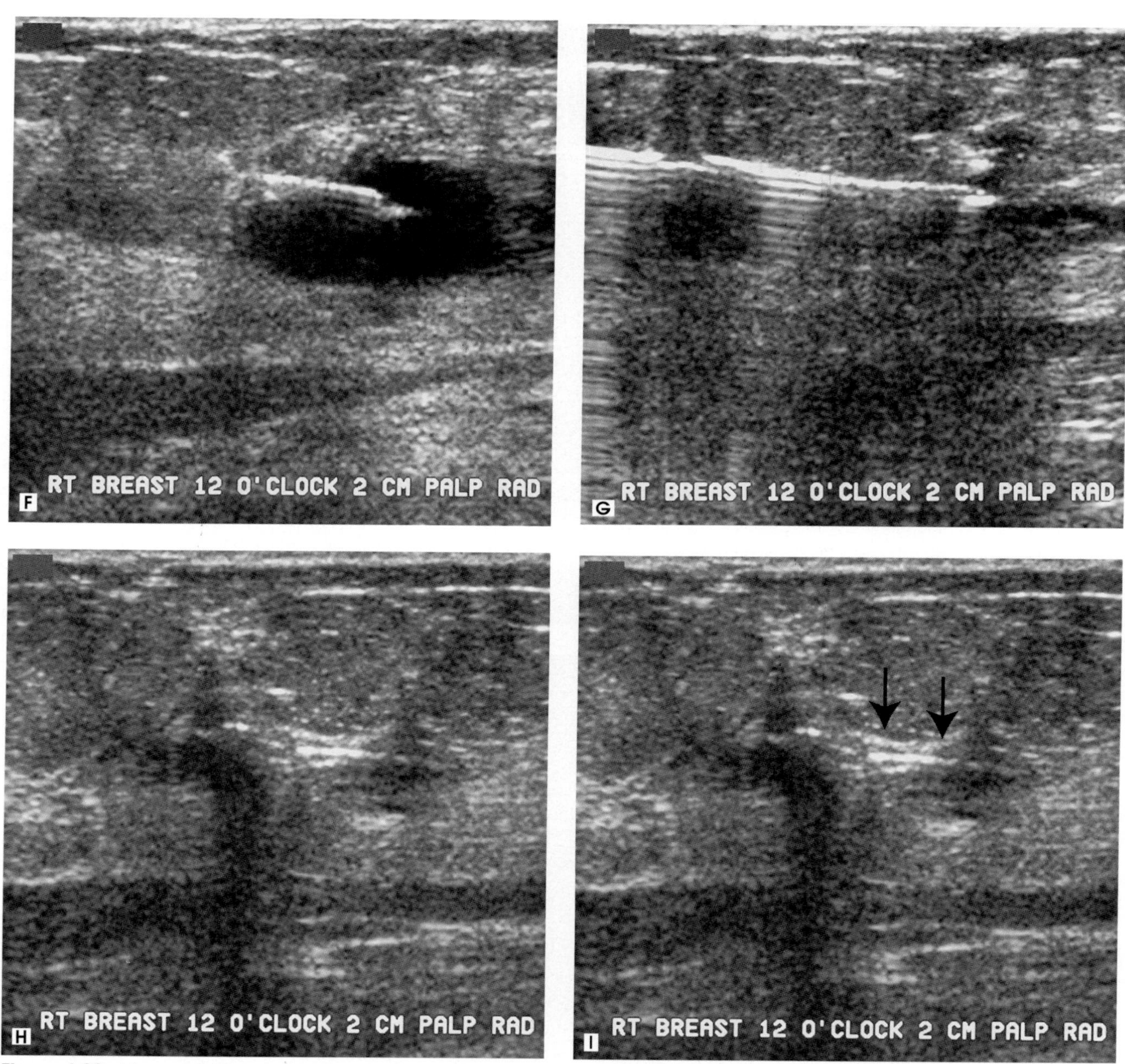

Figure 4.29. (*Continued*) Ultrasound images of aspiration. Preaspiration image, documenting needle positioning in the cyst **(F)**, postaspiration image demonstrating no residual abnormality **(G)** surrounding the needle, and image obtained following the injection of air **(H)**. Ultrasound image following air injection **(I)**. Air is seen as an echogenic line (*arrows*).

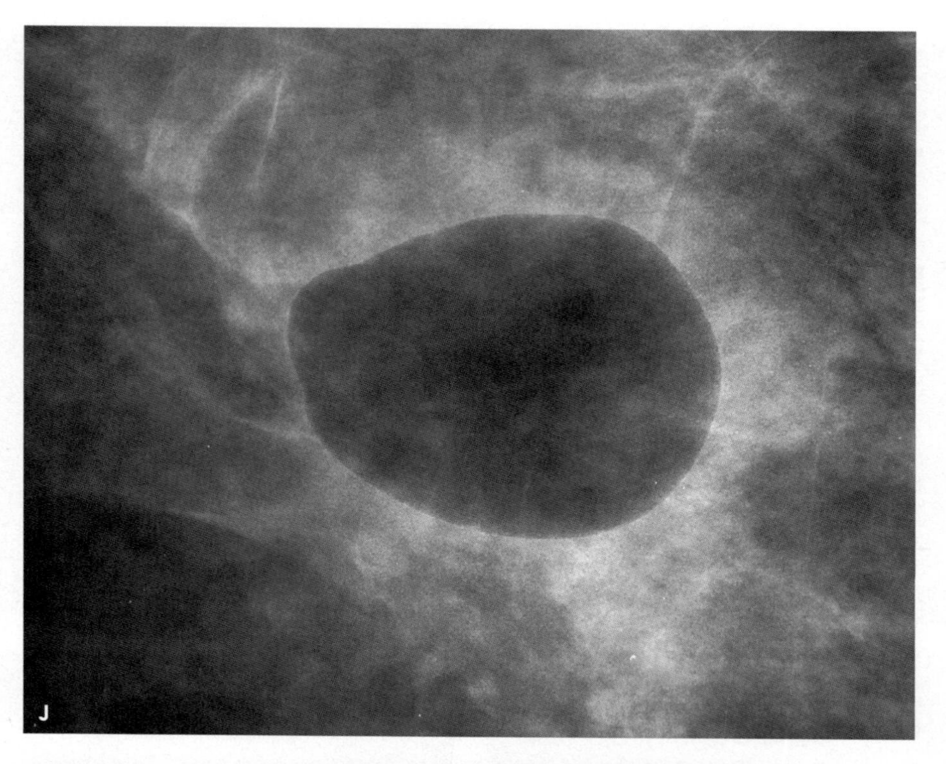

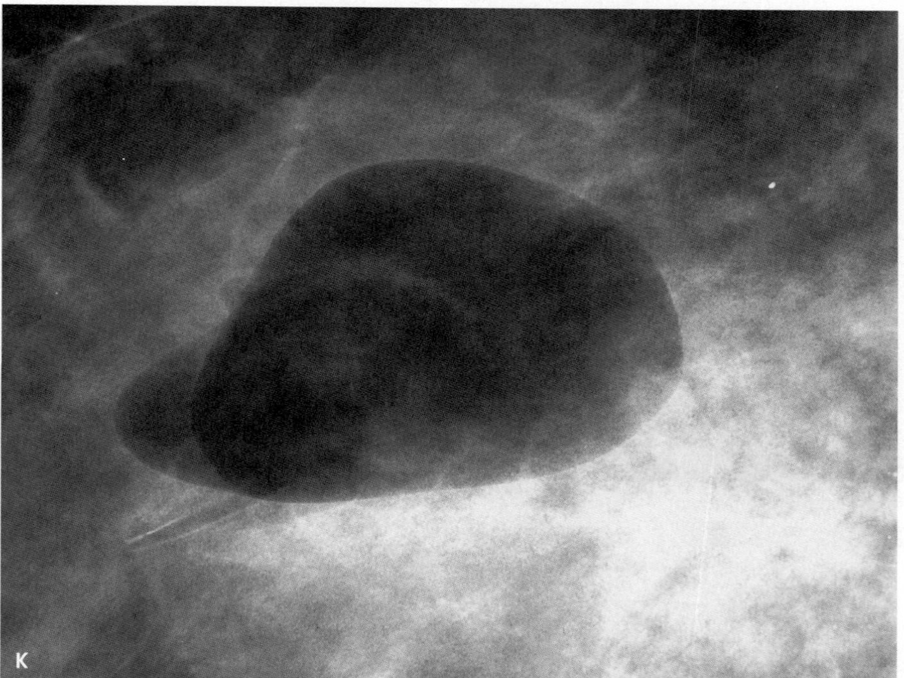

Figure 4.29. (*Continued*) Pneumocystogram films. Spot compression magnification views of air-filled cyst, craniocaudal **(J)** and mediolateral oblique **(K)** projections.

PATIENT 30

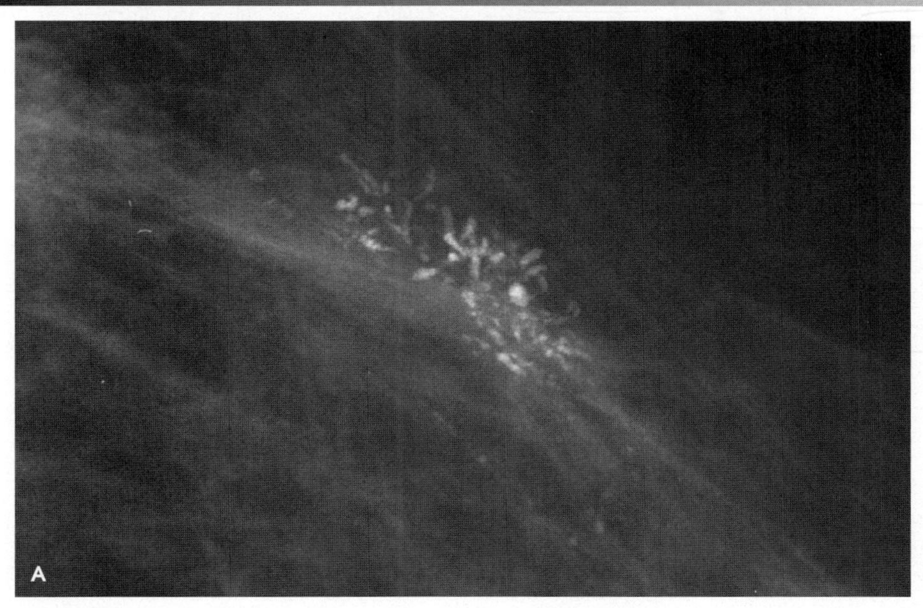

Figure 4.30. Diagnostic evaluation, 55-year-old patient called back for evaluation of a cluster of calcifications in the left breast detected on her screening mammogram. Double spot compression magnification view **(A)**, craniocaudal projection.

What is your working diagnosis, and what is your recommendation?

The magnification views confirm a cluster of calcifications with linear forms having irregular margins, clefts, and demonstrating linear orientation. The main consideration with calcifications having these features is ductal carcinoma in situ with central necrosis, likely high nuclear grade. Biopsy is indicated.

As described previously (see discussion with Figs. 4.18 and 4.19), these types of calcifications are closely associated with the malignant cells. Targeting the calcifications targets the malignant cells. If calcifications are removed in the cores, the diagnosis is established. Consequently, I evaluate patients having a tight cluster of this type of calcifications with ultrasound. Although in some of these patients a mass is identified sonographically in association with the calcifications, the primary reason for doing the ultrasound is not to detect or further characterize the calcifications, but rather to determine whether I can use ultrasound guidance for the biopsy. My preference is to do ultrasound-guided core biopsies because patients are more comfortable in a supine position with no breast compression, and no radiation is needed. If I can see the calcifications with ultrasound, I can target them.

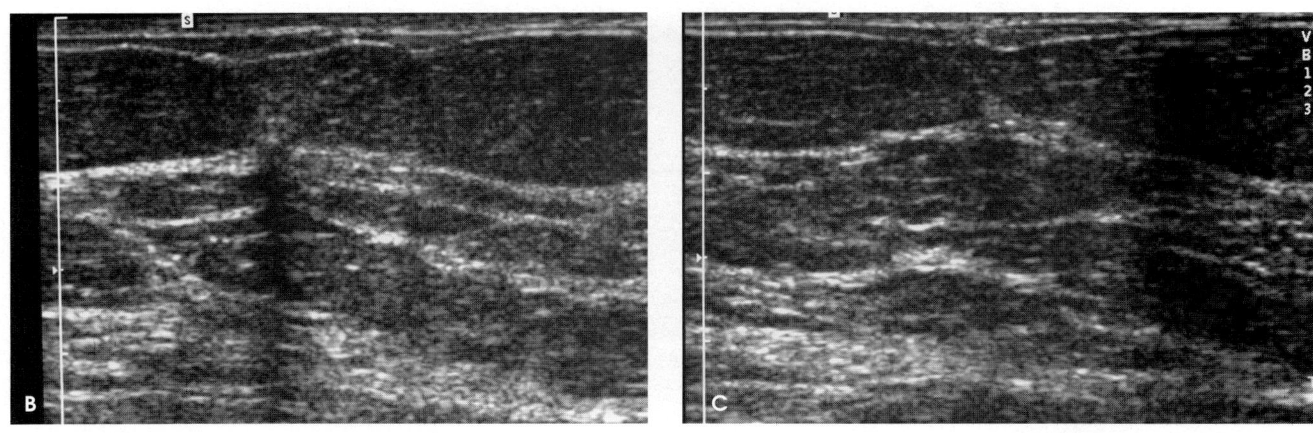

Figure 4.30. (*Continued*) Ultrasound images **(B, C)** done in the upper outer quadrant of the left breast at the expected location of the calcifications.

What do you think?

Multiple spicular echoes (large arrows, Fig. 4.30D, E) some with associated shadowing (Fig. 4.30D, small arrows) are imaged at the expected location of the calcifications seen mammographically in the upper outer quadrant of the left breast. Three 14G core samples are done through this area, and core radiographs are obtained. If calcifications are confirmed on the cores, nothing further is done (remember that with this type of calcification, removing calcifications targets the malignant cells directly). If no calcifications are seen, additional cores are obtained.

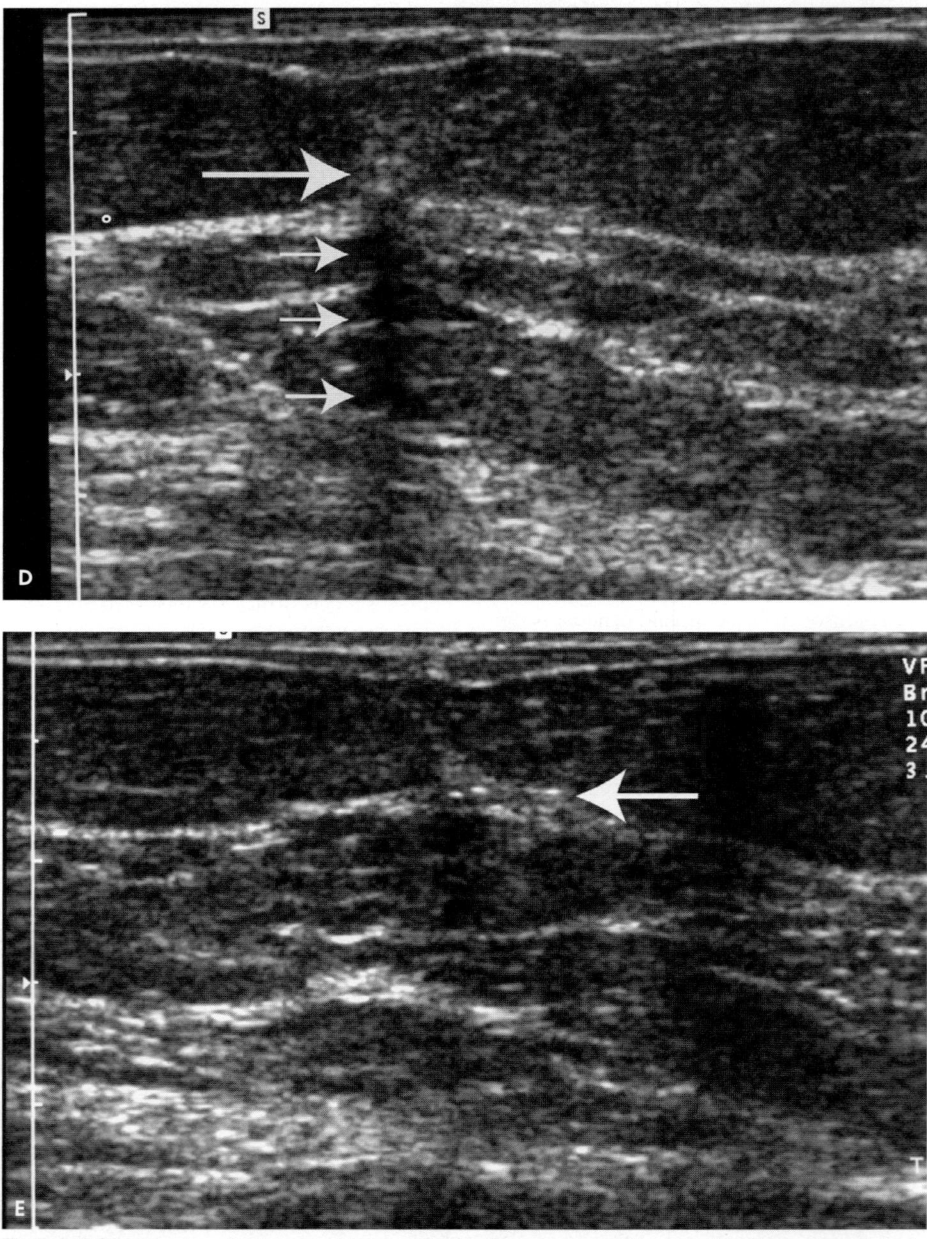

Figure 4.30. (*Continued*) Ultrasound images **(D, E)** demonstrating echogenic foci (large arrows) in the tissue consistent with the presence of calcifications. Shadowing (small arrows) can be seen associated with some of the echogenic foci.

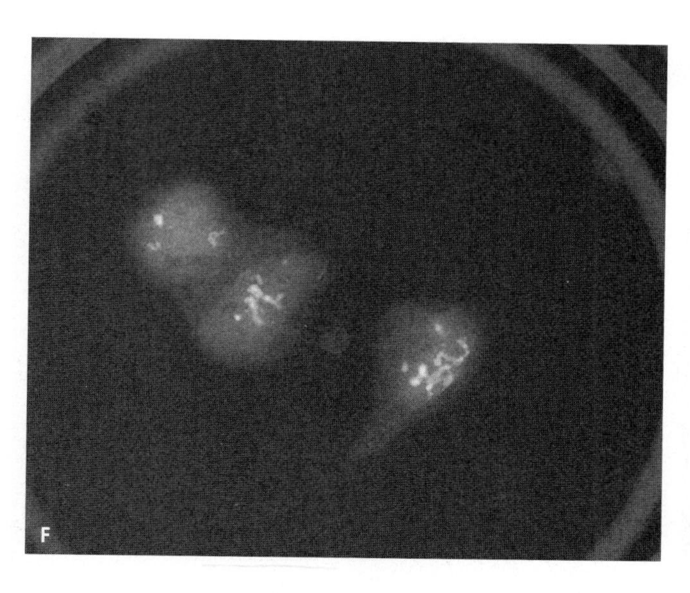

Figure 4.30. (*Continued*) Radiograph of three cores **(F)** obtained using ultrasound guidance.

What do you think?

Calcifications are present in all of the cores. A high-nuclear-grade ductal carcinoma in situ with central necrosis is diagnosed on the cores.

My approach to patient care is to do whatever I need to do to arrive at the correct diagnosis as simply, easily, and efficiently as I can. This is in the context of complete, high-quality imaging workups; I am not suggesting or advocating cutting corners or accepting suboptimal work—quite the opposite. Although I am sure that percutaneous treatment of small breast cancers is the future, at this time that is not what I am trying to do. When I do a breast biopsy, I am trying to arrive at a correct diagnosis in the easiest, least invasive, and most efficient way possible for my patient. If the correct diagnosis can be established with a fine-needle aspiration or one or two cores using a 14G needle, why do more? If there is no chance that I will remove a lesion in its entirety during the biopsy, why deploy a clip? Just because I can? I challenge you to think methodically about what and how you do things to patients. Step back and ask yourself: What do I absolutely need to do to take care of this patient optimally, and what is the easiest way to accomplish the goal? Keep it simple!

PATIENT 31

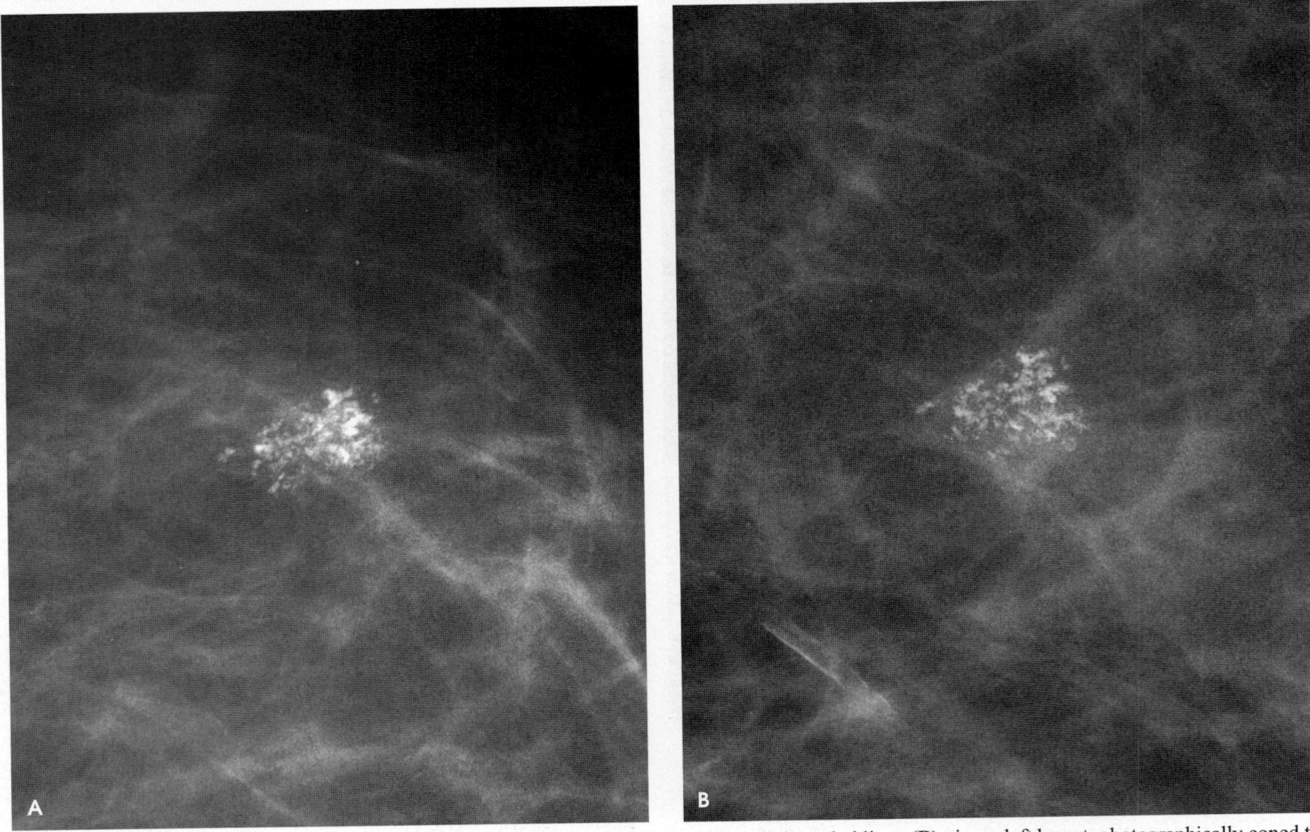

Figure 4.31. Screening mammogram, 73-year-old woman. Craniocaudal **(A)** and mediolateral oblique **(B)** views, left breast, photographically coned to an area of calcifications.

What do you think? Are magnification views indicated?

These are dense, coarse calcifications, most likely dystrophic in etiology. Magnification views are not indicated. In looking through the patient's jacket, prior studies provide an explanation for the calcifications. Vascular calcifications are also present.

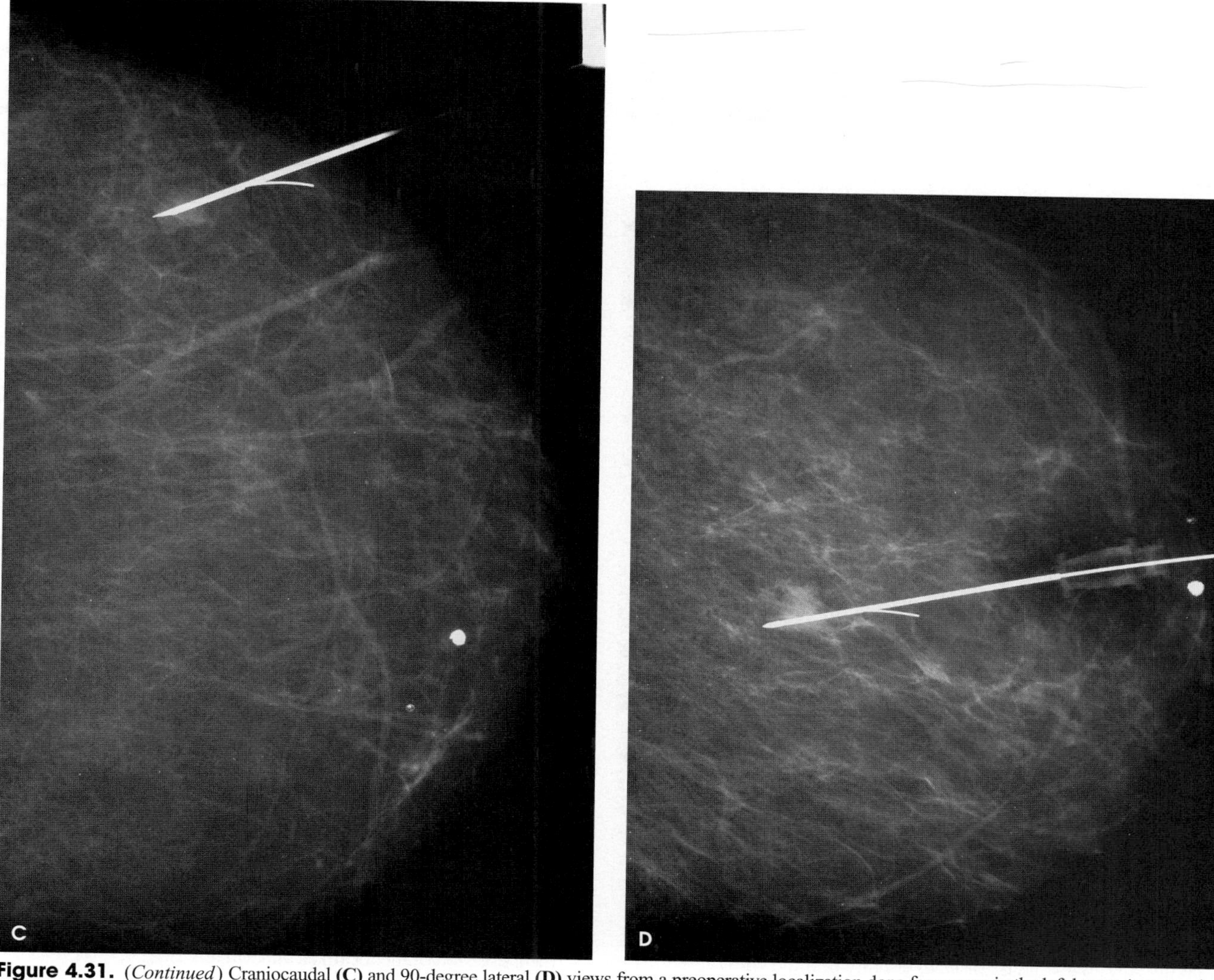

Figure 4.31. (*Continued*) Craniocaudal **(C)** and 90-degree lateral **(D)** views from a preoperative localization done for a mass in the left breast 4 years prior to **(A)** and **(B)**.

What approach was used for the localization, and what are the limitations and possible complications inherent in this approach? What are the alternative options for preoperative wire localizations?

In this patient, the calcifications are dystrophic and localized to the prior site. They require no further evaluation, intervention, or short-interval follow-up. Annual screening mammography is recommended for the patient.

A free-hand anteroposterior, or frontal, approach was used to localize the mass in the left breast. This is an acceptable method for preoperative localizations; however, it is more of a challenge to localize lesions precisely using this approach. Also, because the needle is advanced toward the chest wall, care should be exercised to minimize the possibility of a pneumothorax, particularly in thin patients with small breasts.

The main challenge in using this method is that it requires you to establish the location of a lesion in the breast, based on images with the breast compressed and pulled out away from the body, and transpose this to a breast that is uncompressed and in its natural position when the needle is advanced in the breast. After you position the needle in the breast free-hand, craniocaudal (Fig. 4.31C) and 90-degree lateral (Fig. 4.31D) views are obtained. In this patient the needle is through the lesion in both images (Fig. 4.31C, D). However, this degree of accuracy is difficult to obtain and often requires serial approximations. Depending on the relationship of the needle to the lesion on the initial images, free-hand adjustments are made to the position of the needle. The images are repeated and, based on the new position of the needle, additional adjustments may be indicated. This is done as many times as necessary to position the needle as close to the lesion as possible (Fig. 4.31E–G). Depending on the size of the breast, the size and location of the lesion being localized, and the experience and persistence of the breast imager, having the needle consistently through or within 5 mm of the lesion is hard to achieve with this method. The issue then becomes what you are willing to accept as an adequate position (distance) for the wire relative to the lesion: Is it acceptable if the wire is 1 cm or 1.5 cm from the lesion? Ideally, you want the wire to be within 5 mm of the lesion, and you do not want the wire to be short of the lesion.

A more accurate method involves using breast compression with an alphanumeric grid and an approach for needle placement that is parallel to the chest wall. This is a simple and safe approach that enables precise localization of even the smallest of lesions. Because the needle is advanced in the breast parallel to the chest wall, the possibility of a pneumothorax is eliminated. The possible routes for needle entry using this approach include craniocaudal, caudocranial (i.e., from below), lateromedial, or mediolateral. The shortest distance from the skin to the lesion is determined on craniocaudal and 90-degree lateral views (Fig. 4.31H) of the breast, and this dictates the route taken for needle entry. The shortest distance to the lesion on the example provided is "s" cm using a mediolateral approach for the localization. A needle that is long enough to go 1 cm beyond the lesion is selected (i.e., 1 cm + "s" cm).

The breast is positioned for a 90-degree mediolateral view using the alphanumeric grid to compress the medial aspect of the breast (Fig. 4.31I). The patient's breast is kept in compression after this image is taken. The coordinates for the lesion are established on the image ("B" and "3") and using the collimator light (or laser light) a shadow of the lesion coordinates is cast on the breast. After anesthetizing the skin entry site with lidocaine, the needle is advanced in the breast at the intersection point for the coordinates. If the patient has not moved from the time the initial image is done to the time you introduce the needle, and you selected a needle long enough to go beyond the lesion, you will have skewered the lesion. At this point, we do another 90-degree mediolateral view (Fig. 4.31J) to document needle and, after deployment, wire positioning in this projection and release compression. A craniocaudal view using the spot compression paddle (Fig. 4.31J) is done next, and the breast is kept in compression after this view is obtained. On the 90-degree mediolateral view, the hub of the needle should be superimposed on the lesion, and on the CC view, the needle should be through or within 5 mm of the lesion and extend 1 cm beyond the lesion. If the needle is correctly positioned on the orthogonal views, the wire is advanced through the needle and the needle is pulled out, making sure that you do not inadvertently pull the wire out with the needle. A repeat CC view is done to document final positioning. Compression is released and the portion of the wire external to the breast is secured on the skin.

After the wire is deployed, we do not compress the breast in a perpendicular direction to the wire because this can result in unwanted changes in the position of the wire (e.g., the wire can be pulled out and end up short of the lesion, or the wire can be advanced significantly beyond the lesion). Because the wire is placed through the needle, the position of the needle in the initial projection (Fig. 4.31J, 90-degree mediolateral view in this example) describes the eventual position of the wire in this projection. There is no need, therefore, to repeat this projection (requiring you to compress the breast perpendicular to the wire) after the wire is deployed.

Lastly, preoperative wire localizations can be done using ultrasound guidance. My general rule is that if I can see the lesion with ultrasound, I prefer to use ultrasound guidance for biopsies and preoperative wire localizations. In order to see the needle (and subsequently the wire) in its entirety, I establish an approach that allows me to advance the needle in the breast parallel to the transducer. I use a 25G, 1.5-in needle to inject lidocaine at the skin entry site and in the expected trajectory of the needle up to the lesion. I then advance the needle through the breast and into the lesion and verify that the needle is through the lesion longitudinally and in cross section (via orthogonal ultrasound images of the needle). Preferably with the tip of the needle 1 cm beyond the lesion, I deploy the wire, remove the needle, making sure that I do not inadvertently pull the wire out with the needle, and obtain orthogonal ultrasound images of the wire (Fig. 4.31L). I measure the distance from the skin directly down to the location of the lesion/wire for the surgeon and I place an "X" on the skin surface directly over the lesion. A single mammographic image is obtained of the wire (Fig. 4.31M). The view used is selected so that compression of the breast occurs parallel (and not perpendicular) to the wire. After the wire is deployed, we do not compress the breast perpendicular to the wire because this might result in changing the final wire positioning (see Fig. 4.32). A radiograph or ultrasound of the specimen is always obtained following preoperative wire localizations to document excision of the localized abnormality (Fig. 4.31N).

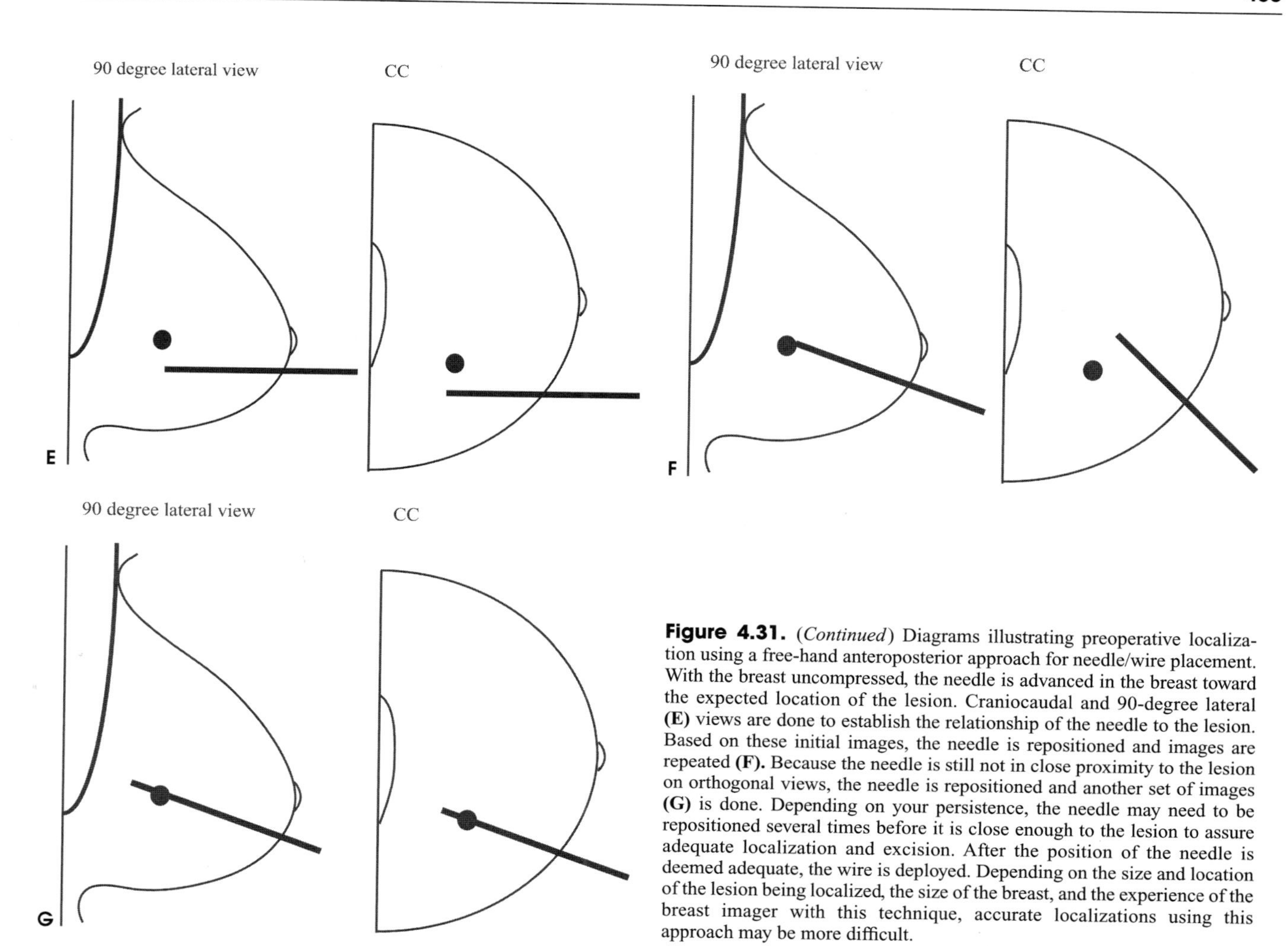

Figure 4.31. (*Continued*) Diagrams illustrating preoperative localization using a free-hand anteroposterior approach for needle/wire placement. With the breast uncompressed, the needle is advanced in the breast toward the expected location of the lesion. Craniocaudal and 90-degree lateral **(E)** views are done to establish the relationship of the needle to the lesion. Based on these initial images, the needle is repositioned and images are repeated **(F).** Because the needle is still not in close proximity to the lesion on orthogonal views, the needle is repositioned and another set of images **(G)** is done. Depending on your persistence, the needle may need to be repositioned several times before it is close enough to the lesion to assure adequate localization and excision. After the position of the needle is deemed adequate, the wire is deployed. Depending on the size and location of the lesion being localized, the size of the breast, and the experience of the breast imager with this technique, accurate localizations using this approach may be more difficult.

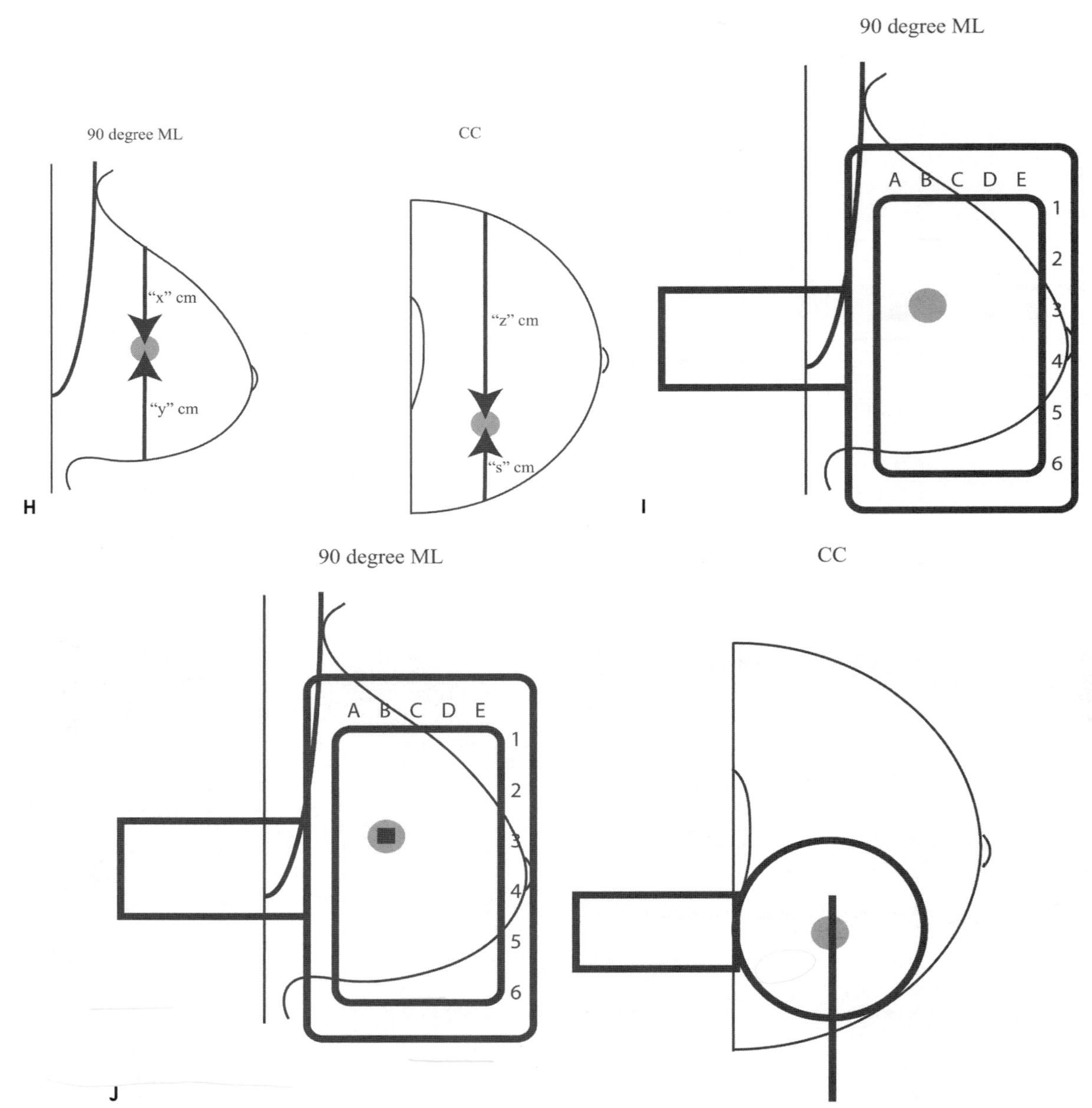

Figure 4.31. (*Continued*) Diagrams illustrating concepts of preoperative wire localization using breast compression with an alphanumeric grid for a parallel-to-chest-wall approach. Ninety-degree and craniocaudal views of the breast **(H)** are reviewed, and the distances from the various skin surfaces to the lesion are measured. The distance from the superior aspect of the breast to the lesion in this example is "x" cm, the distance from the inferior aspect of the breast to the lesion in this example is "y" cm, the distance from the lateral aspect of the breast in this example is "z" cm, and the distance from the medial aspect of the breast is "s" cm. The shortest distance from the skin to the lesion dictates the approach used for needle placement. In this example, the lesion is closest to the medial aspect of the breast, so a mediolateral approach is used. A needle long enough to go 1 cm beyond the lesion is selected. Using a compression paddle that has a central fenestration surrounded by an alphanumeric grid, a 90-degree mediolateral view is done **(I).** The coordinates for the center of this lesion are "B" and "3". Using the collimator light, a shadow of these coordinates is cast on the patient's breast, lidocaine is used at the intersection point of these coordinates, and the needle is advanced in the breast. A second 90-degree mediolateral view is done **(J).** Because the wire is placed through the needle, this view describes the eventual trajectory and relationship of the wire to the lesion in this plane. The hub of the needle *(black square superimposed on the mass)* is superimposed on the lesion. Next, using the spot compression paddle, a craniocaudal view **(J)** is done to document the relationship of the needle to the lesion in the orthogonal projection. The breast is kept in compression in this projection until after the wire is deployed.

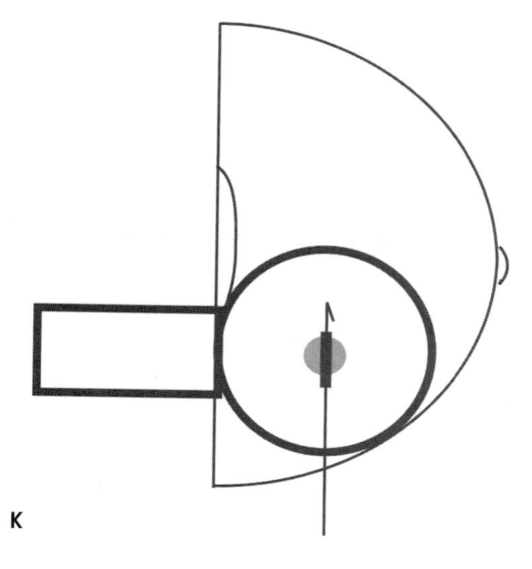

Figure 4.31. (*Continued*) The needle should be through or within 5 mm of the mass and 1 cm beyond the lesion. If the tip of the needle is more than 1 cm beyond the lesion, the needle is pulled out as much as needed for the tip to be 1 cm beyond the lesion. If the needle is associated with the lesion on the orthogonal views (as in this example), the wire is deployed and another craniocaudal view **(K)** is done to document final wire positioning. After the wire is deployed, the breast is not compressed again in a projection that is perpendicular to the wire (the lateral projection in this example).

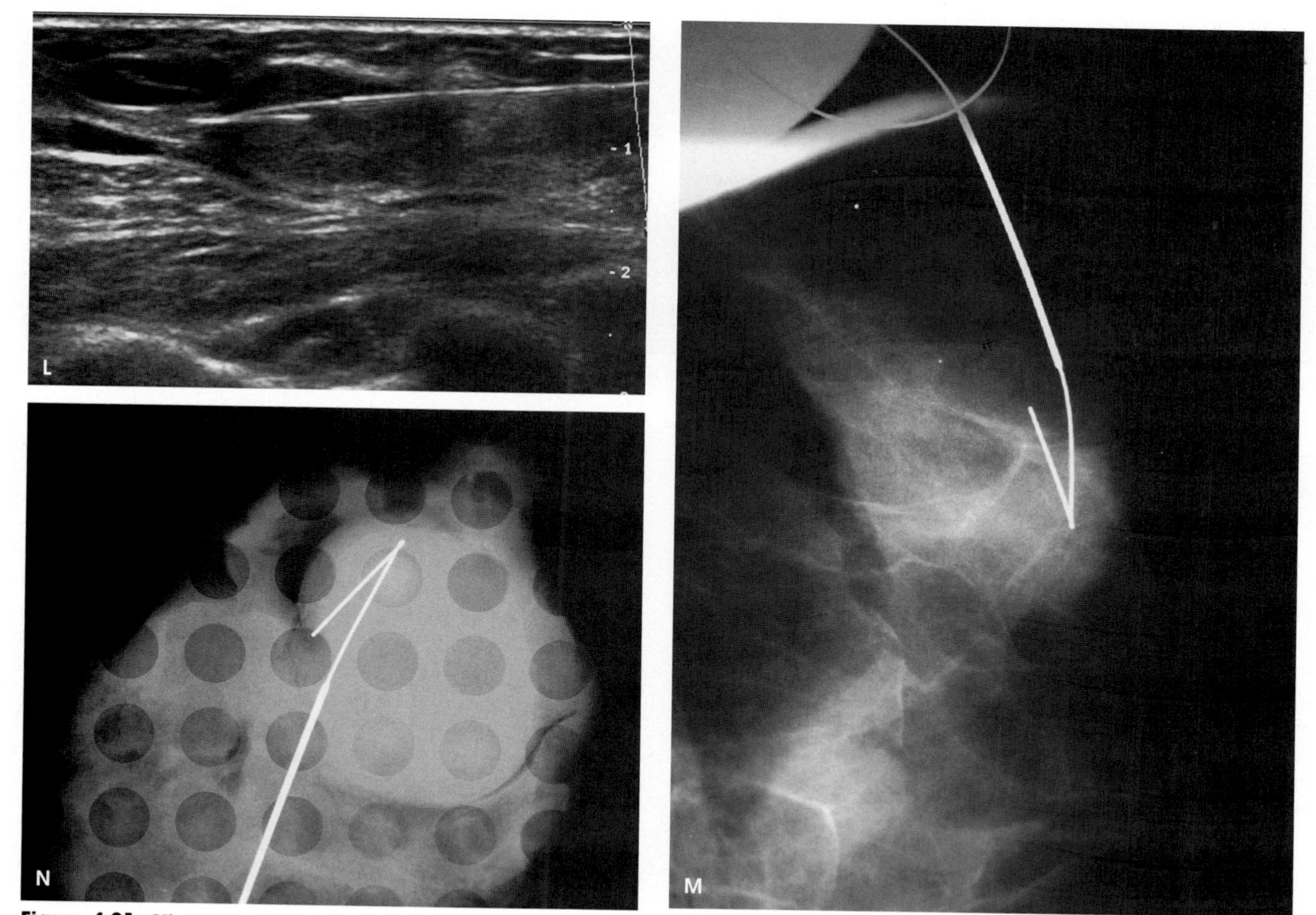

Figure 4.31. Ultrasound image **(L)** obtained after the wire is deployed in a hypoechoic mass in the left breast. If the trajectory of the needle (and consequently the wire) is parallel to the orientation of the transducer, the needle and wire can be seen in their entirety. In this patient, you can see the hook of the wire and a portion of the reinforced wire segment in the mass. The distance from the skin to the mass is measured, and using an indelible marker, an "X" is placed on the skin directly over the mass/wire as an additional guide for the surgeon. A mammographic image **(M)** obtained with compression applied parallel to the course of the wire is obtained to document the position of the wire in the lesion. A radiograph of the specimen **(N)** is obtained to verify excision of the localized lesion and localization wire and to mark the location of the lesion for the pathologist. Alternatively, sonography of the specimen can be done to document excision of the lesion and is indicated when the lesion is seen on ultrasound only (i.e., it is not seen mammographically).

PATIENT 32

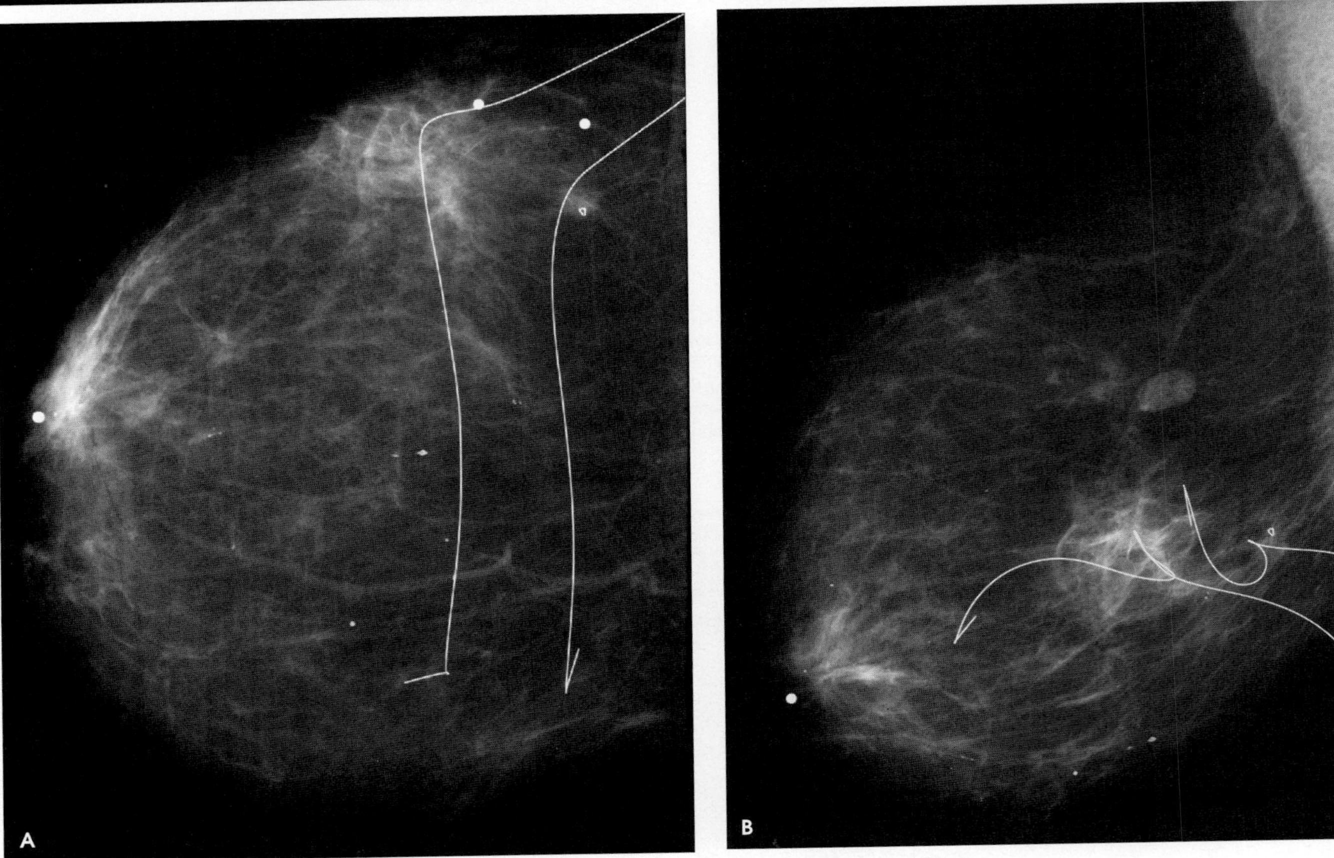

Figure 4.32. Preoperative wire localization, 47-year-old patient. Craniocaudal **(A)** and 90-degree lateral **(B)** views.

How was this localization approached, and what do you think about the final position of the wires?

In this patient, two lesions in the right breast (a clip deployed after a stereotactically guided biopsy is evident in one of the lesions) are localized using a 90-degree lateromedial approach. The shortest distance from the skin to the lesion being localized, as measured on craniocaudal (CC) and 90-degree lateral views, dictates the approach that is taken when the parallel-to-the-chest-wall approach using an alphanumeric grid is the method selected for preoperative wire localizations. In this patient, the lesions are closest to the lateral aspect of the breast on the CC view. Consequently, the needles/wires are placed in the breast correctly using a 90-degree lateromedial approach.

The problem with this wire localization is that the wires ended up significantly beyond the lesions, as seen on the CC view. This can occur if, after the wire is deployed, the breast is compressed perpendicular to the direction in which the wire is deployed (Fig. 4.32C, D). In this patient the lateral view (Fig. 4.32B) was done after the wires were deployed, resulting in the inadvertent repositioning of the wires.

An image is always done after the needle is placed in the breast in the initial projection (see Fig. 4.31J). Because the wire is placed through this needle, the position of the needle describes the eventual position of the wire in the initial projection. There is no need, therefore, to repeat this projection (requiring you to compress the breast perpendicular to the wire) after the wire is deployed.

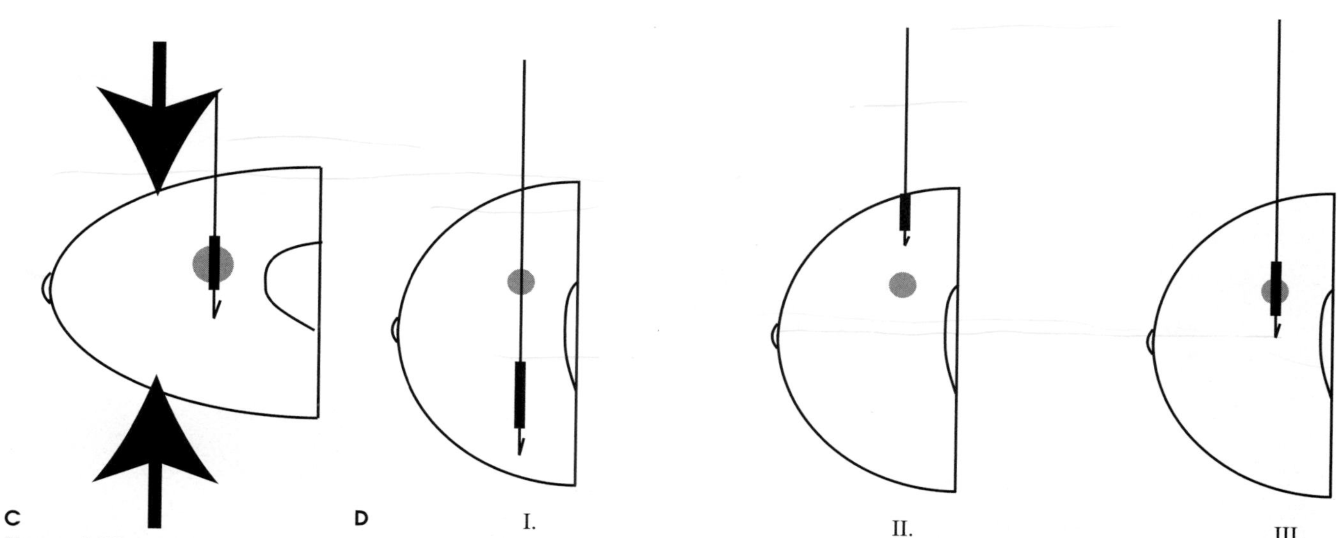

Figure 4.32. Diagram illustrating the inadvertent repositioning of the wire that can result when breast compression is applied perpendicular to the direction of wire deployment **(C).** This can have an accordion effect so that the wire is advanced in, or pulled out, of the breast. After compression is released, and the orthogonal view is obtained **(D),** the wire may have been advanced significantly beyond the lesion (I.), pulled out of the lesion (II.), or it may remain appropriately positioned (III.). While it is acceptable (though not desirable) to have the wire beyond the lesion, it is not acceptable for the wire to be short of the lesion (II.).

PATIENT 33

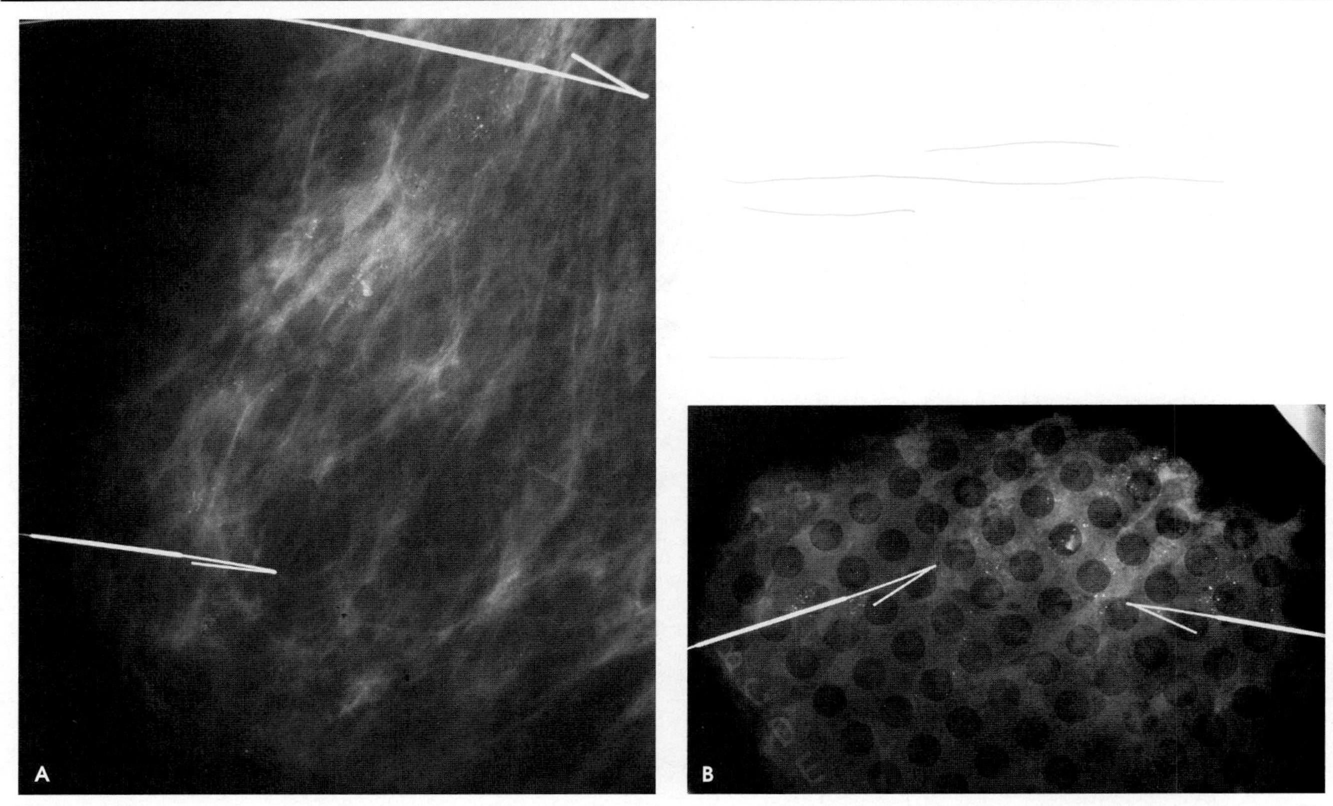

Figure 4.33. Preoperative wire localization, 56-year-old patient. Ninety-degree lateral view **(A)** obtained after wire placement. Specimen radiograph **(B)**.

How was this localization done, and why were two wires used? After reviewing the specimen radiograph, what will you tell the surgeon?

This patient has pleomorphic calcifications in a segmental distribution extending for approximately 6 to 7 cm in the upper outer (craniocaudal view not shown) quadrant of the right breast. Two wires are used for the localization to bracket the location of the calcifications for the surgeon. To excise a lesion completely, the use of two or more wires is recommended in some patients when the lesion spans several centimeters or when dealing with multifocal or multicentric disease.

On the specimen radiograph, calcifications are noted extending to the edges of the specimen. This is discussed directly with the surgeon at the time of the surgery so that additional tissue can be obtained. Although the specimen is a two-dimensional representation of a three-dimensional structure, if the lesion of interest approximates one of the margins, this is discussed with the surgeon. With the patient still in the operating room, additional tissue can be taken in an effort to minimize the likelihood that a second operative procedure will be needed to obtain clear margins.

Following preoperative wire localizations, the specimen is placed in a container that allows for compression of the specimen with an alphanumeric grid. However, based on recent reports in the literature suggesting that vigorous specimen compression may result in "false positive" histologic interpretations of tumor extending to the margins, we apply only a minimal amount of compression. The specimen radiograph is done using magnification technique on a mammographic unit, or a dedicated specimen radiography unit. The use of an alphanumeric grid enables us to place a pin through the center of the lesion, or four pins can be used to delineate the margins of larger lesions for the pathologist. This assures that the area of mammographic concern is fully evaluated histologically.

The specimen radiograph is done to confirm that the localized lesion is excised, assess gross margin involvement, document removal of the localization wire, potentially identify additional unsuspected lesions, and mark the area of concern for the pathologist.

Because of the extent (6 to 7 cm) of the lesion in this patient, and the difficulty in obtaining clear margins with an acceptable resulting cosmetic effect, she went on to have a simple mastectomy. She also had a sentinel lymph node biopsy. Although sentinel lymph node biopsies are not done routinely in patients diagnosed with ductal carcinoma in situ (DCIS) on core biopsy, they are usually done in patients in whom an extensive area of DCIS is suspected based on the imaging findings. In these patients, the likelihood of microinvasive disease is increased and, because of the extent of the disease, it is possible that not all of the tissue will be evaluated histologically. In this patient, high-nuclear-grade ductal carcinoma in situ with central necrosis is diagnosed extensively involving the upper outer quadrant of the right breast. No invasion is identified in the tissue examined. The excised sentinel lymph nodes are normal [Tis, pN0(sn) (i−), pMX, Stage 0].

PATIENT 34

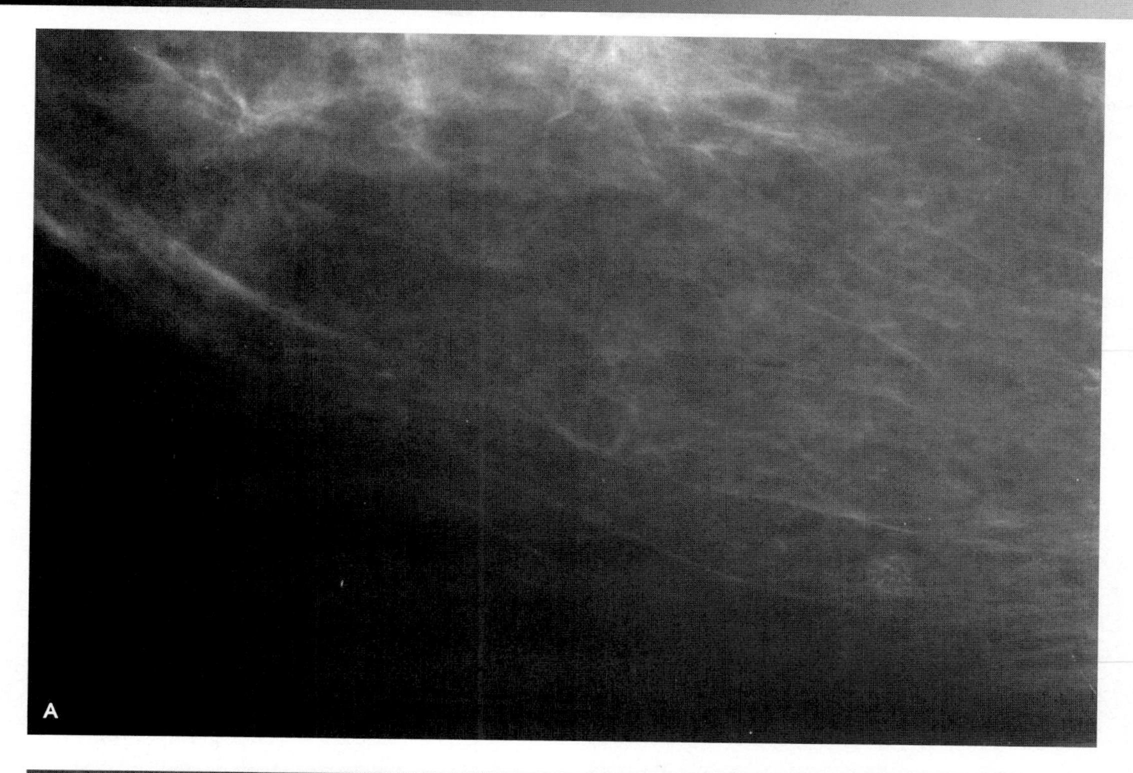

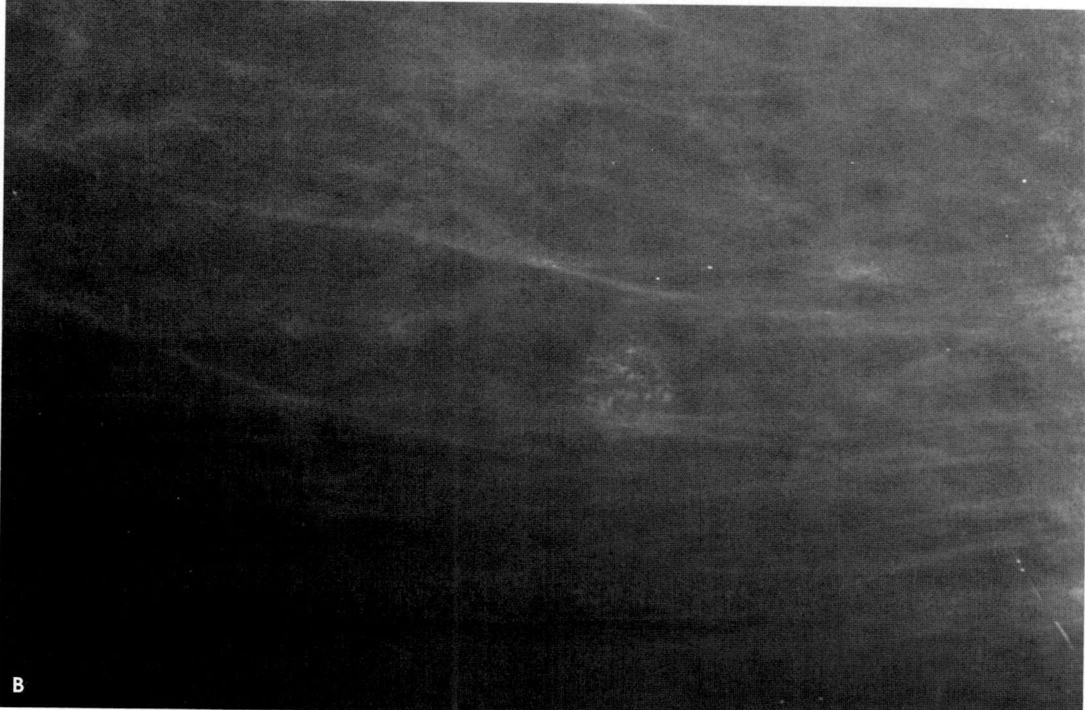

Figure 4.34. Diagnostic evaluation, 55-year-old patient being evaluated for a cluster of calcifications, posteromedially in the right breast. Craniocaudal **(A)** view, right breast. Craniocaudal **(B)** view, photographically coned to the cluster of calcifications.

Although no lucent-centered calcifications are identified in the cluster, because of the close proximity to the skin, a skin location for these calcifications is suspected. What can you do to prove that these calcifications are on the skin and that biopsy is not needed?

If these calcifications are in the skin, a tangential view of the skin containing the calcifications should show that these are dermal. To obtain the tangential view, a "skin localization" is done. Craniocaudal and oblique views are reviewed to establish the shortest distance from the skin to the calcifications. In this patient, the calcifications are closest to the skin on the medial aspect of the breast, so a 90-degree mediolateral approach is taken. Normally, a regular, full compression paddle with an alphanumeric grid is used to compress the breast for localization. However, having a spot compression paddle with an alphanumeric grid is helpful in reaching lesions in hard-to-access locations including the axillary tail or anywhere posteriorly in the breast. The spot compression paddle facilitates the inclusion of tissue that may otherwise be difficult to include on an image with a full paddle.

A 90-degree mediolateral view using the spot compression paddle with an alphanumeric grid is obtained so that coordinates for the calcifications can be determined (Fig. 4.34C). The patient is maintained in compression until the coordinates for the calcifications are determined. A metallic BB is placed at C.5 and 2.5. Compression is released and a tangential view of the metallic BB is obtained. If the calcifications are in the skin, they will be imaged in tangent to the x-ray beam and in close association with the metallic BB (Fig. 4.34D). If they are not on the skin, they will be imaged in the breast parenchyma, not in tangent to the x-ray beam and at a distance from the metallic BB. In this patient, the calcifications are dermal in location, and further intervention or short-term follow-up is not indicated. Annual screening mammography is recommended.

BI-RADS® category 2: benign finding.

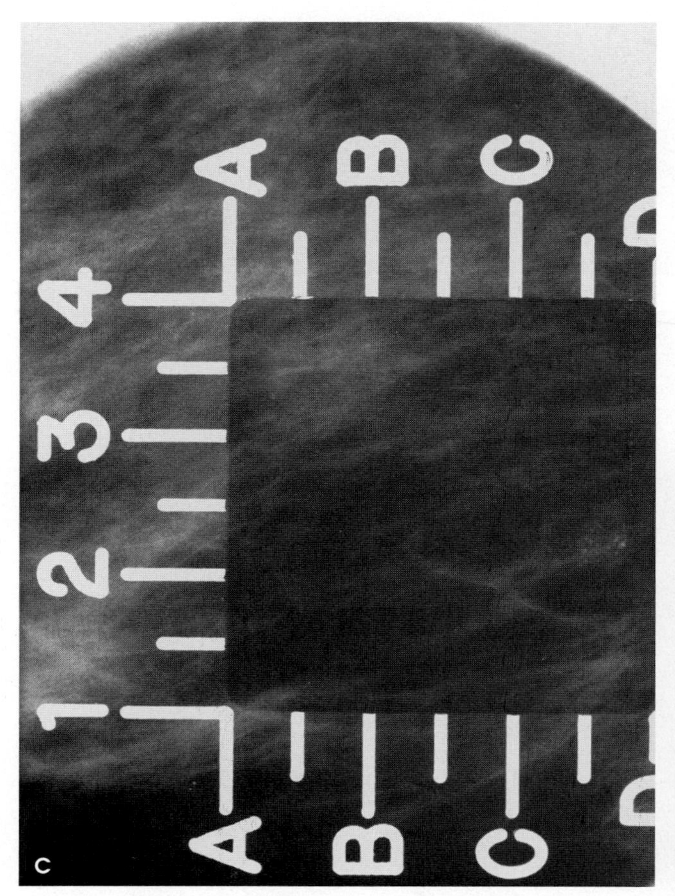

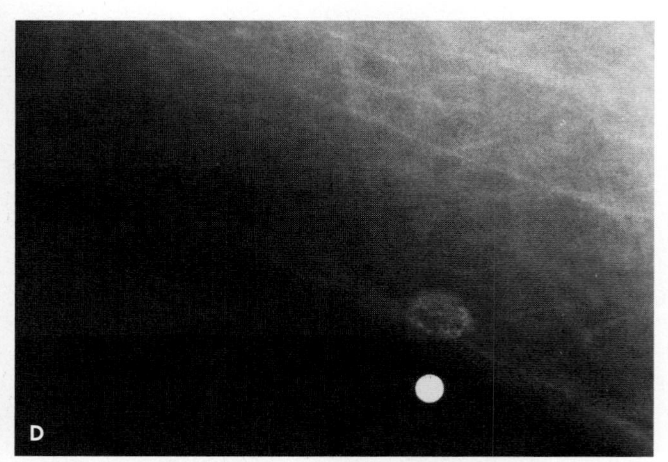

Figure 4.34. (*Continued*). Image **(C)** of the right breast using a fenestrated, alphanumeric spot compression paddle to determine the coordinates for the calcifications seen mammographically. Spot tangential **(D)** view of the metallic BB placed at the coordinates for the calcifications confirming that these are skin calcifications.

BIBLIOGRAPHY

Agoff SN, Lawton TJ. Papillary lesions of the breast with and without atypical ductal hyperplasia. *Am J Clin Pathol.* 2004;122: 440–443.

Asoglu O, Ugurlu MM, Blanchard K, et al. Risk factor for recurrence and death after primary surgical treatment of malignant phyllodes tumors. *Ann Surg Oncol.* 2004;11:1011–1017.

Berg WA. Image-guided breast biopsy and management of high-risk lesions. *Radiol Clin N Am.* 2004;42:935–946.

Berg WA, Mrose HE, Ioffe OB. Atypical lobular hyperplasia or lobular carcinoma in situ at core-needle biopsy. *Radiology.* 2001;218:503–509.

Brenner RJ, Jackman RJ, Parker SH, et al. Percutaneous core needle biopsy of radial scars of the breast: when is excision necessary? *AJR Am J Roentgenol.* 2002;179:1179–1184.

Carder PJ, Garvican J, Haigh I, Liston JC. Needle core biopsy can reliably distinguish between benign and malignant papillary lesions of the breast. *Histopathology.* 2004;46:320–327.

Carder PJ, Murphy CE, Liston JC. Surgical excision is warranted following a core biopsy diagnosis of mucocele-like lesion of the breast. *Histopathology.* 2004;45:148–154.

Farshid G, Pieterse S, King JM, Robinson J. Mucocele-like lesions of the breast: a benign cause for indeterminate or suspicious mammographic microcalcifications. *Breast J.* 2005;11(1):15–22.

Fasih T, Jain M, Shrimankar J, et al. All radial scars/complex sclerosing lesions seen on breast screening mammograms should be excised. *Eur J Surg Oncol.* 2005;31:1125–1128.

Foster MC, Helvie MA, Gregory NE, et al. Lobular carcinoma in situ or atypical lobular hyperplasia at core needle biopsy: is excisional biopsy necessary? *Radiology.* 2004;231:813–819.

Gill HK, Ioffe OB, Berg WA. When is a diagnosis of sclerosing adenosis acceptable at core biopsy? *Radiology.* 2003;228:50–57.

Glazebrook K, Reynolds C. Mucocele-like tumors of the breast: mammographic and sonographic appearances. *AJR Am J Roentgenol.* 2003;180:949–954.

Greenstein-Orel S, Evers K, Yeh IT, et al. Radial scar with microcalcifications: radiologic-pathologic correlation. *Radiology.* 1992;183:479–482.

Guerra-Wallace MM, Chistensen WN, White RL. A retrospective study of columnar alteration with prominent apical snouts and secretions and the association with cancer. *Am J Surg.* 2004; 188:395–398.

Günhan-Bilgen I, Memis A, Üstün EE, et al. Sclerosing adenosis: mammographic and ultrasonographic findings with clinical and histopathological correlation. *Eur J Radiol.* 2002;44:232–238.

Hamele-Bena D, Cranor ML, Rosen PP. Mammary mucocele-like lesions: benign and malignant. *Am J Surg Pathol.* 1996;20: 1081–1085.

Ivan D, Selinko V, Sabin AA, et al. Accuracy of core needle biopsy diagnosis in assessing papillary breast lesions: histologic predictors of malignancy. *Mod Pathol.* 2004;17:165–171.

Jacobs TW, Byrne C, Colditz G, et al. Radial scars in benign breast biopsy specimens and the risk of breast cancer. *N Engl J Med.* 1999;340:430–436.

Jacobs TW, Chen YY, Guinee DG, et al. Fibroepithelial lesions with cellular stroma on breast core needle biopsy. *Am J Clin Pathol.* 2005;124:342–354.

Jacobs TW, Connolly JL, Schnitt SJ. Nonmalignant lesions in breast core needle biopsies. *Am J Surg Pathol.* 2002;26:1095–1110.

Jacobs TW, Natasha P, George K, Schnitt SJ. Carcinomas in situ of the breast with indeterminate features: role of E-cadherin staining in categorization. *Am J Surg Pathol.* 2001;25:229–236.

Kim JY, Han BK, Choe YH, Ko YH. Benign and malignant mucocele-like tumors of the breast: mammographic and sonographic appearances. *AJR Am J Roentgenol.* 2005;185:1310–1316.

Komenaka IK, El-Tmaer M, Pile-Spellman E, Hibschoosh H. Core needle biopsy as a diagnotic tool to differentiate phyllodes tumor from fibroadenoma. *Arch Surg.* 1003;138:987–990.

Liberman L. Clinical management issues in percutaneous core breast biopsy. *Radiol Clin North Am.* 2000;38:791–807.

Liberman L, Bracero N, Vuolo MA, et al. Percutaneous large-core biopsy of papillary breast lesions. *AJR Am J Roentgenol.* 1999; 172:331–337.

Liberman L, Sama M, Susnik B, et al. Lobular carcinoma in situ at percutaneous breast biopsy: surgical biopsy findings. *AJR Am J Roentgenol.* 1999;173:291–299.

Mercado CL, Hamele-Bena D, Oken SM, et al. Papillary lesions of the breast at percutaneous core-needle biopsy. *Radiology.* 2006; 238:801–808.

Page DL, Schuyler PA, Dupont WD, et al. Atypical lobular hyperplasia as a unilateral predictor of breast cancer risk: a retrospective cohort study. *Lancet.* 2003;361:125–129.

Patterson JA, Scott M, Anderson N, Kirk SJ. Radial scar, complex sclerosing lesion and risk of breast cancer. Analysis of 75 cases in Northern Ireland. *Eur J Surg Oncol.* 2004;30:1065–1068.

Ramsaroop R, Greenberg D, Tracey N, Benson-Cooper D. Mucocele-like lesions of the breast: an audit of 2 years at Breast Screen Auckland (New Zealand). *Breast J.* 2005;11(5): 321–325.

Renshaw AA, Derhagopian RP, Tizol-Blanco DM, Gould EW. Papillomas and atypical papillomas in breast core needle biopsy specimens. *Am J Clin Pathol.* 2004;122:217–221.

Rosai J. Borderline epithelial lesions of the breast. *Am J Surg Pathol.* 1991;15:209–221.

Rosen EL, Bentley RC, Baker JA, et al. Image-guided core needle biopsy of papillary lesions. *AJR Am J Roentgenol.* 2002;179: 1185–1192.

Rosen, PP. *Rosen's Breast Pathology.* 2nd ed. Philadelphia: Lippincott Williams & Wilkins; 2001.

Ung OA, Lee WB, Greenberg ML, Bilous M. Complex sclerosing lesion: the lesion is complex, the management is straightforward. *ANZ J Surg.* 2001;71:35–40.

Appendix: Breast Cancer TNM Classification and Stage Grouping

PRIMARY TUMOR (same for clinical and pathologic classification)

TX	primary tumor cannot be assessed
T0	no evidence of primary tumor
Tis	carcinoma in situ
Tis(DCIS)	ductal carcinoma in situ
Tis(LCIS)	lobular carcinoma in situ
Tis(Paget)	Paget disease of the nipple with no tumor
T1	tumor 2 cm or less in greatest dimension
T1mic	microinvasion 0.1 cm or less in greatest dimension
T1a	tumor >0.1 cm but not >0.5 cm in greatest dimension
T1b	tumor >0.5 cm but not >1 cm in greatest dimension
T1c	tumor >1 cm but not >2 cm in greatest dimension
T2	tumor >2 cm but not >5 cm in greatest dimension
T3	tumor >5 cm in greatest dimension
T4	tumor of any size with direct extension to chest wall or skin
T4a	extension to chest wall but not including pectoral muscle
T4b	edema (*peau d'orange*) or ulceration of the skin of the breast, or satellite skin nodules confined to the same breast
T4c	both T4a and T4b
T4d	inflammatory carcinoma

REGIONAL LYMPH NODE (pathologic, pN)

pNX	regional lymph nodes cannot be assessed (previously removed or not excised)
pN0	No regional lymph node metastasis histologically; no additional examination for isolated tumor cells (ITC)
pN0(i−)	No regional lymph node metastasis histologically, negative immunohistochemical (IHC) studies
pN0(i+)	No regional lymph node metastasis histologically, positive IHC, no IHC cluster >0.2 mm
pN0(mol−)	No regional lymph node metastasis histologically; negative molecular findings (reverse transcriptase/polymerase chain reaction, RT-PCR)
pN0(mol+)	No regional lymph node metastasis histologically; positive molecular reaction (RT-PCR)
pN1	metastasis in 1 to 3 axillary lymph nodes and/or internal mammary lymph nodes with microscopic disease detected by sentinel lymph node dissection but not clinically apparent (not detected by imaging studies or clinical examination)
pN1mi	micrometastasis (>0.2 mm, none >2.0 mm)
pN1a	metastasis in 1 to 3 axillary lymph nodes
pN1b	metastasis in internal mammary lymph nodes with microscopic disease detected by sentinel lymph node but not clinically apparent (not detected by imaging studies or clinical examination)
pN1c	metastasis in 1 to 3 axillary lymph nodes and in internal mammary lymph nodes with microscopic disease detected by sentinel lymph node dissection but not clinically apparent (not detected by imaging studies or clinical examination). If associated with >3 positive axillary lymph nodes, the internal mammary nodes are classified as pN3b
pN2	metastasis in 4 to 9 axillary lymph nodes, or in clinically apparent internal mammary lymph nodes in the absence of axillary lymph node metastasis
pN2a	metastasis in 4 to 9 axillary lymph nodes (at least one tumor deposit >2.0 mm)

pN2b	metastasis in clinically apparent (detected by imaging studies, excluding lymphoscintigraphy or clinical examination) internal mammary lymph nodes in the absence of axillary lymph node metastasis
pN3	metastasis in 10 or more axillary lymph nodes, or in infraclavicular lymph nodes, or in clinically apparent ipsilateral internal mammary lymph nodes in the presence of 1 or more positive axillary lymph node; or in >3 axillary lymph nodes with clinically negative microscopic metastasis in internal mammary lymph nodes; or in ipsilateral supraclavicular lymph nodes
pN3a	metastasis in 10 or more axillary lymph nodes (at least one tumor deposit >2.0 mm), or metastasis to the infraclavicular lymph nodes
pN3b	metastasis in clinically apparent ipsilateral mammary lymph nodes in the presence of 1 or more positive axillary lymph nodes; or in >3 axillary lymph nodes and in internal mammary lymph nodes with microscopic disease detected by sentinel lymph node dissection but not clinically apparent
pN3c	metastasis in ipsilateral supraclavicular lymph nodes

(sn) = sentinel lymph node

If surgery occurs after the patient has received neoadjuvant chemotherapy, hormonal therapy, immunotherapy, or radiation therapy, the prefix "y" is used with the TNM classification

DISTANT METASTASIS

MX	distant metastasis cannot be assessed
M0	no distant metastasis
M1	distant metastasis

Stage 0	Tis	N0	M0
Stage I	T1	N0	M0
Stage IIA	T0	N1	M0
	T1	N1	M0
	T2	N0	M0
Stage IIB	T2	N1	M0
	T3	N0	M0
Stage IIIA	T0	N2	M0
	T1	N2	M0
	T2	N2	M0
	T3	N1	M0
	T3	N2	M0
Stage IIIB	T4	N0	M0
	T4	N1	M0
	T4	N2	M0
Stage IIIC	Any T	N3	M0
Stage IV	Any T	Any N	M0

Patient List

CHAPTER 1: MY AUNT MINNIE

PATIENT 1: Neurofibromatosis
PATIENT 2: Seborrheic keratoses
PATIENT 3: Lymph nodes
PATIENT 4: Fibroadenolipomas
PATIENT 5: Lipomas
PATIENT 6: Oil cysts
PATIENT 7: Oil cysts
PATIENT 8: Oil cysts, reduction mammoplasty
PATIENT 9: Fibroadenomas, popcorn calcifications
PATIENT 10: Fibroadenomas, popcorn calcifications
PATIENT 11: Fibroadenomas, developing calcifications
PATIENT 12: Fibroadenoma, coarse calcifications
PATIENT 13: Vascular calcification
PATIENT 14: Vascular calcification
PATIENT 15: Large rodlike calcifications
PATIENT 16 Milk of calcium
PATIENT 17: Dystrophic calcifications
PATIENT 18: Fibroadenoma, coarse, dystrophic calcifications
PATIENT 19 Skin calcifications
PATIENT 20: Implant rupture
PATIENT 21: Implant rupture
PATIENT 22: Collapsed saline implant
PATIENT 23: Implant rupture
PATIENT 24: Hair
PATIENT 25: Artifact, Desitin
PATIENT 26: Hickman catheter cuff
PATIENT 27: Retained wire fragment
PATIENT 28: Retained needle tip
PATIENT 29: Skin folds craniocaudal views
PATIENT 30: Skin folds, mediolateral oblique views
PATIENT 31: Sternalis muscle
PATIENT 32: Nail crimp
PATIENT 33: Finger prints
PATIENT 34: Poor film screen contact
PATIENT 35: Nipple rings
PATIENT 36: Static
PATIENT 37: Deodorant
PATIENT 38: Parasites, calcified
PATIENT 39: Pectoral lipoma
PATIENT 40: Keloids
PATIENT 41: Shrapnel, bullet fragments

CHAPTER 2: SCREENING

PATIENT 1: Technical issues, posterior nipple line
PATIENT 2: Normal variant, global parenchymal asymmetry
PATIENT 3: Normal mammogram, pseudolesion
PATIENT 4: Normal mammogram, pseudolesion
PATIENT 5: Normal variant, focal parenchymal asymmetry
PATIENT 6: Fat necrosis, postoperative distortion
PATIENT 7: Invasive ductal carcinoma, not otherwise specified
PATIENT 8: Ductal carcinoma in situ
PATIENT 9: Invasive ductal carcinoma with tubular features
PATIENT 10: Effects of weight loss
PATIENT 11: Invasive ductal carcinoma not otherwise specified
PATIENT 12: Invasive ductal carcinoma not otherwise specified
PATIENT 13: Arterial and large rodlike calcifications
PATIENT 14: Invasive mammary carcinoma, apocrine type
PATIENT 15: Normal mammogram, pseudolesion
PATIENT 16: Ductal carcinoma in situ
PATIENT 17: Normal variant, focal parenchymal asymmetry
PATIENT 18: Invasive lobular carcinoma
PATIENT 19: Invasive ductal carcinoma, not otherwise specified
PATIENT 20: Invasive ductal carcinoma with apocrine features
PATIENT 21: Reduction mammoplasty
PATIENT 22: Edema, congestive heart failure
PATIENT 23: Arterial, large rodlike and dystrophic calcifications

PATIENT 24: Tubular carcinoma, lesion triangulation
PATIENT 25: Global parenchymal asymmetry secondary to surgery
PATIENT 26: Invasive lobular carcinoma
PATIENT 27: Invasive ductal carcinoma, grade I with metastasis to axilla
PATIENT 28: Synchronous, bilateral breast cancers
PATIENT 29: Changes following implant removal
PATIENT 30: Normal variant, focal parenchymal asymmetry
PATIENT 31: Invasive ductal carcinoma with prominent lobular features
PATIENT 32: Invasive ductal carcinoma, not otherwise specified
PATIENT 33: Invasive lobular carcinoma
PATIENT 34: Normal mammogram, global parenchymal asymmetry
PATIENT 35: Invasive mammary carcinoma, micropapillary type
PATIENT 36: Invasive ductal carcinoma with mucinous features
PATIENT 37: Ductal carcinoma in situ
PATIENT 38: Normal mammogram, global parenchymal asymmetry
PATIENT 39: Invasive ductal carcinoma not otherwise specified; cyst
PATIENT 40: Invasive ductal carcinoma, not otherwise specified
PATIENT 41: Synchronous bilateral breast cancers
PATIENT 42: Poland's syndrome
PATIENT 43: Edema, congestive heart failure
PATIENT 44: Mondor's disease, varix, healed
PATIENT 45: Cysts

CHAPTER 3 DIAGNOSTIC BREAST IMAGING

PATIENT 1: Complex fibroadenoma; use of spot compression and rolled views
PATIENT 2: Invasive ductal carcinoma with tubular features, use of spot tangential view
PATIENT 3: Mucinous carcinoma, use of ultrasound
PATIENT 4: Ductal carcinoma in situ; use of double spot compression magnification views
PATIENT 5: Invasive mammary carcinoma with apocrine differentiation, use of spot compression views
PATIENT 6: Complex fibroadenoma and metaplastic carcinoma, lesion location and triangulation
PATIENT 7: Invasive ductal carcinoma, not otherwise specified, use of spot tangential view
PATIENT 8: Invasive ductal carcinoma not otherwise specified, axillary lymph node dissection and sentinel lymph node biopsy
PATIENT 9: Hematoma, post-traumatic changes
PATIENT 10: Lactational adenoma
PATIENT 11: Granular cell tumor
PATIENT 12: Mucinous carcinoma
PATIENT 13: Papillary carcinoma
PATIENT 14: Abscess (peripheral)
PATIENT 15: Synchronous bilateral invasive lobular carcinomas
PATIENT 16 Medullary carcinoma
PATIENT 17: Mastitis
PATIENT 18: Cyst
PATIENT 19: Fibromatosis (extraabdominal desmoid)
PATIENT 20: Ductal carcinoma in situ
PATIENT 21: Invasive ductal carcinoma, not otherwise specified
PATIENT 22: Gold in axillary lymph nodes
PATIENT 23: Gynecomastia
PATIENT 24: Complex sclerosing lesion
PATIENT 25: Fibrocystic complex with milk of calcium
PATIENT 26: Invasive lobular carcinoma
PATIENT 27: Changes related to a portable catheter (Port-A-Cath)
PATIENT 28: Cat scratch disease
PATIENT 29: Diabetic fibrous mastopathy
PATIENT 30: Invasive ductal carcinoma, not otherwise specified in male patient
PATIENT 31: Trauma
PATIENT 32: Invasive ductal carcinoma, not otherwise specified, neoadjuvant therapy
PATIENT 33: Tubulolobular carcinoma
PATIENT 34: Ductal carcinoma in situ
PATIENT 35: Galactocele
PATIENT 36: Invasive ductal carcinoma, not otherwise specified
PATIENT 37: Fibroadenoma
PATIENT 38: Sclerosing adenosis
PATIENT 39: Lipoma and cyst
PATIENT 40: Invasive ductal carcinoma, not otherwise specified
PATIENT 41: Columnar alteration with prominent apical snouts and secretions
PATIENT 42: Tubular adenoma
PATIENT 43: Metaplastic carcinoma
PATIENT 44: Multiple peripheral papillomas
PATIENT 45: Lymphoma, left axilla
PATIENT 46: Metastatic lung carcinoma
PATIENT 47: Fat necrosis
PATIENT 48: Sebaceous cyst, inflamed

CHAPTER 4: MANAGEMENT

PATIENT 1: Fat necrosis, post surgical
PATIENT 2: Invasive ductal carcinoma, not otherwise specified
PATIENT 3: Multicentric disease: invasive ductal carcinoma, not otherwise specified and ductal carcinoma in situ
PATIENT 4: Invasive ductal carcinoma, not otherwise specified, correlation of mammographic and sonographic findings
PATIENT 5: Abscess (subareolar)
PATIENT 6: Cyst
PATIENT 7: Cyst
PATIENT 8: Cyst, enlarging
PATIENT 9: Fat necrosis
PATIENT 10: Intracystic papillary carcinoma
PATIENT 11; Papillomas, nipple discharge
PATIENT 12: Ductal carcinoma in situ, nipple discharge
PATIENT 13: Multicentric disease, use of MRI

PATIENT 14: Fibroadenoma, enlarging
PATIENT 15: Phyllodes tumor
PATIENT 16: Mucocele-like lesion and papilloma
PATIENT 17: Atypical ductal hyperplasia, ductal carcinoma in situ apocrine type
PATIENT 18: Atypical ductal hyperplasia
PATIENT 19: Ductal carcinoma in situ
PATIENT 20: Columnar alteration with prominent apical snouts and secretions and associated atypia and atypical lobular hyperplasia
PATIENT 21: Complex sclerosing lesion
PATIENT 22: Complex sclerosing lesion and adenosis tumor
PATIENT 23: Multiple peripheral papillomas and ductal carcinoma in situ
PATIENT 24: Atypical ductal hyperplasia
PATIENT 25: Sclerosing adenosis
PATIENT 26: Ipsilateral breast tumor recurrence
PATIENT 27: Invasive ductal carcinoma not otherwise specified, metastasis to axilla, neoadjuvant therapy and postoperative seroma
PATIENT 28: Breast bud development
PATIENT 29: Cyst, pneumocystogram
PATIENT 30: Ductal carcinoma in situ
PATIENT 31: Dystrophic calcifications; approaches to preoperative wire localizations
PATIENT 32: Preoperative wire localization, inadvertent repositioning of wires
PATIENT 33: Preoperative wire localization: bracketing the lesion
PATIENT 34: Skin calcifications, skin localization

Index